Introductory Pathophysiology

Course Notes

2012-2013 Edition

Kraig Chugg

Jim Hutchins

Kathryn Newton

Weber State University

Health Sciences

WILEY Custom
LEARNING SOLUTIONS

To order books or for customer service, please call 1(800)-CALL-WILEY (225-5945).

Printed in the United States of America.

ISBN 978-1-118-51020-9

Printed and Bound by Courier Digital Solutions

10 9 8 7 6 5 4 3 2 1

Prerequisite Material

Study Guide Objectives - Introductory Pathophysiology (HTHS 2230)

Prerequisite Learning Material

Chapter 1 – Cellular Biology

1. Describe the eight major cellular functions: movement, conductivity, absorption, secretion, excretion, respiration, reproduction, and communication. (pp. 2-3)

2. Identify and describe the three principal parts of a typical eukaryotic cell. (p. 3)

3. Describe the function of the nucleus and the cytoplasmic organelles. (pp. 2-3)

4. Describe the structure, composition, and function of the plasma membrane. (pp. 3-7)

5. Compare and contrast the mechanisms that bind cells together and to the extracellular matrix: desmosomes, tight junctions, and gap junctions. (pp. 8-9)

6. Describe the modes of cellular communication and signal transduction: direct linkup, neurotransmitter, hormonal, neurohormonal, paracrine, and autocrine. (pp. 9-13)

7. Describe the production of ATP by glycolysis, the citric acid cycle, and oxidative phosphorylation. (pp. 13-14)

8. Compare and contrast passive and active transport. Classify passive and active transport mechanisms: diffusion, facilitated diffusion, endocytosis, active transport (primary and secondary), and osmosis. (pp. 14-21)

9. State the electrical properties of the cell membrane in excitable cells (muscle and nerve cells), resting membrane potential and action potential. (pp. 21-22)

10. Explain the phases of the cell cycle. Relate growth factors to the cell cycle. (pp. 22-24)

11. Identify and describe the phases of mitosis and cytokinesis. (pp. 23)

12. State the four tissue types and give examples of each. (pp. 24-30)

13. Classify the different types of epithelial tissue. (pp. 25-26)

14. Classify the different types of connective tissue. (pp. 27-29)

1

Prerequisite Learning Material
Chapter 1
Cellular Biology

2

Important Relationships

- Anatomy vs. Physiology
  - Structure determines function
- Pathophysiology
  - Diseases mess up structure and/or function

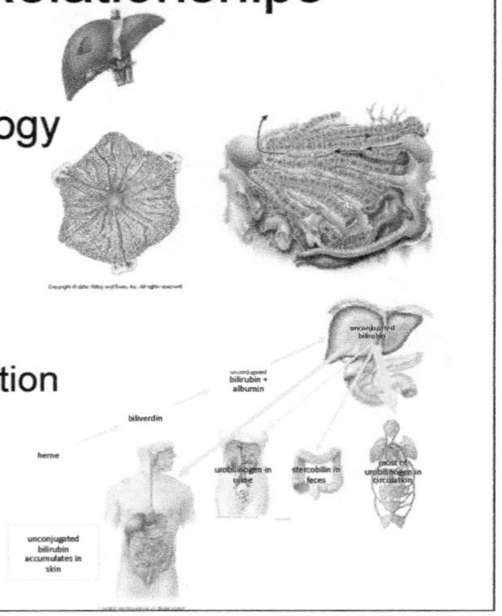

unconjugated bilirubin + albumin
biliverdin
heme
urobilinogen in urine
stercobilin in feces
unconjugated bilirubin accumulates in skin

3

Major Cellular Functions

- Movement — structure.
  - Skeletal and smooth muscle — actin / myosin.
- Conductivity — axon.
  - Nerve and muscle cells
- Metabolic Absorption — microvilli
  - Epithelial cells of the GI and urinary tracts
- Secretion – product — excretion = waste
  - Cells of endocrine glands, mucous glands, and reproductive organs — ? ↑ vacuoles?

1-1

4

Major Cellular Functions

- Excretion — Lysosomes
  - Release of waste products
- Respiration — thin membrane.
  - Cells absorb oxygen to transform nutrients (glucose) into ATP (energy) (accepts Hydrogen. at end of electron transport H- e- produces water. metabolic water.)
- Reproduction
  - Tissue growth to enlarge or just for tissue maintenance
- Communication
  - Communication (local or distant) between cells to maintain homeostasis

1-1

The Three Principal Parts of the Cell

1) Nucleus
- Control center of the cell
- The envelope has nuclear pores that allow movement of substances in and out of the nucleus by both active and passive transport
- Groups of coiled DNA during replication are called chromosomes
- Uncoiled DNA is called chromatin
- The nucleus contains hereditary factors (**genes**) that control a cell and direct a cell's activities.

1-2

The Three Principal Parts of the Cell
Nucleus

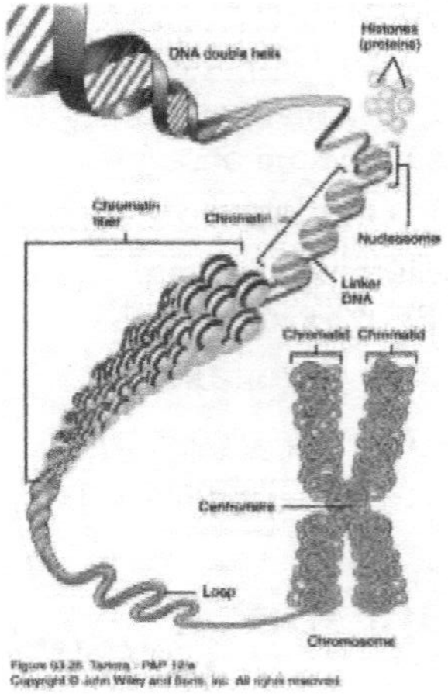
DNA double helix
Histones (proteins)
Chromatin fiber
Chromatin
Nucleosome
Linker DNA
Chromatid
Chromatid
Centromere
Loop
Chromosome

Figure 03.28 Tortora - PAP 12/e

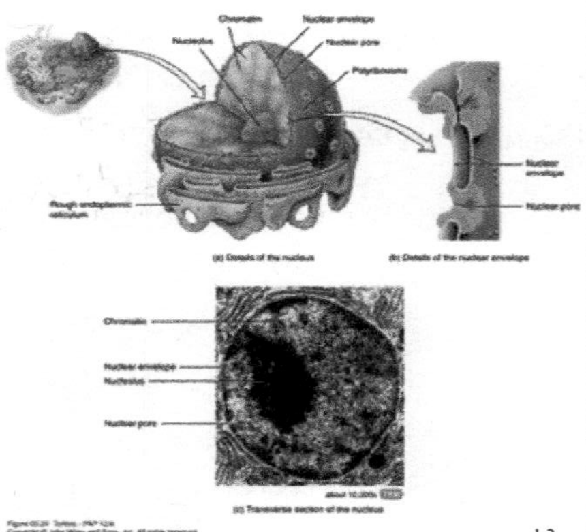

1-3

The Three Principal Parts of the Cell

- 2) Cytoplasm
  - All of the cellular contents between the plasma membrane and the nucleus
    - Organelles (cytoskeleton, ribosome, Golgi, etc.)
    - Cytosol - aqueous solution making up about half of a cell's volume

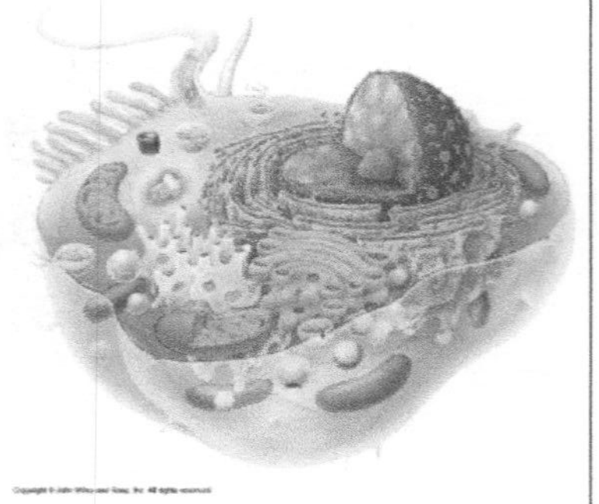

1-2

Organelles
Ribosomes

- Ribosomes
  - Ribosomes are sites of protein synthesis.
  - Ribosomes can be free, attached to ER, or in the mitochondria.
  - Ribosomes are constructed of two subunits created in the nucleolus and assembled in the cytosol.

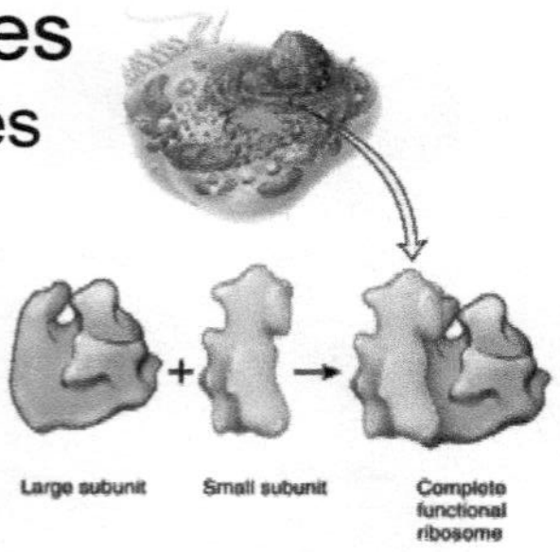
Large subunit
Small subunit
Complete functional ribosome

Details of ribosomal subunits

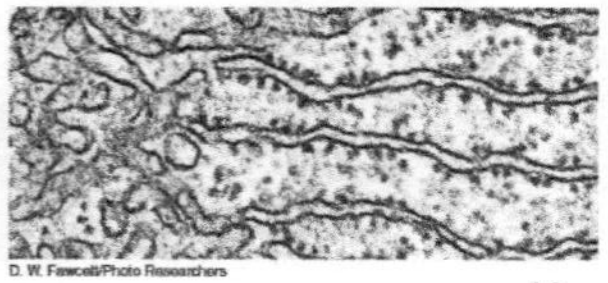

D. W. Fawcett/Photo Researchers

1-3

Organelles
Endoplasmic Reticulum

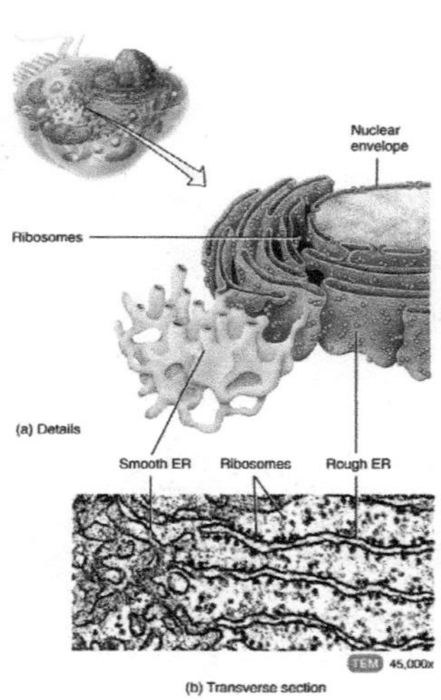

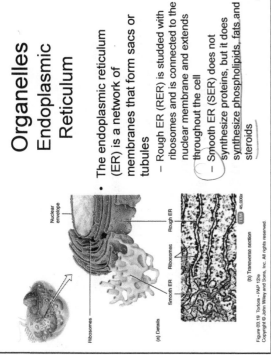

Nuclear envelope
Ribosomes
(a) Details
Smooth ER
Ribosomes
Rough ER
TEM 45,000x
(b) Transverse section

Figure 03.19 Tortora - PAP 12/e

- The endoplasmic reticulum (ER) is a network of membranes that form sacs or tubules
  - Rough ER (RER) is studded with ribosomes and is connected to the nuclear membrane and extends throughout the cell
  - Smooth ER (SER) does not synthesize proteins, but it does synthesize phospholipids, fats and steroids

Organelles
Golgi Complex

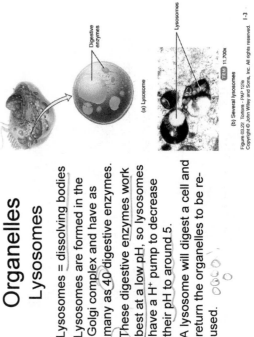

- Proteins that are synthesized at ribosomes attached to ER are transported to the Golgi complex
- In the Golgi complex, the proteins are modified and packaged for excretion and transport to their end destinations

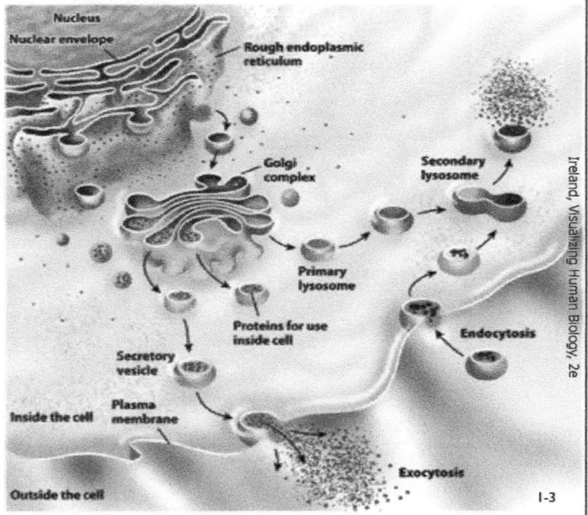

Nucleus
Nuclear envelope
Rough endoplasmic reticulum
Golgi complex
Secondary lysosome
Primary lysosome
Proteins for use inside cell
Endocytosis
Secretory vesicle
Inside the cell
Plasma membrane
Exocytosis
Outside the cell

Ireland, Visualizing Human Biology, 2e

Organelles
Lysosomes

- Lysosomes = dissolving bodies
- Lysosomes are formed in the Golgi complex and have as many as 40 digestive enzymes.
- These digestive enzymes work best at a low pH, so lysosomes have a H^+ pump to decrease their pH to around 5.
- A lysosome will digest a cell and return the organelles to be re-used.

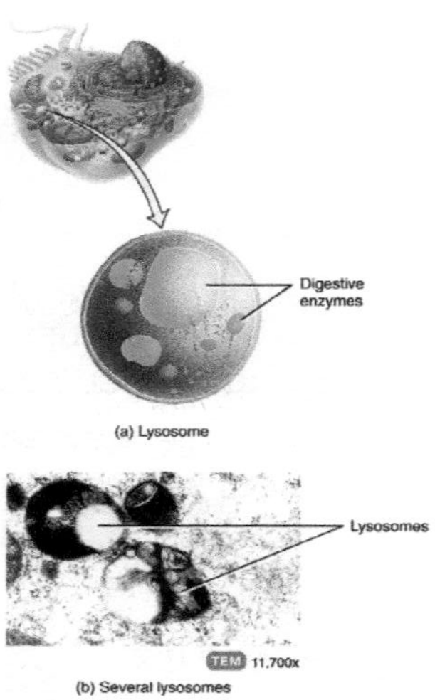

Digestive enzymes
(a) Lysosome
Lysosomes
TEM 11,700x
(b) Several lysosomes

Figure 03.22 Tortora - PAP 12/e

Organelles
Peroxisomes

- Like lysosomes, they destroy materials for the cell
- Like lysosomes, they are membrane-bound
- Unique properties:
  - they can replicate themselves
  - they make hydrogen peroxide (H_2O_2), which is itself toxic and needs to be inactivated by *catalase* and other enzymes
- Common in liver and kidney ("detox" function of these organs)
- They break down fatty acids in *β-oxidation* (using fats for energy)
- Peroxisomes create free radicals

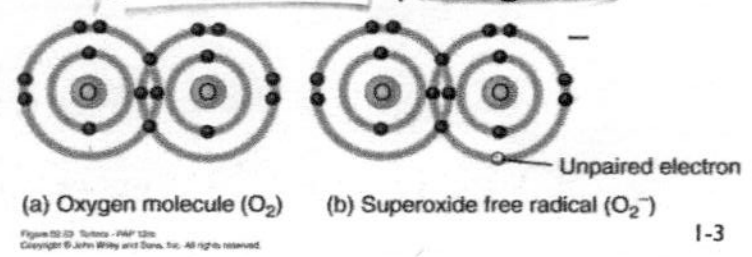

Unpaired electron
(a) Oxygen molecule (O_2)
(b) Superoxide free radical (O_2^-)

Organelles
Mitochondria

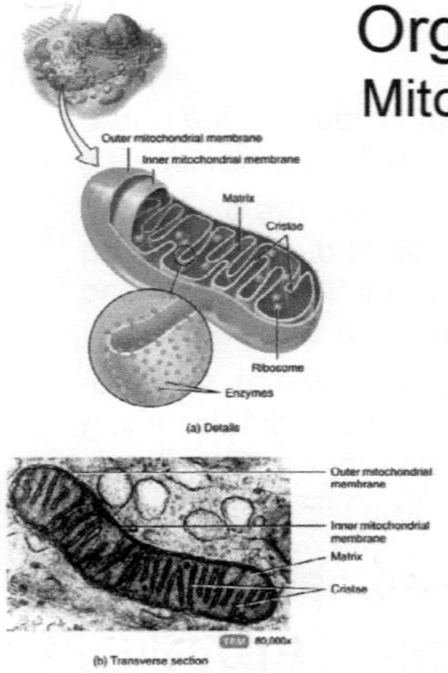

Outer mitochondrial membrane
Inner mitochondrial membrane
Matrix
Cristae
Ribosome
Enzymes
(a) Details
Outer mitochondrial membrane
Inner mitochondrial membrane
Matrix
Cristae
TEM 80,000x
(b) Transverse section

Figure 03.23 Tortora - PAP 12/e

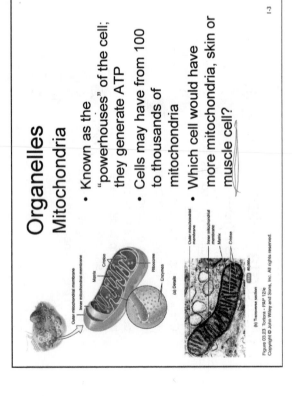

- Known as the "powerhouses" of the cell; they generate ATP
- Cells may have from 100 to thousands of mitochondria
- Which cell would have more mitochondria, skin or muscle cell?

Kato K *et al. Biol Crystallogr* **D64**:525, 2008.

Organelles
Vaults

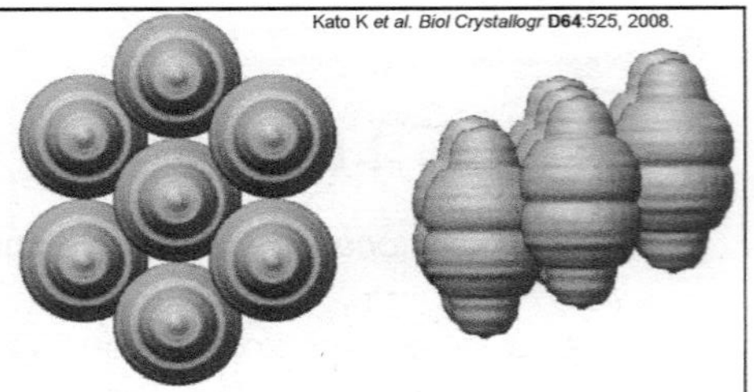

- Ribonucleoproteins RNA
- "Trucks" associated with nuclear pores
- Implicated in resistance to cancer chemotherapy

Cytosol

- Cytosol is the solvent (water) and solutes (salts and dissolved proteins) that make up the soluble part of the cytoplasm
  - Using a fruitcake analogy, it's the cake part of a fruitcake dissolved salt + sugar in batter
- Cytoplasm is the cytosol plus organelles
  - organelles are the fruits and nuts in the fruitcake

Organelles
Cytoskeleton

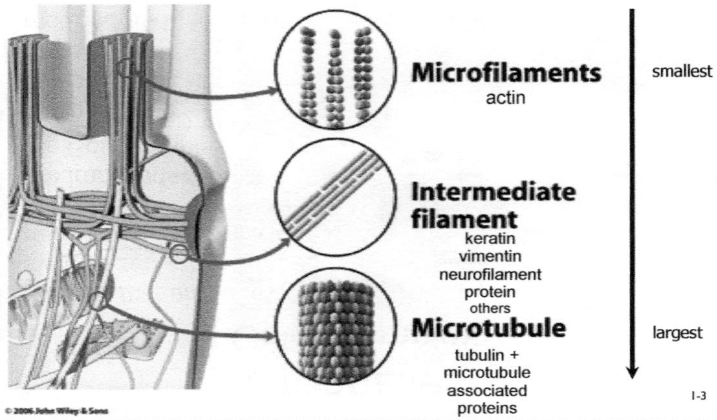

Microfilaments
actin
Intermediate filament
keratin
vimentin
neurofilament protein
others
Microtubule
tubulin + microtubule associated proteins
smallest
largest

Pruitt, Bioinquiry: Making Connections in Biology, 3/e

Organelles

Cytoskeleton & Axonal Transport

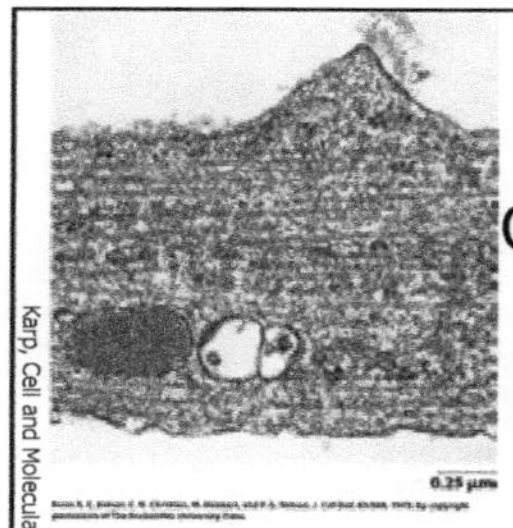

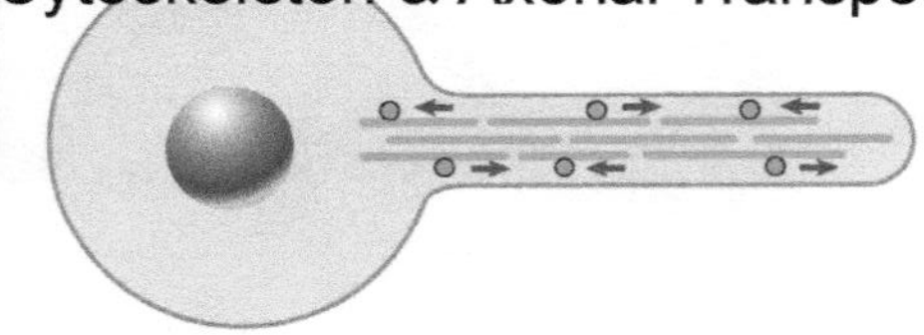

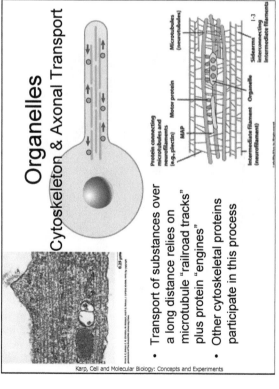

- Transport of substances over a long distance relies on microtubule "railroad tracks" plus protein "engines"
- Other cytoskeletal proteins participate in this process

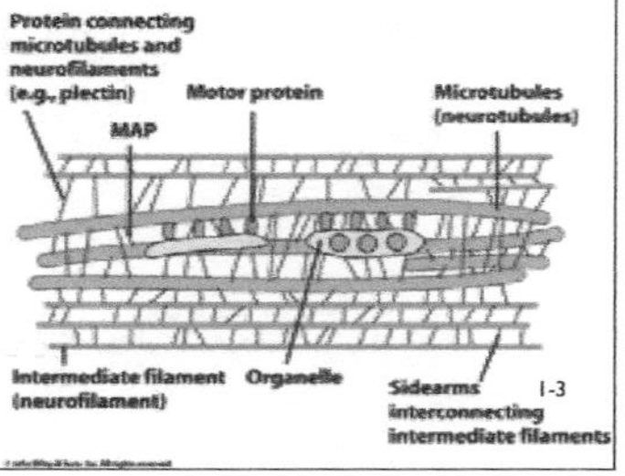

Protein connecting microtubules and neurofilaments (e.g., plectin)
MAP
Motor protein
Microtubules (neurotubules)
Intermediate filament (neurofilament)
Organelle
Sidearms interconnecting intermediate filaments

Karp, Cell and Molecular Biology: Concepts and Experiments

1-3

The Three Principal Parts of the Cell

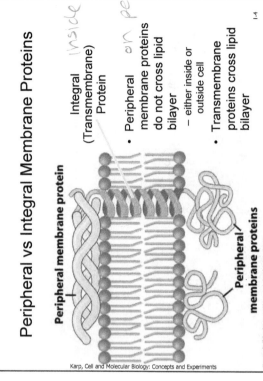

3) Plasma Membrane

- Separates the cell's internal environment from the external environment
- Selective, semipermeable barrier
- The basic frame of the plasma membrane is the lipid bilayer
- The plasma membrane is made of 3 types of lipids.
  - Phospholipids, cholesterol, and glycolipids
- The lipid bilayer is amphipathic (polar and non-polar parts)

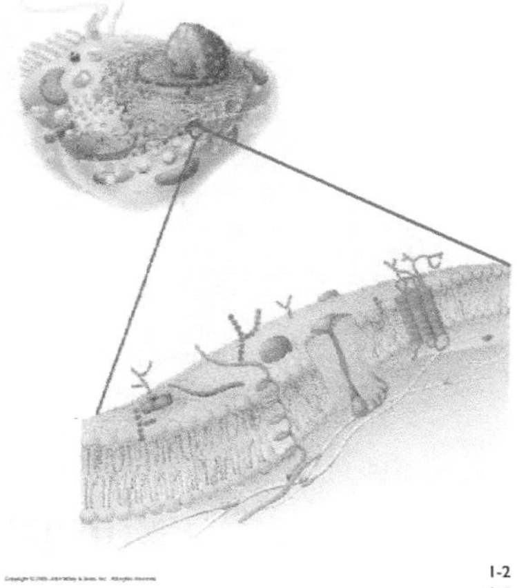

1-2
1-4

Molecules of the Cell Membrane

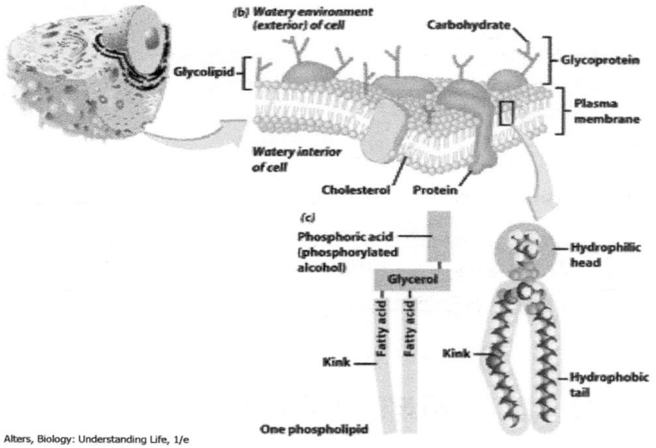

(b) Watery environment (exterior) of cell
Carbohydrate
Glycolipid
Glycoprotein
Plasma membrane
Watery interior of cell
Cholesterol
Protein
(c)
Phosphoric acid (phosphorylated alcohol)
Glycerol
Fatty acid
Fatty acid
Kink
Kink
Hydrophilic head
Hydrophobic tail
One phospholipid

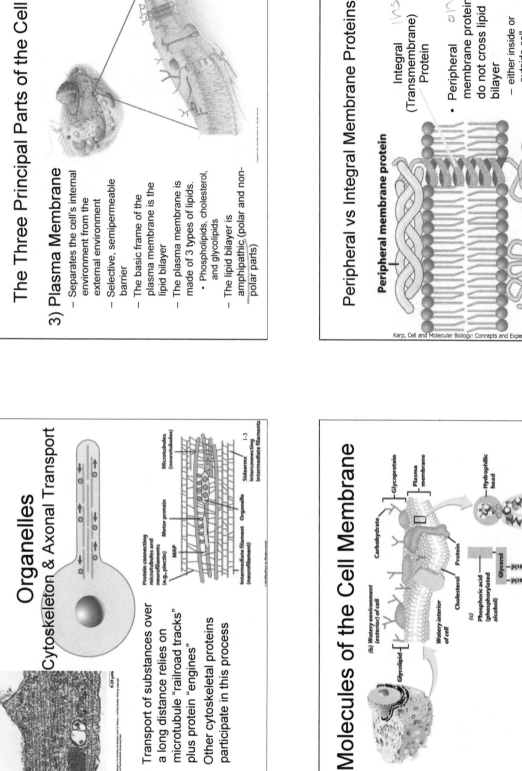

Alters, Biology: Understanding Life, 1/e

1-4

Peripheral vs Integral Membrane Proteins

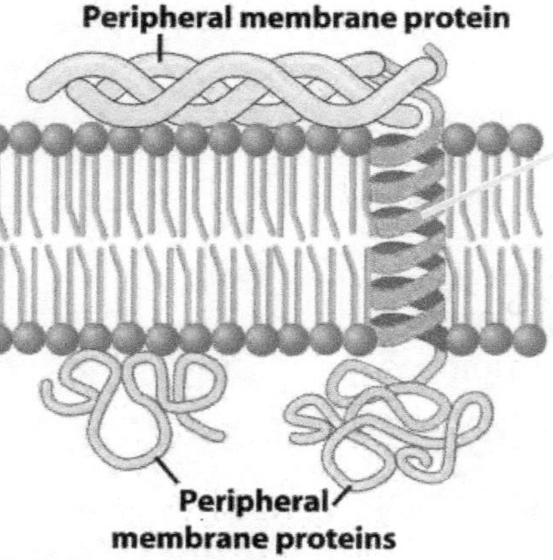

Peripheral membrane protein
Peripheral membrane proteins

Integral (Transmembrane) Protein inside

- Peripheral on perimeter membrane proteins do not cross lipid bilayer
  - either inside or outside cell
- Transmembrane proteins cross lipid bilayer

Karp, Cell and Molecular Biology: Concepts and Experiments

Figure 4-12b Cell and Molecular Biology, 5/e (© 2008 John Wiley & Sons)

1-4

The Three Principal Parts of the Cell

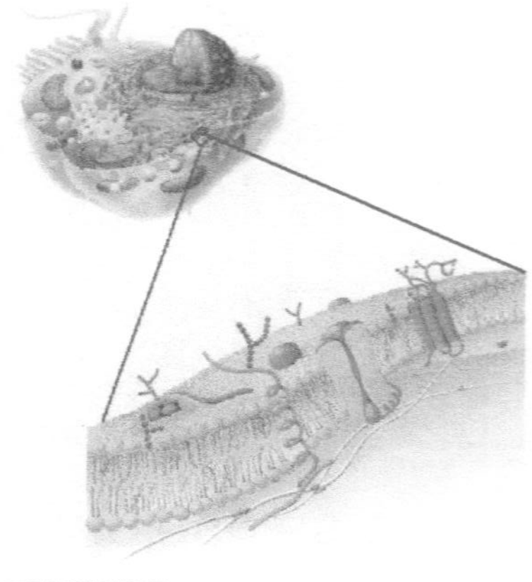

- Functions of the Plasma Membrane
  - Separate the cellular components from the surrounding environment
  - Facilitate recognition of the cell
  - Provides receptors and enzymes
  - Regulate entry and exit of substances
  - Provides an anchor for the cytoskeleton

1-4

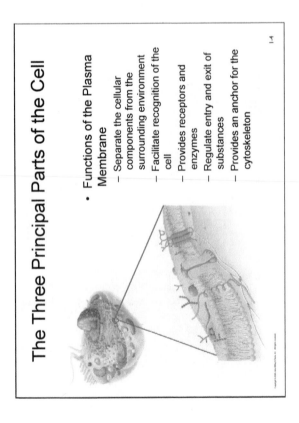

Membrane Protein Function

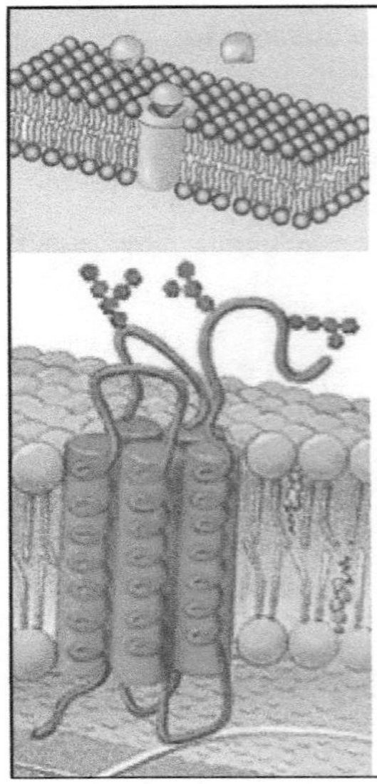

- Receptors
  - Cellular recognition sites that bond to a specific substance for a certain cellular function
  - Ligands: hormones, antigens, neurotransmitters, drugs, and infectious agents

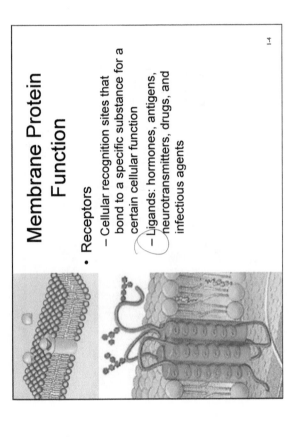

1-4

Plasma Membrane Receptors

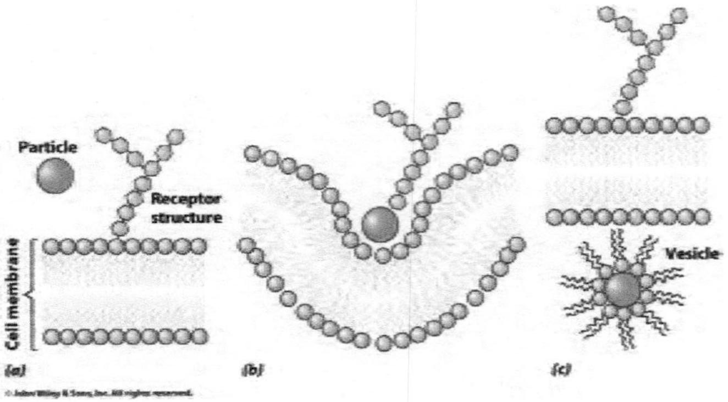
Particle
Receptor structure
Cell membrane
Vesicle
(a)
(b)
(c)

Trefil, The Sciences, 6e

1-4

Extracellular Matrix Proteins

<u>ECM components</u>

Fibronectin

Laminin

Proteoglycans

(Proteoglycans are 1:6 protein:sugar)

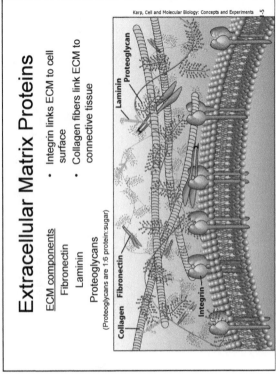

- Integrin links ECM to cell surface
- Collagen fibers link ECM to connective tissue

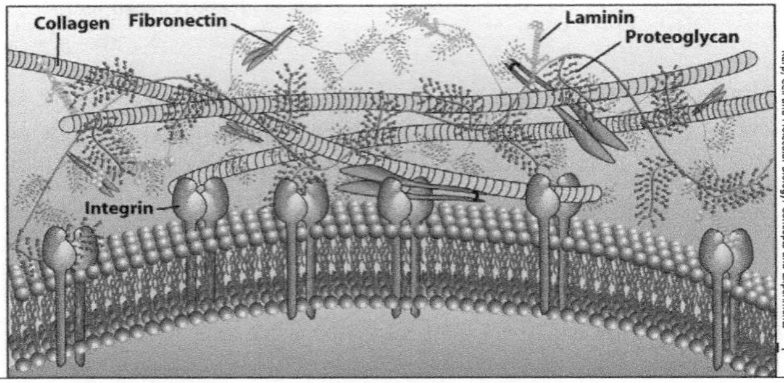
Collagen
Fibronectin
Laminin
Proteoglycan
Integrin

Karp, Cell and Molecular Biology: Concepts and Experiments

1-5

Extracellular Matrix Fibers

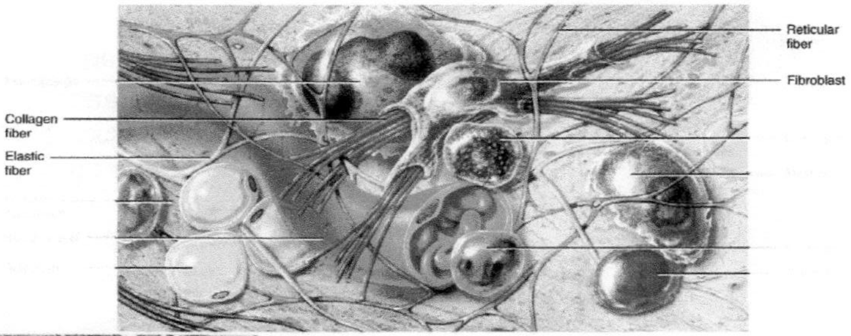
Reticular fiber
Fibroblast
Collagen fiber
Elastic fiber

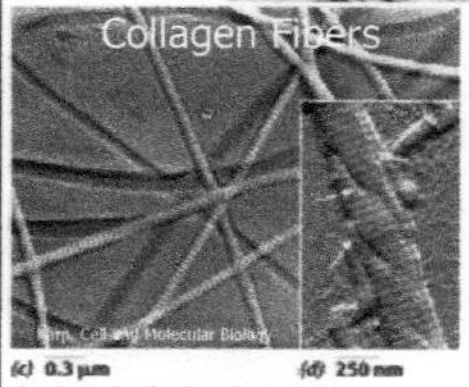
Collagen Fibers
(c) 0.3 µm
(d) 250 nm

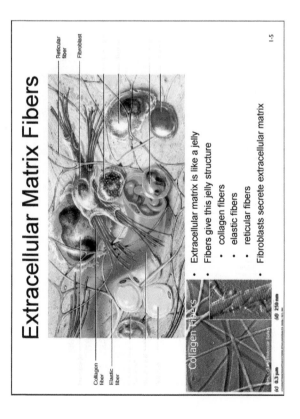

- Extracellular matrix is like a jelly
- Fibers give this jelly structure
  - collagen fibers
  - elastic fibers
  - reticular fibers
- Fibroblasts secrete extracellular matrix

1-5

Specialized Cell Junctions

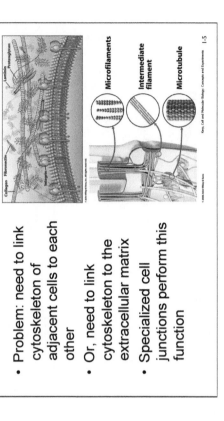

- Problem: need to link cytoskeleton of adjacent cells to each other
- Or, need to link cytoskeleton to the extracellular matrix
- Specialized cell junctions perform this function

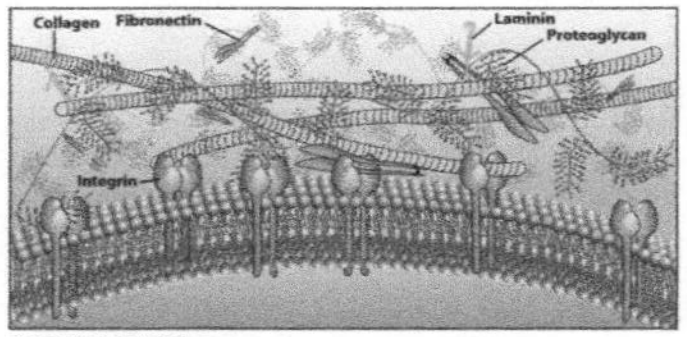
Collagen
Fibronectin
Laminin
Proteoglycan
Integrin

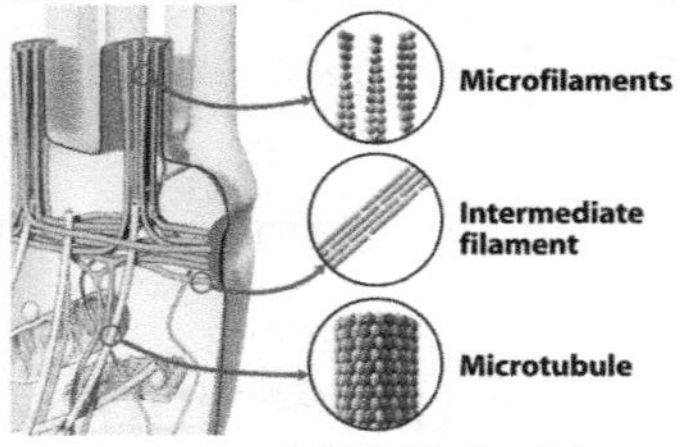
Microfilaments
Intermediate filament
Microtubule

Karp, Cell and Molecular Biology: Concepts and Experiments

1-5

Desmosomes

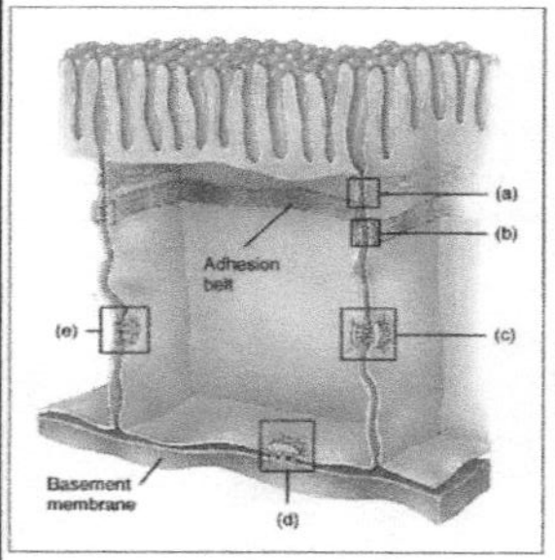
(a)
(b)
Adhesion belt
(e)
(c)
Basement membrane
(d)

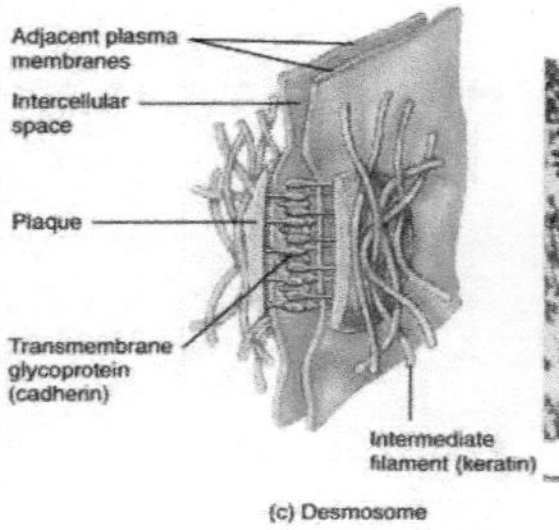
Adjacent plasma membranes
Intercellular space
Plaque
Transmembrane glycoprotein (cadherin)
Intermediate filament (keratin)

(c) Desmosome

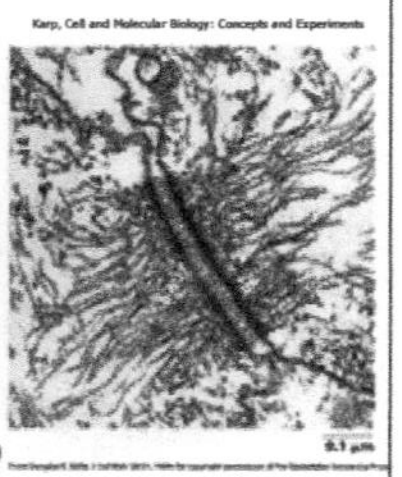
Karp, Cell and Molecular Biology: Concepts and Experiments

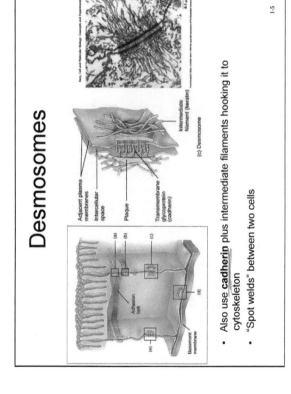

- Also use **cadherin** plus intermediate filaments hooking it to cytoskeleton
- "Spot welds" between two cells

1-5

Tight Junctions

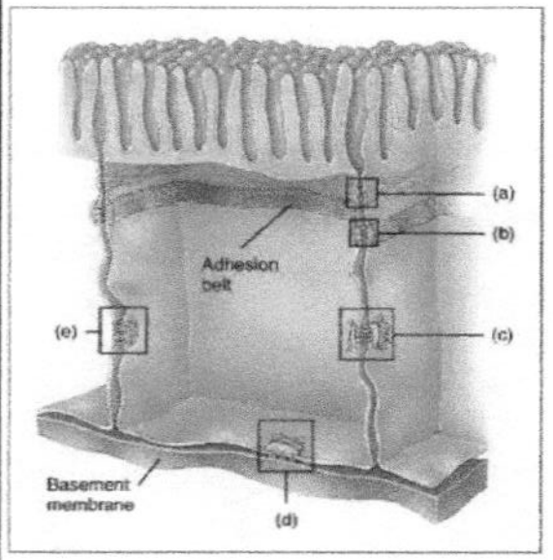
(a)
(b)
Adhesion belt
(e)
(c)
Basement membrane
(d)

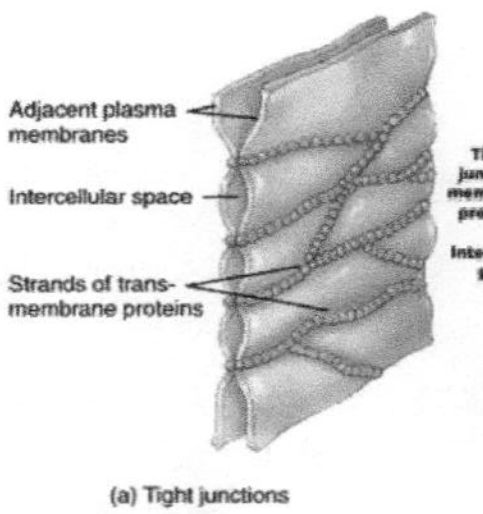
Adjacent plasma membranes
Intercellular space
Strands of trans-membrane proteins

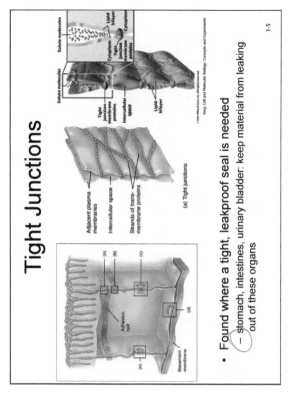

(a) Tight junctions

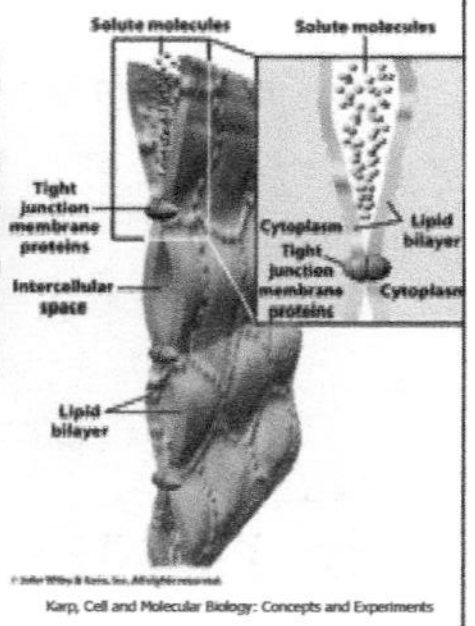
Solute molecules
Solute molecules
Tight junction membrane proteins
Intercellular space
Lipid bilayer
Cytoplasm
Tight junction membrane proteins
Lipid bilayer
Cytoplasm

Karp, Cell and Molecular Biology: Concepts and Experiments

- Found where a tight, leakproof seal is needed
  - stomach, intestines, urinary bladder: keep material from leaking out of these organs

1-5

Gap Junctions

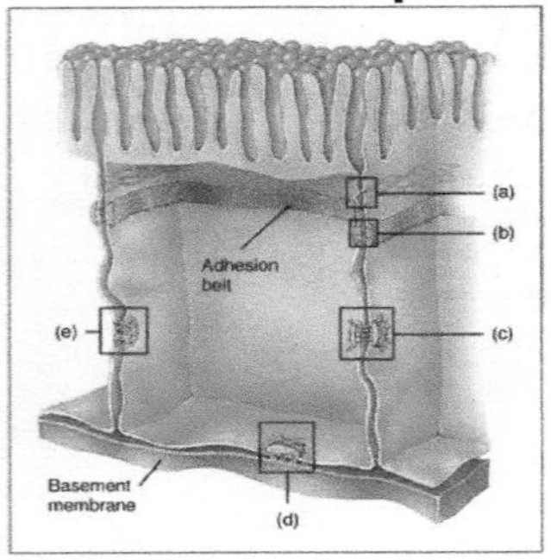
(a)
(b)
(c)
(d)
(e)
Adhesion belt
Basement membrane

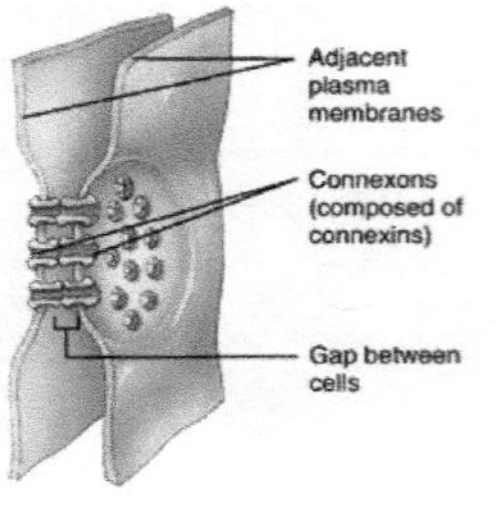
Adjacent plasma membranes
Connexons (composed of connexins)
Gap between cells

(e) Gap junction

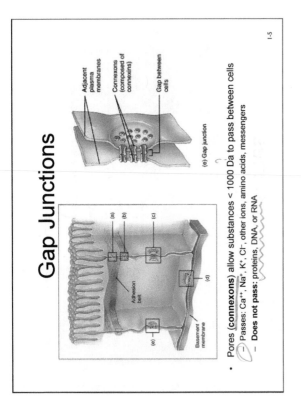

- Pores (**connexons**) allow substances < 1000 Da to pass between cells
  - Passes: Ca^{++}, Na^{+}, K^{+}, Cl^{-}, other ions, amino acids, messengers
  - **Does not pass:** proteins, DNA, or RNA

I-5

Gap Junctions

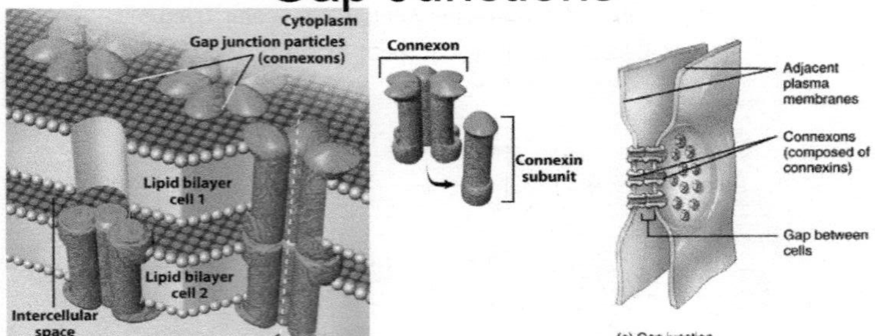
Cytoplasm
Gap junction particles (connexons)
Lipid bilayer cell 1
Lipid bilayer cell 2
Intercellular space
Cytoplasm
Hydrophilic channel
Connexon
Connexin subunit
Adjacent plasma membranes
Connexons (composed of connexins)
Gap between cells

(e) Gap junction

 Karp, Cell and Molecular Biology: Concepts and Experiments

- Calcium and other small, hydrophilic ions can pass through the channel formed by connexons
- Cells are **electrically coupled**
- If one of the cells gets sick or dies, then [Ca^{++}] increases and these seal like a hatch

I-5

Cellular Communication

- The nervous system and the endocrine system "blend together", sharing the same neurotransmitters / hormones, receptors, and signaling pathways
- The difference is in the distance that information travels

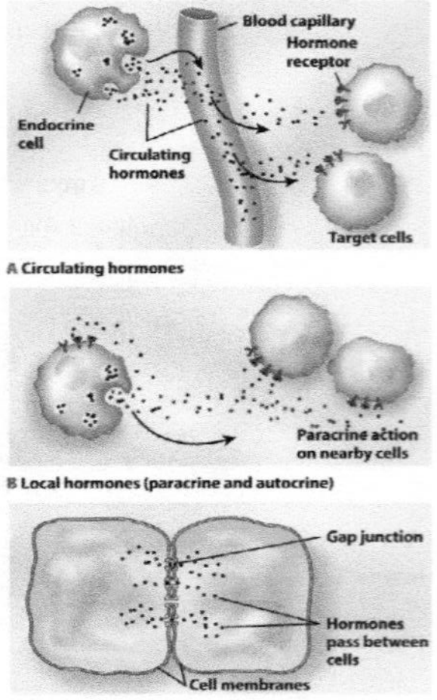
Blood capillary
Hormone receptor
Endocrine cell
Circulating hormones
Target cells
Paracrine action on nearby cells
Gap junction
Hormones pass between cells
Cell membranes

A Circulating hormones

B Local hormones (paracrine and autocrine)

C Gap junctions

Ireland, Visualizing Human Biology, 2e

I-6

Cellular Communication

- Autocrine: cells signaling themselves
- Paracrine: cells signaling neighbors
- Hormonal and Neurohormonal: cells signaling distant targets use blood

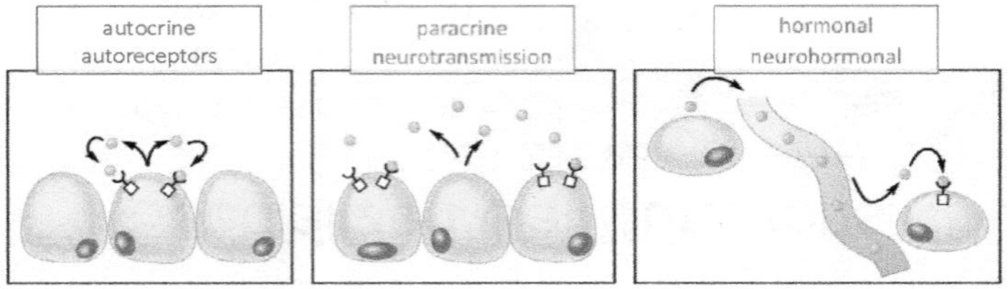
autocrine
autoreceptors
paracrine
neurotransmission
hormonal
neurohormonal

Karp, Cell and Molecular Biology: Concepts and Experiments

I-6

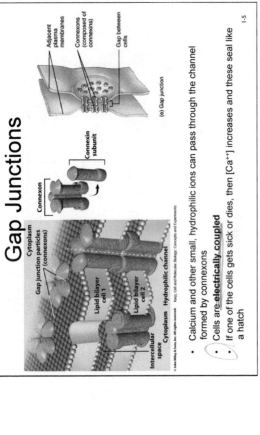

Signal Transduction

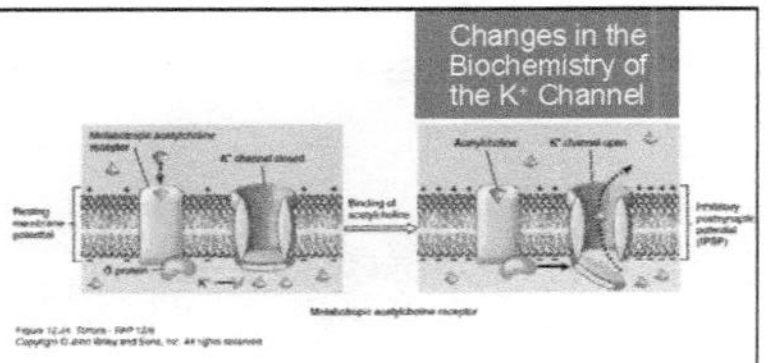
Changes in the Biochemistry of the K⁺ Channel

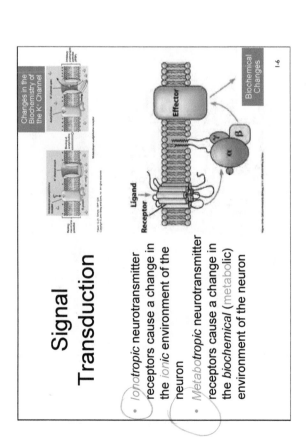

- *Ionotropic* neurotransmitter receptors cause a change in the *ionic* environment of the neuron
- *Metabotropic* neurotransmitter receptors cause a change in the *biochemical* (metabolic) environment of the neuron

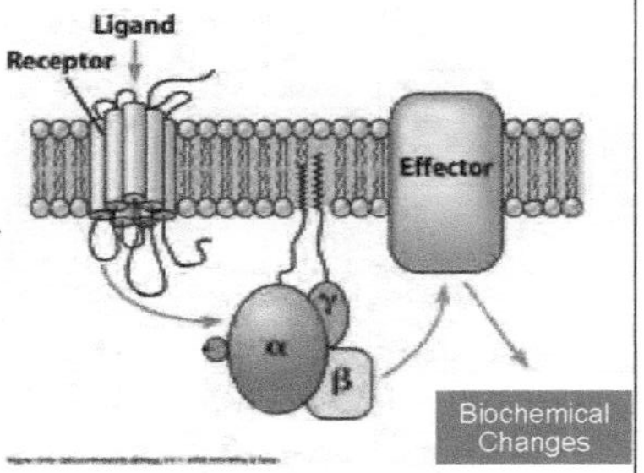
Ligand
Receptor
Effector
α
β
γ
Biochemical Changes

1-6

Second Messengers

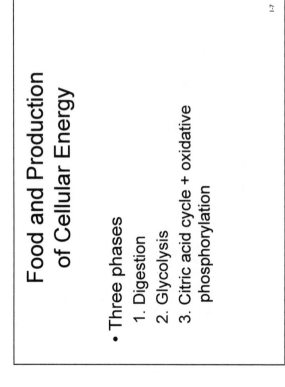

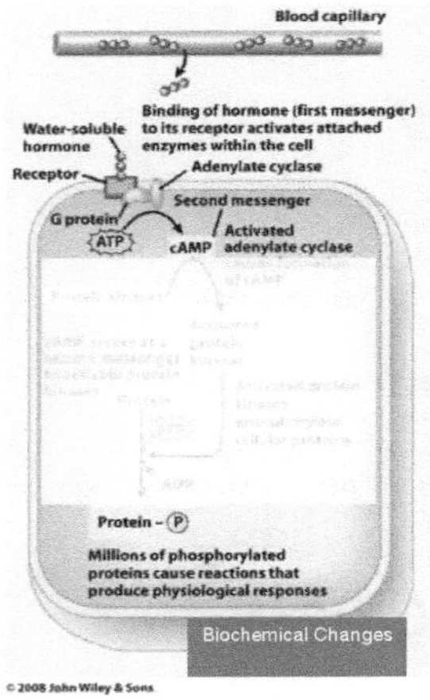
Blood capillary
Water-soluble hormone
Binding of hormone (first messenger) to its receptor activates attached enzymes within the cell
Receptor
Adenylate cyclase
G protein
ATP
Second messenger
cAMP
Activated adenylate cyclase
Protein - P
Millions of phosphorylated proteins cause reactions that produce physiological responses
Biochemical Changes
© 2008 John Wiley & Sons

- A wide variety of hormones, neurotransmitters and other factors activate these metabotropic receptors
- Two major second messenger pathways:
  - cyclic adenosine monophosphate (cyclic AMP, cAMP)
    - middleman: G protein that carries GTP or GDP
  - calcium (Ca^{++})
    - also use G protein middleman
    - activates phospholipase C

1-6

Food and Production of Cellular Energy

- Three phases
  1. Digestion
  2. Glycolysis
  3. Citric acid cycle + oxidative phosphorylation

1-7

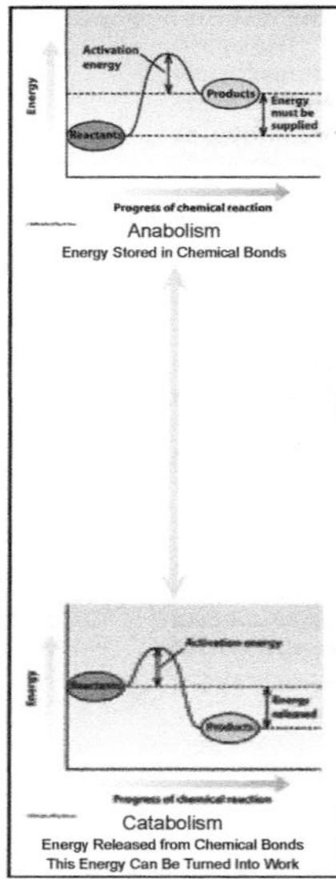
Activation energy
Reactants
Products
Energy must be supplied
Progress of chemical reaction
Anabolism
Energy Stored in Chemical Bonds
Activation energy
Energy released
Catabolism
Energy Released from Chemical Bonds
This Energy Can Be Turned Into Work

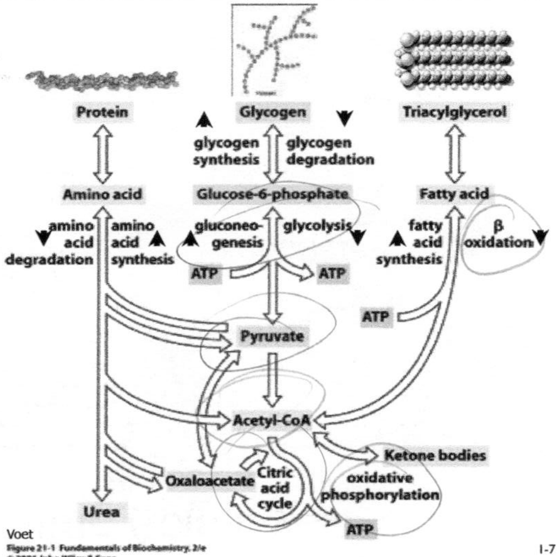
Protein
Glycogen
Triacylglycerol
glycogen synthesis
glycogen degradation
Amino acid
Glucose-6-phosphate
Fatty acid
amino acid degradation
amino acid synthesis
gluconeo-genesis
glycolysis
fatty acid synthesis
β oxidation
ATP
ATP
ATP
Pyruvate
Acetyl-CoA
Ketone bodies
Oxaloacetate
Citric acid cycle
oxidative phosphorylation
Urea
ATP

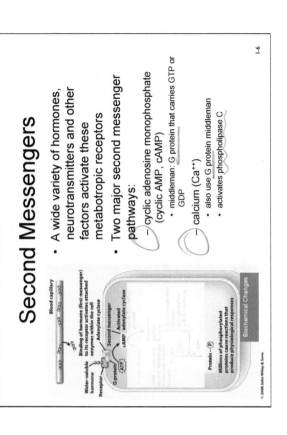

Voet
Figure 21-1 Fundamentals of Biochemistry, 2/e
© 2006 John Wiley & Sons

1-7

Glycolysis
Phase 2

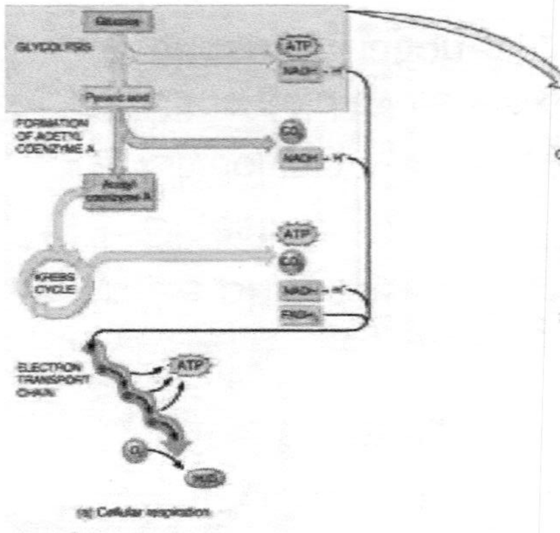
ATP
ELECTRON TRANSPORT CHAIN
(a) Cellular respiration

Note:
no O_2 needed
no CO_2 made

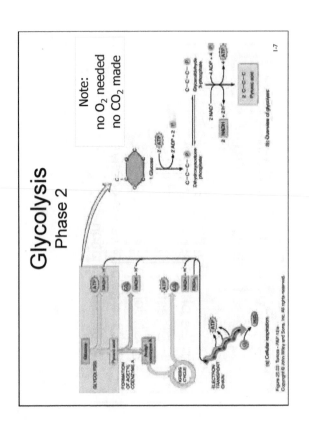

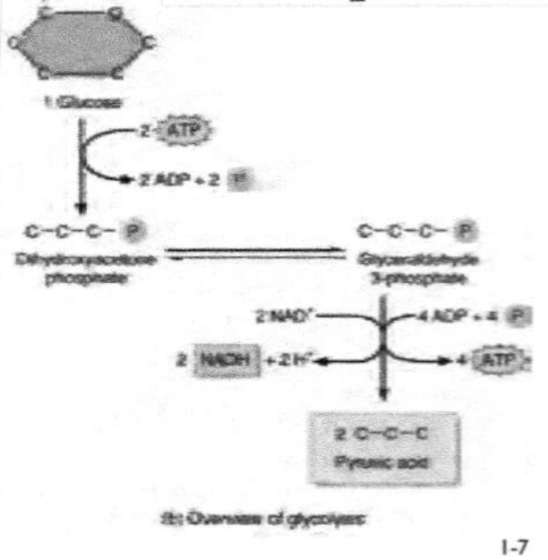
(b) Overview of glycolysis

Figure 25.22 Tortora - PAP 12/e
Copyright © John Wiley and Sons, Inc. All rights reserved.

I-7

Citric Acid Cycle
Phase 3a

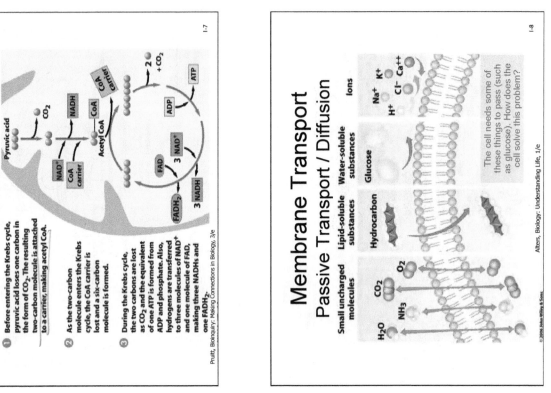

1. Before entering the Krebs cycle, pyruvic acid loses one carbon in the form of CO_2. The resulting two-carbon molecule is attached to a carrier, making acetyl CoA.
2. As the two-carbon molecule enters the Krebs cycle, the CoA carrier is lost and a six-carbon molecule is formed.
3. During the Krebs cycle, the two carbons are lost as CO_2 and the equivalent of one ATP is formed from ADP and phosphate. Also, hydrogens are transferred to three molecules of NAD^+ and one molecule of FAD, making three NADHs and one $FADH_2$.

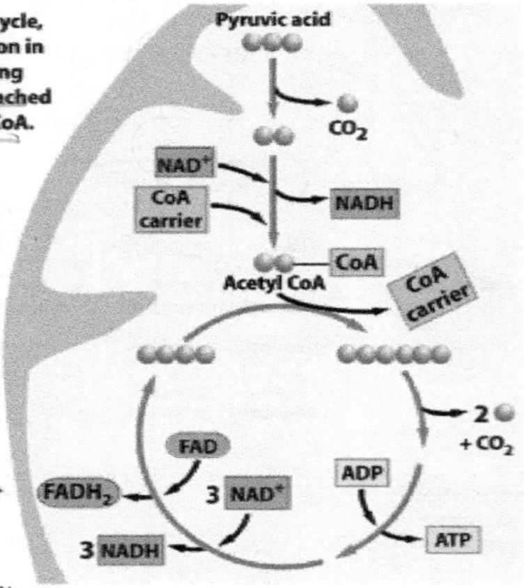
Pyruvic acid
CO2
NAD+
CoA carrier
NADH
CoA
Acetyl CoA
CoA carrier
2
+ CO2
FAD
FADH2
3 NAD+
3 NADH
ADP
ATP

Pruitt, Bioinquiry: Making Connections in Biology, 3/e

I-7

Oxidative Phosphorylation
Phase 3b

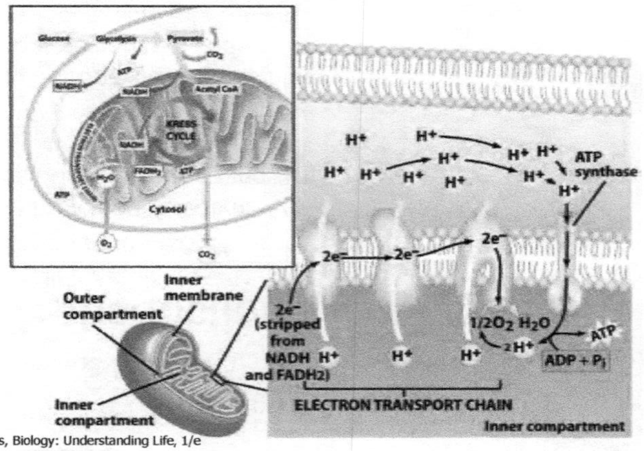
Outer compartment
Inner membrane
Inner compartment
2e−
(stripped from NADH H+ and FADH2)
H+
2e−
ATP synthase
1/2O2 H2O
2H+
ATP
ADP + Pi
ELECTRON TRANSPORT CHAIN
Inner compartment

Alters, Biology: Understanding Life, 1/e
© 2006 John Wiley & Sons

I-7

Membrane Transport
Passive Transport / Diffusion

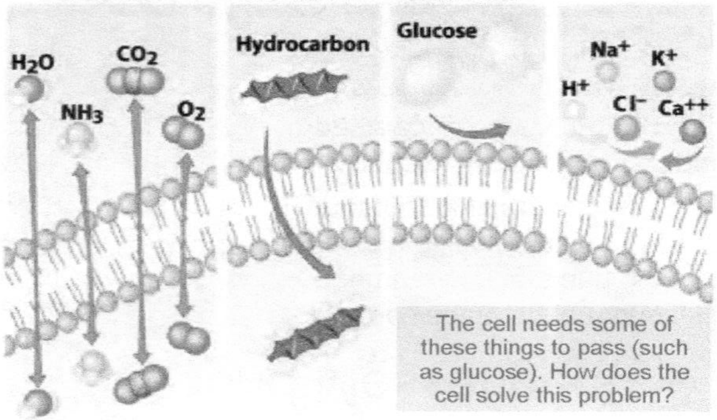
Small uncharged molecules
Lipid-soluble substances
Water-soluble substances
Ions
H2O
CO2
NH3
O2
Hydrocarbon
Glucose
Na+
K+
H+
Cl−
Ca++

The cell needs some of these things to pass (such as glucose). How does the cell solve this problem?

© 2006 John Wiley & Sons

Alters, Biology: Understanding Life, 1/e

I-8

Membrane Transport

Passive Transport / Mediated Transport / Facilitated Diffusion

- Facilitated diffusion is similar to diffusion but it requires the assistance of a carrier molecule because the substance is too polar or too big to pass on its own.

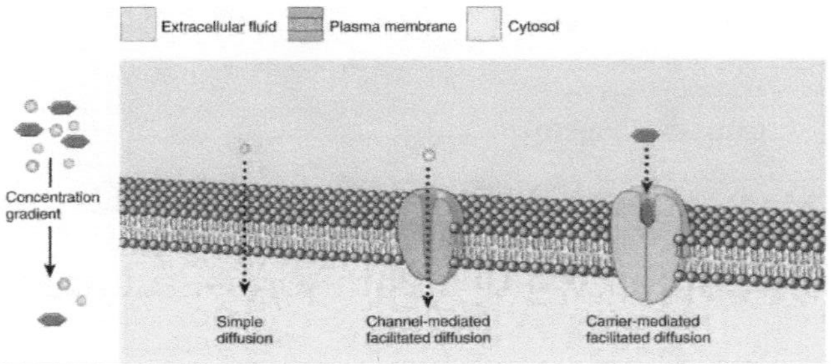

Extracellular fluid
Plasma membrane
Cytosol
Concentration gradient
Simple diffusion
Channel-mediated facilitated diffusion
Carrier-mediated facilitated diffusion

I-8

Membrane Transport

Passive Transport / Mediated Transport / Ion Channels

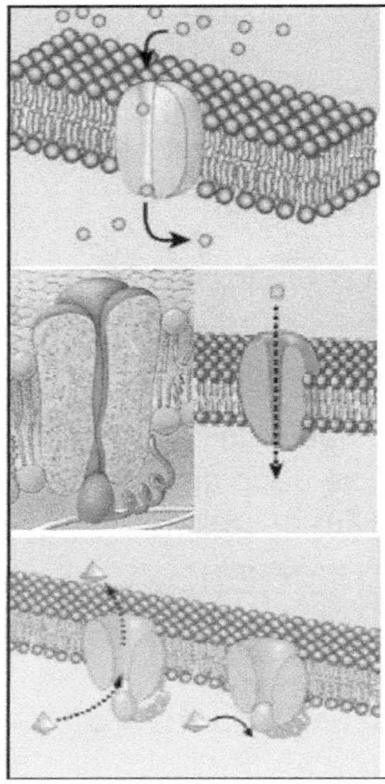

- Remember that the non-polar tails of lipid molecules prevent charged molecules, like ions, from crossing the cell membrane
- Ion channels allow ions to pass down their concentration gradient (from high concentration areas to low)
- Some are open all the time
- Some are *gated*: open and close on demand

I-8

Membrane Transport

Active Transport / Na^+/K^+ pump

- Active transport: requires ATP as energy source
- Found in virtually all cells

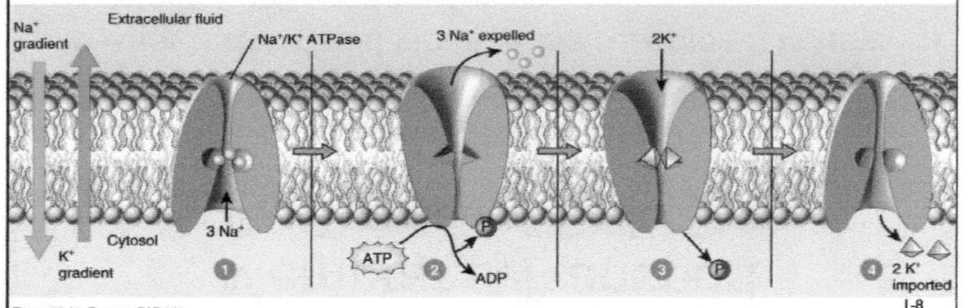

Na⁺ gradient
Extracellular fluid
Na⁺/K⁺ ATPase
3 Na⁺ expelled
2K⁺
Cytosol
K⁺ gradient
3 Na⁺
1
ATP
2
ADP
3
4
2 K⁺ imported

Figure 03.10 Tortora - PAP 12/e

I-8

Membrane Transport

Active Transport / Mediated Transport / Symport and Antiport

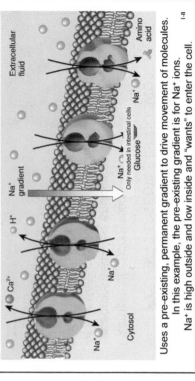

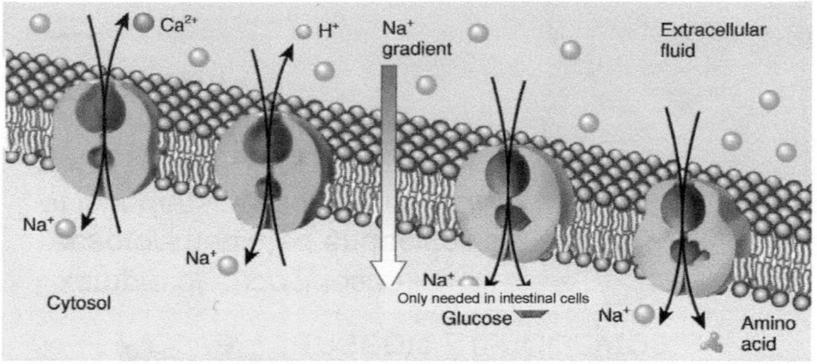

Ca²⁺
H⁺
Na⁺ gradient
Extracellular fluid
Na⁺
Na⁺
Cytosol
Na⁺
Only needed in intestinal cells
Glucose
Na⁺
Amino acid

Uses a pre-existing, permanent gradient to drive movement of molecules. In this example, the pre-existing gradient is for Na^+ ions. Na^+ is high outside and low inside and "wants" to enter the cell.

I-8

Membrane Transport
Active Transport / Endocytosis

- Cell surface proteins (receptors) can bind molecules the cell wants to take in
- After the material binds to the receptor, it is taken into the cell (**endocytosis**)
- **Exocytosis** is the same process in reverse

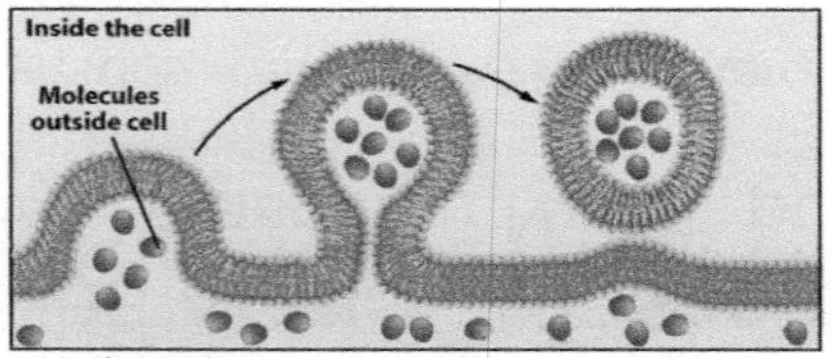

Inside the cell
Molecules outside cell

***(a)* Endocytosis** Pruitt, Bioinquiry: Making Connections in Biology, 3/e

1-8

Membrane Transport
Active Transport / Endocytosis

- Example of endocytosis: receptor-mediated endocytosis of low-density lipoprotein (LDL)
- Remember that LDL is one of the forms of lipid in the bloodstream

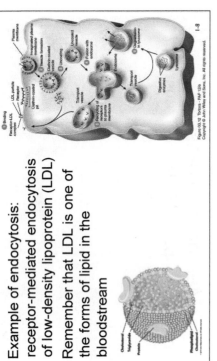

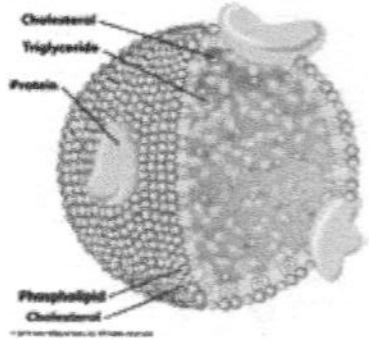

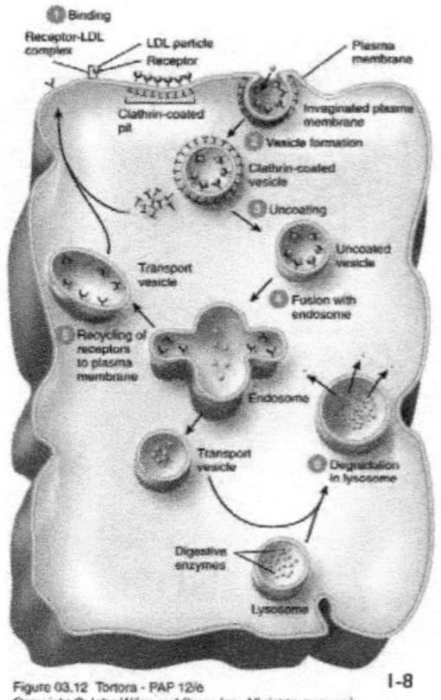

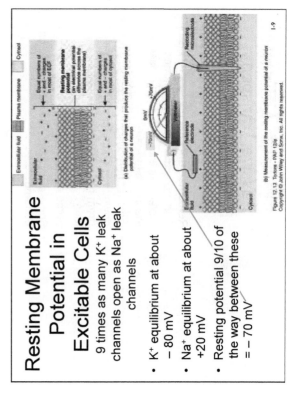

Figure 03.12 Tortora - PAP 12/e

1-8

Membrane Potentials in Excitable Cells
(Nerve & Muscle)

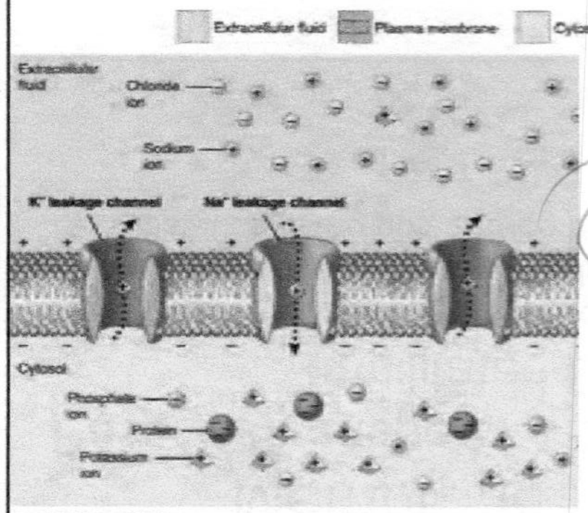

Extracellular fluid
Plasma membrane
Cytosol

- Resting Potential
  - Resting (not conducting an impulse)
  - Potential (a difference in the electrical charge)
- A resting membrane: inside (negative) the membrane is negatively charged compared with the outside (positive)

Figure 12.14 Tortora - PAP 12/e

1-9

Resting Membrane Potential in Excitable Cells

9 times as many K^+ leak channels open as Na^+ leak channels

- K^+ equilibrium at about – 80 mV
- Na^+ equilibrium at about +20 mV
- Resting potential 9/10 of the way between these = – 70 mV

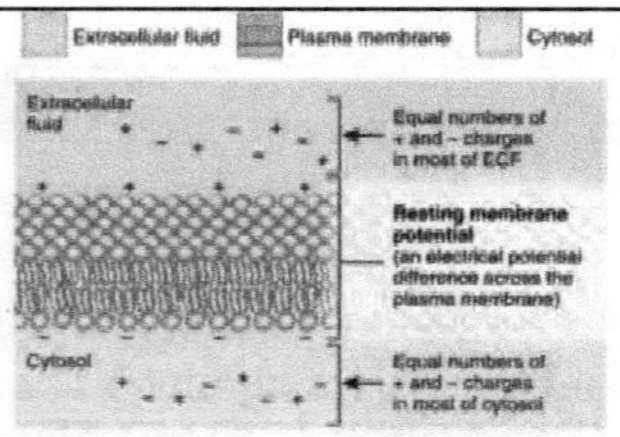

Extracellular fluid
Plasma membrane
Cytosol
Equal numbers of + and – charges in most of ECF
Resting membrane potential (an electrical potential difference across the plasma membrane)
Equal numbers of + and – charges in most of cytosol

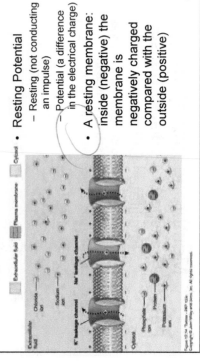

(a) Distribution of charges that produce the resting membrane potential of a neuron

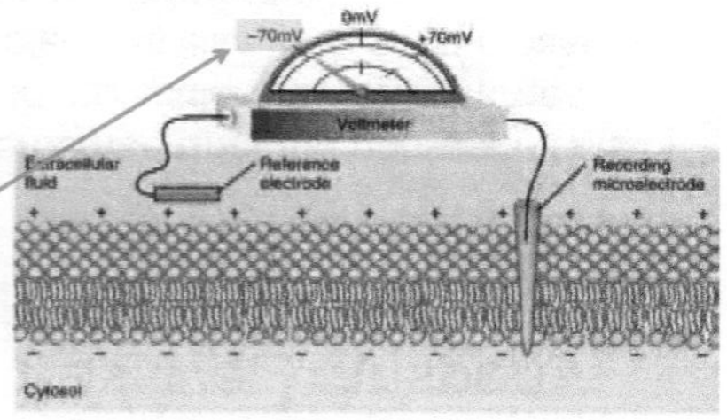

–70mV
0mV
+70mV
Voltmeter
Reference electrode
Recording microelectrode
Extracellular fluid
Cytosol

(b) Measurement of the resting membrane potential of a neuron

Figure 12.13 Tortora - PAP 12/e

1-9

The Action Potential in Excitable Cells (Nerve & Muscle)

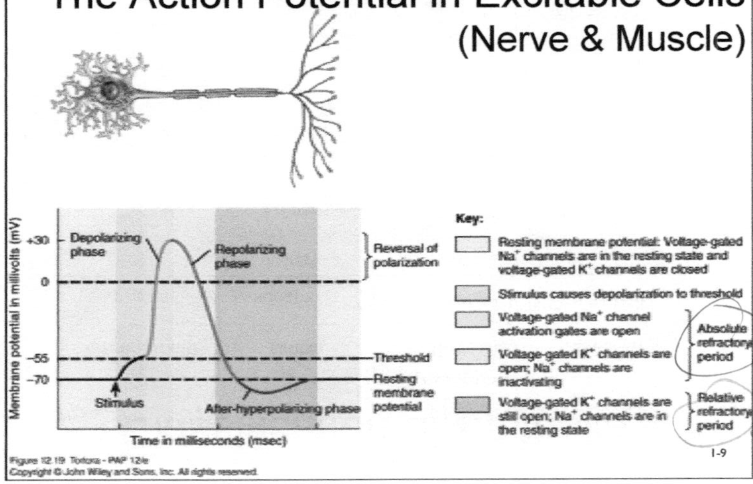
Membrane potential in millivolts (mV)
+30
0
–55
–70
Depolarizing phase
Repolarizing phase
Reversal of polarization
Threshold
Resting membrane potential
Stimulus
After-hyperpolarizing phase
Time in milliseconds (msec)
Key:
Resting membrane potential: Voltage-gated Na⁺ channels are in the resting state and voltage-gated K⁺ channels are closed
Stimulus causes depolarization to threshold
Voltage-gated Na⁺ channel activation gates are open
Voltage-gated K⁺ channels are open; Na⁺ channels are inactivating
Voltage-gated K⁺ channels are still open; Na⁺ channels are in the resting state
Absolute refractory period
Relative refractory period

Figure 12.19 Tortora - PAP 12/e

1-9

cannot B stimulated during this phase

can be triggerd by BIG stimulus

Cell Cycle

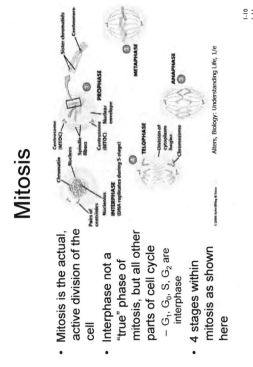

- When cells become damaged, diseased, or simple worn out, they must be replaced. Cells have to divide to repair and replace old or damaged cells.
- In somatic (non-reproductive) cell division both the nucleus (mitosis) and the cytoplasm (cytokinesis) divide.
- For a cell to divide it must receive a stimulatory signal from a cytokine called a growth factor. Specific cells respond to specific growth factors.

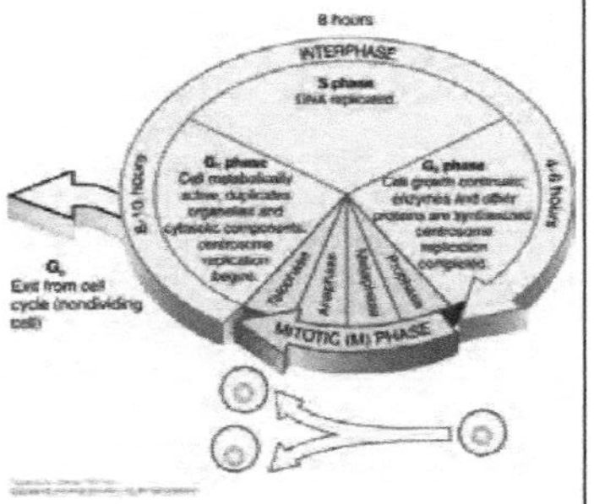
8 hours
INTERPHASE
S phase
8-10 hours
4-6 hours
G_1 phase
G_2 phase
MITOTIC (M) PHASE
G_0
Exit from cell cycle (nondividing cell)

1-10

Growth Factors (Cytokines)

- Transmit signals within and between cells
- Regulate checkpoints in the cell cycle
  - Platelet-derived growth factor (PDGF)
    - Encourages proliferation of connective tissue
  - Nerve growth factor (NGF)
    - Encourages proliferation of nerve cells
  - Insulin-like growth factors I & II (IGF I&II)
    - Works with PDGF to encourage proliferation of fat cells and connective tissue
  - Erythropoietin
    - Encourages proliferation of red cell precursor cells
  - Others

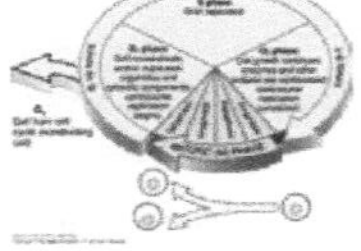

1-10

Mitosis

- Mitosis is the actual, active division of the cell
- Interphase not a "true" phase of mitosis, but all other parts of cell cycle
  - G_1, G_0, S, G_2 are interphase
- 4 stages within mitosis as shown here

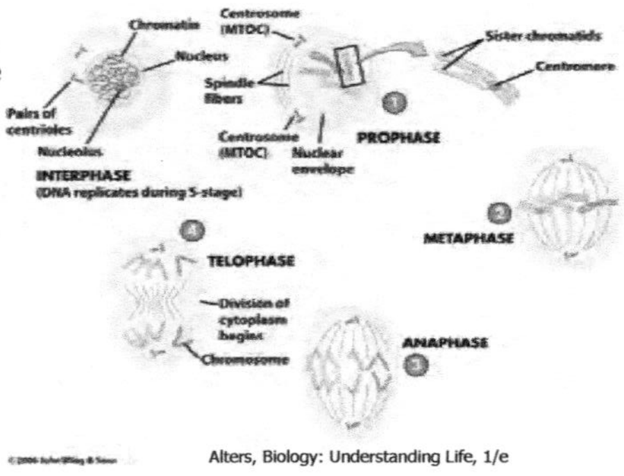
Chromatin
Centrosome (MTOC)
Nucleus
Spindle fibers
Sister chromatids
Centromere
Pairs of centrioles
Nucleolus
Centrosome (MTOC)
Nuclear envelope
PROPHASE
INTERPHASE (DNA replicates during S-stage)
METAPHASE
TELOPHASE
Division of cytoplasm begins
Chromosome
ANAPHASE

Alters, Biology: Understanding Life, 1/e

1-10
1-11

The Four Tissue Types

1. Epithelial tissue
   - Forms coverings protecting the body from the outside world
   - Remember that the lumen (opening) of the gut tube is "outside"
2. Connective tissue
   - Holds structure of body
3. Muscular tissue
   - Moves body parts
4. Nervous tissue
   - Sensation, information processing, and control of body parts

Features of an Epithelium

- One free surface (*apical surface*)
- One surface attached to *basement membrane*
  - *basal lamina*
  - *reticular lamina*
- Underlying connective tissue
- Locations:
  1. Barriers to keep outside out and inside in
  2. Barriers that secrete substances
  3. Barriers for protection

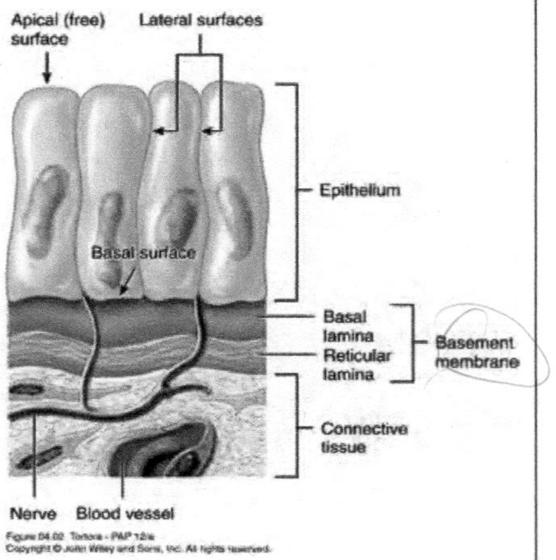

Apical (free) surface
Lateral surfaces
Epithelium
Basal surface
Basal lamina
Reticular lamina
Basement membrane
Connective tissue
Nerve
Blood vessel

Classification of Epithelia

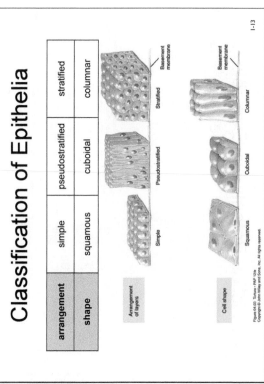

arrangement	simple	pseudostratified	stratified
shape	squamous	cuboidal	columnar

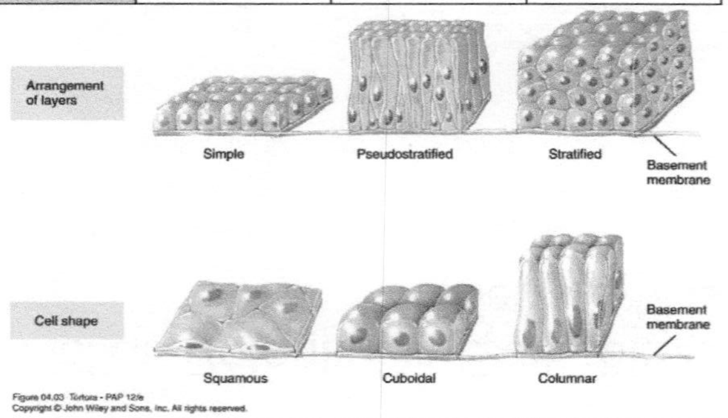

Arrangement of layers
Simple
Pseudostratified
Stratified
Basement membrane
Cell shape
Squamous
Cuboidal
Columnar
Basement membrane

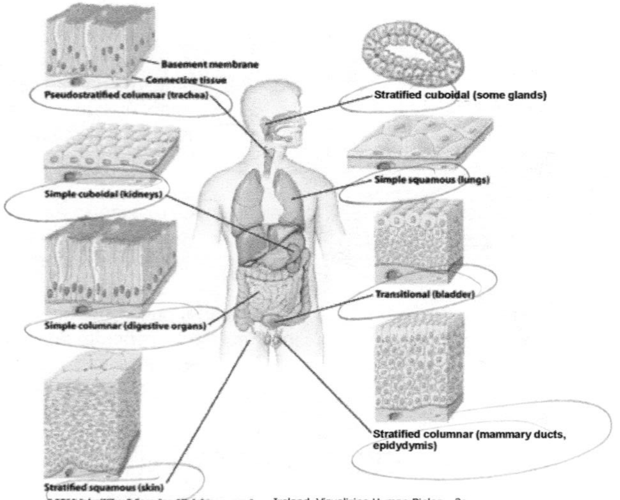

Basement membrane
Connective tissue
Pseudostratified columnar (trachea)
Simple cuboidal (kidneys)
Simple columnar (digestive organs)
Stratified squamous (skin)
Stratified cuboidal (some glands)
Simple squamous (lungs)
Transitional (bladder)
Stratified columnar (mammary ducts, epidydymis)

 Ireland, Visualizing Human Biology, 2e

Connective Tissue Classification

- Embryonic connective tissue
  - Mesenchyme
  - Mucous connective tissue
- Mature connective tissue
  - Loose connective tissue
  - Dense connective tissue
  - Cartilage
  - Bone
  - Liquid

1-14

Review: Types of Connective Tissue

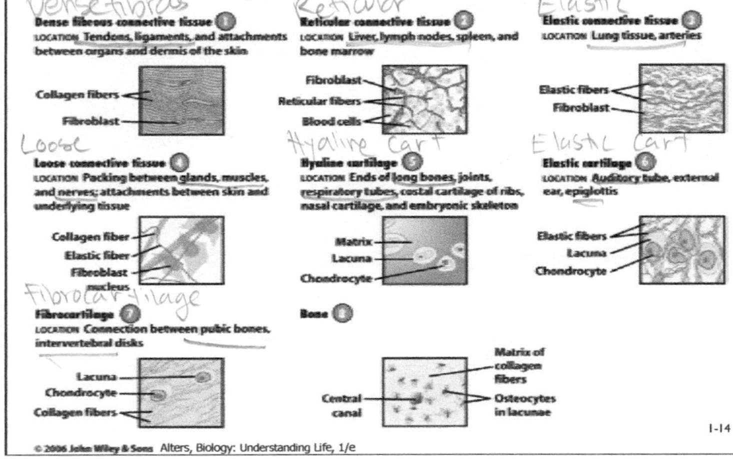
Dense fibrous connective tissue 1
LOCATION Tendons, ligaments, and attachments between organs and dermis of the skin
Collagen fibers
Fibroblast
Reticular connective tissue 2
LOCATION Liver, lymph nodes, spleen, and bone marrow
Fibroblast
Reticular fibers
Blood cells
Elastic connective tissue 3
LOCATION Lung tissue, arteries
Elastic fibers
Fibroblast
Loose connective tissue 4
LOCATION Packing between glands, muscles, and nerves; attachments between skin and underlying tissue
Collagen fiber
Elastic fiber
Fibroblast nucleus
Hyaline cartilage 5
LOCATION Ends of long bones, joints, respiratory tubes, costal cartilage of ribs, nasal cartilage, and embryonic skeleton
Matrix
Lacuna
Chondrocyte
Elastic cartilage 6
LOCATION Auditory tube, external ear, epiglottis
Elastic fibers
Lacuna
Chondrocyte
Fibrocartilage 7
LOCATION Connection between pubic bones, intervertebral disks
Lacuna
Chondrocyte
Collagen fibers
Bone 8
Central canal
Matrix of collagen fibers
Osteocytes in lacunae

© 2006 John Wiley & Sons Alters, Biology: Understanding Life, 1/e

1-14

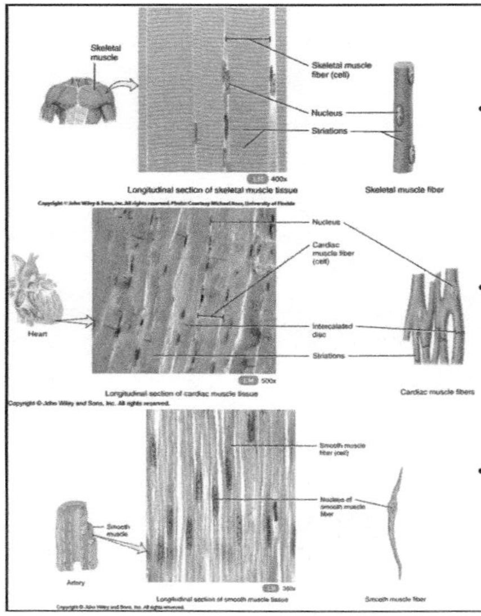

Muscle Tissue

- Skeletal muscle
  - also called **voluntary muscle**
  - under our voluntary control
  - moves body at joints
  - multiple cells fuse to form long muscle fibers, so it has multiple, eccentric nuclei
- Cardiac muscle
  - found only in heart
  - not under voluntary control
  - striated appearance like skeletal
  - **intercalated discs**
  - branched structure
- Smooth muscle
  - single cells, central nucleus
  - not under voluntary control
  - arteries, gut tube

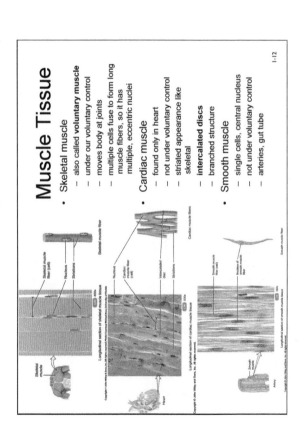

1-12

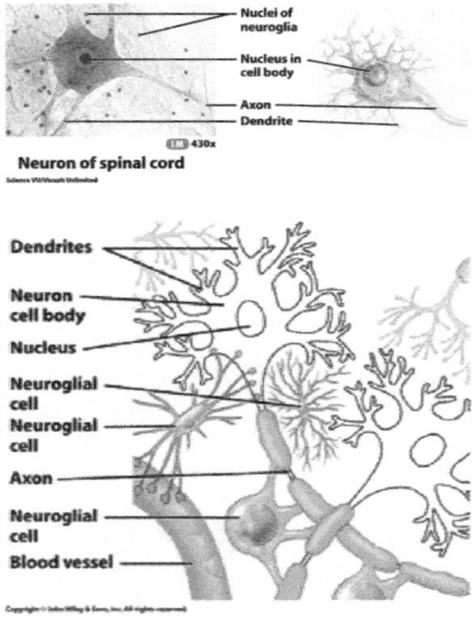
Nuclei of neuroglia
Nucleus in cell body
Axon
Dendrite
Neuron of spinal cord
Dendrites
Neuron cell body
Nucleus
Neuroglial cell
Neuroglial cell
Axon
Neuroglial cell
Blood vessel

Nervous Tissue

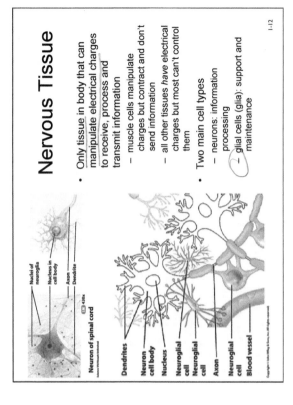

- Only tissue in body that can manipulate electrical charges to receive, process and transmit information
  - muscle cells manipulate charges but contract and don't send information
  - all other tissues *have* electrical charges but most can't control them
- Two main cell types
  - neurons: information processing
  - glial cells (glia): support and maintenance

1-12

UNIT 1

Study Guide Objectives - Introductory Pathophysiology (HTHS 2230)

Unit 1

Chapter 3 – Altered Cellular and Tissue Biology

1. Compare and contrast the adaptive and maladaptive cellular adaptations: atrophy, hypertrophy, hyperplasia, dysplasia and metaplasia. (pp. 60-62)

2. State the three common forms of cell injury: hypoxic injury, reactive oxygen species and free radicals, and chemical injury. Compare and contrast these. (pp. 62-73)

3. Compare and contrast injuries from blunt force injuries (contusions, abrasions, and lacerations); sharp force injuries (incised wounds and stab wounds); gunshot wounds; asphyxiation; and other sources of injury. (pp. 73-79)

4. Discuss the manifestations of cellular injury including accumulation of substances characteristic of cellular damage. (pp. 80-84)

5. Compare and contrast different forms of necrosis: coagulative, liquefactive, caseous, fat and gangrenous. (pp. 85-87)

6. Compare and contrast necrosis and apoptosis. (pp. 85-88)

7. Characterize the process of aging. (pp. 90-93)

8. Describe the signs of somatic death. (pp. 93-94)

Chapter 4 –Fluids and Electrolytes, Acids and Bases

1. Describe the distribution of body fluids between intracellular and extracellular compartments. (pp. 98-99)

2. State and describe the forces responsible for the distribution of water and the movement of nutrients and wastes between the capillary and interstitial compartments (Starling forces). Be able to use this information to determine the direction of water movement. (pp. 99-100)

3. Explain edema formation. (pp. 100-101)

4. Describe the important features of sodium, chloride, and water balance. Name signs and symptoms associated with imbalances. (pp. 102-109)

5. Describe the important features of potassium, calcium, phosphate, and magnesium balance, and name signs and symptoms associated with imbalances. (pp. 105-109)

6. Compare and contrast the important features of acid-base balance: acidosis vs. alkalosis, and metabolic vs respiratory causes. Given a patient's arterial blood values, be able to state the exact description of the acid-base imbalance (i.e. "uncompensated metabolic acidosis"). (pp. 109-114)

Unit 1
Chapter 3
Altered Cellular and Tissue Biology

1

Cellular Adaptation

- Cells change to
  - Adapt to a new environment
  - Escape
  - Protect themselves
- Cell types adapt in very specific ways
  - Muscle vs epithelium
  - Nerves
  - Connective tissue
- Can cellular adaptation be a pathological response, functional response, or both? yes
- Cellular adaptation vs cellular injury

2-1

2

Cell Adaptation:
Variation in Size & Shape

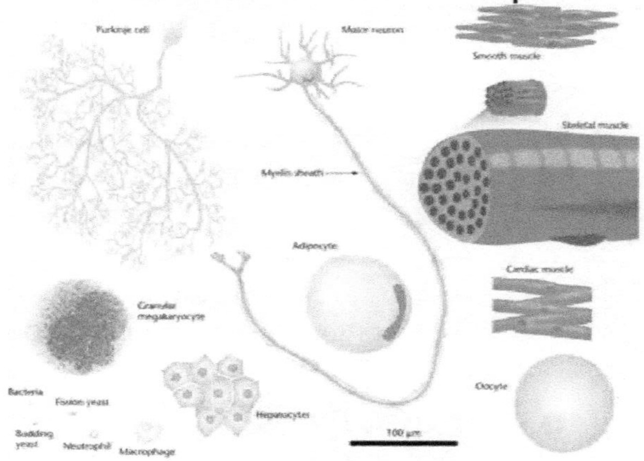

Guertin DA & Sabatini DM. Cell Size Control. *Encyclopedia of Life Sciences*, 2005.

2-1

3

Atrophy

"a–" = not, loss of
"–trophy" = size

- Atrophy is a decrease in cell size
  - may even result in the complete loss of cells
  - it is a sign of pathophysiology rather than a successful adaptation
- Usually caused by disease or ischemia – obstruction of blood flow
  - reduced blood supply → reduced oxygen and glucose to tissues → cellular shrinkage and death
- May also result from:
  - diminished nerve stimulation
  - poor nutrition
  - other diseases (e.g. Alzheimer disease in brain)

2-1

slow twitch? red fibers. endurance more O2

white fibers sprint less O2 fast twitch?

Hypertrophy

- Increase in the **mass** of the cell but not the number of cells
- Increase in the number of muscle proteins (not fluid) to allow muscle fibers to do more work
- Common tissues
  - Cardiac muscle enlarged
  - Skeletal muscle exercise.
  - Kidneys

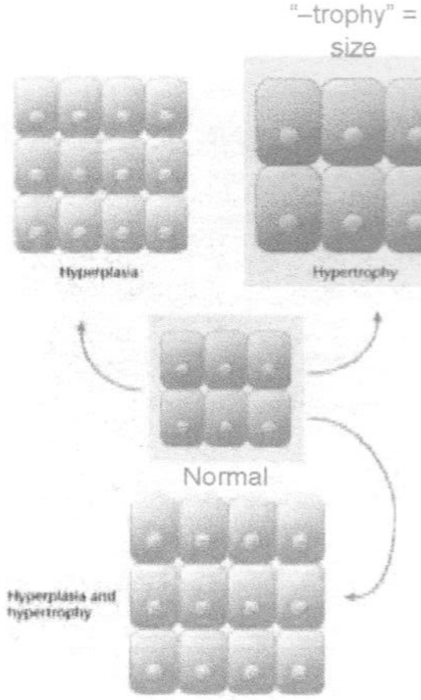
"–trophy" = size
Hyperplasia
Hypertrophy
Normal
Hyperplasia and hypertrophy

Guertin DA & Sabatini DM. Cell Size Control. *Encyclopedia of Life Sciences*, 2005.

2-1

Hyperplasia

- Increase in the **number** of cells of a tissue or organ from an increased rate of cell division
- The cells involved must have mitotic ability
- In any given organ, it's possible for **both hyperplasia and hypertrophy** to occur
  - Uterine muscle enlargement during pregnancy (hypertrophy)
  - Hyperplasia of the uterine endometrium during pregnancy (and also during every menstrual cycle)

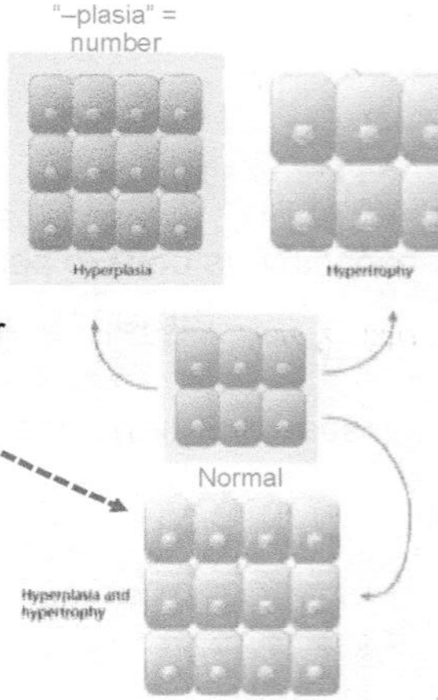
"–plasia" = number
Hyperplasia
Hypertrophy
Normal
Hyperplasia and hypertrophy

Guertin DA & Sabatini DM. Cell Size Control. *Encyclopedia of Life Sciences*, 2005.

2-1

Metaplasia

- An **adaptive** substitution to a **different**, "hardier" cell line
  - Usually changes to a hypertrophied or hyperplastic tissue

    ~~tougher~~? ? in #
- Example:
  - Replacement of ciliated columnar epithelium with stratified squamous epithelium in the respiratory tract of a smoker

- the stem cells that switched to squamous can switch back to columnar. fixable.

2-1

Dysplasia

- A change to an abnormal cell line
  - Dysplastic cells are not normal and not found anywhere in the body
  - This is a **precancerous** change
- Characterized by atypical changes in the size, shape, and appearance, and of the cells (*atypical hyperplasia*)
- Caused by persistent injury or irritation progressing towards neoplasia (new, abnormal proliferation of cells)
- Examples of the precancerous changes of dysplasia
  - cervical dysplasia from *human papilloma virus* (HPV)
  - bronchial dysplasia from smoking

2-1

8

Example: Cervical Dysplasia

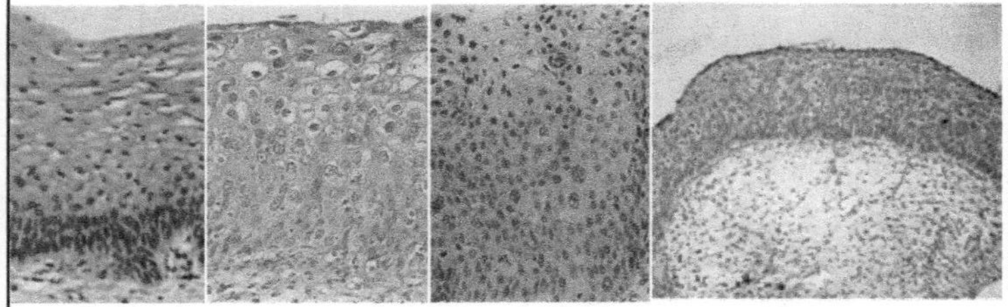

Nelson JH *et al. CA Cancer J Physicians* **39**:157, 1989.

good ⟶ bad

Good:
normal shapes and sizes of cells (this is skin, so basal cells dark and round, mature cells clear and squamous)

Bad:
Lots of mitotic figures (dividing cells), abnormal shapes and sizes of cells (no longer resembles skin)

2-1

9

Cellular Injury

stimulus exceeds coping mechanism

- Cells become injured in many ways:
  - Membrane permeabilty changes
  - Interruption of oxidative metabolism (ATP production)
  - Diminished protein synthesis
  - Leakage of digestive enzymes
- If two people are exposed to the same stimulus, will they incur the same degree of cellular damage? maybe.

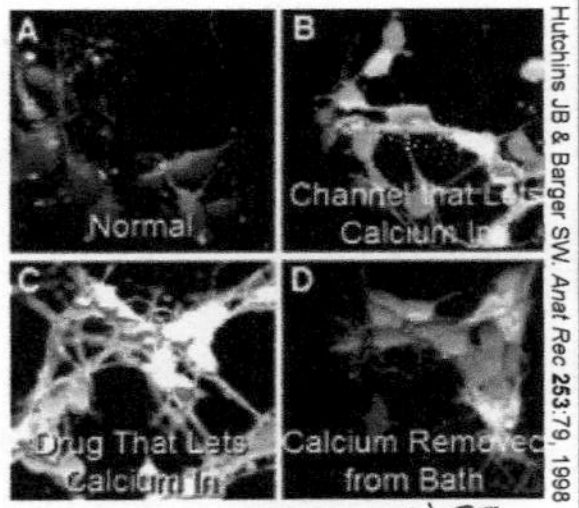
A
Normal
B
Channel That Lets Calcium In
C
Drug That Lets Calcium In
D
Calcium Removed from Bath

Hutchins JB & Barger SW. *Anat Rec* **253**:79, 1998

but people r diff.
-genetics
-amt, length damage.

2-2

= prevent Edema etc. swelled swell

29

- most comen form of cell damage
- ischemia #1 cause.

10

Hypoxia

- Tissue hypoxia is when cells are deprived of oxygen
  - *hyp[o]–* = low
  - *–oxia* = oxygen
- It is probably the most common cause of a non-adaptive cellular injury
- Hypoxia can be caused by:
  - Low levels of oxygen in the air
  - Poor or absent hemoglobin function
    - *hyp[o]–* + *–ox–* + *–emia* = low oxygen blood
  - Respiratory or cardiovascular diseases
  - Ischemia
    - reduced supply of blood, which carries oxygen

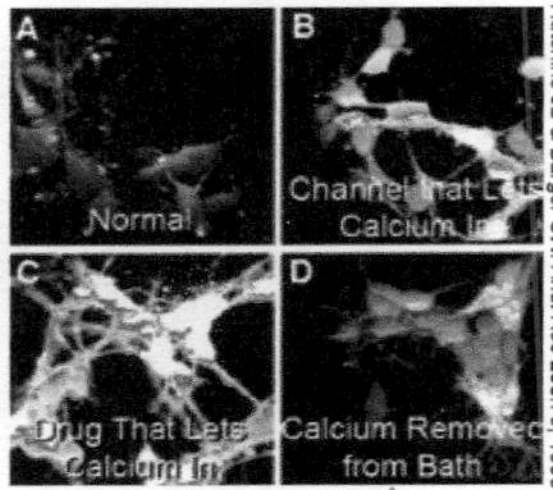
A
Normal
B
Channel That Lets Calcium In
C
Drug That Lets Calcium In
D
Calcium Removed from Bath

Hutchins JB & Barger SW. *Anat Rec* **253**:79, 1998

spleen etc not tolerant of crappy hemoglobin & will rip it out of circulation causing ↓ O_2 anyway.

2-2

11

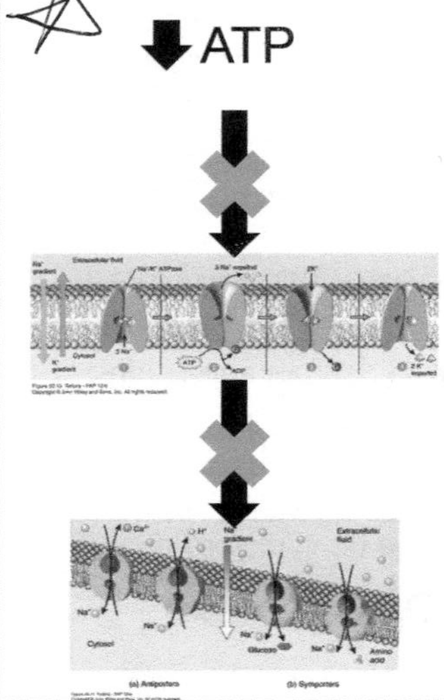
↓ATP

Hypoxia

- Because of the reduction of oxidative metabolism, ATP levels decline
  - this causes decreased Na^+/K^+ pump activity
  - Na^+ begins to accumulate in cells
  - Water follows Na^+ and also accumulates in cells
  - Intracellular K^+ decreases, approaching levels outside the cell
    - decreased protein synthesis
    - decreased membrane transport (symport and antiport systems which depend on normal Na^+ and K^+ levels are disrupted)
    - increased lipids (*lipogenesis*)

2-2

maintain = concentration gradient

oxygen = H^- e^- acceptor in ET chain.

ATP mostly used for Active transport.

$3Na^+$ + H_2O · Na^+/K^+ pumps; ECF / ICF $2K^+$

Ca++ also ↓ cell to cell communication.

12

Hypoxia

- Change in membrane permeability
  - ↑ intracellular Ca^{++}
  - this impairs mitochondrial function
- Cellular accumulations
  - abnormal ↑ water, ↑ lipids, ↑ proteins
- ↓ Protein synthesis
  - as ribosomes are separated from endoplasmic reticulum by increased fluid levels
- ↑ Glycolysis (*anaerobic metabolism*) because of ↓ O_2
  - lactic acid accumulates and causes low cellular pH (acidosis)
  - lysosomes swell and dump, chromatin clumps, proteins denature

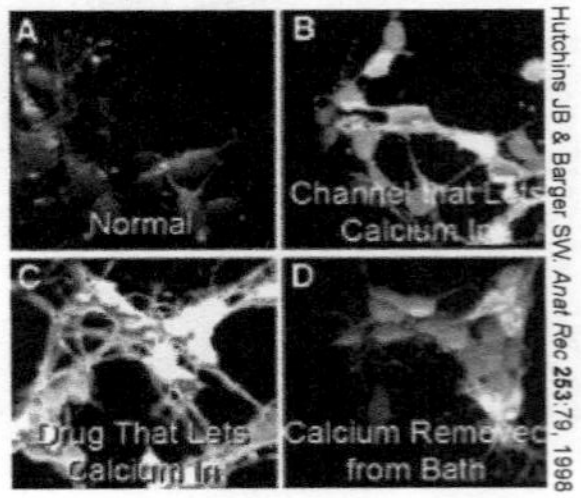
A
Normal
B
Channel that Lets Calcium In
C
Drug That Lets Calcium In
D
Calcium Removed from Bath

Hutchins JB & Barger SW. *Anat Rec* **253**:79, 1998

2-2

Free rad steals an e⁻, then that molecule goes & does same thing to another molecule and on and on.

13

Free Radicals

- A free radical is an atom or molecules that has an unpaired electron. This radical makes the atom very unstable and active.
- To gain stability, the radical gives up or steals an electron
- Superoxide ion (O_2^-)
- Hydroxyl ($OH^{\cdot}$)
- Peroxinitrite ion ($ONOO^-$)

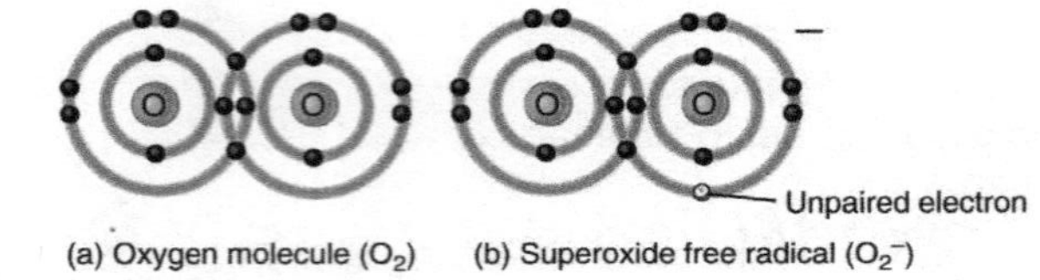
Unpaired electron

(a) Oxygen molecule (O_2) (b) Superoxide free radical (O_2^-)

2-2

reactive oxygen species. (ROS) all oxygen species.

14 oxidation / reduction

molecule antioxidant

Free Radical Formation

- Formation of free radicals
  - Normal metabolism, ionizing radiation, drug metabolism
- Mechanisms of injury: ~~unsaturated fa~~
  - Lipid peroxidation
    - Destruction of unsaturated fatty acids by free radicals (cell membrane)
  - Protein destruction
    - Fragmentation of polypeptide chains and denaturation
  - DNA alteration
    - Breakage of DNA strands

free radicals damage these

2-2

15

Free Radical Inactivation

- **Antioxidants**
  - Block synthesis or inactive free radicals
  - Vitamin E, Vitamin C, albumin, ceruloplasmin (carries copper), and transferrin (carries iron)
- **Enzymes**
  - Superoxide dismutase (SOD)
    - This is usually inactivated by the enzyme *superoxide dismutase* (SOD)
    - SOD converts superoxide to H_2O_2.
  - Catalase
    - SOD makes H_2O_2
    - Catalase then converts $2H_2O_2 \rightarrow O_2 + 2H_2O$
  - Glutathione peroxidase (GPx)

2-2

- insulin a protein. stomach absorbs amino acids ∅ proteins
- insulin needs to B in blood.

°reperfusion injury - too much O_2 poured in extras become free rads.

16

Lead Poisoning

- Key: acts like iron, calcium and zinc
- Interferes with neurotransmitters in the CNS.
  - May cause wrist, finger and foot paralysis in the peripheral nervous system.
- Interferes with hemoglobin synthesis
- Accounts for a significant number of childhood poisonings
  - Sources include paint, dust and soil, contaminated tap water, dyes, pottery glazes, gasoline

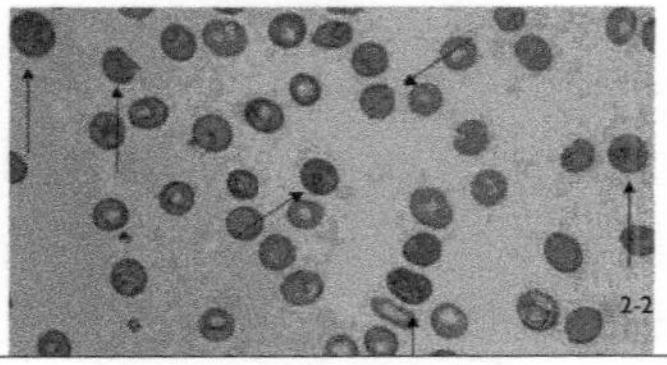

Dedeken GM *et al. J Gen Internal Med* **21**:C1, 2006.

2-2

17

Toxic Chemical Agents

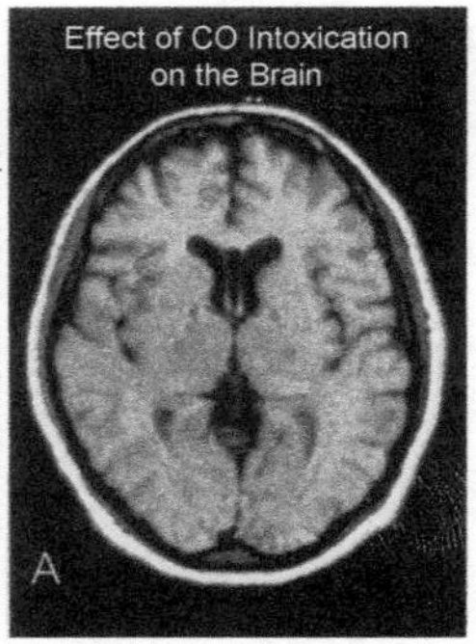
Effect of CO Intoxication on the Brain
A

Bruno A *et al. Acta Neurol Scand* **87**:205, 1993.

- Cellular injury by chemical agents can be caused by direct contact of the chemical, with molecular components of the cell, formation of free radicals, or lipid peroxidation
  - For example, carbon monoxide (CO) has a very high affinity for Hgb
    - CO is colorless and odorless
    - CO causes nausea and vomiting, headache, weakness, & tinnitus (ringing in the ears)

2-2

hemoglobin has a higher affinity for CO but then O let go

18

Ethanol

- Form of alcohol found in mood-altering beverages
- In the liver, ethanol is converted to acetaldehyde which is toxic to the liver (free radical damage)
  - This toxicity leads to deposition of fat, hepatomegaly, interruption of protein transport, decreased fatty acid oxidation, increased membrane rigidity, and liver cell necrosis

2-2

with ethanol O absorb 100 of the alcohol with it.

if metabolism of alcohol to acetaldehyde to next step is fast: effects short. if is slow effects longer. but the longer acetaldehyde stays the worse hangover u get.

19

Trauma

- Blunt-force injuries are mechanical injuries resulting in tearing, shearing, or crushing of tissues
- The most common blunt injuries are caused by falls and auto accidents
- **Contusion:** Bleeding into the skin or underlying tissue
- **Hematoma:** A collection of blood in an enclosed space
  - subdural & epidural hematomas in the skull
  - *compartment syndrome* shown here

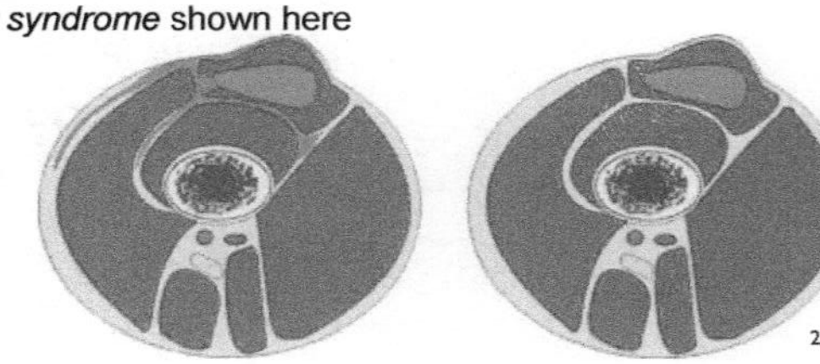

Beyer R. *et al. Haemophilia* 1, 2010.

2-3

20

Trauma

- **Abrasion**
  - Removal of the superficial layers of the skin caused by contact between the skin and the injuring object.
- **Laceration**
  - A rip or tear when the elasticity of the skin or tissue will not hold up to the pressure applied by injuring object

2-3

21

Trauma

- **Incised Wound**
  - A cut that is longer than it is deep
- **Stab Wound**
  - A cut that is deeper than it is long
  - How does it compare with a puncture wound? teared edges.
- **Gunshot Wound (GSW)**
  - Can be penetrating: bullet remains in the body
  - Or perforating: bullet exits the body

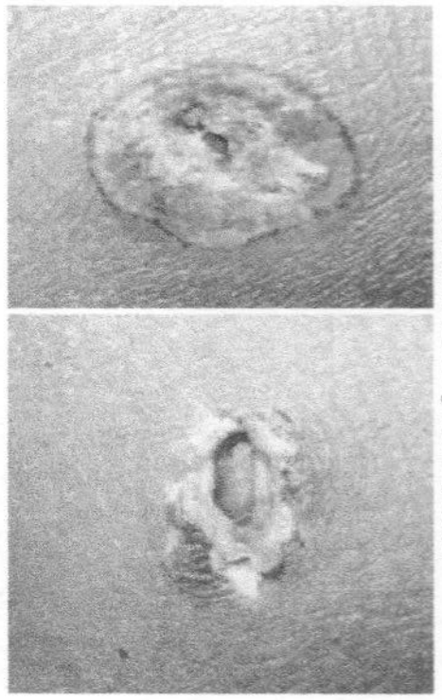

Guest GD *et al.* *ANZ J Surg* **75**:220, 2005.

2-3

22

Asphyxia as a Means to Hypoxia

- Asphyxial injuries occur because of a failure of airflow (oxygen) to the lungs
  - Suffocation barrier
  - Strangulation obstruction
  - Chemical no available
  - Drowning water.

2-3

23

Nutritional Imbalances

- For adequate cellular function and integrity, adequate amounts of proteins, lipids & carbohydrates are required
  - Low levels of plasma proteins, like albumin, encourages movement of water into the tissues, thereby causing edema
  - Hyperglycemia and hypoglycemia
  - Vitamin deficiencies

2-3

24

Physical Agents

- **Extreme Temperatures**
  - Hypothermia
    - vasoconstriction
    - ice crystal formation causing cellular swelling
  - Hyperthermia
    - loss of fluids and plasma proteins
- **Atmospheric Pressure**
  - Blast injuries
    - Compressed waves of air
    - Thorax collapses; organs hemorrhage and rupture
- **Water pressure**
  - Causes nitrogen to dissolve in blood
  - When pressure removed, nitrogen released and forms gas emboli

thawing cells start to burst.

sodden.

like soda bubbles escap into air your blood bubbles want to escape. "nitrogen bends" need to redesolve.

2-3

25

Physical Agents

- Ionizing Radiation xray
  - Electron removal from active cells
  - DNA is the most vulnerable target
    - When? during reproducton?
- Noise
  - Acute loud noise or cumulative effect

5 psi

2-3

26

Cellular Accumulations

- Water
- Lipids
- Carbohydrates
- Glycogen eating too much sugar. harding.
- Protein
- Pigments
- Calcium
- Urate

2-4

27

Five Types of Necrosis

- *Necrosis* is local cell death and is irreversible
- Necrosis involves the process of self/auto digestion and lysis
- Five types
  1. Coagulative
  2. Liquefactive
  3. Caseous
  4. Fat necrosis
  5. Gangrenous

2-5

Coagulative Necrosis

- Common in kidneys, heart, and adrenal glands
- Coagulation is caused by protein denaturation
  - Albumin is changed from a gelatinous, transparent state to a firm, opaque state. Compare what happens when an egg is cooked.
- It is suspected that high levels of intracellular calcium play a role in coagulative necrosis

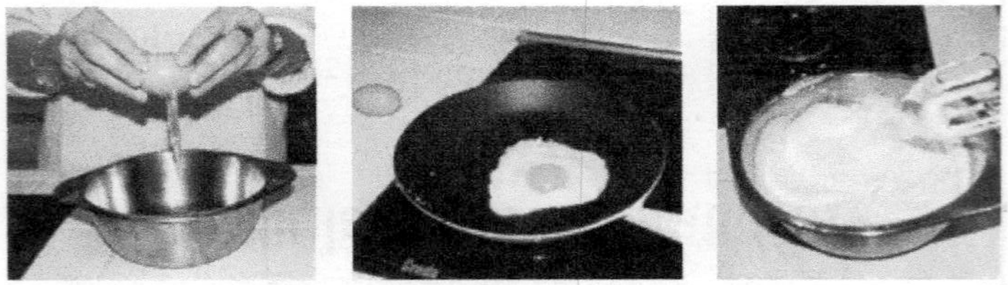

Hein, *Introduction to General, Organic and Biochemistry*, 9e, fig. 29.12

2-5

Liquefactive Necrosis

- Occurs in neurons and glial cells of the CNS
  - Brain cells have a large amount of digestive enzymes (hydrolases). These enzymes cause the neural tissue to become soft and liquefy.
- Liquefactive necrosis can also occur with certain infections.
  - Hydrolytic enzymes are released from neutrophils to fight an invading pathogen

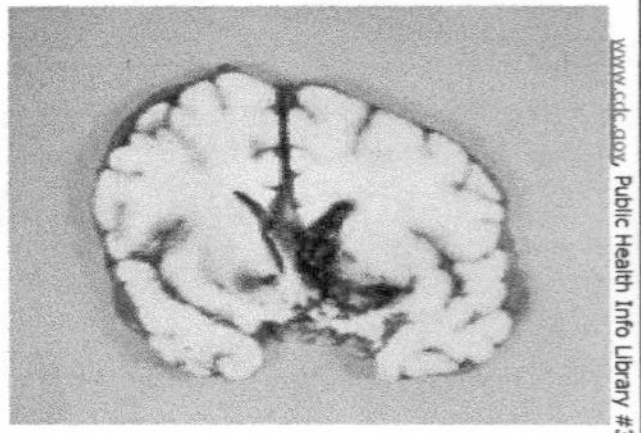

www.cdc.gov, Public Health Info Library #3976

2-5

Caseous Necrosis

- Combination of coagulative and liquefactive necrosis
- Results from pulmonary infection with *Mycobacterium tuberculosis*
  - The tissue is destroyed, but it is not completely digested
  - The remaining tissue resembles clumped cheese

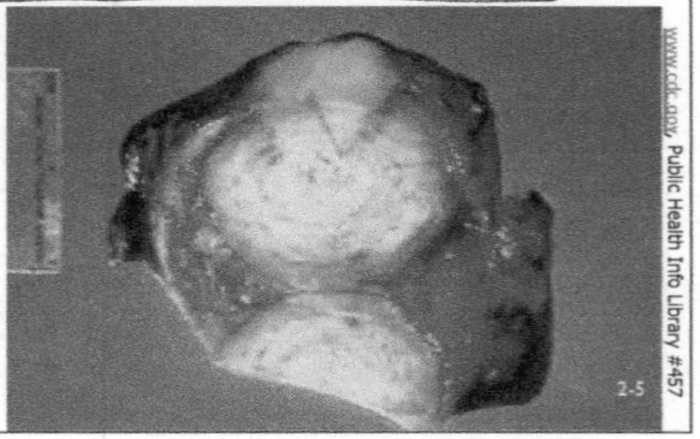

www.cdc.gov, Public Health Info Library #457

2-5

Fat Necrosis

- Occurs in breast, pancreas, and abdominal tissues
- Caused by lipases, which are found in very high levels in "lipo" (fat) tissues
- Lipases break down triglycerides, releasing free fatty acids
- The fatty acids combine with calcium, magnesium, and sodium to form soaps

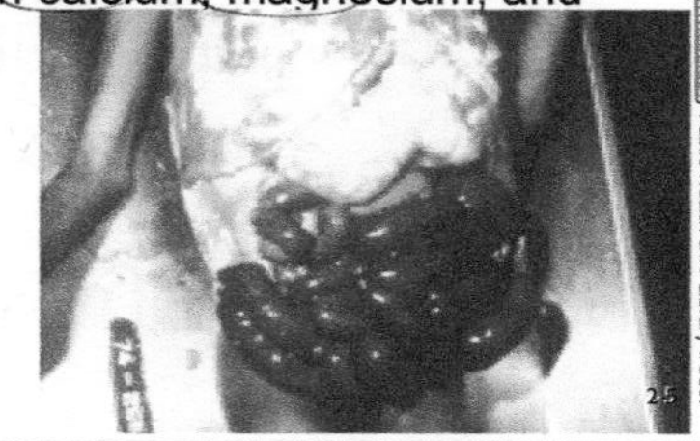

This patient died of shigellosis, with bowel necrosis

www.cdc.gov, Public Health Info Library #5167

2-5

snake bites · can activate coagulation factors. clot – ↓ O_2 – necrosis

Gangrenous Necrosis

(widespread)

- Term used in clinical practice that refers to wide-spread death of tissue due to hypoxia
  - Wet (liquefactive)
  - Dry (coagulative)
  - Gas Gangrene
    - Infection caused by many species of *Clostridium* bacteria (anaerobic)
    - The enzymes and toxins released by these bacteria cause bubbles of gas to form

enables it to move very fast across tissues.

clostridium deficile tetanus

gas gangrene.

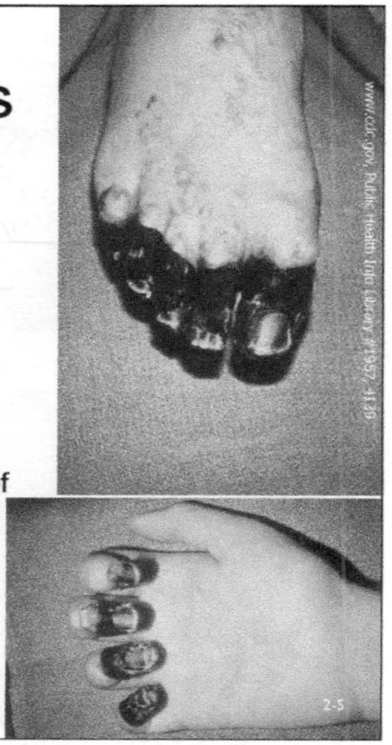

www.cdc.gov, Public Health Info Library #1957, 4139

2-5

MRSA - methyl resistant staph

VRSA - vancomycin resistent staph.

Cellular Death

- Apoptosis
  - Cell death involved in normal & pathologic conditions
  - Apoptosis depends on cellular signals
  - These signals cause protein cleavage (proteases) within the cell, causing cell death
  - Apoptosis is different from necrosis:
    - it is an active process
      - apoptosis: the cell is a "suicide victim"
      - necrosis: the cell is a "homicide victim"
    - it affects scattered, individual cells
      - apoptosis: gene activation in "chosen" cells
      - necrosis: death is widespread
    - it results in cell shrinkage, not lysis and swelling
      - apoptosis: cells shrink
      - necrosis: cells swell and lyse

2-6

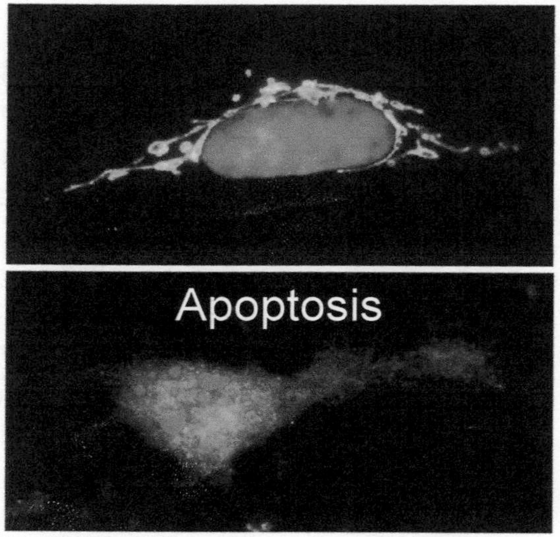

Apoptosis

Courtesy of S. E. Wiley, USCD/Walther Cancer Institute

Karp, Cell and Molecular Biology: Concepts and Experiments

2-6

Apoptosis:
Send in the Macrophages

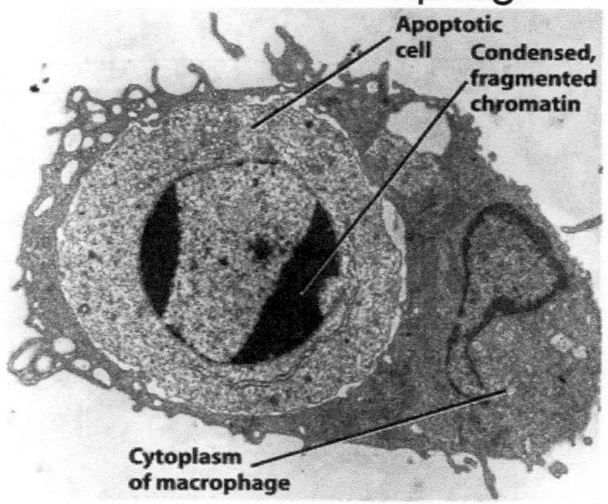

Apoptotic cell
Condensed, fragmented chromatin
Cytoplasm of macrophage

Reprinted with permission from Peter M. Henson, Donna L. Bratton, and Valerie A. Fadok, Curr. Biol. 11:R796, 2001.

Karp, Cell and Molecular Biology: Concepts and Experiments

2-6

Aging and Cellular Death

- Theories
  - Aging is caused by accumulations of injurious events (environment)
  - Aging is the result of a genetically-controlled developmental program
- Mechanisms
  - Genetic, environmental, and behavioral
  - Changes in regulatory mechanisms
  - Degenerative alterations

2-7

Somatic Death

- Death of an entire organism
- Cessation of respiration and circulation
- **Algor mortis**
  - Skin becomes pale and the body temperature falls
- **Livor mortis**
  - purplish discoloration in peripheral tissues
- **Rigor mortis**
  - Depletion of ATP keeps contractile proteins from detaching causing muscle stiffening
  - Within 12-14 hours, rigor mortis gradually diminishes
- **Postmortem autolysis** breaks down muscle and other tissues

2-8

Framaldyhyde – slows decompose. locks proteins. freezes them

Rigor Mortis

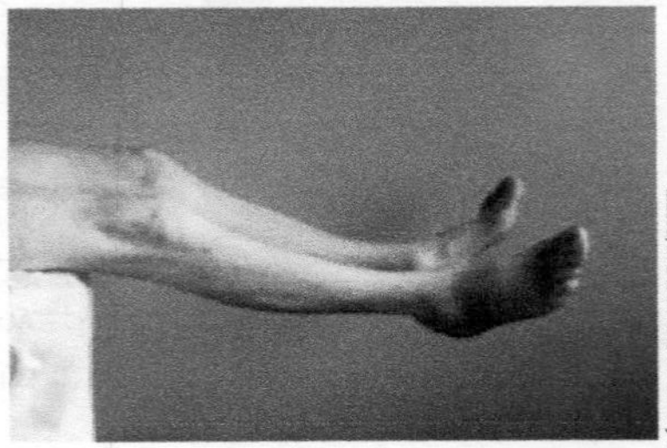

Madea, B. Death: Time of. In: *Wiley Encyclopedia of Forensic Science*, 2010.

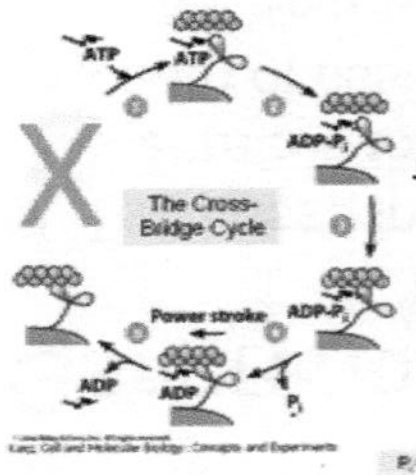

ATP
ADP-Pi
The Cross-Bridge Cycle
Power stroke
ADP
Pi

Pi = phosphate group

- What happens if ATP is absent?
- Myosin remains permanently bound to actin, muscles cannot move
  - muscle stuck between step 5 and step 1
- **Rigor mortis** results
- Eventually, enzymes and microbes destroy muscle structure and corpse becomes "loose" again

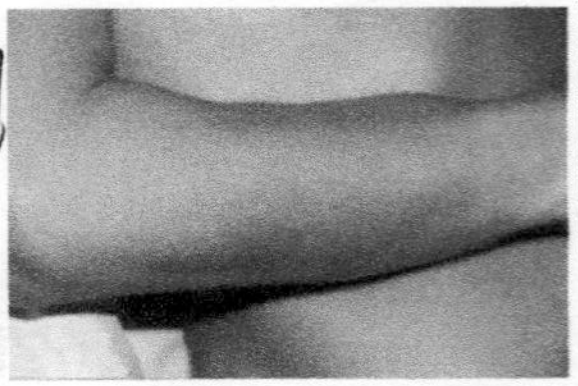

Postmortem gooseflesh due to rigor mortis in arrectores pilorum

2-8

Unit 1
Chapter 4
Fluids and Electrolytes, Acids and Bases

mm tissue - is hydrophilic
fat tissue is hydrophobic

caffeine - pee salt. Diuretics cuz water follows.
Diabetic - pee sugar

Distribution of Body Fluids

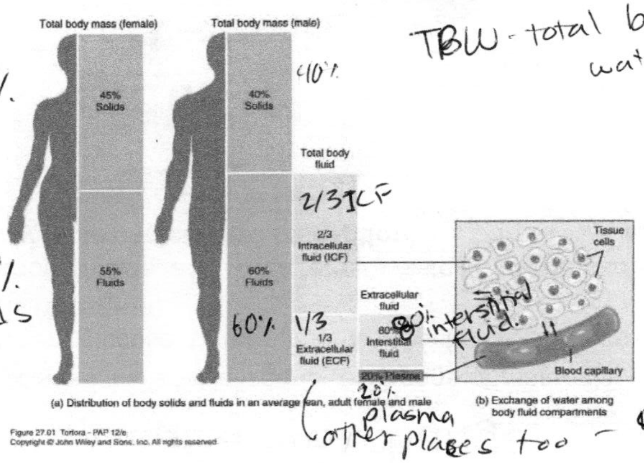

Total body mass (female)
Total body mass (male)
45% Solids
55% Fluids
40% Solids
60% Fluids
Total body fluid
2/3 Intracellular fluid (ICF)
1/3 Extracellular fluid (ECF)
Extracellular fluid
80% Interstitial fluid
20% Plasma
Tissue cells
Blood capillary

(a) Distribution of body solids and fluids in an average lean, adult female and male

(b) Exchange of water among body fluid compartments

Figure 27.01 Tortora - PAP 12/e
Copyright © John Wiley and Sons, Inc. All rights reserved.

TBW - total body water
45% solid
55% fluids
40%
60%
2/3 ICF
1/3
80% interstitial fluid
20% plasma
other places too - CSF, aqueous, sinus, serous fluid etc.

equilibrium is dependent on concentration not volume.

3-1

Water Gains and Losses

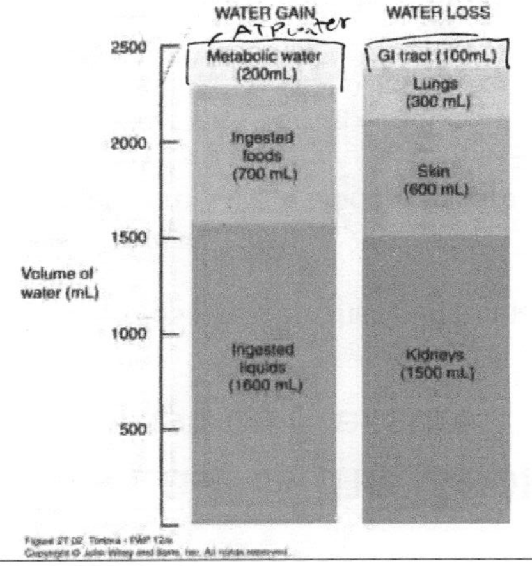

WATER GAIN
WATER LOSS
Volume of water (mL)
2500
2000
1500
1000
500
Metabolic water (200mL)
Ingested foods (700 mL)
Ingested liquids (1600 mL)
GI tract (100mL)
Lungs (300 mL)
Skin (600 mL)
Kidneys (1500 mL)

Figure 27.02 Tortora - PAP 12/e
Copyright © John Wiley and Sons, Inc. All rights reserved.

ATP water

3-1

37

Osmotic Forces

- **Isosmotic** – Concentrations of two fluids separated by a membrane are equal.

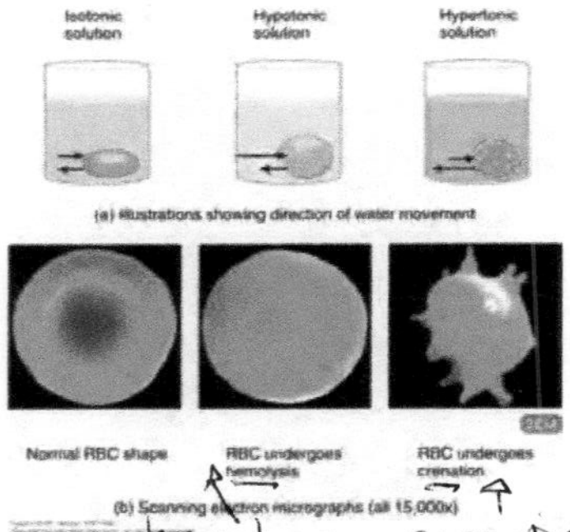

Isotonic solution
Hypotonic solution
Hypertonic solution
(a) Illustrations showing direction of water movement
Normal RBC shape
RBC undergoes hemolysis
RBC undergoes crenation
(b) Scanning electron micrographs (all 15,000x)

hemolysis
crenation

3-1

isotonic IVs - same concentration as tissues
hypertonic - ↑ concentration
hypo - ↓ concentration

Osmotic Forces

- **Hyperosmotic** – The concentration of the ECF is higher than the ICF. The net movement of water is from the ICF to the ECF.

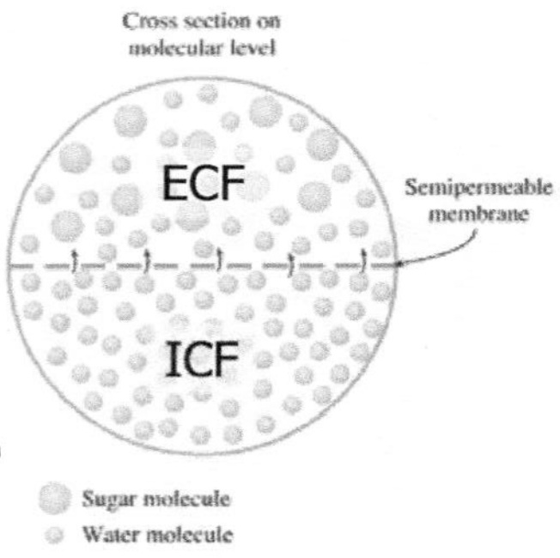

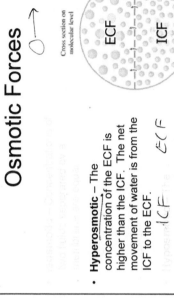

Cross section on molecular level
ECF
ICF
Semipermeable membrane
Sugar molecule
Water molecule

Hein, *Introduction to General, Organic and Biochemistry*, 9e fig. 14.9

ICF 300 mOsm → ECF 500 mOsm

3-1

6.023×10^{23} = mole   mmol
# of parts.   osmole   mOsm
osmosis
↑ 300 mOsm → 500 mOsm ↓ until equal.
this concentration goes up | this concentration dilutes goes down

when i'm sample fluid it ECF
so a hyperosmotic its the ECF

Osmotic Forces

ECF 300 mOsm, ICF 500 mOs
ICF 500 mOsm, ECF 300 mOs

- **Hyposmotic** – The concentration of the ICF is higher than the ECF. The net movement of water is from the ECF to the ICF.

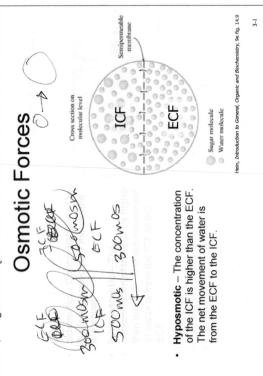

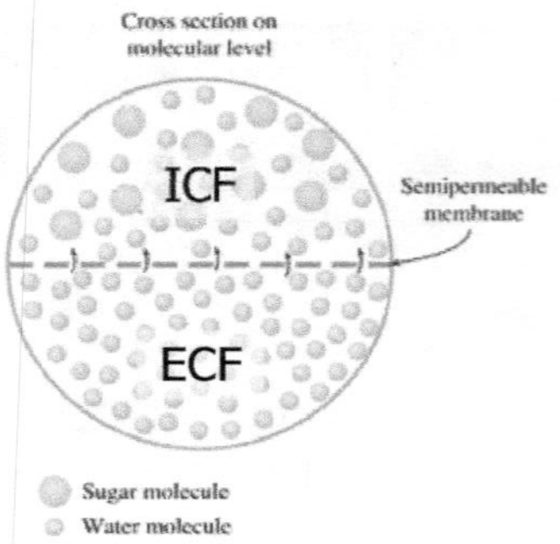
Cross section on molecular level
ICF
ECF
Semipermeable membrane
Sugar molecule
Water molecule

Hein, *Introduction to General, Organic and Biochemistry*, 9e fig. 14.9

in diabetics it is thicker. ↓ exchange.
basement membrane - connective tissue.
endothelium - simple squamous.

Capillaries

- **Capillaries** join arterioles (smallest arteries) and venules (smallest veins)
- Capillaries occur as capillary beds of interconnected vessels
- Capillaries small enough that RBCs must fold to pass through
- **Precapillary sphincters** are smooth muscle cuffs that regulate flow of blood through capillary bed

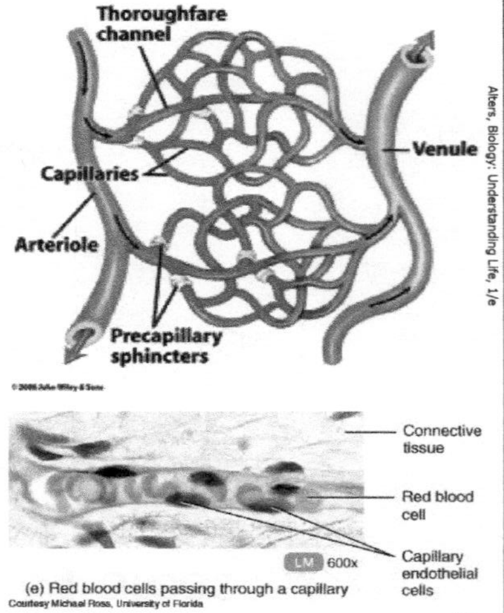
Thoroughfare channel
Venule
Capillaries
Arteriole
Precapillary sphincters
Connective tissue
Red blood cell
Capillary endothelial cells
LM 600x

(e) Red blood cells passing through a capillary
Courtesy Michael Ross, University of Florida

Alters, Biology: Understanding Life, 1/e

BOP - blood osmotic pressure
IOP - interstitial osmotic pressure

4-6 liters blood. control distribution by sympathetic + parasymp nervous system.

Capillary Exchange

- Capillaries are specialized for exchange of materials
- Oxygen, glucose, other nutrients must be delivered to cells **(filtration)**
- Carbon dioxide, acid, urea, other wastes must be carried away to be excreted **(reabsorption)**

3L/day lymphatic system inspects blood sends WBCs PRN to areas.

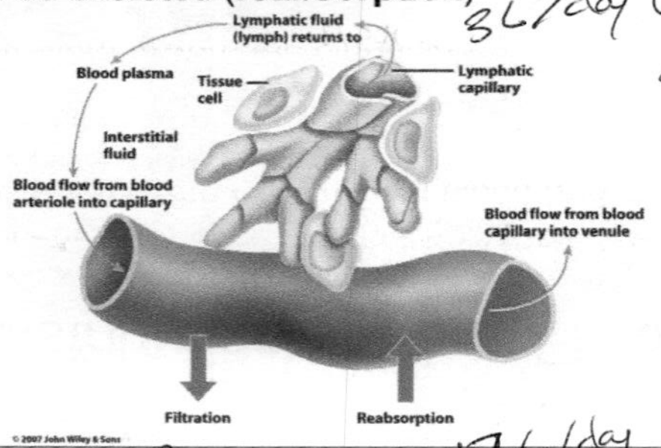
Lymphatic fluid (lymph) returns to
Blood plasma
Tissue cell
Lymphatic capillary
Interstitial fluid
Blood flow from blood arteriole into capillary
Blood flow from blood capillary into venule
Filtration
Reabsorption

BP pushes it out 20 L per day
17 L/day

BHP - blood hydrostatic pressure
IHP - interstitial hydrostatic pressure

Starling's Law of the Capillary
Hydrostatic Pressure

- Hydrostatic pressure
- This is simply the pressure from the "pump" that pushes blood around
  - like water pressure in pipes
- That is: hydrostatic pressure = blood pressure

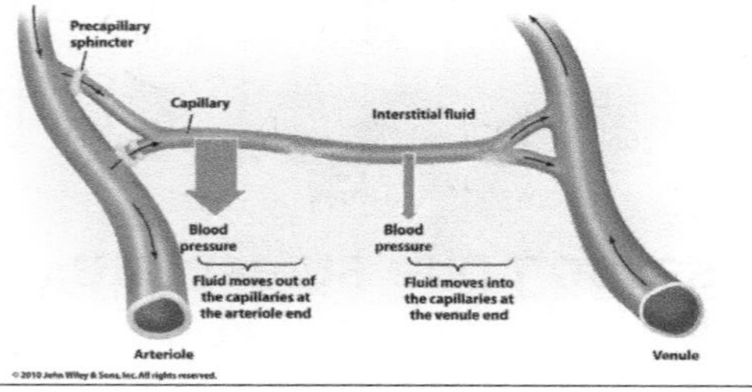
Precapillary sphincter
Capillary
Interstitial fluid
Blood pressure
Blood pressure
Fluid moves out of the capillaries at the arteriole end
Fluid moves into the capillaries at the venule end
Arteriole
Venule

Ireland, Visualizing Human Biology, 2e

Starling's Law of the Capillary
Osmotic Pressure

- The concentration force of water trying to dilute out higher concentration of solutes in blood (**net osmotic pressure**)
- This forces water from the tissues (lower solute concentration) toward the bloodstream (higher solute concentration)

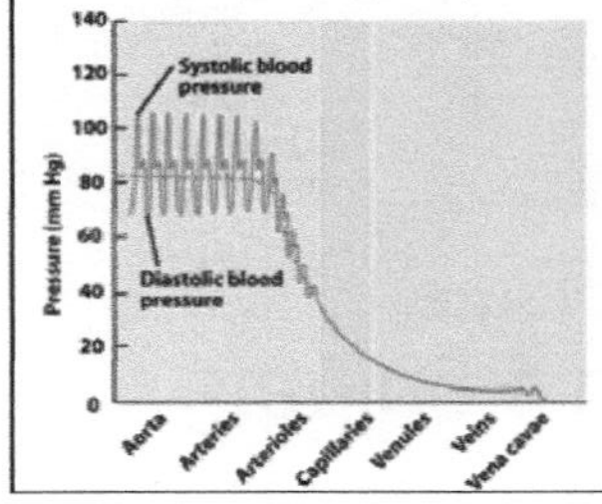

Pressure (mm Hg)
140
120
100
80
60
40
20
0
Systolic blood pressure
Diastolic blood pressure
Aorta
Arteries
Arterioles
Capillaries
Venules
Veins
Venae cavae

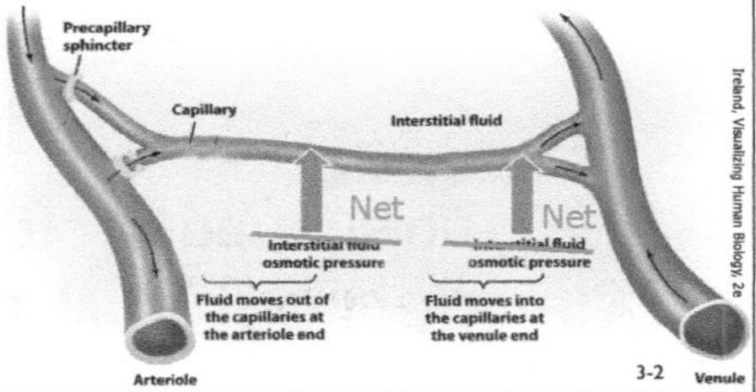

Precapillary sphincter
Capillary
Interstitial fluid
Net
Net
Interstitial fluid osmotic pressure
Interstitial fluid osmotic pressure
Fluid moves out of the capillaries at the arteriole end
Fluid moves into the capillaries at the venule end
Arteriole
Venule

Ireland, Visualizing Human Biology, 2e

3-2

Starling's Law of the Capillary
Permeability

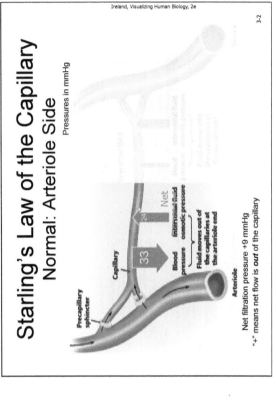

- This is how many holes are in the capillaries, and how large those holes are
- Disease conditions can increase the size and number of holes in the capillaries
  - e.g. inflammation, burns, allergies

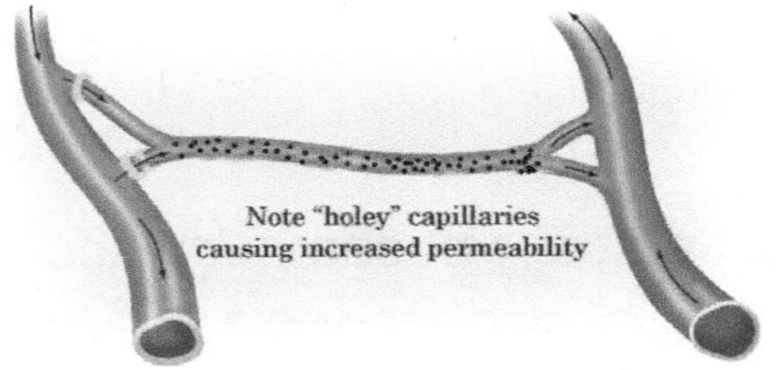

Note "holey" capillaries causing increased permeability

Ireland, Visualizing Human Biology, 2e

3-2

Starling's Law of the Capillary

Three Factors

1. Hydrostatic pressure
2. Osmotic (oncotic) pressure
3. Permeability

- The balance between these forces is called the **Starling forces** and the equation which relates them is called **Starling's Law of the Capillary**
- Interstitial fluid osmotic pressure about the same throughout capillary, but hydrostatic pressure drops
- This means the capillary *delivers nutrients on the arteriole side, and picks up wastes on the venule side*

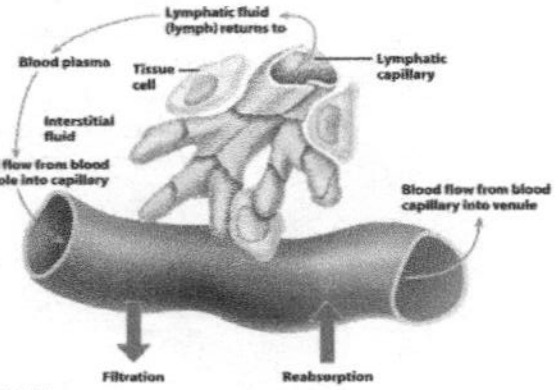

Lymphatic fluid (lymph) returns to
Blood plasma
Tissue cell
Lymphatic capillary
Interstitial fluid
Blood flow from blood arteriole into capillary
Blood flow from blood capillary into venule
Filtration
Reabsorption

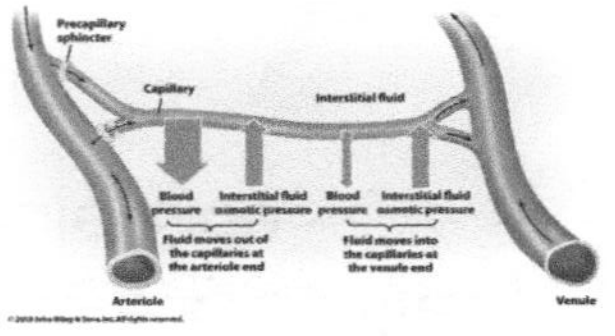

Precapillary sphincter
Capillary
Interstitial fluid
Arteriole
Venule

Ireland, Visualizing Human Biology, 2e

3-2

Starling's Law of the Capillary
Normal: Arteriole Side

Pressures in mmHg

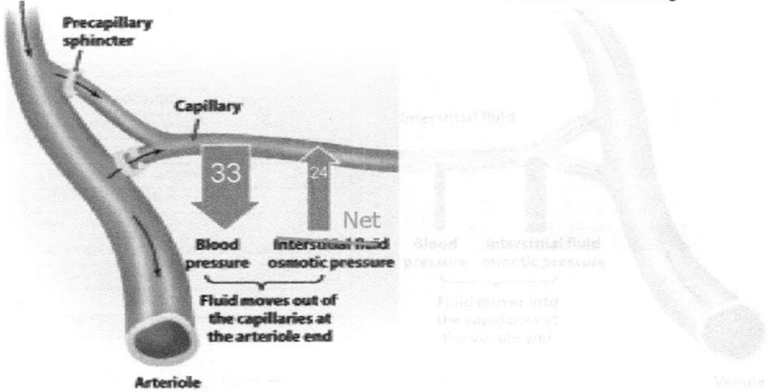

Precapillary sphincter
Capillary
33
24
Net
Blood pressure
Interstitial fluid osmotic pressure
Fluid moves out of the capillaries at the arteriole end
Arteriole

Net filtration pressure +9 mmHg
"+" means net flow is *out* of the capillary

Ireland, Visualizing Human Biology, 2e

3-2

Starling's Law of the Capillary

Normal: Venule Side

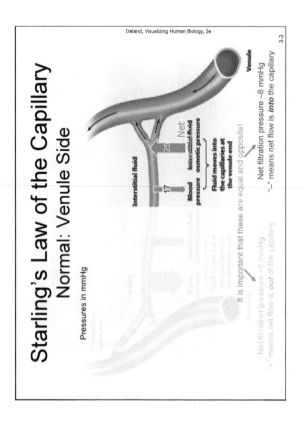

Pressures in mmHg

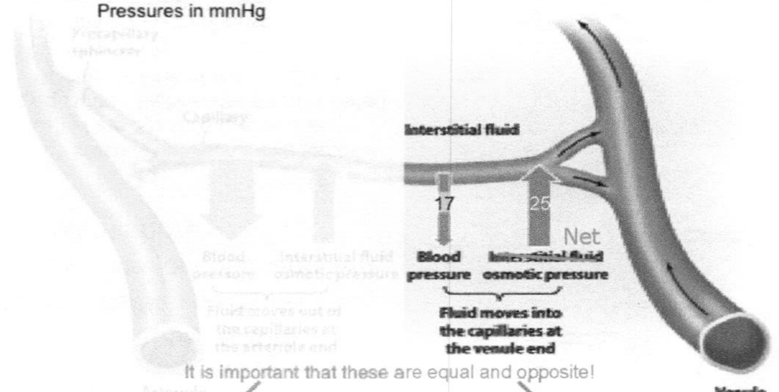

Interstitial fluid
17
25
Net
Blood pressure
Interstitial fluid osmotic pressure
Fluid moves into the capillaries at the venule end
Venule

It is important that these are equal and opposite!

Net filtration pressure +9 mmHg
"+" means net flow is *out* of the capillary

Net filtration pressure –8 mmHg
"–" means net flow is ***into*** the capillary

Ireland, Visualizing Human Biology, 2e

3-2

Edema: Causes

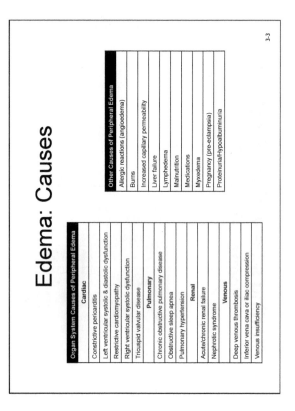

Organ System Causes of Peripheral Edema
Cardiac
Constrictive pericarditis
Left ventricular systolic & diastolic dysfunction
Restrictive cardiomyopathy
Right ventricular systolic dysfunction
Tricuspid valvular disease
Pulmonary
Chronic obstructive pulmonary disease
Obstructive sleep apnea
Pulmonary hypertension
Renal
Acute/chronic renal failure
Nephrotic syndrome
Venous
Deep venous thrombosis
Inferior vena cava or iliac compression
Venous insufficiency

Other Causes of Peripheral Edema
Allergic reactions (angioedema)
Burns
Increased capillary permeability
Liver failure
Lymphedema
Malnutrition
Medications
Myxedema
Pregnancy (pre-eclampsia)
Proteinuria/Hypoalbuminuria

3-3

Starling's Law of the Capillary

Pathology: Hypertension

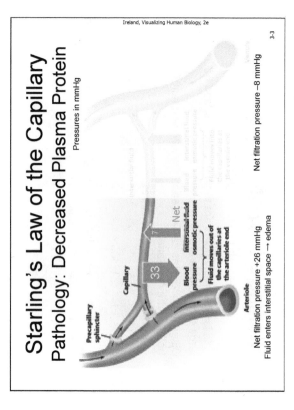

Pressures in mmHg

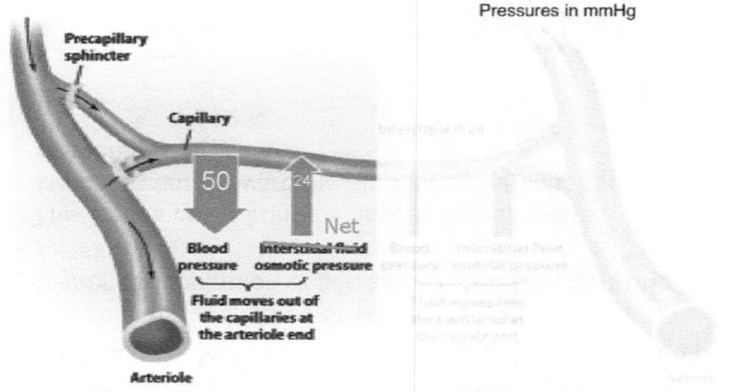

Precapillary sphincter
Capillary
50
24
Net
Blood pressure
Interstitial fluid osmotic pressure
Fluid moves out of the capillaries at the arteriole end
Arteriole

Net filtration pressure +26 mmHg
Fluid enters interstitial space → edema

Net filtration pressure –8 mmHg

Ireland, Visualizing Human Biology, 2e

3-3

Starling's Law of the Capillary

Pathology: Decreased Plasma Protein

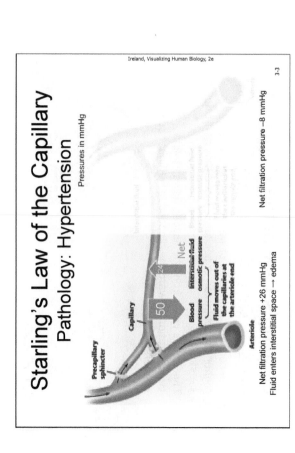

Pressures in mmHg

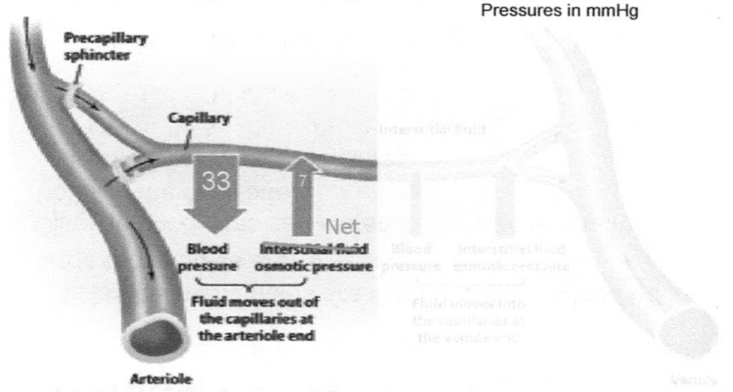

Precapillary sphincter
Capillary
33
7
Net
Blood pressure
Interstitial fluid osmotic pressure
Fluid moves out of the capillaries at the arteriole end
Arteriole

Net filtration pressure +26 mmHg
Fluid enters interstitial space → edema

Net filtration pressure –8 mmHg

Ireland, Visualizing Human Biology, 2e

3-3

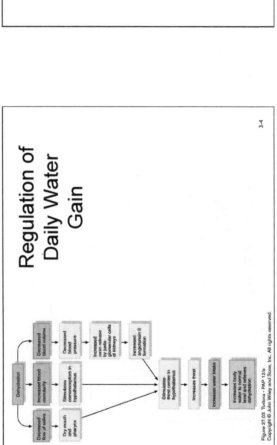

Starling's Law of the Capillary
Pathology: Increased Vascular Permeability

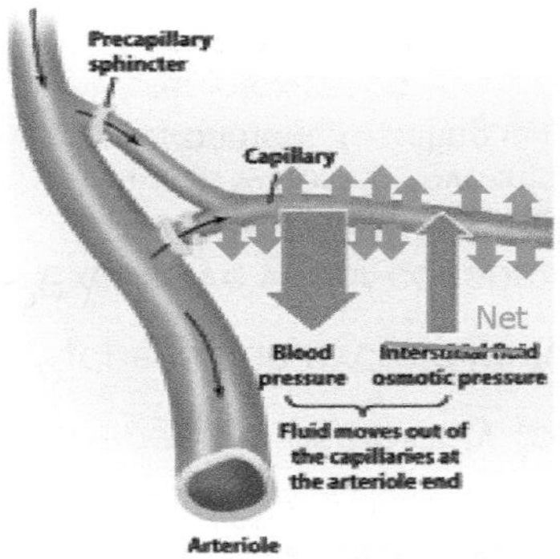
Precapillary sphincter
Capillary
Net
Blood pressure
Interstitial fluid osmotic pressure
Fluid moves out of the capillaries at the arteriole end
Arteriole

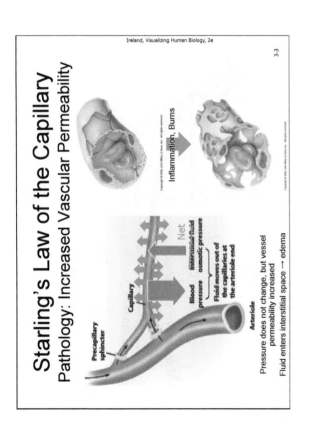

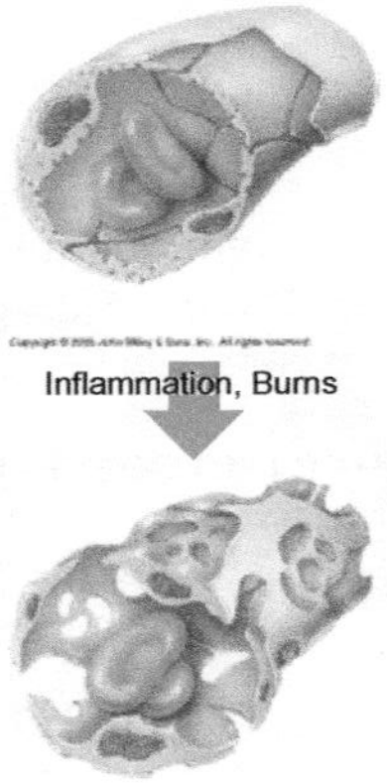
Inflammation, Burns

Pressure does not change, but vessel permeability increased

Fluid enters interstitial space → edema

Ireland, Visualizing Human Biology, 2e

3-3

Regulation of Daily Water Gain

- Thirst center is located in the hypothalamus
  - Detects increases in the blood osmolarity
- Dehydration
  - Water loss exceeds gains
  - Decreases blood pressure
  - Increases blood osmolarity
- Other receptors for dehydration include the kidneys, baroreceptors in the arteries, and neurons in the mouths that detect dryness.

3-4

Regulation of Daily Water Gain

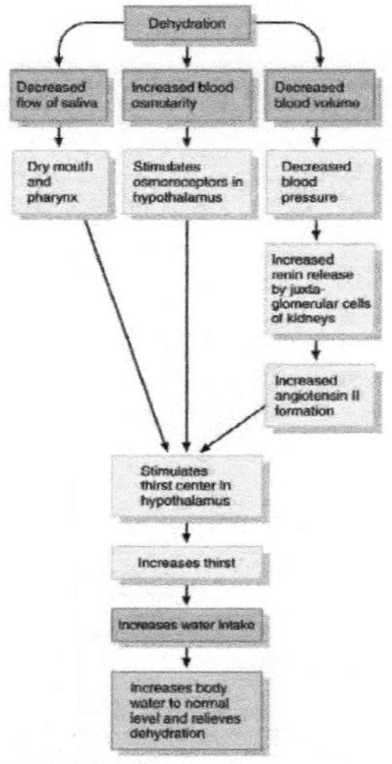
Dehydration
Decreased flow of saliva
Increased blood osmolarity
Decreased blood volume
Dry mouth and pharynx
Stimulates osmoreceptors in hypothalamus
Decreased blood pressure
Increased renin release by juxta-glomerular cells of kidneys
Increased angiotensin II formation
Stimulates thirst center in hypothalamus
Increases thirst
Increases water intake
Increases body water to normal level and relieves dehydration

Figure 27.03 Tortora - PAP 12/e

3-4

Renin-Angiotensin-Aldosterone System (RAAS)

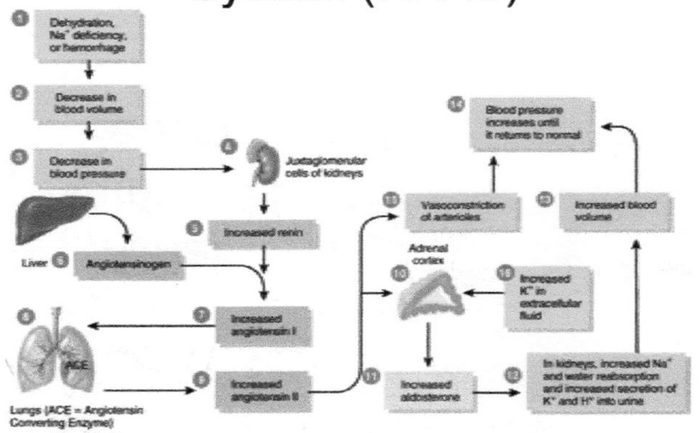
Dehydration, Na+ deficiency, or hemorrhage
Decrease in blood volume
Decrease in blood pressure
Juxtaglomerular cells of kidneys
Increased renin
Liver
Angiotensinogen
Increased angiotensin I
ACE
Increased angiotensin II
Lungs (ACE = Angiotensin Converting Enzyme)
Vasoconstriction of arterioles
Adrenal cortex
Increased K+ in extracellular fluid
Increased aldosterone
In kidneys, increased Na+ and water reabsorption and increased secretion of K+ and H+ into urine
Increased blood volume
Blood pressure increases until it returns to normal

Figure 18.16 Tortora - PAP 12/e

3-4

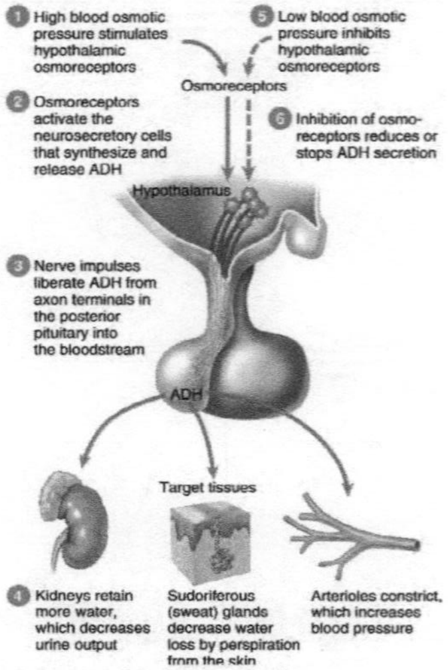
1 High blood osmotic pressure stimulates hypothalamic osmoreceptors
5 Low blood osmotic pressure inhibits hypothalamic osmoreceptors
Osmoreceptors
2 Osmoreceptors activate the neurosecretory cells that synthesize and release ADH
6 Inhibition of osmo-receptors reduces or stops ADH secretion
Hypothalamus
3 Nerve impulses liberate ADH from axon terminals in the posterior pituitary into the bloodstream
ADH
Target tissues
4 Kidneys retain more water, which decreases urine output
Sudoriferous (sweat) glands decrease water loss by perspiration from the skin
Arterioles constrict, which increases blood pressure
Figure 18.09 Tortora - PAP 12/e

Antidiuretic Hormone (ADH)

3-4

Atrial Natriuretic Peptide

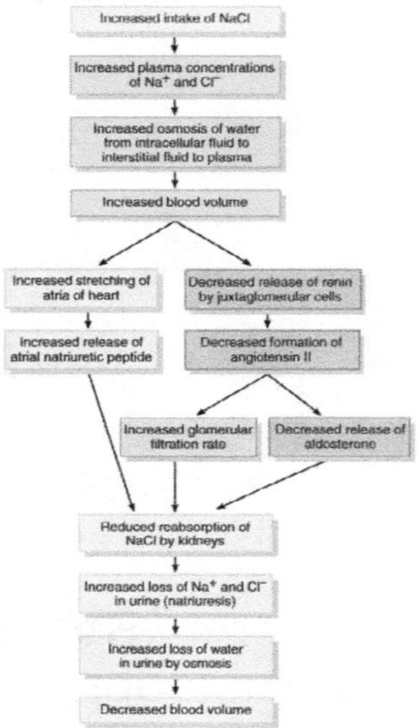
Increased intake of NaCl
Increased plasma concentrations of Na+ and Cl−
Increased osmosis of water from intracellular fluid to interstitial fluid to plasma
Increased blood volume
Increased stretching of atria of heart
Decreased release of renin by juxtaglomerular cells
Increased release of atrial natriuretic peptide
Decreased formation of angiotensin II
Increased glomerular filtration rate
Decreased release of aldosterone
Reduced reabsorption of NaCl by kidneys
Increased loss of Na+ and Cl− in urine (natriuresis)
Increased loss of water in urine by osmosis
Decreased blood volume

3-4

Water Movement

- Changes in osmolarity (concentration)
- Kidneys can excrete water at a rate of 15 ml/min
- Excessive water consumption
  - A decrease in plasma and interstitial osmolarity causes water to move into the intracellular environment, resulting in cellular swelling.
  - Water intoxication
    - Can one really drink too much water?

3-4

What is an Electrolyte?

- A substance that dissociates into ions in aqueous solution, and conductions.
- Common electrolytes are
  - cations: Na^+, K^+, Ca^{++}, Mg^{++}
  - anions: Cl^-, HCO_3^-, PO_4^{-3}
- Functions
  - Volume and osmotic regulation, myocardial function, enzyme cofactors, acid-base balance, etc.
- When any electrolyte is measured, is it the ECF or the ICF that is measured?

3-4/5

TABLE 2.3

Percentage and Molarity

DEFINITION	EXAMPLE
Percentage (mass per volume)	
Number of grams of a substance per 100 milliliters (mL) of solution.	To make a 10% NaCl solution, take 10 gm of NaCl and add enough water to make a total of 100 mL of solution.
Molarity = moles (mol) per liter	
A 1 molar (1 M) solution = 1 mole of a solute in 1 liter of solution.	To make a 1 molar (1 M) solution of NaCl, dissolve 1 mole of NaCl (58.44 gm) in enough water to make a total of 1 liter of solution.

3-4/5

Equivalent Weight

- 1 mole is Avogadro's number (6.023 x 10^{23}) of something (molecules, atoms, ions, donuts)
- The term **equivalent** is only used for ionic compounds: acids, bases and salts
- In water, these compounds ionize into cations and anions
- An equivalent weight of something is the amount of that compound that will liberate one mole of charge as cations or anions

3-4/5

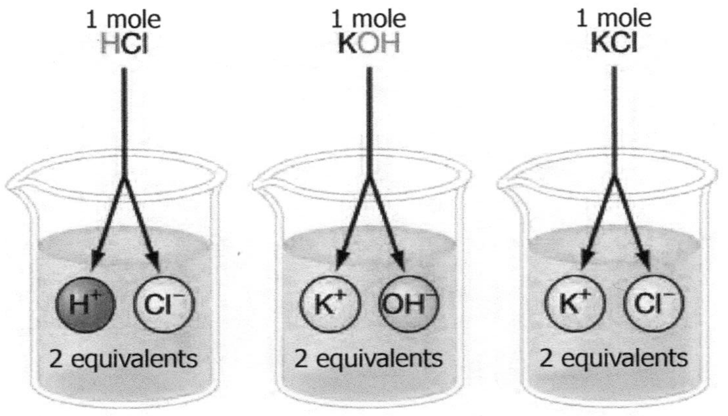
1 mole
HCl
H+
Cl−
2 equivalents
1 mole
KOH
K+
OH−
2 equivalents
1 mole
KCl
K+
Cl−
2 equivalents

(a) Acid (b) Base (c) Salt

3-4/5

Equivalent and Milliequivalents

- In the body, there are very small amounts (by weight) of ions, so they are listed on **mOsm/L or mEq/L**
  - Simply move the decimal like you do for liters to milliliters
- Examples
  - Na^+ = 0.14 M = 0.14 moles/L = 140 mmoles/L = 136-146 mEq/L
  - K^+ = 3.4-5.0 mEq/L

3-4/5

Normal Analyte Levels

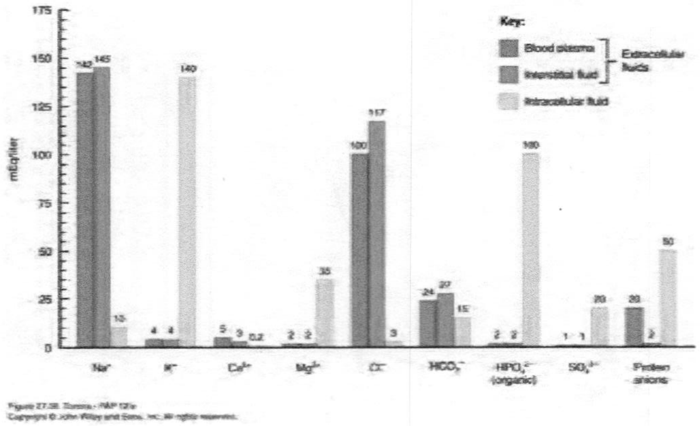
Key:
Blood plasma
Interstitial fluid
Intracellular fluid
Extracellular fluids
mEq/liter
175
150
125
100
75
50
25
0
142 145 13
4 4 140
5 3 0.2
2 2 35
100 117 3
24 27 15
2 2 100
1 1 20
20 2 50
Na^+
K^+
Ca^{2+}
Mg^{2+}
Cl^-
HCO_3^-
HPO_4^{2-} (organic)
SO_4^{2-}
Protein anions

3-4

Abnormal Analyte Levels

- Hypernatremia
- Hyperkalemia
- Hypermagnesemia
- Hyperphosphatemia
- Hypercalcemia

- Hyponatremia
- Hypokalemia
- Hypomagnesemia
- Hypophosphatemia
- Hypocalcemia

3-4

Sodium

- The plasma concentration of sodium is kept within a very narrow range (136-146 mEq/L)
- The body's sodium concentration is maintained primarily by the kidney
  1. **glomerular filtration**
  2. **renin – angiotensin – aldosterone system**
- Aided by hormones produced by the heart, brain, and kidney that also influence sodium reabsorption/excretion
  3. **natriuretic peptides**

3-4

As Goes Sodium…

- Sodium accounts for 90% of the **ECF cations**
- Sodium together with choloride (Cl^-) and the bicarbonate ion regulates **osmotic forces** and therefore regulates water balance.
- **In ECF : *"As sodium goes, so goes water"***
- Sodium also works with potassium to maintain neuromuscular "irritability" for conduction of nerve impulses and muscle contraction.

3-4

Abnormal Levels of Sodium

- Hypernatremia
  (>146 mEq/L)
  - **Cellular shrinking**
  - **Hypertension**
  - **Thrist**
  - **Oliguria and Anuria**
- Hyponatremia
  (<135 mEq/L)
  - **Cellular swelling**
  - **Edema**
  - **Hypotension**

3-4

Potassium

- Potassium has a major influence on ICF osmolality and maintenance of electroneutrality in relation to Na^+ and H^+
- Potassium is required for maintaining the resting membrane potential, transmission and conduction of nerve impulses, maintaining normal cardiac rhythms, and muscle contraction
- The kidney plays the largest role in maintaining potassium levels
- Normal plasma potassium: **3.4 – 5.0 mEq/L**

3-5

Potassium

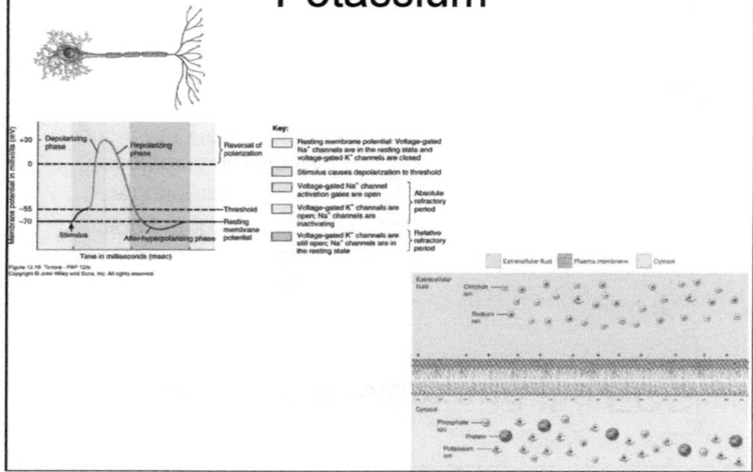
Depolarizing phase
Repolarizing phase
Reversal of polarization
Threshold
Resting membrane potential
Stimulus
After-hyperpolarizing phase
Time in milliseconds (msec)
Key:

Abnormal Potassium

Hyperkalemia (> 5.5 mEq/L)

- Altered conductivity in the heart
- **Cell membrane is depolarized** (i.e. more positive than normal)
  - Mild attacks (muscular irritability)
  - Severe (muscle weakness)
- Can be caused by blood transfusions
- Associated with metabolic acidosis (K^+ for H^+)
- Lethal injections (big dose of potassium)

Hypokalemia (< 3.5 mEq/L)

- Muscle cramping progressing to muscle weakness
- Dysrhythmias
- **Cell membrane is hyperpolarized**
- Polyuria (diuresis) leads to K^+ loss in the urine

3-5

Abnormal Potassium and the ECG

- Normal ECG at top
- Hypokalemia causes a reversal of the cardiac action potential
- Hyperkalemia (depolarization) slows, and even stops, the heart

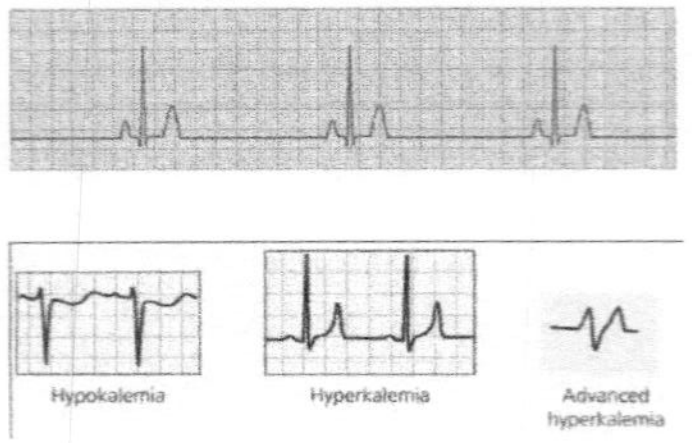
Hypokalemia
Hyperkalemia
Advanced hyperkalemia

Stouffer GA. *Practical ECG Interpretation.* 2009

3-5

Calcium and Phosphate

- **Calcium** (8.6 – 10.5 mg/dl) is necessary in many metabolic processes
  - Main cation in bones and teeth
  - Cofactor in the clotting pathways
  - **Key: calcium blocks sodium channels**
- **Phosphate** (2.5 – 4.5 mg/dl) is found throughout the body
  - Bone (calcium phosphate = hydroxyapatite)
  - Phospholipids
  - Creatine phosphate (brain and muscle energy source)
  - ATP (energy currency)
- The concentrations of calcium and phosphate are inversely related; if one increases, the other decreases
  - The renal system maintains these levels

3-5

Bone is a Calcium Reservoir:
Hormonal Control of Blood [Ca^{++}]

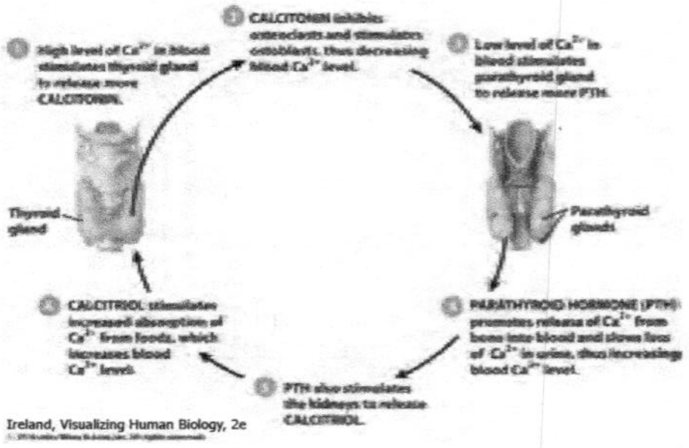
Thyroid gland
Parathyroid glands

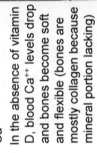

Ireland, Visualizing Human Biology, 2e

Three hormones involved in this process

1. Calcitonin
   - inhibits osteoclasts
   - stimulates osteoblasts
   - decreases blood [Ca^{++}]
   - increases bone formation
2. Parathyroid hormone (PTH)
   - stimulates osteoclasts
   - inhibits osteoblasts
   - increases blood [Ca^{++}]
   - decreases bone formation
3. Calcitriol (active vit. D)
   - not directly involved with bone
   - however, PTH stimulates kidneys to release calcitriol, which increases absorption of Ca^{++} from foods

3-5

Hormonal Control of Bone

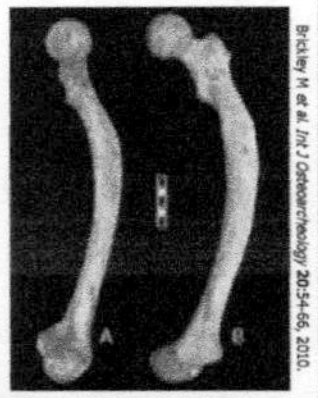

Brickley M *et al. Int J Osteoarcheology* 20:54-66, 2010.

- Vitamin D also important in intestinal absorption of Ca^{++}
- In the absence of vitamin D, blood Ca^{++} levels drop and bones become soft and flexible (bones are mostly collagen because mineral portion lacking)
- In children, **rickets** result

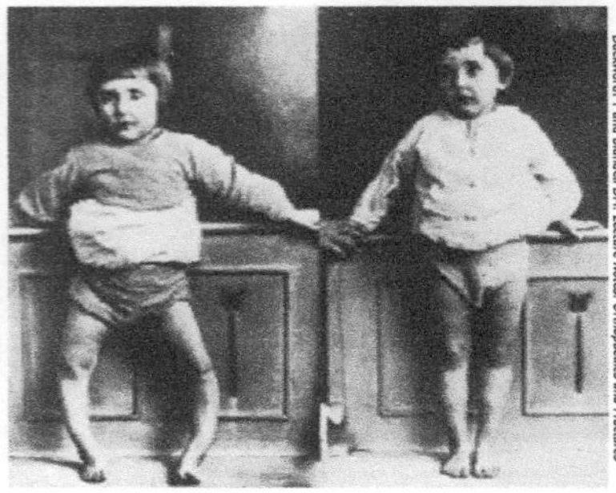

Duckworth T and Blundell DM. *Lecture Notes: Orthopaedics and Fractures*

3-5

Abnormal Levels of Calcium

- **Hypercalcemia**
  (>12.0 mg/dl)
- **Hypophosphatemia**
  (<2.0mg/dl)
  - Decreased neuromuscular excitability (hyperpolarization)
  - Increased bone fractures
  - Kidney stones
- **Hypocalcemia**
  (<8.5 mg/dl)
- **Hyperphosphatemia**
  (>4.5 mg/dl)
  - Increased neuromuscular excitability (partial depolarization)
  - Muscle cramps

3-5

Abnormal Calcium and the ECG

- Abnormal calcium has an effect on the electrocardiogram, but it is much more subtle than the effects of abnormal potassium

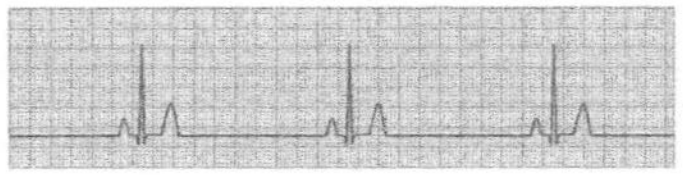

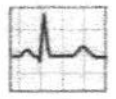

Hypocalcemia

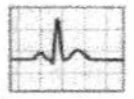

Hypercalcemia

Stouffer GA. *Practical ECG Interpretation*. 2009

3-5

Magnesium

- Intracellular cation
- Plasma concentration 1.8 – 2.4 mEq/L
- Acts as a cofactor in cellular reactions
  - important for protein & nucleic acid synthesis
- Required for ATPase activity
- **Key: decreased acetylcholine release at the neuromuscular junction (NMJ)**
  - Example: given in pre-eclampsia

3-5

Abnormal Levels of Mg^{++}

- **Hypermagnesemia**
  (> 2.5 mEq/L)
  - Skeletal muscle depression
  - Bradycardia
  - Muscle weakness
- **Hypomagnesemia**
  (< 1.5 mEq/L)
  - Neuromuscular irritability
  - Hyperactive reflexes

3-5

pH

pH < 7.0 is acidic (more H+ than OH⁻)

pH = 7.0 is neutral (equal amounts H+ and OH⁻)

pH > 7.0 is alkaline/basic (more OH⁻ than H+)

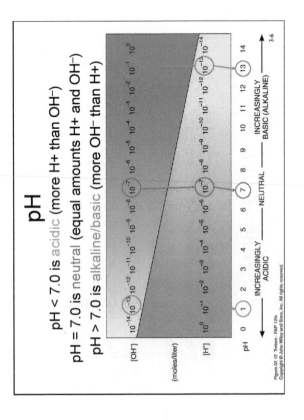

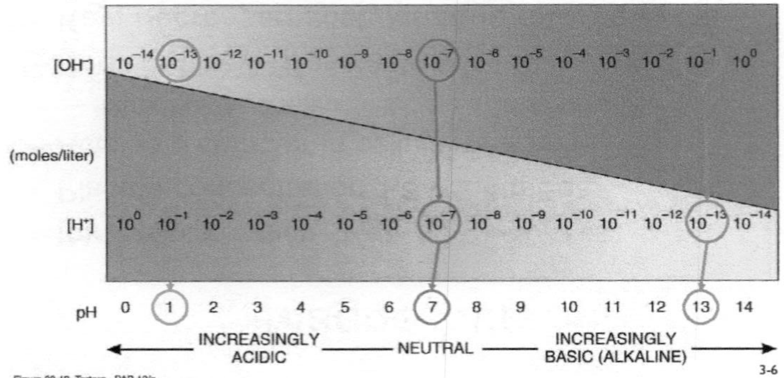

[OH⁻]
10⁻¹⁴ 10⁻¹³ 10⁻¹² 10⁻¹¹ 10⁻¹⁰ 10⁻⁹ 10⁻⁸ 10⁻⁷ 10⁻⁶ 10⁻⁵ 10⁻⁴ 10⁻³ 10⁻² 10⁻¹ 10⁰
(moles/liter)
[H⁺]
10⁰ 10⁻¹ 10⁻² 10⁻³ 10⁻⁴ 10⁻⁵ 10⁻⁶ 10⁻⁷ 10⁻⁸ 10⁻⁹ 10⁻¹⁰ 10⁻¹¹ 10⁻¹² 10⁻¹³ 10⁻¹⁴
pH 0 1 2 3 4 5 6 7 8 9 10 11 12 13 14
INCREASINGLY ACIDIC
NEUTRAL
INCREASINGLY BASIC (ALKALINE)

3-6

Buffers in the Human Body

- A buffer acts as a H+ and/or OH⁻ "sponge" so that pH is kept relatively constant

The most important buffer system in human biology is the carbonic acid–bicarbonate buffer system

when H⁺ is abundant (acidic conditions), excess H⁺ is "sponged up" by HCO_3^- to form H_2CO_3

← reaction goes this way

$H_2O + CO_2 \longleftrightarrow H_2CO_3 \longleftrightarrow H^+ + HCO_3^-$

Water, Carbon dioxide, Carbonic acid, Hydrogen ion, Bicarbonate ion (weak base)

reaction goes this way →

when H⁺ is scarce (alkaline conditions), excess H⁺ is released by H_2CO_3 to form HCO_3^- and H⁺

3-6

Buffers in the Human Body

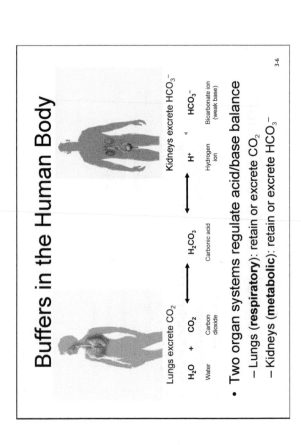

Lungs excrete CO_2 — Kidneys excrete HCO_3^-

$H_2O + CO_2 \longleftrightarrow H_2CO_3 \longleftrightarrow H^+ + HCO_3^-$

Water, Carbon dioxide, Carbonic acid, Hydrogen ion, Bicarbonate ion (weak base)

- Two organ systems regulate acid/base balance
  - Lungs (**respiratory**): retain or excrete CO_2
  - Kidneys (**metabolic**): retain or excrete HCO_3^-

3-6

Acidosis and Alkalosis

- The **respiratory system** and **renal system** must work together to maintain an appropriate pH for the body
  - The **respiratory system** affects pH by changing the **P_{CO2} level**
    - P_{CO2} is the same thing as carbonic acid (H_2CO_3)
    - As the equation below says, they're interchangeable
  - The **kidneys** affect pH by retaining or dumping **HCO_3^-**

3-6

Acidosis and Alkalosis

Four Categories of Acid/Base Imbalance		
Respiratory	Acidosis	elevation of P_{CO2}
	Alkalosis	depression of P_{CO2}
Metabolic	Acidosis	depression of HCO_3^-
	Alkalosis	elevation of HCO_3^-

3-6

Acidosis and Alkalosis

- **Respiratory Acidosis**
  - Hypoventilation
  - Asthma, Emphysema
  - Pneumonia
  - Coma
  - Snickers stuck in throat
- The kidneys will compensate (over a period of hours) by conserving HCO_3^- and excreting H^+ ions

- **Respiratory Alkalosis**
  - Hyperventilation
  - Drugs
  - Excitement
  - Anxiety
- The kidneys will compensate (over a period of hours) by retaining H^+ and excreting HCO_3^- ions

3-6

Acidosis and Alkalosis

- **Metabolic Acidosis**
  - Renal failure
  - Shock
  - Ketoacidosis
  - Lactic acidosis
  - Salicylate overdose
- The lungs will **immediately** begin to compensate by "wasting" CO_2 (hyperventilation)

- **Metabolic Alkalosis**
  - Ingestion of bicarbonate
  - Vomiting (losing gastric juice high in H^+ ions)
  - Chloride depletion
  - Diuretic therapy
- The lungs will **immediately** begin to compensate by holding on to CO_2 (hypoventilation)

3-6

Normal Acid/Base Values

pH	7.35 – 7.45
P_{O2}	68 – 72 mmHg
P_{CO2}	35 – 45 mmHg
HCO_3^-	22 – 26 mEq/L

this is not used to determine pH, but will give us clues to lung function (→ P_{O2})

3-6

Acid/Base Rubric

- To determine which category the patient fits into, follow these steps:
  - First, look at the pH. Is it acidosis or alkalosis?
    - For purposes of figuring this out:
    - anything above 7.40 is alkalotic
    - anything below 7.40 is acidotic
  - Write that down – **acidosis** or **alkalosis**

3-6

Acid/Base Rubric

- Second, cover up all the rest of the results and just ask: "What P_{CO2} or HCO_3^- level would cause that pH?"
- There are two choices each time:
  - Acidosis
    - too much CO_2: respiratory
    - too little HCO_3^- : metabolic
  - Alkalosis
    - too little CO_2: respiratory
    - too much HCO_3^-: metabolic

3-6

Acid/Base Rubric

- Third, check the "other" value to see if compensation is going on.
  - For instance, if the acidosis is respiratory because the pCO_2 is high, then check the HCO_3^- to see if it is within normal range **("uncompensated"),** or if it has gone outside the normal range because it is trying to re-establish homeostasis **("compensated"** to one degree or another).

3-6

Acid/Base Rubric

- Last, if there is compensation going on, determine if it is "partially" or "fully" compensated
- Is the pH is back into the normal 7.35 – 7.45 range?
- "**Fully compensated**"
  - pH within normal 7.35 – 7.45 range
  - never goes beyond 7.40
    - in acidosis it remains slightly acidic (7.35 – 7.39)
    - in alkalosis it remains slightly alkaline (7.41 – 7.45)
- "**Partially compensated**"
  - pH is not back into the normal range
  - Note that this will still throw P_{CO2} or $[HCO_3^-]$ outside normal limits

3-6

Acid/Base Rubric

- Write down the whole triple/ quadruple-barreled name
- Examples:
  - Partially-compensated metabolic acidosis
  - Uncompensated respiratory alkalosis
  - Compensated respiratory acidosis

3-6

Examples

Patient A	
pH	7.55
P_{O2}	70 mmHg
P_{CO2}	40 mmHg
$[HCO_3^-]$	36 mEq/L

Normal Values	
pH	7.35 – 7.45
P_{O2}	68 – 72 mmHg
P_{CO2}	35 – 45 mmHg
$[HCO_3^-]$	22 – 26 mEq/L

? alkalosis
metabolic
non compensated

3-6

Examples

Patient A, Later	
pH	7.44
P_{O2}	60 mmHg
P_{CO2}	55 mmHg
$[HCO_3^-]$	36 mEq/L

Normal Values	
pH	7.35 – 7.45
P_{O2}	68 – 72 mmHg
P_{CO2}	35 – 45 mmHg
$[HCO_3^-]$	22 – 26 mEq/L

? respiratory acidosis
compensated

3-6

Examples

Patient B	
pH	7.28
P_{O2}	50 mmHg
P_{CO2}	60 mmHg
$[HCO_3^-]$	25 mEq/L

Normal Values	
pH	7.35 – 7.45
P_{O2}	68 – 72 mmHg
P_{CO2}	35 – 45 mmHg
$[HCO_3^-]$	22 – 26 mEq/L

? respiratory acidosis
non compensated

3-6

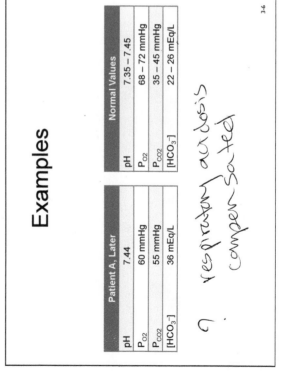

Examples

Patient B, Later	
pH	7.36
P_{O2}	50 mmHg
P_{CO2}	60 mmHg
$[HCO_3^-]$	34 mEq/L

Normal Values	
pH	7.35 – 7.45
P_{O2}	68 – 72 mmHg
P_{CO2}	35 – 45 mmHg
$[HCO_3^-]$	22 – 26 mEq/L

? respiratory acidosis
compensated

3-6

Examples

Patient C	
pH	7.22
P_{O2}	70 mmHg
P_{CO2}	40 mmHg
$[HCO_3^-]$	14 mEq/L

Normal Values	
pH	7.35 – 7.45
P_{O2}	68 – 72 mmHg
P_{CO2}	35 – 45 mmHg
$[HCO_3^-]$	22 – 26 mEq/L

metabolic acidosis
non compensated

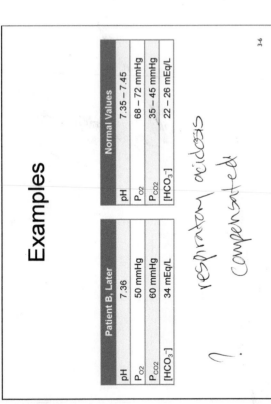

3-6

Examples

Patient C, Later	
pH	7.30
P_{O2}	80 mmHg
P_{CO2}	20 mmHg
$[HCO_3^-]$	14 mEq/L

Normal Values	
pH	7.35 – 7.45
P_{O2}	68 – 72 mmHg
P_{CO2}	35 – 45 mmHg
$[HCO_3^-]$	22 – 26 mEq/L

metabolic acidosis? or resp alkalosis?

compensated

3-6

UNIT 2

Study Guide Objectives - Introductory Pathophysiology (HTHS 2230)

Unit 2

Chapter 2 – Genes and Genetic Diseases

1. Explain each of the steps in the transfer of genetic information from DNA to RNA to protein. (pp. 34-38)

2. Identify the salient features of DNA that make it suitable for replication. Explain the process of replication. (pp. 35-36)

3. Define the types of mutation that affect the sequence of DNA bases at a single site (silent, missense, nonsense) and those that affect downstream DNA sequences (frameshift mutations). Give examples of mutagens. Define mutational hot spots. (p. 37)

4. Compare and contrast normal and abnormal chromosome numbers: euploidy and aneuploidy, including haploid, diploid, triploid, and tetraploid. In each case, identify a normal cell type (if present) that corresponds to each type of ploidy. (pp. 41-42)

5. Subdivide the aneuploidies into monosomies and trisomies of the autosomes and sex chromosomes. Explain the process of nondisjunction which gives rise to aneuploidies. Give examples of diseases which involve these aneuploidies. (pp. 42-44)

6. Describe changes in chromosome structure, including deletions, duplications, inversions and translocations. Define reciprocal and Robertsonian translocations. Explain fragile sites. (pp. 44-46)

7. Define gene, locus, allele, polymorphism, heterozygous and homozygous. Compare and contrast phenotype and genotype. (pp. 46-47)

8. Recognize symbols used in pedigree charts. Define: carrier, proband. (pp. 46-47)

9. Recognize autosomal dominant pedigree charts. State recurrence risk for autosomal dominant pedigrees, and factors which alter the recurrence risk for this type of pedigree. (pp. 47-48)

10. Define and be able to apply the concepts of penetrance and expressivity. (pp. 48-49)

11. Recognize autosomal recessive pedigree charts. State recurrence risk for autosomal recessive pedigrees, and factors which alter the recurrence risk for this type of pedigree. (pp. 47-48)

12. Recognize X-linked inheritance pedigree charts. State recurrence risk for sex-linked pedigrees, and factors which alter the recurrence risk for this type of pedigree. (pp. 47-48)

13. Define multifactorial inheritance. Define and apply the terms liability distribution and threshold of liability as they relate to the threshold model of multifactorial disease. (pp. 53-54)

Chapter 9 – Biology, Clinical Manifestations, and Treatment of Cancer

1. Define and contrast tumor, neoplasm, and cancer. (pp. 222-223)

2. Compare characteristics of benign and malignant tumors. (p. 223)

3. Cite the method for naming and classifying tumors; provide examples. (p. 223)

4. Define and describe carcinoma in situ (CIS); contrast with invasive carcinomas. (p. 223)

5. Describe how cancer cells are classified based on histological features and gene expression. (pp. 223-224)

6. Describe the advantages and limitations of tumor markers; cite marker examples that suggest the existence of cancer. Define paraneoplastic syndromes and give examples. (pp. 225-227, 244).

7. Name key features of cancer cells in the laboratory. (p. 227)

8. Compare and contrast the gene products of proto-oncogenes, oncogenes, and tumor-suppressor genes (anti-oncogenes). (p. 229)

9. Define loss of heterozygosity. (pp. 231-232)

10. Explain why cancer seems to "run in families". Give examples of gene alterations in cancer and explain their pathophysiology: growth signals, angiogenesis, telomeres, cancer metabolism, and oncogene addiction. (pp. 234-238)

11. Describe the characteristics of the cancer stem cell, and explain why targeting stem cells may be important in cancer treatment. (pp. 238-239)

12. Describe the interactions between cancer cells and the underlying stroma. (pp. 239-240)

13. Relate chronic inflammation to cancer cell development. (p. 240)

14. Describe the carcinogenesis of oncogenic viruses and bacteria, citing examples. (pp. 240-241)

15. Describe the mechanisms and steps for metastatic spread: detachment, invasion, intravasation, adherence in favorable sites, extravasation, and colonization. (pp. 241-243)

16. Describe the location and cellular characteristics related to the staging of cancers. (pp. 243-244)

17. Identify and describe the common clinical manifestations of cancer: anemia, leukopenia, thrombocytopenia, infection, fatigue, and pain. (pp. 245-248)

18. Compare and contrast the modalities for the treatment of cancer: chemotherapy, to include new-era anticancer drugs, surgery, and radiation. (pp. 248-249)

Unit 2
Chapter 2
Genes and Genetic Diseases

Genetics

- In the nineteenth century, scientists still only suspected that inheritance was contained in the nucleus of the cell.
- They had noticed that in a dividing cell the granular appearing chromatin condensed to form chromosomes.
- At the turn of the century, Gregor Mendel's experiments had helped describe the outward expression of hereditable traits without yet knowing where in cells the information was contained.

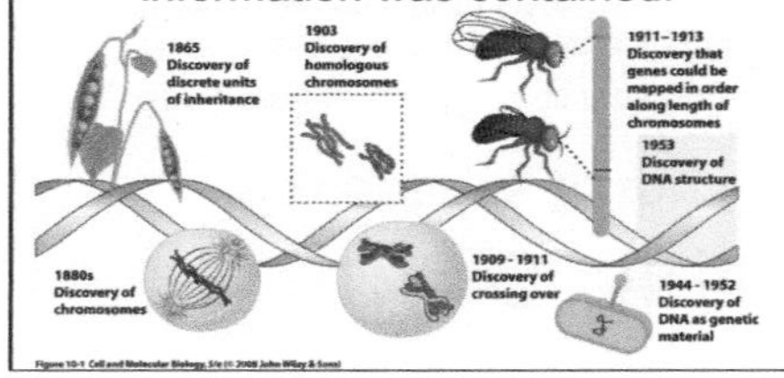

1865 Discovery of discrete units of inheritance
1903 Discovery of homologous chromosomes
1911–1913 Discovery that genes could be mapped in order along length of chromosomes
1953 Discovery of DNA structure
1880s Discovery of chromosomes
1909–1911 Discovery of crossing over
1944–1952 Discovery of DNA as genetic material

2-1

Genetics

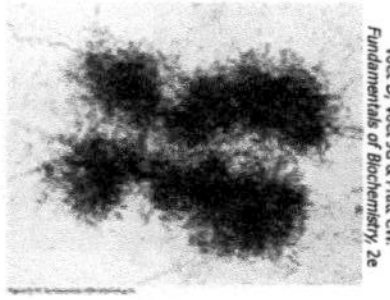

Voet D, Voet JG & Pratt CW. *Fundamentals of Biochemistry*, 2e

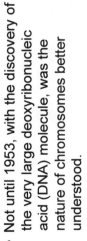

- Not until 1953, with the discovery of the very large deoxyribonucleic acid (DNA) molecule, was the nature of chromosomes better understood.
- Mendel's "inherited traits" turned out to be what we now call genes, specific sequences of DNA that dictate the makeup of proteins.

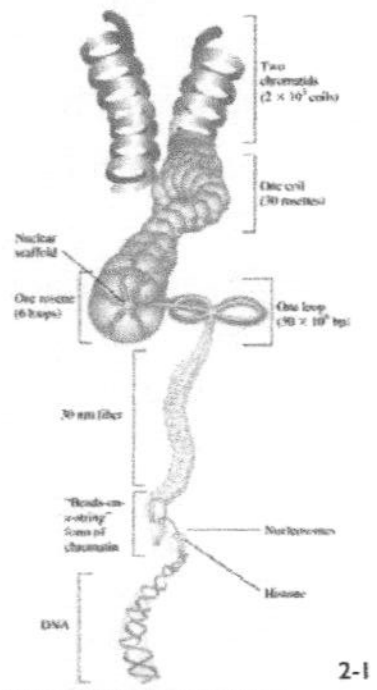

Figure 10-24 Concepts in Biochemistry, 3/e © 2006 John Wiley & Sons

2-1

Genetics: The Central Dogma

DNA

↓ transcription

RNA

↓ translation

protein

DNA
makes
RNA
makes
protein

2-1

Genetics: The Central Dogma

DNA → transcription → RNA → translation → protein

- DNA to RNA is called *transcription*
  - Your friend wants to borrow your class notes. You say, "All I have is a recording. You have to transcribe them."
  - Same language, different format
  - Language: sequence of A, C, G, T
- RNA to protein is called *translation*
  - Your Brazilian friend wants to borrow your class notes.
  - You say, "Mas eles esteja em inglês, nao português. Você terá que traduzi-los."
    - "But they are in English, not Portugese. You will have to translate them."
  - Different language: sequence of A, C, G, U converted to amino acids (glycine, glutamate, lysine, etc.)

2-1

DNA → transcription → RNA → translation → protein

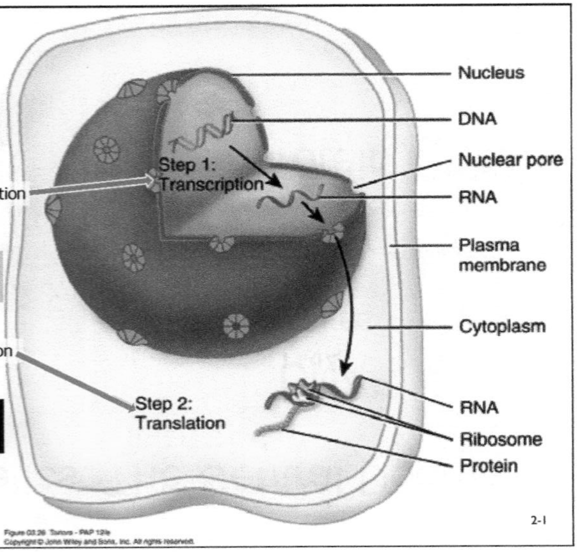

Nucleus
DNA
Nuclear pore
RNA
Plasma membrane
Cytoplasm
RNA
Ribosome
Protein
Step 1: Transcription
Step 2: Translation

2-1

Genetics: The Central Dogma

DNA → transcription → RNA → translation → protein

- Is the Central Dogma ever "violated"? yes, virus
- Does protein ever make RNA? no
- Does RNA ever make DNA? yes

retro virus use RNA as genetic material

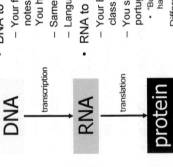

2-1

The Central Dogma

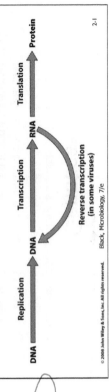

Exceptions to the Central Dogma

- Some viruses use RNA as their genetic material
- These carry the code for an enzyme called **reverse transcriptase** that converts RNA to DNA
- For this reason, these viruses are called **retroviruses**
- DNA is then inserted into the host cell
- This is a destructive process for the host cell; damage to the host cell DNA is common and results in diseases such as cancer

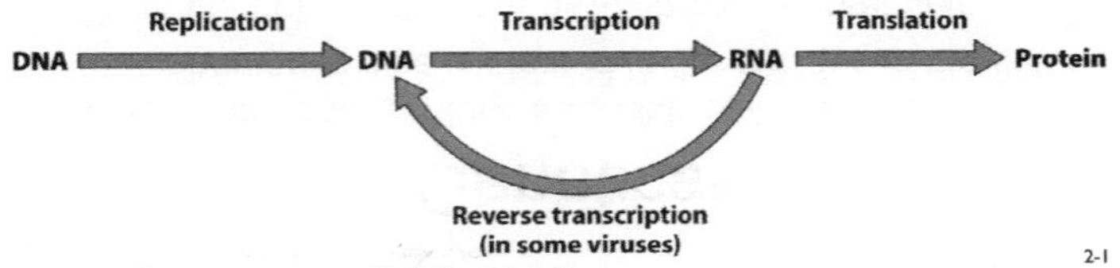

Replication
Transcription
Translation
DNA
DNA
RNA
Protein
Reverse transcription (in some viruses)

 Black, Microbiology, 7/e

2-1

The Human Genome Project

- **The Human Genome Project (HGP),** completed in 2003, accomplished its goal to determine the sequences of base pairs that make up human DNA.
- Of the approximately **30,000** genes thus identified by the Human Genome Project, only a portion have been linked to specific genetic conditions.

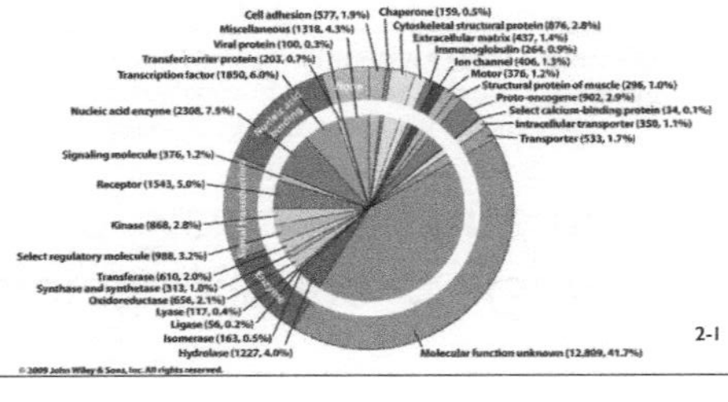

2-1

S phase

- DNA replication during S phase
- All DNA must be duplicated, in preparation for cell division

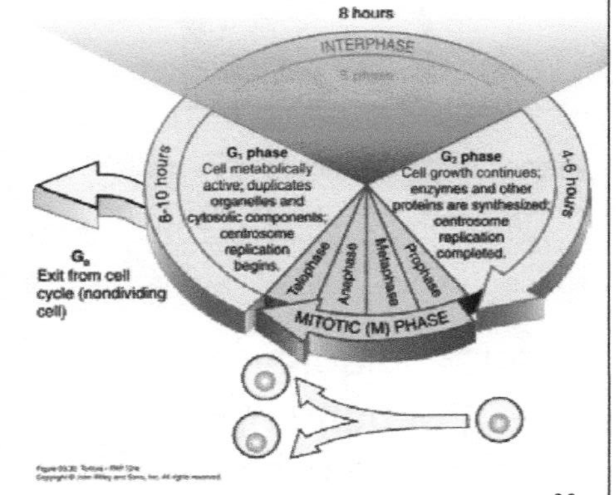
8 hours
INTERPHASE
6-10 hours
G_1 phase
Cell metabolically active; duplicates organelles and cytosolic components; centrosome replication begins.
G_2 phase
Cell growth continues; enzymes and other proteins are synthesized; centrosome replication completed.
4-6 hours
Telophase
Anaphase
Metaphase
Prophase
MITOTIC (M) PHASE
G_0
Exit from cell cycle (nondividing cell)

2-2

DNA Replication

- DNA strands separated
- Two new DNA strands (teal) constructed using original strands (purple) as templates
- Same base-pairing rules allow new strands to be made with exact fidelity

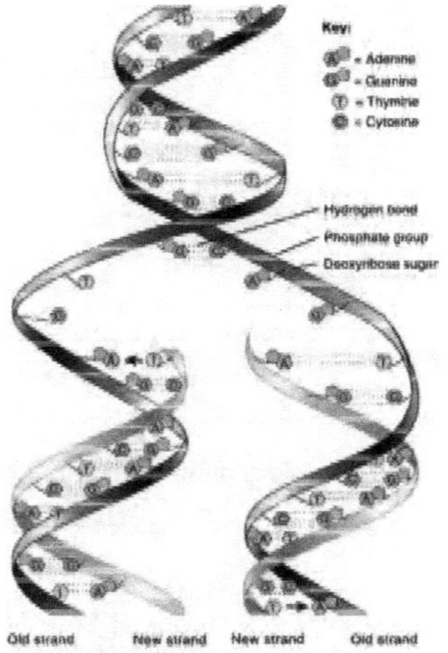
Key:
= Adenine
= Guanine
= Thymine
= Cytosine
Hydrogen bond
Phosphate group
Deoxyribose sugar
Old strand
New strand
New strand
Old strand

Figure 03.31 Tortora - PAP 12/e

2-2

Gene Polymorphism Mutation

- A change in the sequence of DNA which then results in a change in the sequence of mRNA is a **gene polymorphism**
- Most polymorphisms are silent, that is, they do not change the primary protein sequence
- Some polymorphisms cause noticeable changes in the organism; these are called **mutations**

2-3

A Mutation

- Any **inherited alteration** of genetic material
  - Any change to the nucleotide sequence of genetic material
- Chromosome changes (mutations) causing **congenital** defects are **easier to observe**
  - However, some mutations are very subtle, and are either difficult or impossible to observe
- Mutations can be favorable or unfavorable

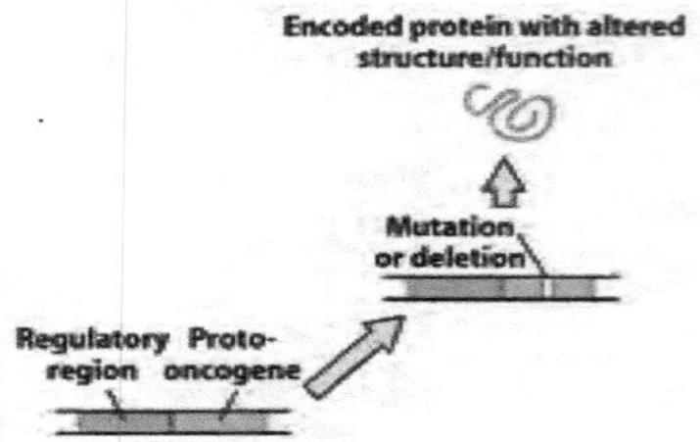

Encoded protein with altered structure/function
Mutation or deletion
Regulatory region
Proto-oncogene

Karp G. *Cell & Molecular Biology*, 6e

2-3

Types of Mutation

- **Reading frame**: 3 bases at a time are read
  - e.g. CAT CAT CAT CAT
- **Point mutations** do not change the reading frame
  - These change only a single base (CAA CAT CAT CAT)
  - Sometimes these do not change the protein sequence
    - **silent mutations**
  - Sometimes these do change the protein sequence
    - **missense mutations**: change one amino acid to another
    - **nonsense mutations**: change codon that codes for an amino acid to a stop codon, resulting in abnormally short protein
- **Frameshift mutations** change the reading frame

2-3

A Missense Mutation in the β –Globin Gene Results in Sickle Cell Anemia

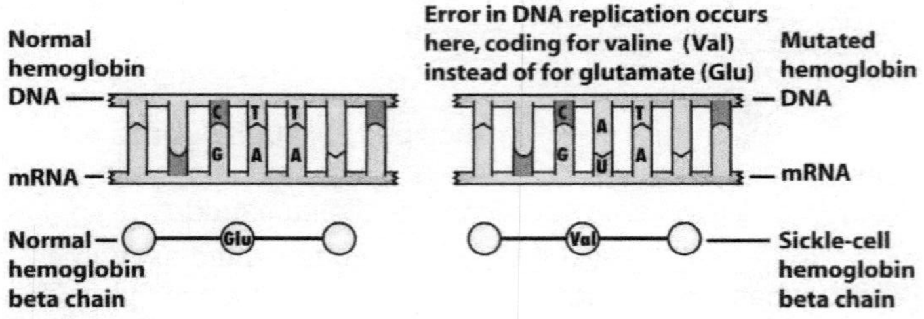

Normal hemoglobin DNA
mRNA
Normal hemoglobin beta chain
Glu
Error in DNA replication occurs here, coding for valine (Val) instead of for glutamate (Glu)
Mutated hemoglobin
DNA
mRNA
Val
Sickle-cell hemoglobin beta chain

© 2006 John Wiley & Sons
Pruitt, Bioinquiry: Making Connections in Biology, 3/e

GUU Val	GCU Ala	GAU Asp	GGU Gly
GUC Val	GCC Ala	GAC Asp	GGC Gly
GUA Val	GCA Ala	GAA Glu	GGA Gly
GUG Val	GCG Ala	GAG Glu	GGG Gly

2-3

The Sickle Cell Mutation in the β -Globin Gene

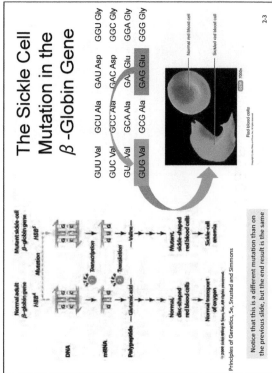

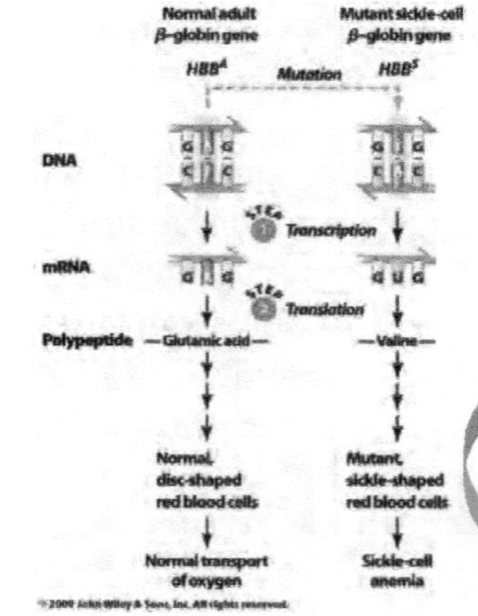

Normal adult β-globin gene
Mutant sickle-cell β-globin gene
Mutation
DNA
Transcription
mRNA
Translation
Polypeptide
Glutamic acid
Valine
Normal, disc-shaped red blood cells
Mutant, sickle-shaped red blood cells
Normal transport of oxygen
Sickle-cell anemia

© 2009 John Wiley & Sons, Inc. All rights reserved.
Principles of Genetics, 5e, Snustad and Simmons

GUU Val	GCU Ala	GAU Asp	GGU Gly
GUC Val	GCC Ala	GAC Asp	GGC Gly
GUA Val	GCA Ala	GAA Glu	GGA Gly
GUG Val	GCG Ala	GAG Glu	GGG Gly

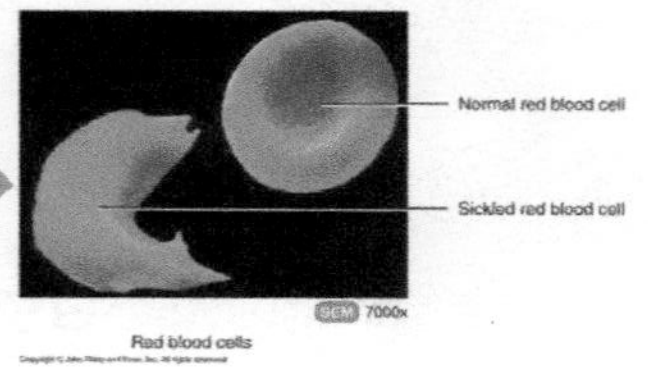

Normal red blood cell
Sickled red blood cell
7000x
Red blood cells

Notice that this is a different mutation than on the previous slide, but the end result is the same

2-3

Types of Mutations

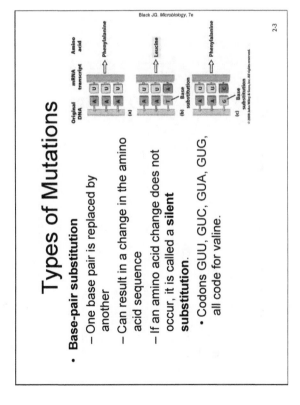

- **Base-pair substitution**
  - One base pair is replaced by another
  - Can result in a change in the amino acid sequence
  - If an amino acid change does not occur, it is called a **silent substitution**.
    - Codons GUU, GUC, GUA, GUG, all code for valine.

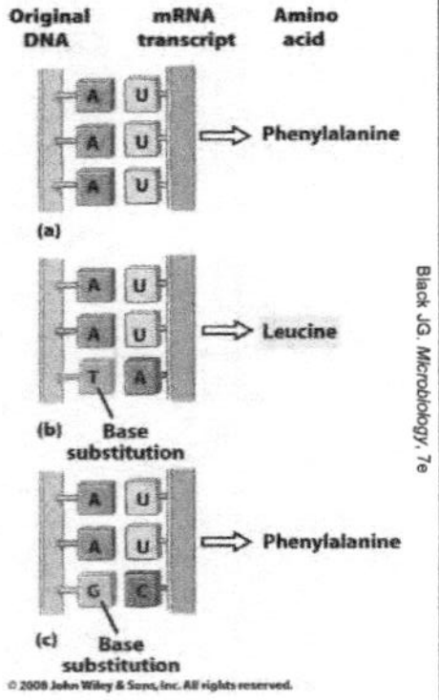
Original DNA
mRNA transcript
Amino acid
Phenylalanine
(a)
Leucine
(b) Base substitution
Phenylalanine
(c) Base substitution

Black JG. *Microbiology*, 7e

2-3

Types of Mutations

- **Frameshift mutation**
  - Insertion or deletion of one or more base pairs in the DNA molecule.

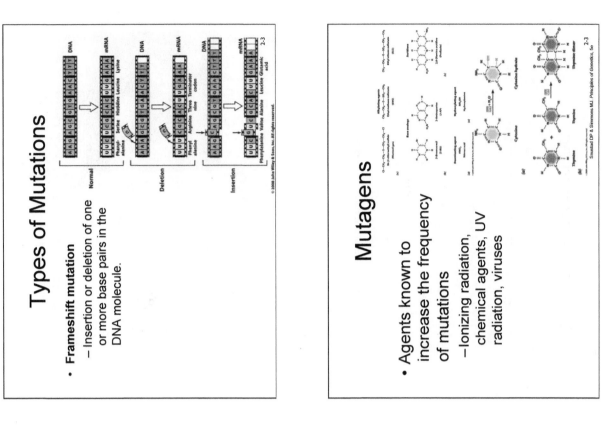

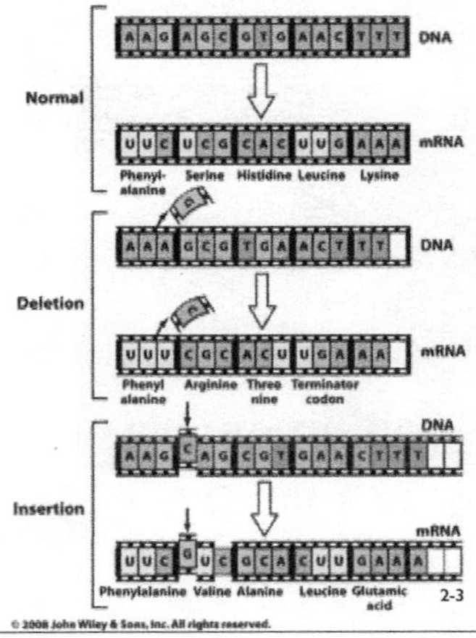
Normal
DNA
mRNA
Phenyl-alanine Serine Histidine Leucine Lysine
Deletion
DNA
mRNA
Phenyl alanine Arginine Threonine Terminator codon
Insertion
DNA
mRNA
Phenylalanine Valine Alanine Leucine Glutamic acid

2-3

Types of Frameshift Mutation

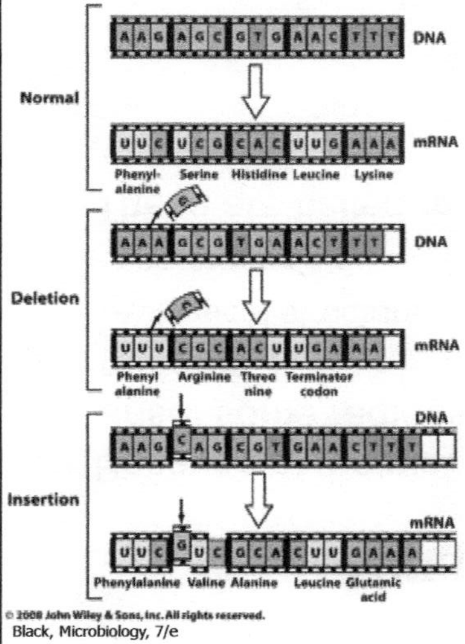
Normal
DNA
mRNA
Phenyl-alanine Serine Histidine Leucine Lysine
Deletion
DNA
mRNA
Phenyl alanine Arginine Threonine Terminator codon
Insertion
DNA
mRNA
Phenylalanine Valine Alanine Leucine Glutamic acid

Black, Microbiology, 7/e

- Frameshift mutations change the reading frame
- 3 bases at a time are read
  - e.g. CAT CAT CAT CAT
  - Deletion mutations
    - one base removed
    - CAT C|TC ATC ATC
  - Insertion mutation
    - one base added
    - CAT CCA TCA TCA

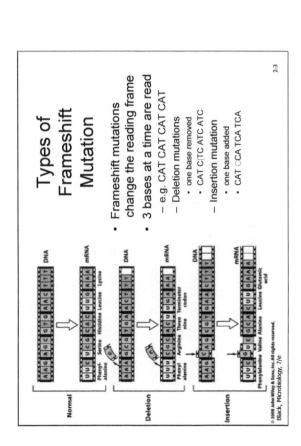

2-3

Mutagens

- Agents known to increase the frequency of mutations
  - Ionizing radiation, chemical agents, UV radiation, viruses

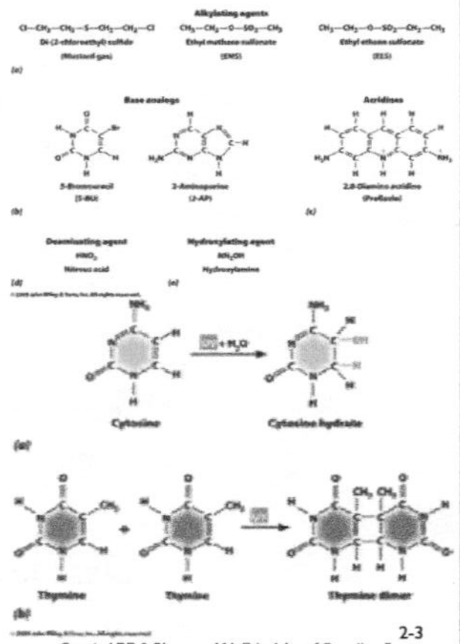
Cytosine
Cytosine hydrate
Thymine
Thymine
Thymine dimer

2-3

Snustad DP & Simmons MJ. *Principles of Genetics*, 5e

Mutational Hot Spots

- Because of the way in which mutations arise, some regions of DNA are often mutated
  - physical structure?
  - sequence?
- These are called **mutational hot spots**

2-3

Two Kinds of Human Cells

- There are 2 basic types of human cells
  - **Somatic cells** are almost all of the 10 trillion cells that make up our body
    - They are **diploid cells**
      - **23 pairs of chromosomes** for **46 total chromosomes**
    - Formed by the process of **mitosis**
  - **Gametes**
    - Specialized sex cells
      - ♂ spermatozoa; ♀ eggs
      - these are **haploid cells** (23 total chromosomes)
    - Formed by the process of **meiosis**

2-4

Haploid and Diploid Cells

- **Somatic cells** make up the majority of the body's cells
  - somatic cells use mitosis to divide
  - these are **diploid (2N)**
  - two copies of each numbered chromosome plus two sex chromosomes (XX or XY)
- **Germ cells (gametes)** are the reproductive cells
  - gametes use meiosis to divide
  - sperm in ♂
  - eggs in ♀
  - these cells are haploid (N)
  - when they join, they make a diploid embryo

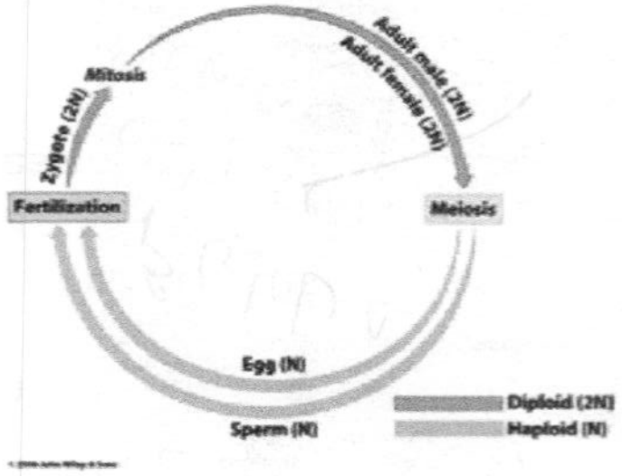

Mitosis
Adult male (2N)
Adult female (2N)
Zygote (2N)
Fertilization
Meiosis
Egg (N)
Sperm (N)
Diploid (2N)
Haploid (N)

Alters, Biology: Understanding Life, 1/e

2-4

Karyotype

- An ordered display of chromosomes is called a karyotype.
  - Image taken during metaphase.
- The homologous chromosomes are paired and displayed according to their size and the position of the centromere in relation to the chromosome bands.
  - Chromosome 1 is the longest and 22 is the shortest.

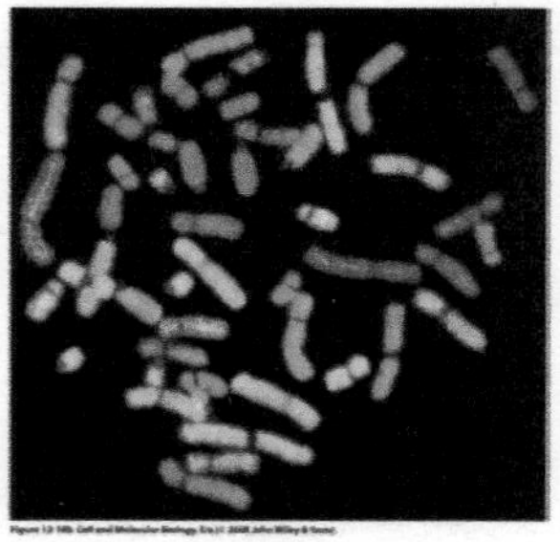

2-4

Chromosomes

- Homologous chromosomes
  - Nearly identical chromosomes
  - The two chromosomes that pair during meiosis
  - Each member of a pair is inherited from one parent
- Non-homologous
  - Non-identical chromosomes
  - An example would be chromosomes 9 and 22

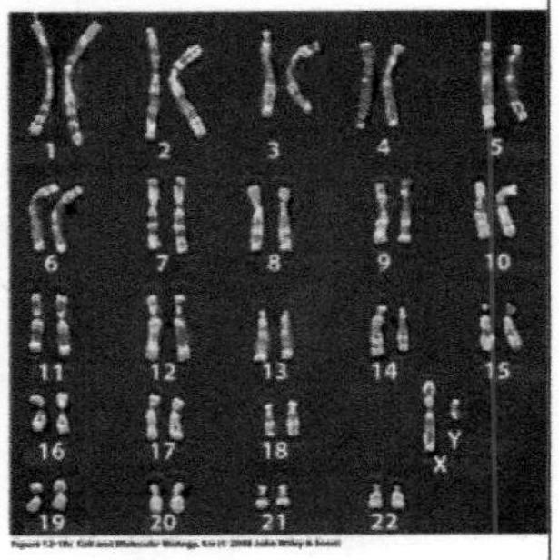

1
2
3
4
5
6
7
8
9
10
11
12
13
14
15
16
17
18
X
Y
19
20
21
22

2-4

Chromosomes

- In humans, numbered chromosomes (1-22) are called **autosomes**
- The remaining pair are **sex chromosomes**.
  - ♀ homologous pair (XX)
  - ♂ non-homologous pair (XY)

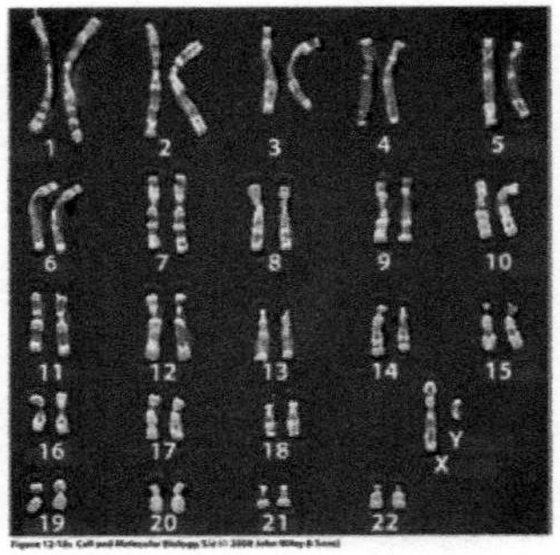

1
2
3
4
5
6
7
8
9
10
11
12
13
14
15
16
17
18
X
Y
19
20
21
22

2-4

Chromosomal Aberrations

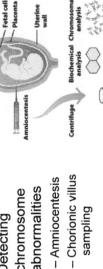

- Detecting chromosome abnormalities
  - Amniocentesis
  - Chorionic villus sampling

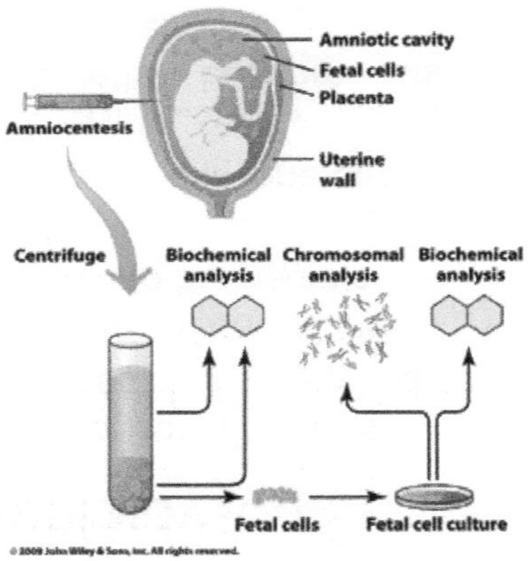

Amniotic cavity
Fetal cells
Placenta
Amniocentesis
Uterine wall
Centrifuge
Biochemical analysis
Chromosomal analysis
Biochemical analysis
Fetal cells
Fetal cell culture
© 2009 John Wiley & Sons, Inc. All rights reserved.

Snustad DP & Simmons MJ. *Principles of Genetics*, 5e

2-4

Polyploidy

- Cells that have a multiple of the normal number/ set (23) of chromosomes are **euploid.**
  - **Is a haploid cell euploid? Yes, 23x1.**
  - **Is a diploid cell euploid? Yes, 23x2.**
- When a euploid cell has more than the **diploid** number, it is called a **polyploid** cell (they still contain a multiple of 23).
  - **Triploid** fetuses have three copies of each chromosome (69 total)
  - **Tetraploid** fetuses have four copies of each (92 each)
  - Neither triploid nor tetraploid fetuses can survive.

2-4

Aneuploidy

- A somatic cell that does not contain an exact multiple of 23 chromosomes is an aneuploid cell.
- A cell containing three copies of one of the chromosome "pairs" is said to be trisomic (trisomy).
- Monosomy is the presence of only one of any of the chromosome "pairs".
- Monosomy is more often lethal, but some infants can survive with trisomy of certain chromosomes.
  - "It is better to have extra than less."

2-4

Disjunction is the Separation of Chromatids at Meiosis

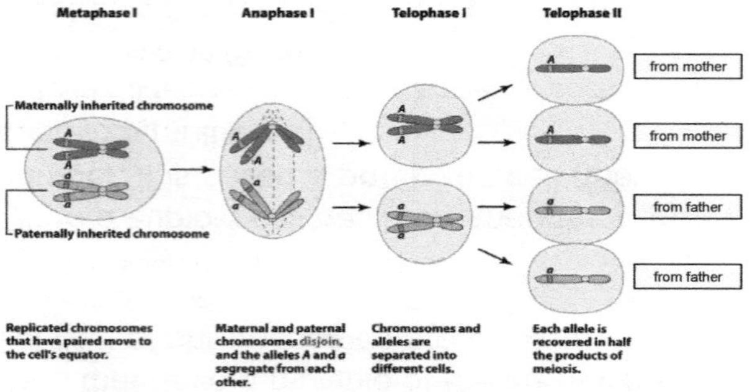
Metaphase I
Anaphase I
Telophase I
Telophase II
Maternally inherited chromosome
Paternally inherited chromosome
from mother
from mother
from father
from father
Replicated chromosomes that have paired move to the cell's equator.
Maternal and paternal chromosomes disjoin, and the alleles A and a segregate from each other.
Chromosomes and alleles are separated into different cells.
Each allele is recovered in half the products of meiosis.

Snustad DP & Simmons MJ. *Principles of Genetics*, 5e

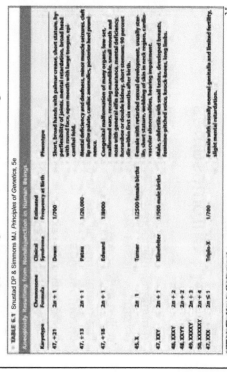

- The purpose of **disjunction** is to distribute equal amounts of genetic material to each gamete
- Normally, one copy of each gene ends up in each gamete
- That is, each normal gamete contains one allele

2-5

Nondisjunction

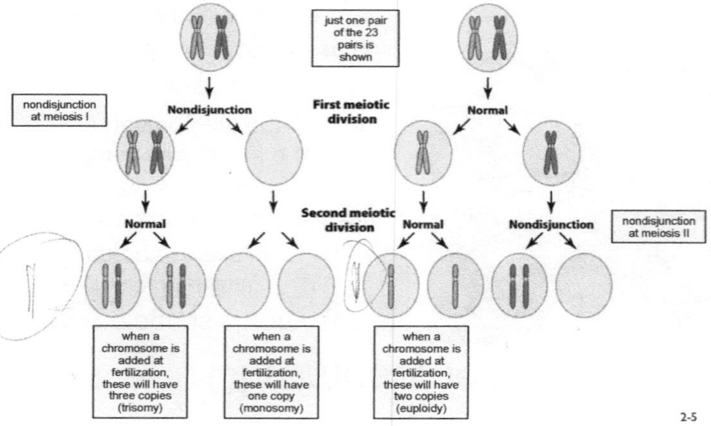
just one pair of the 23 pairs is shown
nondisjunction at meiosis I
Nondisjunction
First meiotic division
Normal
Second meiotic division
Normal
Normal
Nondisjunction
nondisjunction at meiosis II
when a chromosome is added at fertilization, these will have three copies (trisomy)
when a chromosome is added at fertilization, these will have one copy (monosomy)
when a chromosome is added at fertilization, these will have two copies (euploidy)

Snustad DP & Simmons MJ. *Principles of Genetics*, 5e

2-5

Aneuploidy from Nondisjunction

TABLE 6.1 Snustad DP & Simmons MJ. *Principles of Genetics*, 5e

Aneuploidy Resulting from Nondisjunction in Human Beings

Karyotype	Chromosome Formula	Clinical Syndrome	Estimated Frequency at Birth	Phenotype
47, +21	2n + 1	Down	1/700	Short, broad hands with palmar crease, short stature, hyperflexibility of joints, mental retardation, broad head with round face, open mouth with large tongue, epicanthal fold.
47, +13	2n + 1	Patau	1/20,000	Mental deficiency and deafness, minor muscle seizures, cleft lip and/or palate, cardiac anomalies, posterior heel prominence.
47, +18	2n + 1	Edward	1/8000	Congenital malformation of many organs, low-set, malformed ears, receding mandible, small mouth and nose with general elfin appearance, mental deficiency, horseshoe or double kidney, short sternum; 90 percent die within first six months after birth.
45, X	2n 1	Turner	1/2500 female births	Female with retarded sexual development, usually sterile, short stature, webbing of skin in neck region, cardiovascular abnormalities, hearing impairment.
47, XXY	2n + 1	Klinefelter	1/500 male births	Male, subfertile with small testes, developed breasts, feminine-pitched voice, knock-knees, long limbs.
48, XXXY	2n + 2			
48, XXYY	2n + 2			
49, XXXXY	2n + 3			
50, XXXXXY	2n + 4			
47, XXX	2n ≤ 1	Triplo-X	1/700	Female with usually normal genitalia and limited fertility, slight mental retardation.

2-5

Down Syndrome

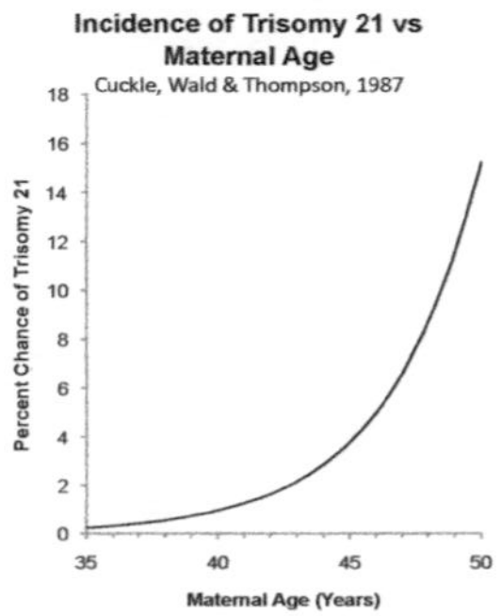
Incidence of Trisomy 21 vs Maternal Age
Cuckle, Wald & Thompson, 1987
Percent Chance of Trisomy 21
Maternal Age (Years)

- **Best-known example of aneuploidy as a result of nondisjunction during fertilization**
- 1/700 live births
- Closely related to maternal age
- Mentally retarded, low nasal bridge, epicanthal folds, protruding tongue, poor muscle tone

Karyotype	Chromosome Formula	Clinical Syndrome	Estimated Frequency at Birth	Phenotype
47, +21	$2n + 1$	Down	1/700	Short, broad hands with palmar crease, short stature, hyperflexibility of joints, mental retardation, broad head with round face, open mouth with large tongue, epicanthal fold.

2-5

Sex Chromosome Aneuploidy

45, X	$2n$ 1	Turner	1/2500 female births	Female with retarded sexual development, usually sterile, short stature, webbing of skin in neck region, cardiovascular abnormalities, hearing impairment.

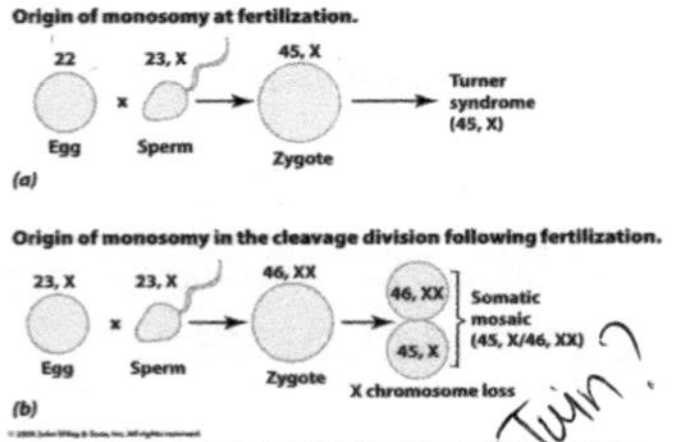
Origin of monosomy at fertilization.
22
23, X
45, X
Egg
Sperm
Zygote
Turner syndrome (45, X)
(a)
Origin of monosomy in the cleavage division following fertilization.
23, X
23, X
46, XX
46, XX
45, X
Somatic mosaic (45, X/46, XX)
Egg
Sperm
Zygote
X chromosome loss
(b)
Twin ?

Snustad DP & Simmons MJ. *Principles of Genetics*, 5e

- **Turner Syndrome (45, X)**
  - Females with only one X chromosome characterized by:
    - Absence of ovaries (sterile)
    - Short stature
    - Webbing of the neck
    - Underdeveloped breasts; wide nipples
    - A high number of fetuses with single X are aborted
    - **The single X is usually inherited from the mother**

2-5

Sex Chromosome Aneuploidy

47, XXX	$2n \leq 1$	Triplo-X	1/700	Female with usually normal genitalia and limited fertility, slight mental retardation.

- Triplo-X (47, XXX)
- Three X chromosomes
- Phenotypically female
  - Sterility, menstrual irregularity and/or mental retardation
  - Symptoms worsen with each additional X

2-5

Sex Chromosome Aneuploidy

47, XXY	$2n + 1$	Klinefelter	1/500 male births	Male, subfertile with small testes, developed breasts, feminine-pitched voice, knock-knees, long limbs.
48, XXXY	$2n + 2$			
48, XXYY	$2n + 2$			
49, XXXXY	$2n + 3$			
50, XXXXXY	$2n + 4$			

- **Klinefelter Syndrome**
  - Individuals with two or more X chromosomes and one Y chromosome (47, XXY) or (48, XXXY) or (49, XXXXY) or (50,XXXXXY)
  - Characteristics
    - Male appearance
    - Develop female-like breasts
    - Small testes
    - Sparse body hair
    - Long limbs
  - **The abnormalities will increase with each "extra" X chromosome**

2-5

Chromosome Structure Abnormalities

- Not a change in chromosome number
- Chromosome alterations at the gene level
  - Breakage
  - Deletions
  - Inversions
  - Duplications
  - Translocations

2-6

Chromosome Structure Abnormality

- **Chromosome breakage**
  - If a chromosome breaks, physiological mechanisms will usually repair it, but the breaks can "heal" in a way that alters the structure of the chromosome.
  - Agents of chromosome breakage are called **clastogens**
    - **Ionizing radiation, chemicals, and certain viruses**

2-6

Deletions

- **Breakage** resulting in loss of DNA
- ***Cri du chat* syndrome**
  - "Cry of the cat"
  - Deletion of short arm of chromosome 5
  - Low birth weight, mental retardation, microcephaly

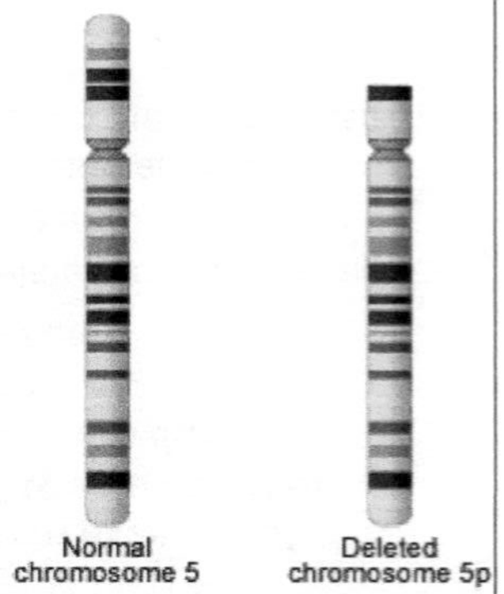
Normal chromosome 5
Deleted chromosome 5p

© Clinical Tools, Inc.

2-6

Inversions

- **Breakage** followed by a reversal of the fragment during re-insertion.
  - ABCDEFGH may become AB**EDC**FGH

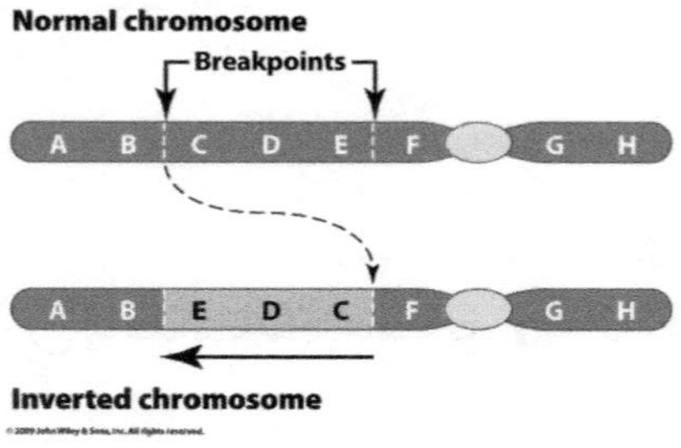
Normal chromosome
Breakpoints
A B C D E F G H
A B E D C F G H
Inverted chromosome

Snustad DP & Simmons MJ. *Principles of Genetics*, 5e

2-6

Duplications

- Replication of a gene sequence resulting in an amino acid sequence being **repeated** multiple times
  - Less serious consequences because it is better to have more genetic material rather than less (deletion)
- The greater the number of repeats, the more severe the manifestation and the earlier the onset
- Duplication in the same region as Cri du chat causes mental retardation but no physical abnormalities

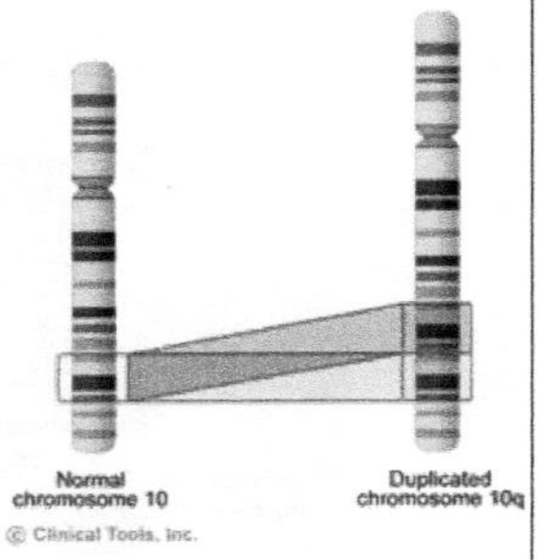
Normal chromosome 10
Duplicated chromosome 10q
© Clinical Tools, Inc.

2-6

Translocations

- The interchanging of material between non-homologous chromosomes (13-14, 2-5)
- Translocation occurs when two chromosomes break and the segments are rejoined in an abnormal arrangement.

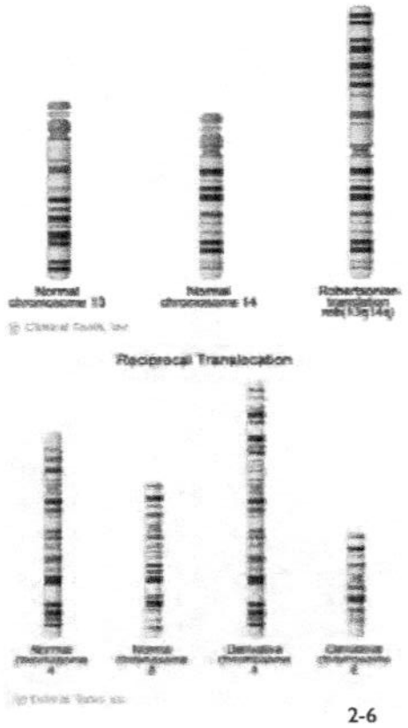
Normal chromosome 13
Normal chromosome 14
Reciprocal Translocation

2-6

Mendelian Genetics

- Because the mother's and father's gametes each contain one copy of each gene, child inherits one copy of a gene from mother and one from father
- In Mendelian terminology, these are called **alleles**
  - Modern molecular genetics: note these are the same as polymorphisms
- Each parent's gametes are haploid and so contain one allele each, but each child has a 50/50 chance of getting each allele
- **Dominant alleles** are those where inheriting one copy will give you a condition or disease
- **Recessive alleles** are those where inheriting one copy makes you a **carrier**, and inheriting two copies will give you a condition or disease

2-7

Punnett Squares

- Punnett squares are used to analyze Mendelian genetics
- Use capital letters for dominant allele
- Use small letters for recessive allele
- If disease or condition is dominant, then individuals with AA or Aa will have disease while those with aa will not
- If disease or condition is recessive, then individuals with AA or Aa will not have disease, but individuals with aa will
  - Aa individuals are called **carriers** because they can pass "bad" gene to their offspring but are not themselves affected

	Father's A	Father's a
Mother's A	AA	Aa
Mother's a	Aa	aa

2-7

Example: Albinism

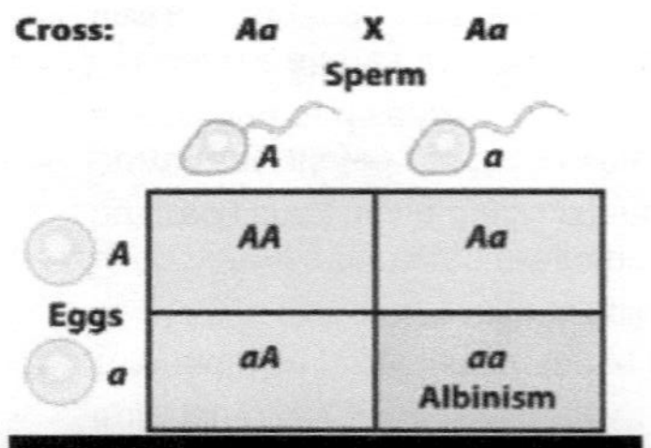

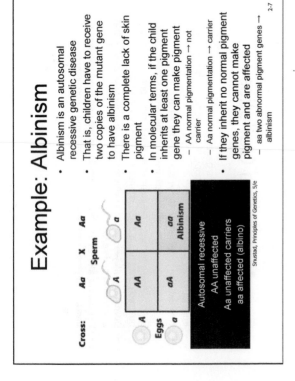

Cross: Aa X Aa
Sperm
A
a
Eggs
A
a
AA
Aa
aA
aa Albinism

Autosomal recessive
AA unaffected
Aa unaffected carriers
aa affected (albino)

Snustad, Principles of Genetics, 5/e

- Albinism is an autosomal recessive genetic disease
- That is, children have to receive two copies of the mutant gene to have albinism
- There is a complete lack of skin pigment
- In molecular terms, if the child inherits at least one pigment gene they can make pigment
  - AA normal pigmentation → not carrier
  - Aa normal pigmentation → carrier
- If they inherit no normal pigment genes, they cannot make pigment and are affected
  - aa two abnormal pigment genes → albinism

2-7

Inheritance of Sickle Trait

- This an example of a **co-dominant** trait
- In molecular terms, the genes for normal Hb and sickle Hb are both transcribed and translated equally
- Father is HbS/HbS: all his Hb is abnormal
- Children are HbA/HbS: on average, about half the Hb in their red blood cells is abnormal

Hemoglobin = Hb
Normal Hb = HbA
Mutated Hb = HbS

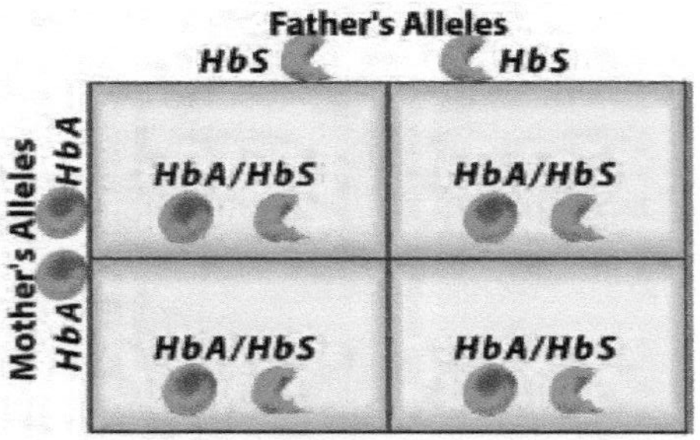

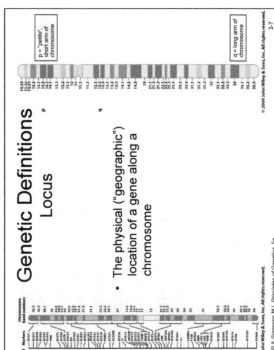

Father's Alleles
HbS
HbS
Mother's Alleles
HbA
HbA
HbA/HbS
HbA/HbS
HbA/HbS
HbA/HbS

Pruitt, Bioinquiry: Making Connections in Biology, 3/e

2-7

Genetic Definitions

Gene

- A segment of DNA that codes for a protein or regulatory molecule
- Synthesis of specific proteins will lead to expression of particular traits
  - e.g. eye color, phosphorylase enzyme, collagen in extracellular matrix

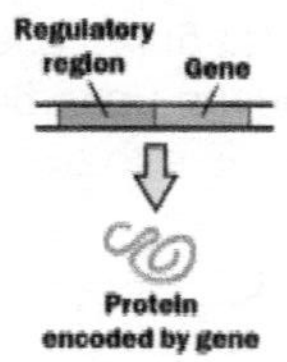

Regulatory region
Gene
Protein encoded by gene

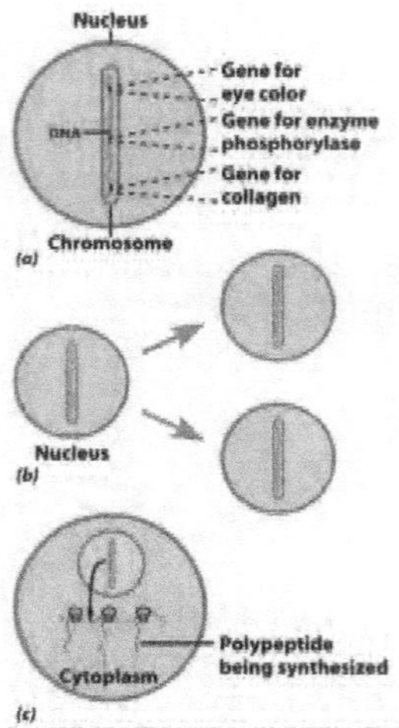

Nucleus
DNA
Gene for eye color
Gene for enzyme phosphorylase
Gene for collagen
Chromosome
(a)
Nucleus
(b)
Cytoplasm
Polypeptide being synthesized
(c)

Figure 10-11 Cell and Molecular Biology, 5/e (© 2008 John Wiley & Sons)

Karp G. *Cell & Molecular Biology*, 6e

2-7

Genetic Definitions

Locus

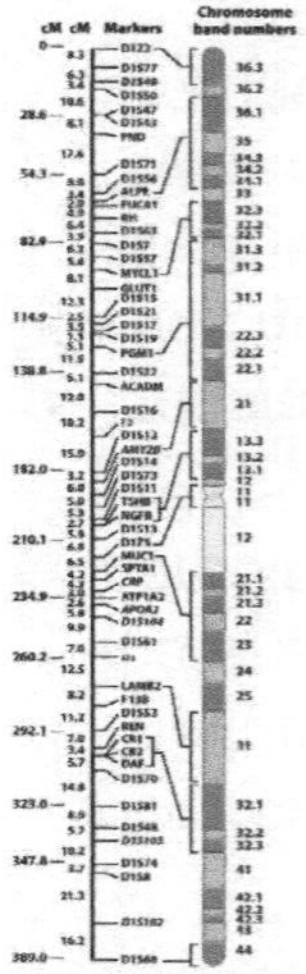

cM cM Markers
Chromosome band numbers

- The physical ("geographic") location of a gene along a chromosome

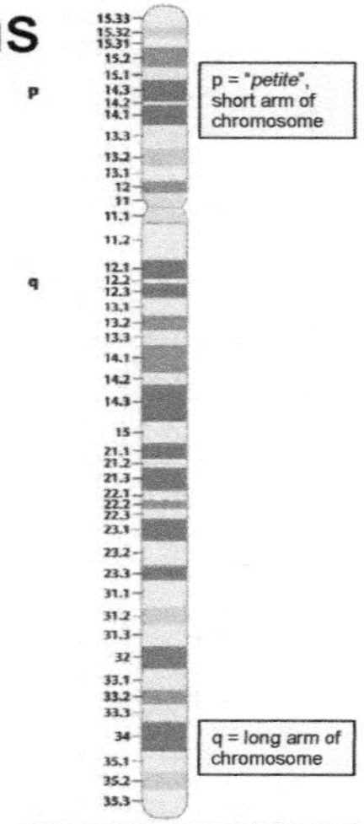

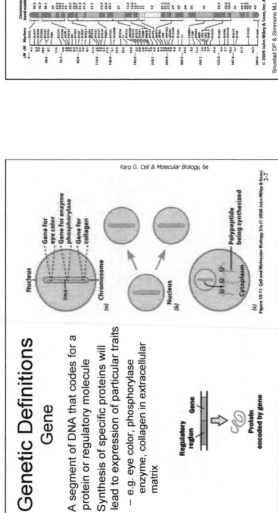

p
q
p = "*petite*", short arm of chromosome
q = long arm of chromosome

Snustad DP & Simmons MJ. *Principles of Genetics*, 5e

2-7

Genetic Definitions

- **Allele**
  - A different form (or copy) of a particular gene
    - For example, there are three alleles for glycolipids found on the surface of red blood cells
      - A glycolipid (I^A), B glycolipid (I^B) or neither (i)

TABLE 4.1

Genotypes, Phenotypes, and Frequencies in the ABO Blood-Typing System

Frequency in Genotype	Blood Type	A Antigen Present	B Antigen Present	U.S. White Population (%)
I^AI^A or I^Ai	A	+	–	41
I^BI^B or I^Bi	B	–	+	11
I^AI^B	AB	+	+	4
ii	O	–	–	44

Snustad DP & Simmons MJ. *Principles of Genetics*, 5e

2-7

Genetic Definitions

- **Homozygous**
  - When the two alleles of a particular gene on a pair of homologous chromosomes are identical
  - One allele inherited from the mother, one from the father
  - e.g. blood genotypes I^AI^A or I^BI^B or ii

TABLE 4.1 Snustad DP & Simmons MJ. *Principles of Genetics*, 5e

Genotypes, Phenotypes, and Frequencies in the ABO Blood-Typing System

Frequency in Genotype	Blood Type	A Antigen Present	B Antigen Present	U.S. White Population (%)
I^AI^A or I^Ai	A	+	–	41
I^BI^B or I^Bi	B	–	+	11
I^AI^B	AB	+	+	4
ii	O	–	–	44

2-7

Genetic Definitions

- **Heterozygous**
  - When the two alleles of a particular gene on a pair of homologous chromosomes are not identical
  - e.g. blood genotypes I^Ai or I^Bi or I^AI^B

TABLE 4.1 Snustad DP & Simmons MJ. *Principles of Genetics*, 5e

Genotypes, Phenotypes, and Frequencies in the ABO Blood-Typing System

Frequency in Genotype	Blood Type	A Antigen Present	B Antigen Present	U.S. White Population (%)
I^AI^A or I^Ai	A	+	–	41
I^BI^B or I^Bi	B	–	+	11
I^AI^B	AB	+	+	4
ii	O	–	–	44

2-7

Genotype vs. Phenotype

Snustad DP & Simmons MJ. *Principles of Genetics*, 5e

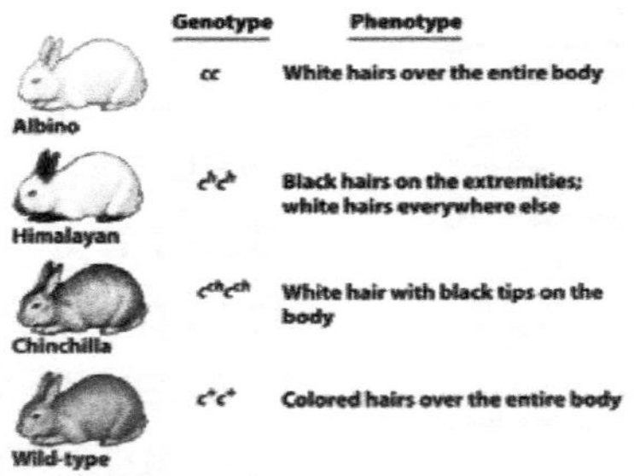

Genotype
Phenotype
Albino
cc
White hairs over the entire body
Himalayan
c^hc^h
Black hairs on the extremities; white hairs everywhere else
Chinchilla
$c^{ch}c^{ch}$
White hair with black tips on the body
Wild-type
c^+c^+
Colored hairs over the entire body

Genotypes, Phenotypes, and Frequencies in the ABO Blood-Typing System

Frequency in Genotype	Blood Type	A Antigen Present	B Antigen Present	U.S. White Population (%)
I^AI^A or I^Ai	A	+	–	41
I^BI^B or I^Bi	B	–	+	11
I^AI^B	AB	+	+	4
ii	O	–	–	44

- **Genotype** ("what they have")
  - **The genetic make-up of an organism**
  - Usually indicated with two letters, one for each allele
- **Phenotype** ("what they demonstrate")
  - This can be a visible observation, or it can be tested for.
  - By observing some phenotypes, you can't necessarily tell what the genotype is
    - e.g. A or B blood group phenotypes each have two possible genotypes

2-7

Genetic Terminology

- An allele that is **observable is dominant**, and the one that is hidden is recessive.
  - In our example, the allele for the "A" blood type is dominant, and the allele for the "O" blood type is recessive.
- Dominant and recessive refer to **which allele is expressed** when the two occur together. There is nothing abnormal or defective implied in the terms.
- Yes, alleles can be co-dominant (AB blood type).
- If letters are used to express alleles, dominant alleles are capitalized; recessive are lower-case.
  - DD, Dd, dd

2-7

Examples of Inherited Conditions Causing Human Disease

TABLE 3.3 Snustad DP & Simmons MJ. *Principles of Genetics*, 5e

Inherited Condition in Human Beings
Dominant Traits
Achondroplasia (dwarfism)
Brachydactyly (short fingers)
Congenital night blindness
Ehler-Danlos syndrome (a connective tissue disorder)
Huntington's disease (a neurological disorder)
Marfan syndrome (tall, gangly stature)
Neurofibromatosis (tumorlike growths on the body)
Phenylthiocarbamide (PTC) tasting
Widow's peak
Woolly hair
Recessive Traits
Albinism (lack of pigment)
Alkaptonuria (a disorder of amino acid metabolism)
Ataxia telangiectasia (a neurological disorder)
Cystic fibrosis (a respiratory disorder)
Duchenne muscular dystrophy
Galactosemia (a disorder of carbohydrate metabolism)
Glycogen storage disease
Phenylketonuria (a disorder of amino acid metabolism)
Sickle-cell anemia (a hemoglobin disorder)
Tay-Sachs disease (a lipid storage disorder)

2-7

Carriers of Genetic Diseases

- A carrier is a person in which one **allele is abnormal**, but the other, normal allele renders them **phenotypically normal**
- So with this in mind, a recessive gene will only be expressed in the absence of a dominant
- In most cases that means that a person must inherit **two diseased alleles** to demonstrate a particular disease.
  - SS = healthy, non-carrier
  - Ss = sickle cell anemia carrier (sickle trait)
  - ss = demonstrates sickle cell disease

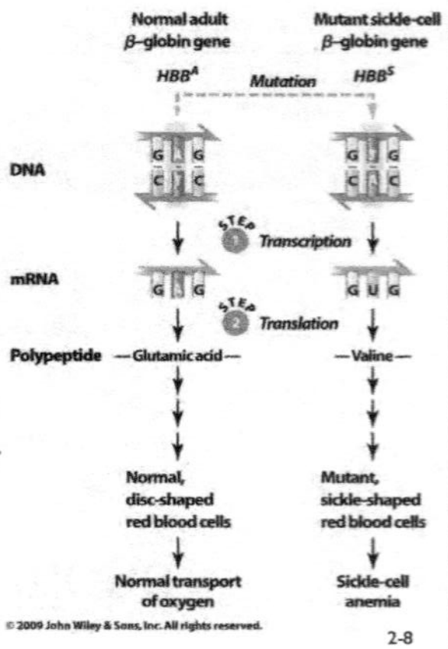

Normal adult β-globin gene
Mutant sickle-cell β-globin gene
HBB^A
Mutation
HBB^S
DNA
Transcription
mRNA
Translation
Polypeptide
—Glutamic acid—
—Valine—
Normal, disc-shaped red blood cells
Mutant, sickle-shaped red blood cells
Normal transport of oxygen
Sickle-cell anemia

2-8

Single-Gene Inheritance

- **Autosomal Dominant Diseases**
  - Abnormal allele is dominant; normal allele is recessive, and the alleles exist on autosomes
- **Autosomal Recessive Diseases**
  - Abnormal allele is recessive and a person must be homozygous for the abnormal alleles to express the disease
  - The trait usually appears in the children, not the parents, and it affects the genders equally because it is present on a pair of autosomes

2-8

Single-Gene Inheritance

Cross: *Aa* X *Aa*

		Male gametes ♂ *A* (1/2)	Male gametes ♂ *a* (1/2)
Female gametes ♀	*A* (1/2)	*AA* (1/4)	*Aa* (1/4)
	a (1/2)	*aA* (1/4)	*aa* (1/4)

Progeny:

Genotype	Frequency	Phenotype	Frequency
AA	1/4	Dominant	3/4
Aa	1/2		
aa	1/4	Recessive	1/4

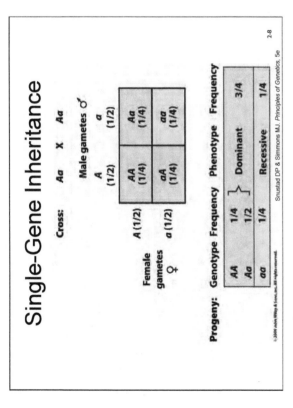

Snustad DP & Simmons MJ. *Principles of Genetics*, 5e

2-8

Recurrence Risk

- The probability (%) of a family with a specific genotype having a child with an expected phenotype
- Each birth to a mating pair is a coin-toss
- For single-gene inheritance, the recurrence risk remains constant
  - Autosomal dominant with one diseased parent: 50%
  - Autosomal recessive with two carrier parents: 25%

2-8

Pedigree Charts

- Charts used to analyze genetic relationships and the number of family member affected by a genetic disease
- **Proband**
  - Usually the initial focus of the pedigree chart because they are the first in the family to be seen in a health care facility and diagnosed

2-8

Symbols Used in Pedigree Charts

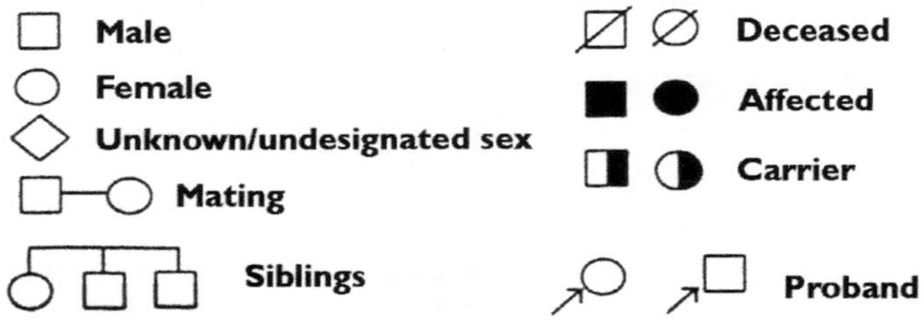

Male
Female
Unknown/undesignated sex
Mating
Siblings
Deceased
Affected
Carrier
Proband

2-8

Reading Pedigrees

Autosomal Dominant

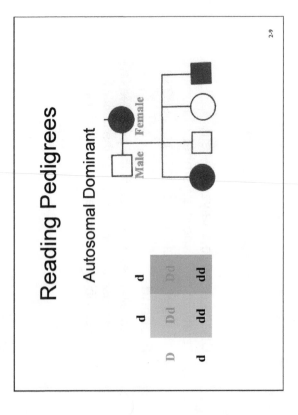

	d	d
D	Dd	Dd
d	dd	dd

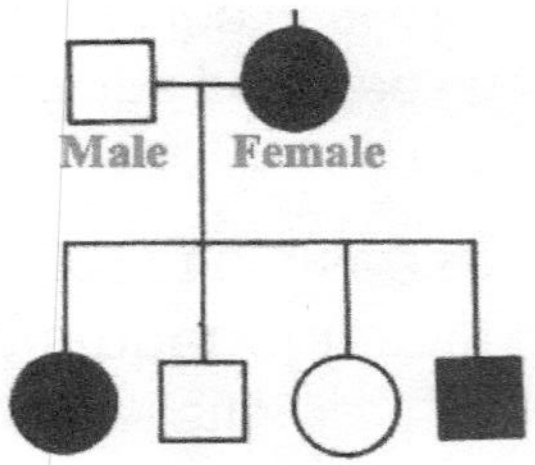

Male
Female

2-9

Penetrance

The proportion of individuals of a particular genotype that express its phenotypic effect in a given environment.
— Merriam-Webster

- Incomplete penetrance
  - Individual who has the gene for a disease but does not express the disease
  - Retinoblastoma (eye tumor in children) demonstrates incomplete penetrance (90%).
  - Huntington disease (CNS disorder) has a 95% penetrance.

2-10

Expressivity

The relative capacity of a gene to affect the phenotype of the organism of which it is a part.
— Merriam-Webster

- Example: **neurofibromatosis** (von Recklinghausen Disease)
- Neurofibromatosis exhibits "expressivity"
  - **Expressivity** is the variable expression of the disease which is caused by modifier genes
  - Disease varies from spots on the skin to malignant neurofibromas, gliomas, and neuromas

2-10

Reading Pedigrees

Autosomal Recessive

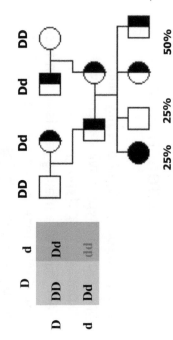

	D	d
D	DD	Dd
d	Dd	dd

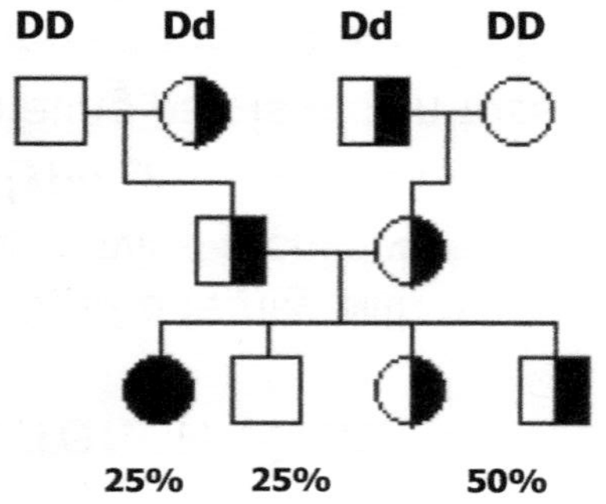

DD
Dd
Dd
DD
25%
25%
50%

2-11

Sex-Linked Inheritance

- **Sex-Linked (X-Linked) Recessive Diseases**
  - **Virtually all sex-linked disorders are recessive**
  - Affected males cannot transmit the genes to sons, but they can to all daughters – who will likely be carriers
  - Sons of female carriers have a 50% risk of getting the disease.
  - These disorders are only expressed by males because females have another X chromosome to mask the abnormal gene
  - Examples of this are **hemophilia A and red-green colorblindness**

2-12

Sex-Linked Inheritance

- **Sex-Linked (X-linked) Dominant Diseases**
  - Presently we know of only a **few rare examples.**
  - Expression in both sexes, but with a **greater incidence in females** due to the greater number of X chromosomes in females.

2-12

Reading Pedigrees

X-linked Recessive

	X	x
Y	XY	xY
X	XX	Xx

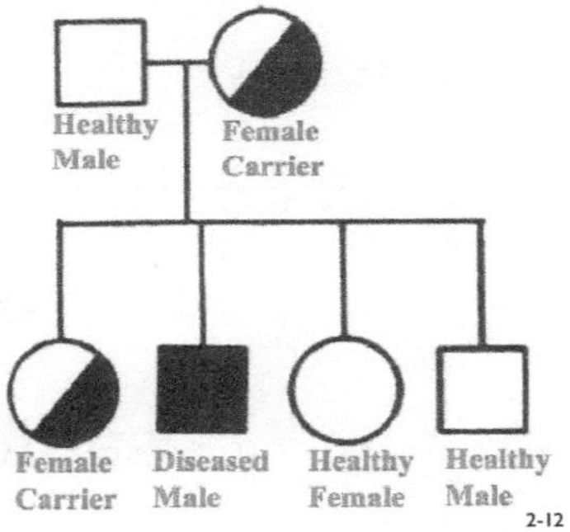
Healthy Male
Female Carrier
Female Carrier
Diseased Male
Healthy Female
Healthy Male

2-12

Hints for Pedigree Charts

- Ask
  - Are there any carriers?
    - If yes, then it's a recessive disease.
    - If there are no carriers, think dominant.
  - Is there an even distribution of the gene or expression of the gene between the genders?
    - Yes, autosomal
    - No, X-linked
  - Are there male carriers?
    - If yes, it can't be X-linked

2-9
2-11
2-12

Pedigrees

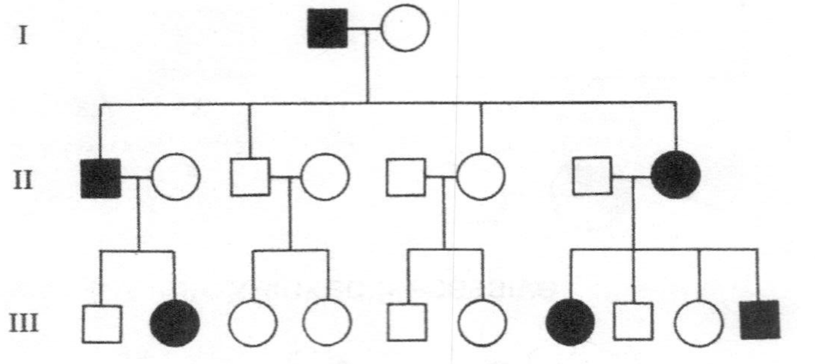

I
II
III

2-9
2-11
2-12

Pedigrees

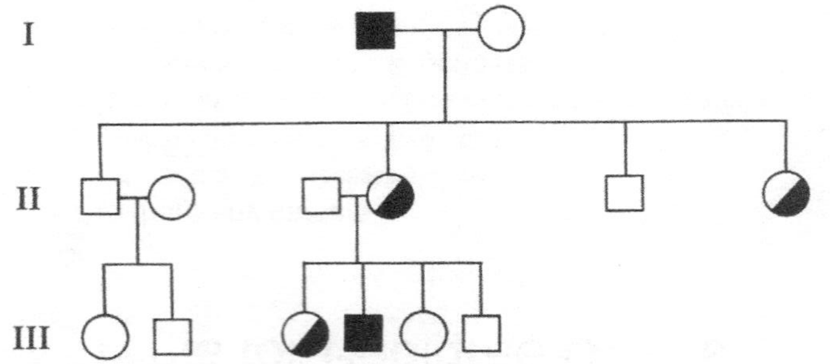

I
II
III

2-9
2-11
2-12

Pedigrees

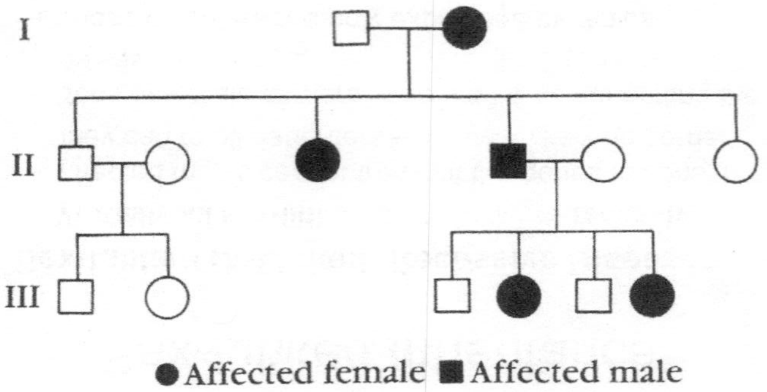

I
II
III
●Affected female ■Affected male

2-9
2-11
2-12

Pedigrees

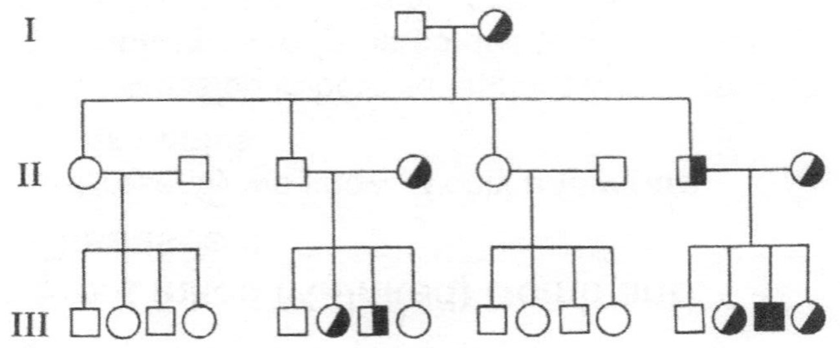

I
II
III

2-9
2-11
2-12

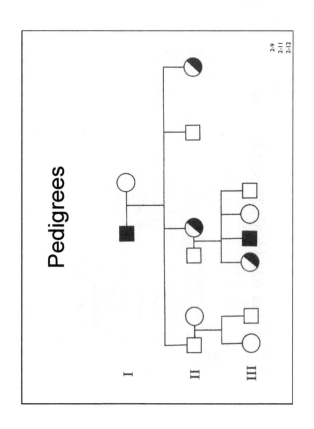

Polygenic Traits

- Traits involving multiple genes
  - Hair color
  - Height
  - Eye color
- If there are two genes (Aa and Bb), each with two alleles for a given trait, how many combinations are there?
  - aabb, aaBb, aaBB, Aabb, AaBb, AaBB, AABb, and AABB

2-13

Environment and Disease

- In addition to genetic alterations, **environment** has a profound influence on a large number of diseases and disorders.
  - **Diets, habits, and exposures**
- If a specific disease-prone population (a certain genetic profile) was moved to a different environment, could that change the prevalence of a specific disease?

2-13

Example of Diseases *Mostly* Due to Environment

- **Colon cancer** is more common in the US
  - Japan: Prevalence 5/100,000
  - US: 30/100,000
- **Stomach cancer** is more common in Japan
  - Japan: 75/100,000
  - US: 10/100,000
- These cancers, with the clear division in populations, **could have genetic causes**

2-13

Stomach, Breast & Colon Cancer in Native Japanese, *Nisei* & *Sansei*

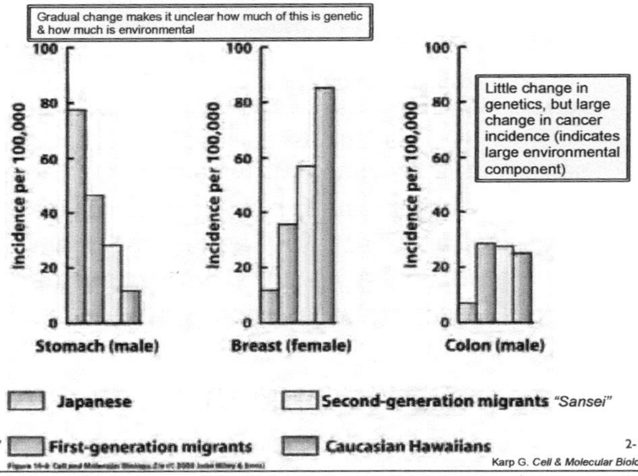

Gradual change makes it unclear how much of this is genetic & how much is environmental
Little change in genetics, but large change in cancer incidence (indicates large environmental component)
Incidence per 100,000
100
80
60
40
20
0
Stomach (male)
Breast (female)
Colon (male)
Japanese
"Nisei" First-generation migrants
Second-generation migrants "Sansei"
Caucasian Hawaiians

2-13

Karp G. *Cell & Molecular Biology*, 5e

Multifactorial Inheritance

- Multifactorial inheritance is responsible for the greatest number of individuals that will need special care or hospitalization because of genetic diseases.
  - Atopic reactions, diabetes, cancer, spina bifida/anencephaly, pyloric stenosis, cleft lip, cleft palate, congenital hip dysplasia, club foot, and a host of other diseases all result from multifactorial inheritance.
  - Some of these diseases occur more frequently in males. Others occur more frequently in females.

2-13

Multifactorial Traits

- A number of **multifactorial traits** follow a **bell-shaped distribution** curve ("Gaussian distribution") because they are influenced by **both** environmental and genetics factors.
  - Blood pressure, serum cholesterol, or all the values reported in a blood chemistry panel.
    - Almost all **quantitative** values in human biology follow this distribution because there is a number (normal value) assigned to them.
    - Normal fasting blood glucose: 70-110 mg/dl
    - Blood pressure: < 120/80
    - Serum cholesterol: <200 mg/dl

2-13

Threshold Model

- "Qualitative" traits are not measured on a numeric scale.
- Multifactorial traits/diseases like hypertension are best explained by the **threshold model.**
- **...you either have them or you don't.**
  - There is a **qualitative threshold** at which the disease manifests.

2-13

Threshold Model

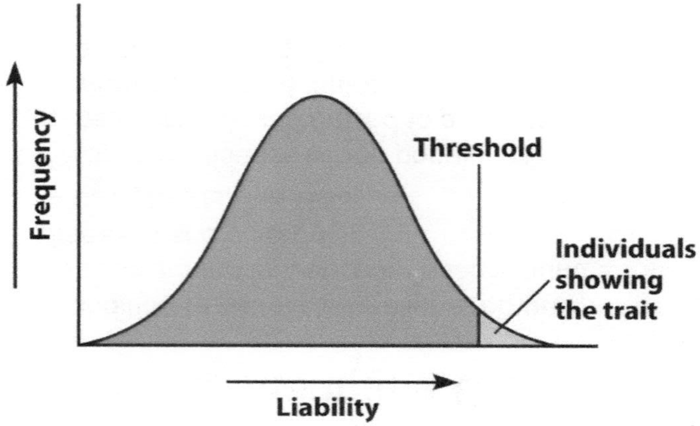

Frequency
Threshold
Individuals showing the trait
Liability

2-13

Blood Pressure

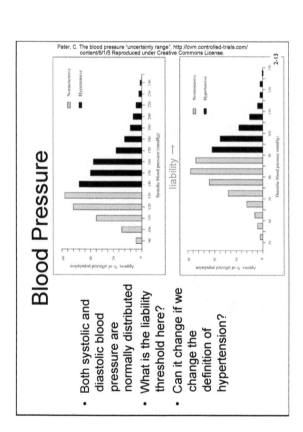

- Both systolic and diastolic blood pressure are normally distributed
- What is the liability threshold here?
- Can it change if we change the definition of hypertension?

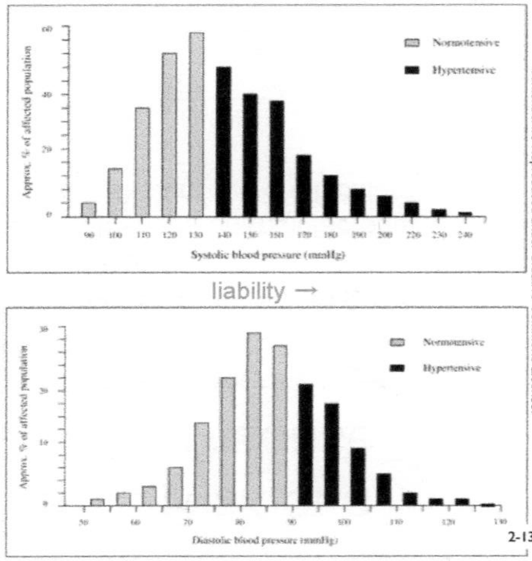

Normotensive
Hypertensive
Systolic blood pressure (mmHg)
liability →
Diastolic blood pressure (mmHg)

Pater, C. The blood pressure "uncertainty range". http://cvm.controlled-trials.com/content/6/1/5 Reproduced under Creative Commons License.

2-13

Blood Glucose

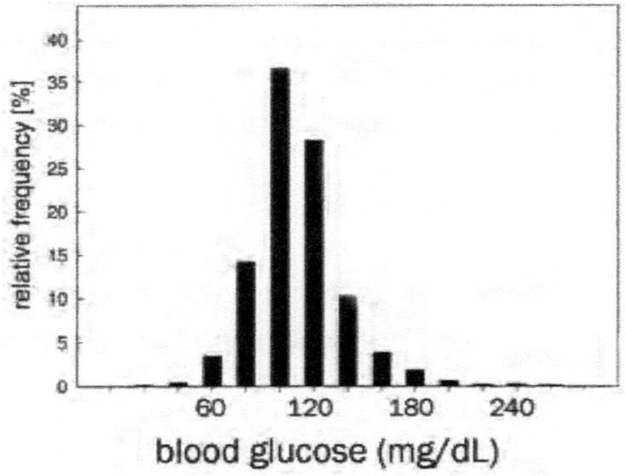

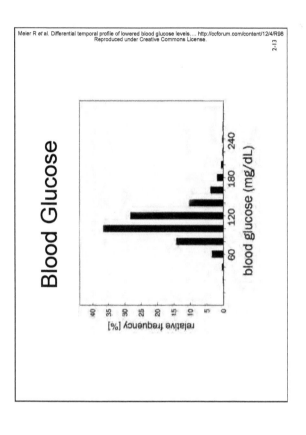

relative frequency [%]
40
35
30
25
20
15
10
5
0
60
120
180
240
blood glucose (mg/dL)

Meier R *et al.* Differential temporal profile of lowered blood glucose levels.... http://ccforum.com/content/12/4/R98 Reproduced under Creative Commons License.

2-13

Threshold Model

- For these diseases, there is said to be an underlying **liability distribution** within a population
- As the number of genetic and/or environmental risk factors increases, so does the **liability** for the disease
- When the **liability** is so great that it reaches a threshold, an abnormality, what we call disease, results

2-13

Threshold Model

- Each factor contributing to the disease **(cards stacked against you)** moves a person closer to the disease threshold.
- Ways to accumulate cards
  - –Genetics
  - –Environment

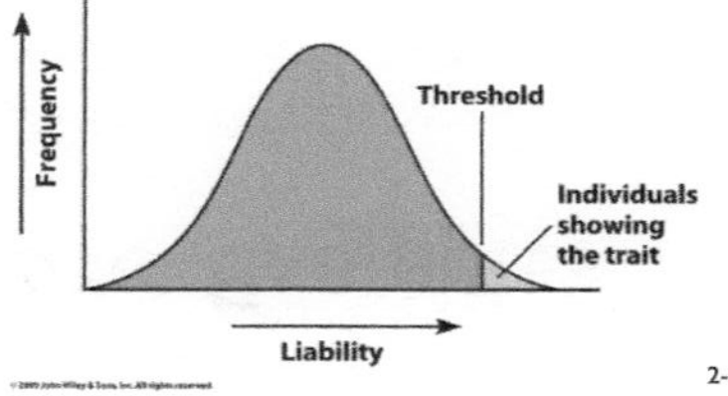

Frequency
Threshold
Individuals showing the trait
Liability

2-13

Threshold Model Examples

- Pyloric stenosis – narrowing or obstruction of the pyloric sphincter
  - 1/200 white males
  - 1/1000 white females
  - Which group has the **lower** liability threshold?

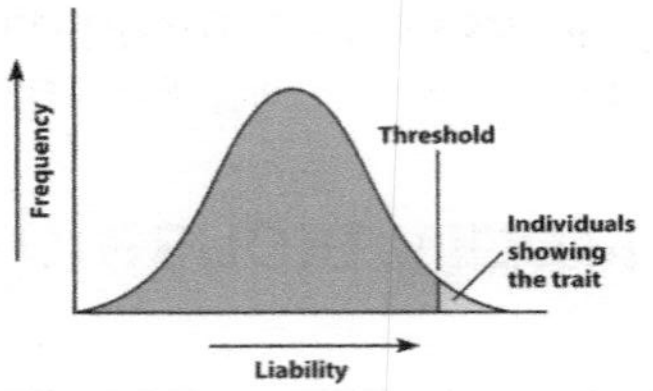

Frequency
Threshold
Individuals showing the trait
Liability

2-13

Threshold Model Examples

- Disease Prevalence
  - White males 1/300
  - Hispanic males 1/400
  - White females 1/1000
  - Hispanic females 1/2000
  - Which of these populations has the highest liability threshold?

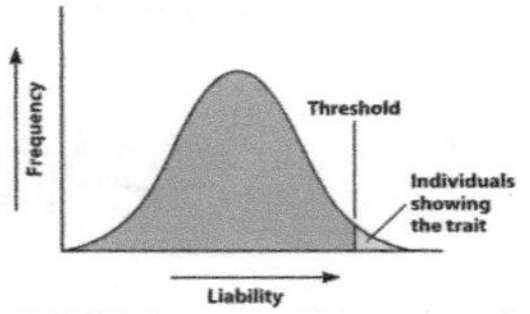

Frequency
Threshold
Individuals showing the trait
Liability

2-13

Recurrence Risk of a Multifactorial Disease

- What would be the recurrence risk for single-gene autosomal dominant diseases?
- What would be the recurrence risk for single-gene autosomal recessive diseases?
- Because of the various influences on multifactorial diseases, the recurrence risks are more difficult to calculate.

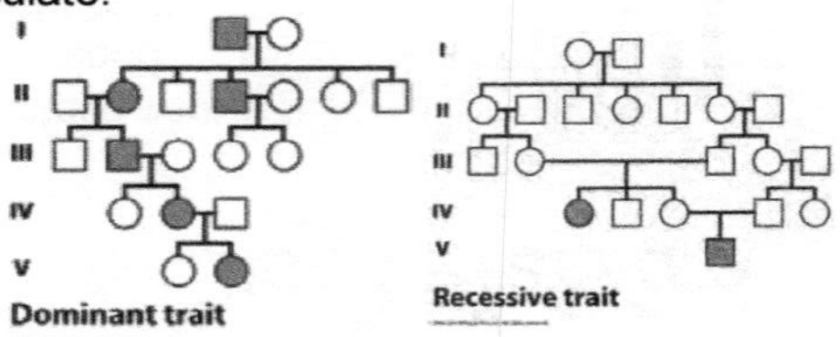

I
II
III
IV
V
Dominant trait
I
II
III
IV
V
Recessive trait

Snustad DP & Simmons MJ. *Principles of Genetics*, 5e

2-13

Recurrence Criteria

- The recurrence risk becomes higher if:
  - More that one family member is affected
    - Sibling risk
  - The expression of the disease in the proband is more severe
  - The proband is of the less commonly affected sex
  - The recurrence risk decreases back towards that of the normal population if the disease is expressed in more remotely-related relatives

2-13

Unit 2
Chapter 9
Biology, Clinical Manifestations, and Treatment of Cancer

Prevalence and Death Rates from Cancer in U.S.

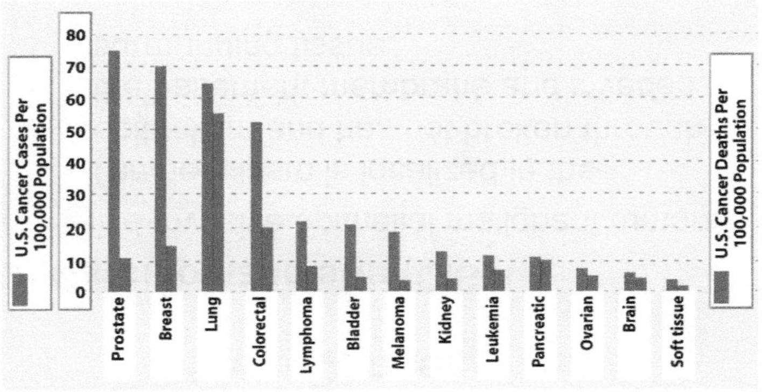

U.S. Cancer Cases Per 100,000 Population
U.S. Cancer Deaths Per 100,000 Population
80
70
60
50
40
30
20
10
0
Prostate
Breast
Lung
Colorectal
Lymphoma
Bladder
Melanoma
Kidney
Leukemia
Pancreatic
Ovarian
Brain
Soft tissue

Karp G. *Cell & Molecular Biology*, 6e

9-1

Kuggles13

Neoplasm, Tumor, and Cancer

- **Neoplasm (Tumor)**
  - New and abnormal development of cells that are unresponsive to normal growth control mechanisms
- Not all neoplasms (tumors) are cancer
  - **Some neoplasms are benign tumors**
    - Cells do not invade the surrounding tissue
  - **Malignant neoplasms are cancer**
    - They invade surrounding tissues and they have the ability to travel to, and proliferate at distant sites (metastasis)

9-1

Benign and Malignant Neoplasms

Benign Neoplasms	Malignant Neoplasms
Slow Growth	Rapid Growth
Encapsulated	Non-encapsulated
Non-invasive	Invade local structures and tissues
Well differentiated	Poorly differentiated
Low mitotic rate	High mitotic rate
Do not metastasize	Metastasize

9-2

Tumor Terminology

- Tumors are named according to their tissue of origin with the suffix "**-oma**"
- Benign tumors have simpler names
  - Lipoma, myoma, adenoma, chondroma
- Names of tumors which have these modifiers: blast, multiple, malignant, carci-, sarc-, are almost always malignant

9-3

Tumor Terminology

- Malignant neoplasms
  - Epithelial tissue **(carcinomas)**
    - Adenocarcinoma, squamous cell carcinoma
  - Connective tissue **(sarcomas)**
    - Chondrosarcoma, osteosarcoma
  - Lymphatic tissue **(lymphosarcomas)**
  - Retinoblastoma and neuroblastoma

9-3

Naming Examples

- Benign
  - Fibroma (fibrous)
  - Chondroma (cartilage)
  - Osteoma (bone)
  - Lipoma (fatty)
  - Hemangioma (vessel)
  - Papilloma (squamous)
  - Meningioma (meninges)
- Malignant
  - Fibrosarcoma
  - Chondrosarcoma
  - Osteosarcoma
  - Liposarcoma
  - Hemangiosarcoma
  - Squamous carcinoma
  - Glioblastoma
  - Retinoblastoma

9-3

Cancer

- **Carcinoma in situ (CIS)**
  - Pre-invasive epithelial malignant tumors
  - The neoplasm is localized in the epithelium and has not broken through the basement membrane and invaded surrounding tissue

9-4

Cancer

- **Transformation**
  - Process by which a normal cell becomes a cancer cell
  - Not a single event
- **Anaplasia**
  - Loss of differentiation
  - Loss of organization

9-5

Histological Features of Cancer Cells

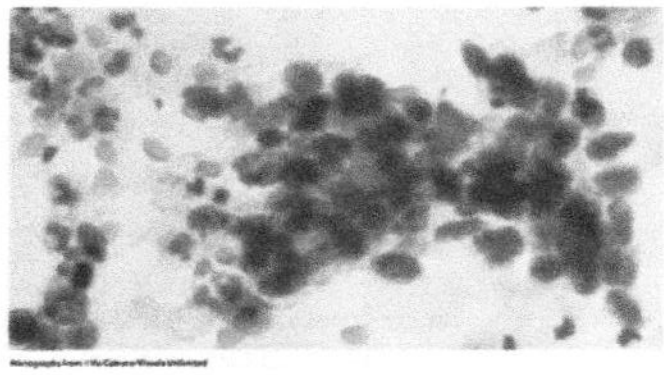

- Bizarre nuclei
  - Cells don't go through normal cell division, or are rapidly dividing
- Bizarre cell shapes or sizes
- Invasion of the basement membrane
- De-differentiation
  - i.e. more like embryonic cells
- Cellular or extracellular accumulations
  - e.g. "mucus lakes" in lung cancer
- Necrotic debris

Abnormal Gene Expression in Cancer Cells

- Turn on genes which:
  - guide the cell through the cell cycle/cell division (violate checkpoints)
  - brings blood vessels to the cell (**angiogenesis**)
  - helps the cancer cell move to places it doesn't belong
    - dissolve connective tissue barriers
    - move into and out of blood vessels
  - collectively, these are called oncogenes ("cancer genes")

9-5

Causes of Cancer
Multi-Hit Model of Carcinogenesis

- Carcinogenesis is a multi-step process characterized by "multiple hits"
  - Age
  - Exposure to environmental agents/ carcinogens

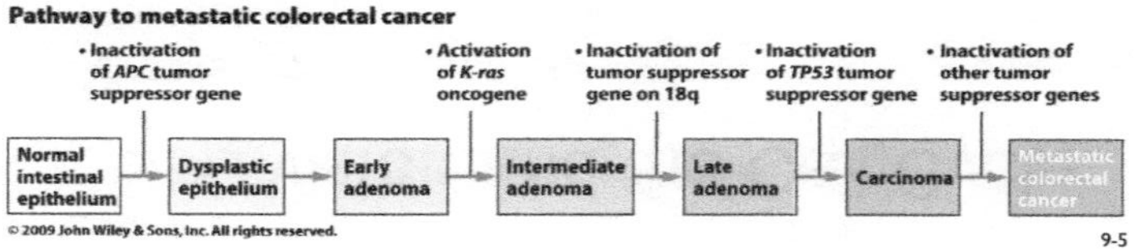

Pathway to metastatic colorectal cancer
• Inactivation of APC tumor suppressor gene
• Activation of K-ras oncogene
• Inactivation of tumor suppressor gene on 18q
• Inactivation of TP53 tumor suppressor gene
• Inactivation of other tumor suppressor genes
Normal intestinal epithelium
Dysplastic epithelium
Early adenoma
Intermediate adenoma
Late adenoma
Carcinoma
Metastatic colorectal cancer

Snustad DP & Simmons MJ. *Principles of Genetics*, 5e

9-5

Multi-Hit Models of Carcinogenesis

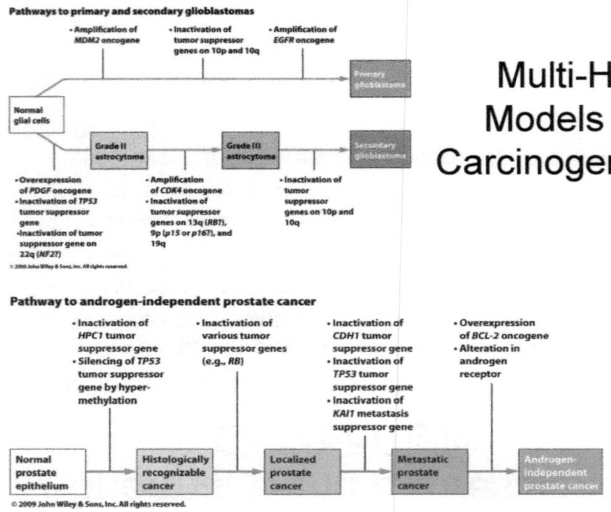

Pathways to primary and secondary glioblastomas
• Amplification of MDM2 oncogene
• Inactivation of tumor suppressor genes on 10p and 10q
• Amplification of EGFR oncogene
Primary glioblastoma
Normal glial cells
Grade II astrocytoma
Grade III astrocytoma
Secondary glioblastoma
• Overexpression of PDGF oncogene
• Inactivation of TP53 tumor suppressor gene
• Inactivation of tumor suppressor gene on 22q (NF2?)
• Amplification of CDK4 oncogene
• Inactivation of tumor suppressor genes on 13q (RB1), 9p (p15 or p16?), and 19q
• Inactivation of tumor suppressor genes on 10p and 10q
Pathway to androgen-independent prostate cancer
• Inactivation of HPC1 tumor suppressor gene
• Silencing of TP53 tumor suppressor gene by hyper-methylation
• Inactivation of various tumor suppressor genes (e.g., RB)
• Inactivation of CDH1 tumor suppressor gene
• Inactivation of TP53 tumor suppressor gene
• Inactivation of KAI1 metastasis suppressor gene
• Overexpression of BCL-2 oncogene
• Alteration in androgen receptor
Normal prostate epithelium
Histologically recognizable cancer
Localized prostate cancer
Metastatic prostate cancer
Androgen-independent prostate cancer

Snustad DP & Simmons MJ. *Principles of Genetics*, 5e

9-5

Cell Division and the Cell Cycle

- All cells make copies of themselves in the growing embryo
- Many adult cell types replace themselves by constant cell division
  - skin, bone marrow, intestinal lining
- Other cells cannot divide after birth
  - muscle, heart muscle, brain

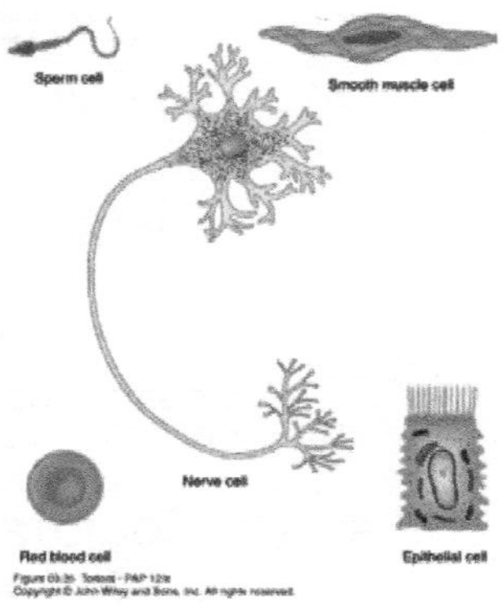

Sperm cell
Smooth muscle cell
Nerve cell
Red blood cell
Epithelial cell

9-5

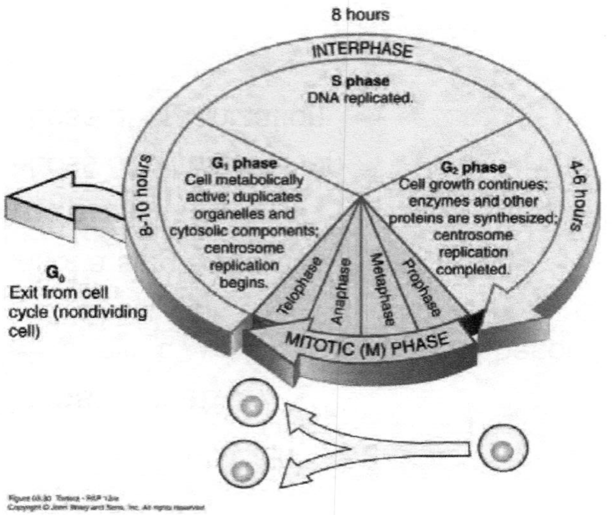

8 hours
INTERPHASE
S phase
DNA replicated.
G₁ phase
Cell metabolically active; duplicates organelles and cytosolic components; centrosome replication begins.
G₂ phase
Cell growth continues; enzymes and other proteins are synthesized; centrosome replication completed.
8-10 hours
4-6 hours
Telophase
Anaphase
Metaphase
Prophase
MITOTIC (M) PHASE
G₀
Exit from cell cycle (nondividing cell)

9-5

Checkpoints

- In order to enter S or M phase, cell must pass a **checkpoint**
- Scientists believe control at these checkpoints is lost in many forms of cancer
- Checkpoints controlled by internal or external signaling molecules

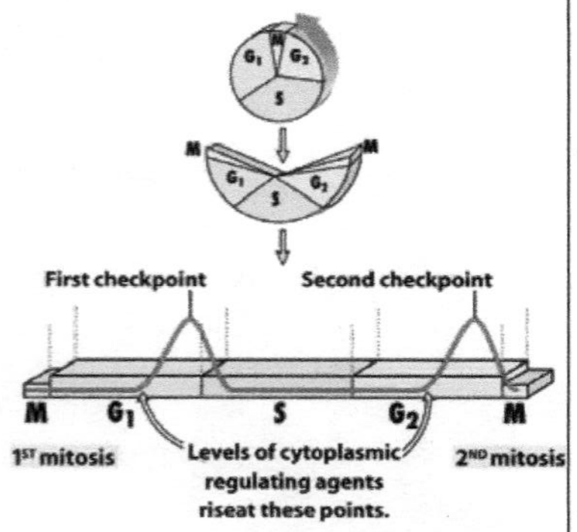

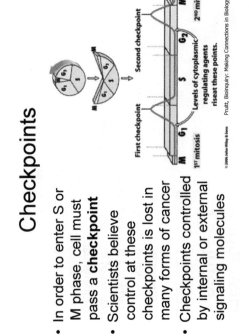

First checkpoint
Second checkpoint
M
G1
S
G2
M
1ST mitosis
2ND mitosis
Levels of cytoplasmic regulating agents riseat these points.

Pruitt, Bioinquiry: Making Connections in Biology, 3/e

9-5

Cytogenetics

- **Philadelphia chromosome** in chronic myelogenous leukemia (CML)
  - –Translocation between chromosomes 9 and 22
  - –Present in 95% of patients with CML

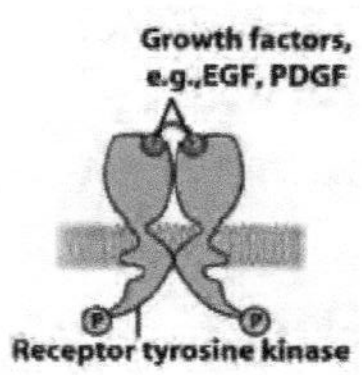
Growth factors, e.g.,EGF, PDGF
Receptor tyrosine kinase

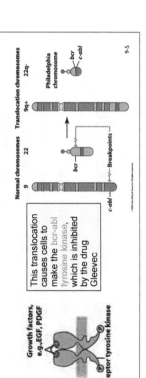

This translocation causes cells to make the bcr-abl tyrosine kinase, which is inhibited by the drug Gleevec

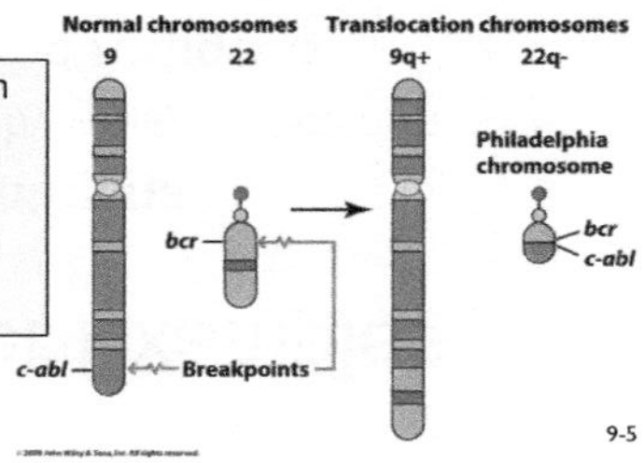
Normal chromosomes
9
22
Translocation chromosomes
9q+
22q-
Philadelphia chromosome
bcr
c-abl
bcr
c-abl
Breakpoints

9-5

Tumor Markers

- Tumor markers are **biological markers** produced by cancer cells:
  - –Any kind of cellular product could be a tumor marker
    - Hormones, antibodies, enzymes
  - –An antigen found on a cancer cell membrane could be a tumor marker
    - Tumor-specific antigen or TSA
  - –An alteration of the genes or chromosomes in the nucleus could be a tumor marker

9-6

Tumor Markers

- If a tumor marker
  - –leaks into the blood, CSF, or urine
  - –or if we could get a sample of the cells from the cancerous tissue
- Then we can use it to **indicate the presence of cancer**

9-6

Tumor Markers

- In this way, tumor markers are used to:
  - –**Screen** and identify individuals at high risk for cancer
  - –**Diagnose** specific types of tumors
  - –**Follow** the clinical course of cancer
- Tumor markers often lack **specificity, sensitivity, predictability, and feasibility**, so there are few ideal tumor markers

9-6

Tumor Marker Examples

- **Hormones**
  - **"Ectopic"** hormone production is the production of hormones by **tumors of non-endocrine origin**
    - ACTH, HCG, HGH, ADH, thyroid-stimulating hormone, epinephrine and norepinephrine from the adrenal medulla
- **Enzymes**
  - Cancers do not produce new or unique enzymes; instead we find the **abnormal levels of normal enzymes**
  - Usually only detected in the blood when the tumor is **very large** or **metastasis** has occurred

9-6

Tumor Marker Examples

- **Antibodies**
  - Produced by some cancers (e.g. **multiple myeloma**)
- **Tumor-specific antigens (TSAs)**
  - Cancer cells express **"non-self"** antigens
  - These TSAs "fly" like a flag
    - Markers from the surface of their cell membranes
      - HER2/*neu* (human epidermal growth factor) in breast cancer

HER is human epidermal growth factor receptor
neu is a gene which is "turned on" in neuroblastoma
these were later discovered to be the same after they were named

9-6

Tumor Marker Examples

- **Viral Tumor-Specific Antigens**
  - Produced and expressed by virally-transformed cells
- **Oncofetal Tumor-Specific Antigens**
  - Expressed by cells during embryonic development but are absent or low in normal adult cells
    - α-fetoprotein in hepatic, pancreatic, and epithelial cancers
    - Carcinoembryonic antigen (CEA) in colonic, pancreatic, and breast tumors

9-6

Tumor Marker Examples

- **Protein Tumor-Specific Antigens**
  - Function in proliferation, enzymatic processes, as receptors, and cellular structures
    - The best example is prostate-specific antigen (PSA)
      - PSA is a glycoprotein produced by the prostate whose values are related to prostate mass
      - it is therefore a tumor cell marker (TCM) used as a screening test for prostate cancer

9-6

Paraneoplastic Syndromes

- Signs and symptoms unrelated to the local effects/presence of the neoplasm
- Caused by substances released from the tumor or an immune response to the tumor
  - Examples:
    - Hypercalcemia in breast and renal carcinomas from PTH-related protein
    - Polycythemia in cerebellar hemangioma and hepatocellular carcinoma from erythropoietin
    - Hypoglycemia in hepatocellular carcinoma from insulin-like substance

9-6

Cancer

- **Anchorage-independence**
  - Continued growth even when unattached from original tissue

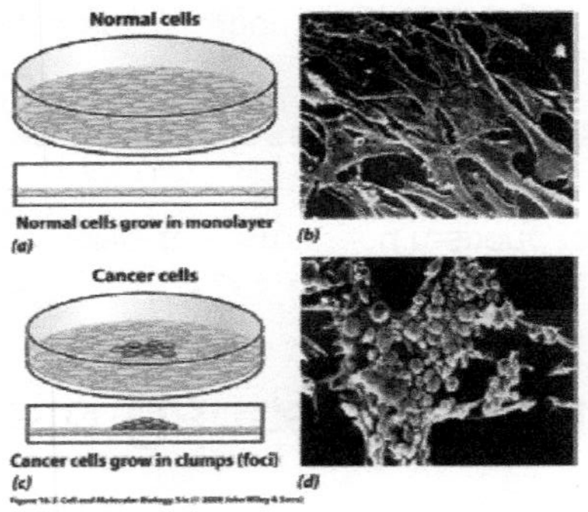

Normal cells
Normal cells grow in monolayer
(a)
(b)
Cancer cells
Cancer cells grow in clumps (foci)
(c)
(d)

9-7

Cancer

- Cancer cells display **autonomy**, which is the cancer cell's independence from normal cellular controls
  - Cell cycle control, repair, cell growth, differentiation factors, and growth factor receptors
  - This would be like a person lacking a social conscience
    - The person demonstrates their own unique behaviors without regard for others

9-7

Retroviral Oncogenes

Oncogene	Host Virus
abl	Abelson murine leukemia virus
erbA	Avian erythroblastosis virus
erbB	Avian erythroblastosis virus
fes	ST feline sarcoma virus
fgr	Gardner-Rasheed feline sarcoma virus
fms	McDonough feline sarcoma virus
fos	FJB osteosarcoma virus
fps	Fuginami sarcoma virus
jun	Avian sarcoma virus 17
mil (mht)	MH2 virus
mos	Moloney sarcoma virus
myb	Avian myeloblastosis virus
myc	MC29 myelocytomatosis virus
raf	3611 murine sarcoma virus
H-ras	Harvey murine sarcoma virus
K-ras	Kirsten murine sarcoma virus
rel	Reticuloendotheliosis virus
ros	URII avian sarcoma virus
sis	Simian sarcoma virus
src	Rous sarcoma virus
yes	Y73 sarcoma virus

Snustad DP & Simmons MJ. *Principles of Genetics*, 5e

Genetic Alterations

Proto-Oncogenes
Oncogenes
Tumor-Suppressor Genes

- **Proto-oncogenes**
  - Unaltered, normal healthy alleles of genes that control/regulate cellular growth and differentiation
- **Oncogene**
  - Is a proto-oncogene that has been altered (mutated) by carcinogenic agent
- **Tumor-suppressor genes** (anti-oncogenes)
  - Encode for proteins that inhibit cell division
- Cancer can occur due to the activation of oncogenes or the inactivation of tumor-suppressor genes.

9-8

Genetic Alterations
Loss of Heterozygosity

- Patient born with one mutated gene
  - *RB* gene in retinoblastoma
  - Recessive, so one copy does not cause disease
  - Heterozygous for *RB*
- Second copy of gene mutates → cancer

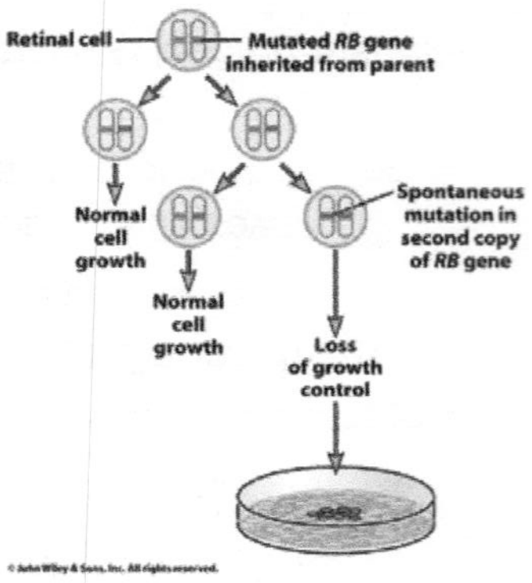

Retinal cell
Mutated *RB* gene inherited from parent
Normal cell growth
Normal cell growth
Spontaneous mutation in second copy of *RB* gene
Loss of growth control

Karp G. *Cell & Molecular Biology*, 6e

Inherited Cancer Syndromes Result from Genetic Alterations

TABLE 22.2 Snustad DP & Simmons MJ. *Principles of Genetics*, 5e

Inherited Cancer Syndromes

Syndrome	Primary Tumor	Gene	Chromosomal Location	Proposed Protein Function
Familial retinoblastoma	Retinoblastoma	*RB*	13q14.3	Cell cycle and transcriptional regulation
Li-Fraumeni syndrome	Sarcomas, breast cancer	*TP53*	17p13.1	Transcription factor
Familial adenomatous polyposis (FAP)	Colorectal cancer	*APC*	5q21	Regulation of β-catenin
Hereditary nonpolyposis colorectal cancer (HNPCC)	Colorectal cancer	*MSH2* *MLH1* *PMS1* *PMS2*	2p16 3p21 2q32 7p22	DNA mismatch repair
Neurofibromatosis type 1	Neurofibromas	*NF1*	17q11.2	Regulation of Ras-mediated signaling
Neurofibromatosis type 2	Acoustic neuromas, meningiomas	*NF2*	22q12.2	Linkage of membrane proteins to cytoskeleton
Wilms' tumor	Wilms' tumor	*WT1*	11p13	Transcriptional repressor
Familial breast cancer 1	Breast cancer	*BRCA1*	17q21	DNA repair
Familial breast cancer 2	Breast cancer	*BRCA2*	13q12	DNA repair
von Hippel-Lindau disease	Renal cancer	*VHL*	3p25	Regulation of transcriptional elongation
Familial melanoma	Melanoma	*p16*	9p21	Inhibitor of CDKs
Ataxia telangiectasia	Lymphoma	*ATM*	11q22	DNA repair
Bloom's syndrome	Solid tumors	*BLM*	15q26.1	DNA helicase

Source: Fearon, E. R. 1997. Human cancer syndromes: clues to the origin and nature of cancer. Science 278:1043–1050.

Genetic Alterations
p53 (Tumor-Suppressor) Gene Mutations

- Normally, if cells are exposed to a hypoxic environment, the p53 is activated to produce the p53 protein
- The p53 protein will activate apoptosis
- In many cancers, the p53 gene is mutated, allowing the abnormal proliferation of cells

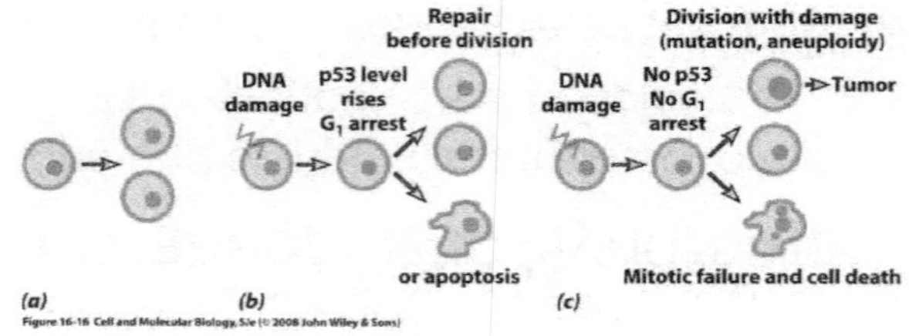

Repair before division
DNA damage
p53 level rises
G1 arrest
or apoptosis
Division with damage (mutation, aneuploidy)
DNA damage
No p53
No G1 arrest
Tumor
Mitotic failure and cell death
(a)
(b)
(c)

Figure 16-16 Cell and Molecular Biology, 5/e (© 2008 John Wiley & Sons)

Contributors to Cancer Growth

- **Autocrine** stimulation
  - Cancers acquire the ability to secrete and respond to their own growth factors
- **Increased expression of growth-factor receptors**
  - Gene amplification allows cancer cells to create numerous copies of genes and expression of gene products
    - HER2/neu in breast cancers
    - bcr/abl receptor tyrosine kinase in CML

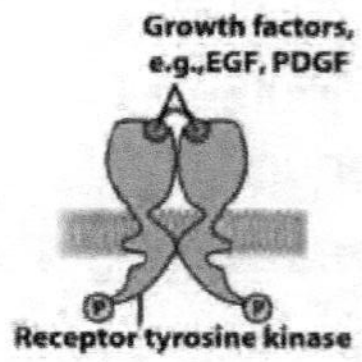

Growth factors, e.g., EGF, PDGF
Receptor tyrosine kinase

Contributors to Cancer Growth

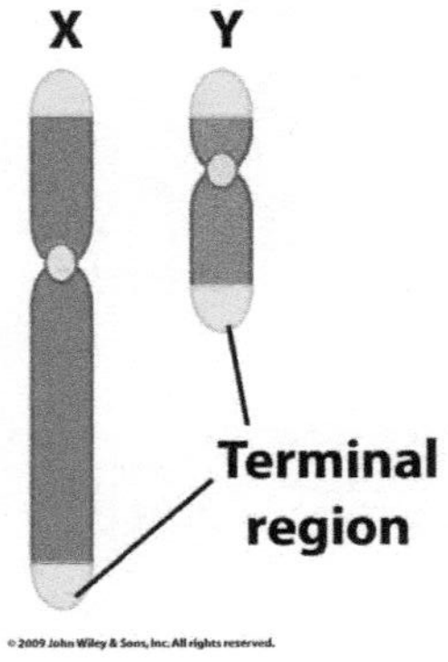
X
Y
Terminal region

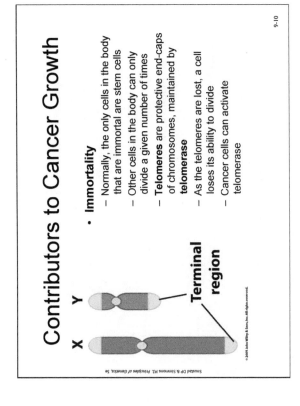

© 2009 John Wiley & Sons, Inc. All rights reserved.

Snustad DP & Simmons MJ. *Principles of Genetics*, 5e

- **Immortality**
  - Normally, the only cells in the body that are immortal are stem cells
  - Other cells in the body can only divide a given number of times
  - **Telomeres** are protective end-caps of chromosomes, maintained by **telomerase**
  - As the telomeres are lost, a cell loses its ability to divide
  - Cancer cells can activate telomerase

9-10

Contributors to Cancer Growth

- **Angiogenesis**
  - Physiological process contributing to the growth of new blood vessels
  - Through secretion of angiogenic factors, cancers can continue to enlarge

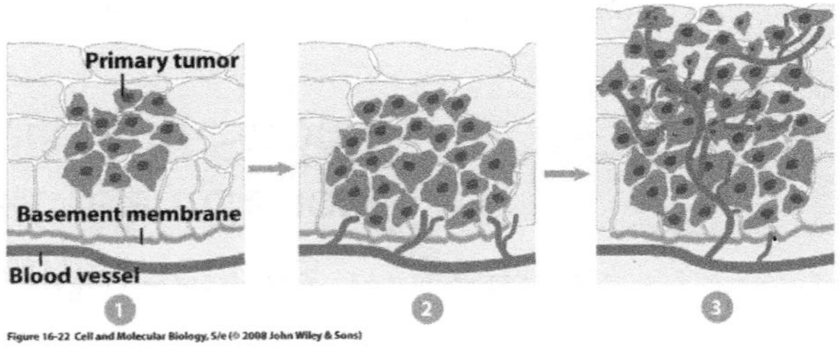
Primary tumor
Basement membrane
Blood vessel
1
2
3

Figure 16-22 Cell and Molecular Biology, 5/e (© 2008 John Wiley & Sons)

9-10

Genetic Alterations
Point Mutations

- A small base-pair change can result in a normal proto-oncogene becoming an unregulated oncogene

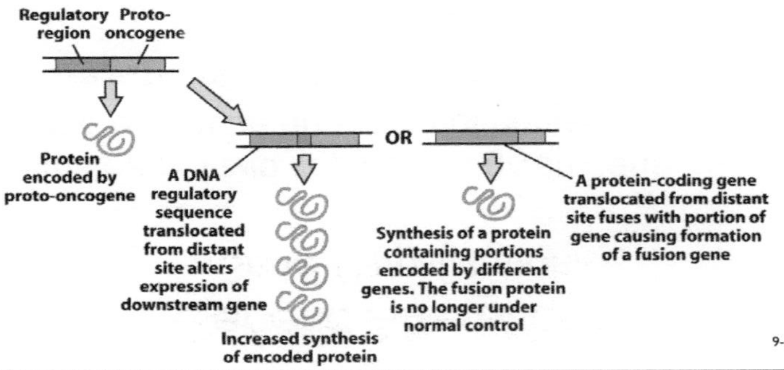
Regulatory region
Proto-oncogene
Protein encoded by proto-oncogene
A DNA regulatory sequence translocated from distant site alters expression of downstream gene
Increased synthesis of encoded protein
OR
Synthesis of a protein containing portions encoded by different genes. The fusion protein is no longer under normal control
A protein-coding gene translocated from distant site fuses with portion of gene causing formation of a fusion gene

Karp G. *Cell & Molecular Biology*, 6e

9-10

Genetic Alterations
Translocations

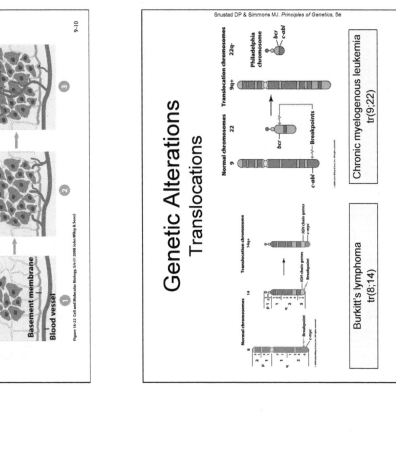

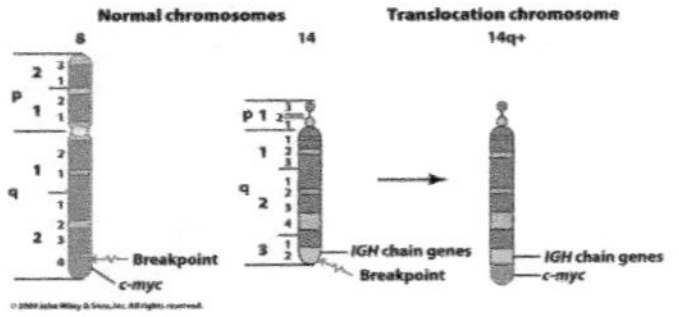
Normal chromosomes
8
14
Translocation chromosome
14q+
Breakpoint
c-myc
IGH chain genes

Burkitt's lymphoma
tr(8;14)

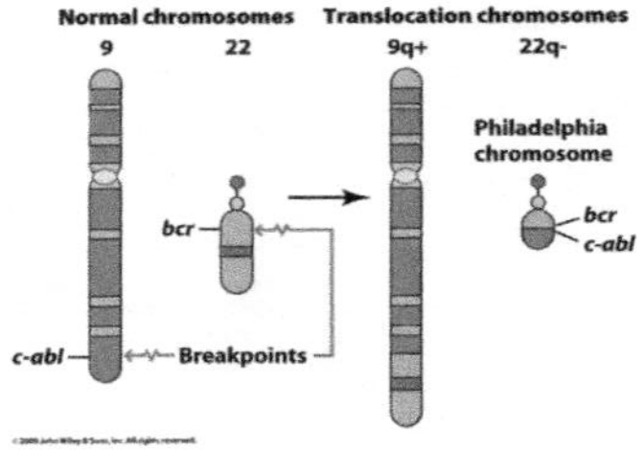
Normal chromosomes
9
22
Translocation chromosomes
9q+
22q-
Philadelphia chromosome
bcr
c-abl
Breakpoints

Chronic myelogenous leukemia
tr(9;22)

Snustad DP & Simmons MJ. *Principles of Genetics*, 5e

9-10

Genetic Alterations
Gene Amplification

- Instead of two copies of a given gene, there may be hundreds of copies
  - e.g. overexpression of an oncogene

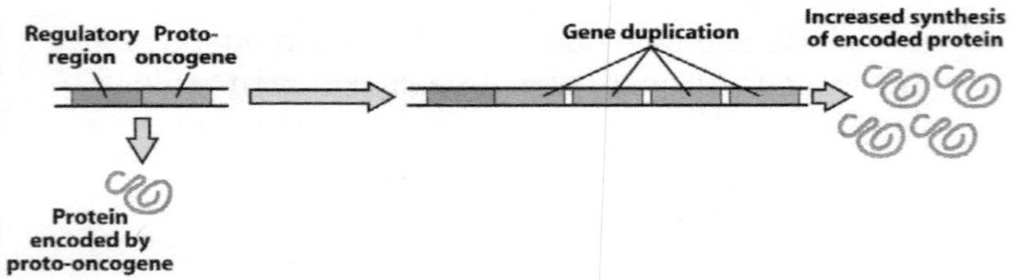

Regulatory region
Proto-oncogene
Protein encoded by proto-oncogene
Gene duplication
Increased synthesis of encoded protein

Karp G. *Cell & Molecular Biology*, 6e

9-10

Genetic Alterations

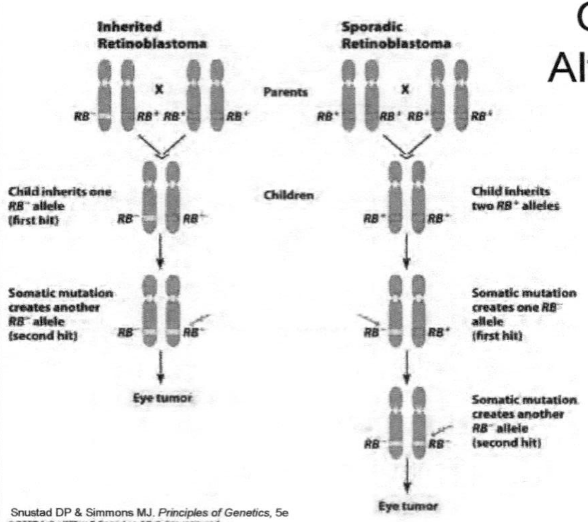

Inherited Retinoblastoma
Sporadic Retinoblastoma
Parents
Children
Child inherits one RB⁻ allele (first hit)
Somatic mutation creates another RB⁻ allele (second hit)
Eye tumor
Child inherits two RB⁺ alleles
Somatic mutation creates one RB⁻ allele (first hit)
Somatic mutation creates another RB⁻ allele (second hit)
Eye tumor

Snustad DP & Simmons MJ. *Principles of Genetics*, 5e

9-10

Cancer Stem Cells

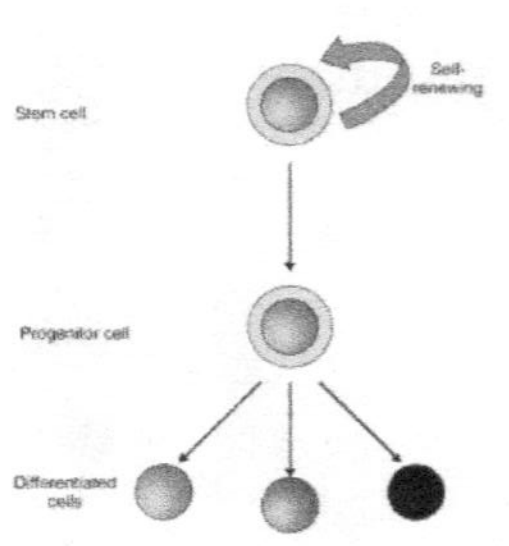

Stem cell
Self-renewing
Progenitor cell
Differentiated cells

Bapat S et al. *Cancer Stem Cells: Identification and Targets*, 2009.

- Cancer stem cells important for identification and treatment of cancer
- These are cells that divide to give rise to more cancer cells
- Often based on cell surface markers called "CD"
- For example:
  - $CD34^+$, $CD38^-$ stem cells in AML
  - $CD133^+$ stem cells in brain, prostate, colon & liver cancer
  - $CD44^+$, $CD24^-$ stem cells in breast cancer

9-11

Interactions Between Cancer Cells and Stroma

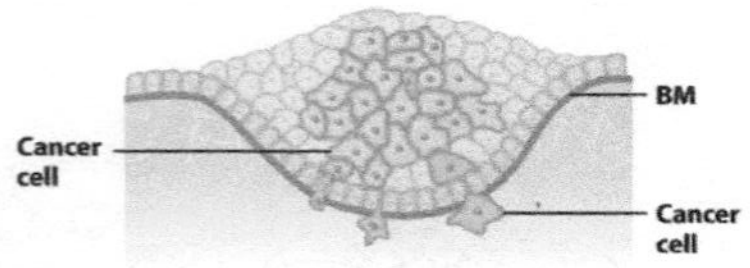

Cancer cell
BM
Cancer cell

Karp G. *Cell & Molecular Biology*, 6e

- Normally, growth factors and adhesive proteins in the surrounding connective tissue and blood vessels (**stroma**) keeps cells from going "off the reservation"
- In cancer, cells begin to express genes that allow them to divide uncontrollably and move freely in stroma
  - Now called carcinoma *in situ* (see 9-4)
- Next step is to "eat through" basement membrane
  - Now called carcinoma

9-12

Chronic Inflammation

- Inflammatory cells release cytokines to:
  - Stimulate cellular proliferation
  - Angiogenesis
  - Promote healing
- Chronic inflammation is an associated risk factor for many types of cancer.
  - Colon cancer with inflammatory bowel diseases
  - Liver cancer with chronic hepatitis
  - Lung cancer with asthmatics

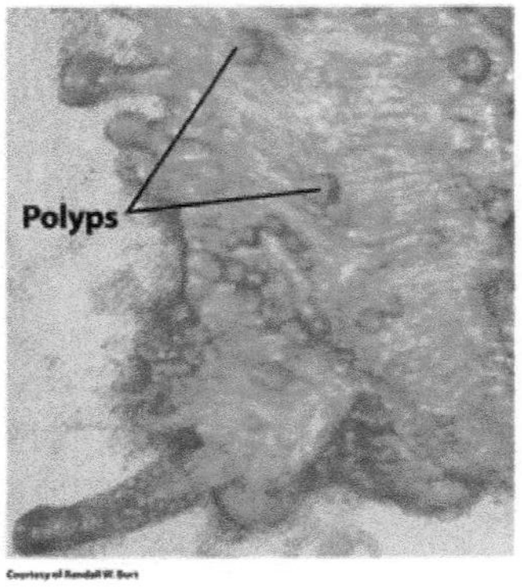

Polyps

Karp G. *Cell & Molecular Biology*, 6e

9-13

Oncogenic Viruses

- Viruses change the genetic makeup of the cell, which results in the alteration of the daughter cells
  - **Epstein-Barr Virus (EBV)**
    - Hodgkin lymphoma, Burkitt lymphoma (B lymphocytes)
  - **Human Papilloma Virus (HPV)**
    - Cervical cancer
  - **HIV**
    - Kaposi sarcoma
      - Associated with immunosuppression and human herpesvirus 8
  - **Hepatitis B Virus (HBV)**
    - Hepatocellular carcinoma

9-14

Oncogenic Bacterium

- Even a bacterium can cause cancer?
- *Helicobacter pylori* is a bacterium that infects the stomach of more than half of the world's population, making it one of the most prevalent infections.
  - Most common cause of peptic ulcer disease, gastric lymphomas, and gastric carcinomas
  - Think chronic inflammation

9-14

Metastasis

- Metastasis is the spread of cancer from the initial site of neoplasm development to distance tissues of the body
- Localized neoplasms are much easier to treat
- Metastasis, similar to the initial cancer development, is a sequence of events

9-15

Metastasis

- **Detachment**
  - Cells break loose from their original location

9-15

Metastasis

- **Invasion**
  - Cellular proliferation
  - Barrier destruction by lytic enzymes
    - **Secretion of proteases and protease activators**
      - Plasminogen activators
      - Type IV collagenase (degrades basement membrane collagen)
  - Down-regulation of cell adhesion molecules
    - Desmosomes, hemidesmosomes, and tight junctions
  - Increased motility
    - Secretion of autocrine motility factors

9-15

Metastasis

- **Intravasation**
  - Passage into vessels (blood or lymph)
  - Lymphatic spread

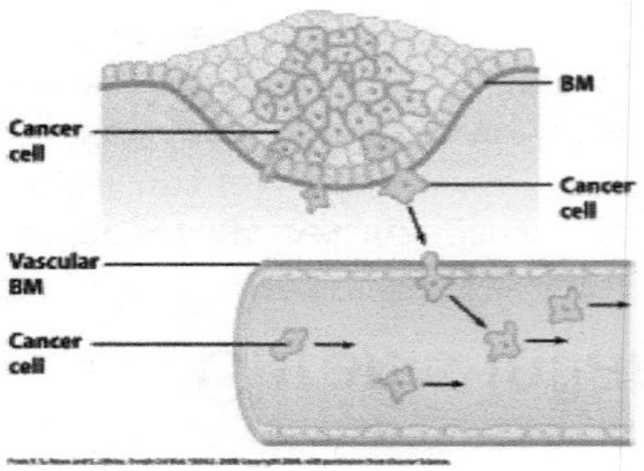

BM
Cancer cell
Cancer cell
Vascular BM
Cancer cell

- Tumors do not usually produce their own lymphatic network
- Lymphatic vessels offer **little resistance** to single cells or clumps of cells
- Once in nearby lymphatics, they may be stopped, or they can remain dormant in the lymphatic system

Karp G. *Cell & Molecular Biology*, 6e

9-15

Metastasis

- **Intravasation**
  - Blood dissemination
    - Tumor cells can form a leukocyte-fibrin-platelet complex to protect themselves from host defenses and help themselves survive mechanical trauma in the bloodstream
    - The cells eventually lodge in the vascular supply of a target organ and invade the tissue of the secondary site

9-15

Metastasis

- **Adherence in favorable sites**
  - Metastatic cancer cells can spread diffusely throughout the body, but certain types of cancerous cells have a preference for specific organs
  - This is often referred to as “organ tropism”
    - Factors encouraging colonization
      - Growth factors from target organ
      - Hormones
      - Presence of tumor receptors on the tissue
      - Route

9-15

Metastasis

- **Extravasation**
  - Leaves blood vessels and invades secondary tissue
- **Colonization**
  - Establishment in new tissue

9-15

Metastasis

- Sequence
  - Local transformation and extension
  - Motility
  - Angiogenesis
  - Invasion
  - Intravasation (blood/lymph penetration)
  - Adherence at a favorable site
  - Extravasation
  - Colonization

9-15

Cancer Staging

Neoplastic cells in original site	Stage 1	Well-differentiated cells
Metastatic cell in original site and local lymphatics	Stage 2	Moderately-differentiated cells
Cells in original site and distant lymphatics	Stage 3	Poorly-differentiated cells
Metastatic cells are found in many body areas	Stage 4	Very poorly-differentiated cells

9-16

Systemic Effects of Neoplasms

- **Vessel** invasion – bleeding
- **Lymphatic** invasion – lymphedema
- **Nerve** invasion – pain, numbness, tingling
- **Bone cortex** invasion – pain and fractures
- **Bone marrow** invasion – pancytopenia, infection, and bleeding
- **Liver** invasion – hepatic insufficiency

9-17

Clinical Manifestations

- **Pain**
  - Little or no pain is associated with early malignancy
  - Pain is influenced greatly by fear, anxiety, sleep loss, and psychological responses
  - Pressure on sensitive structures, obstruction, severe stretching of tissues – all cause pain
  - Patients that have terminal cancer will usually manifest severe pain
    - Bone metastases (periosteal irritation, medullary pressure, and/or fractures)

9-17

Clinical Manifestations

- **Fatigue**
  - Due to:
    - Sleep disturbance
    - Biochemical changes to treatment
    - Diminished activity level
    - Nutritional status
  - Muscle tone loss can be due to lack of activity and/or circulating necrosis factors

9-17

Clinical Manifestations

- **Anemia**
  - Reduction in red blood cell numbers
  - Causes
    - Chronic bleeding
    - Malnutrition
    - Therapies
    - Malignancy in blood-forming organs
  - Malignancy of the bone marrow can also cause leukopenia and thromboycytopenia

9-17

Clinical Manifestations

- **Infection**
  - –This is the most common event leading to the demise of patient with malignancy
  - –Reduction in immunologic functions due to treatment regimens
  - –Poor wound care
  - –Compromised patient care

9-17

Clinical Manifestations

- **Cachexia Syndrome**
  - –State of ill health, wasting, emaciation and decreased quality of life
  - –Symptoms
    - Reduced sweet, sour, and salty sensations
    - Depression of appetite (early filling response)
    - Weight loss and asthenia (marked weakness)
    - Altered metabolism (increased BMR)
    - **Cachexia and anorexia are present in 80% of cancer deaths**

9-17

Cancer Treatments

- **Chemotherapy**
  - –Chemotherapy is intended to destroy cells that are in a stage of vulnerability
    - Mitotically active cells are very vulnerable
  - –The chemotherapy must eliminate enough cells to allow the immune system to destroy the others
  - –Usually a cocktail of drugs

9-18

Cancer Treatments

- **Chemotherapy**
  - –Molecular-era anti-cancer drugs
  - –“Targeted Therapy”
    - Enzyme inhibitors
    - Monoclonal antibodies
      - –Directed at a specific tumor antigen

9-18

Cancer Treatments

- **Radiation**
  - –Radiation damages the DNA of the rapidly dividing neoplastic cells
  - –General and targeted radiation therapy

9-18

Cancer Treatments

- **Surgical therapy**
  - –**Excisional, Debulking, Palliative**
    - Useful when the tumor is accessible and has not passed beyond stage 3 (regional lymph nodes)
    - The tumor and any affected lymph nodes must both be removed
    - Surgery decreases the total number of cancer cells, giving normal immune mechanisms a fighting chance
    - Palliative surgery can relieve symptoms of malignancy

9-18

UNIT 3

Study Guide Objectives – Introductory Pathophysiology (HTHS 2230)

Unit 3

Chapter 19 - Structure and Function of the Hematologic System

1. Identify and describe the constituents of whole blood: formed elements (WBCs, RBCs, platelets), plasma proteins, and solutes (electrolytes, gases, nutrients, and waste products). (pp. 477-480)

2. Identify the structural characteristics and function of red blood cells. (p. 480)

3. Describe the following laboratory tests for red blood cells: hematocrit, hemoglobin, red blood cell count, mean corpuscular volume (MCV), mean corpuscular hemoglobin (MCH), and mean corpuscular hemoglobin concentration (MCHC). (p. 494)

4. Identify the characteristics and functions of the various types of white blood cells (leukocytes): neutrophils, basophils, eosinophils, lymphocytes, monocytes, and macrophages. (pp. 480-481)

5. Identify and describe the primary and secondary lymphoid organs. (pp. 482-483)

6. Describe the process of hematopoiesis. (pp. 483-389)

7. Describe the effects of colony-stimulating factors. (pp. 484-485)

8. Identify the characteristics and functions of platelets. (p. 481)

9. Describe the sequence of events in hemostasis. (pp. 489-490).

10. Describe specific substances that activate the intrinsic and extrinsic pathways of the coagulation system. Describe stages of coagulation. (pp. 491-493).

11. Describe the role of the fibrinolytic system. (p. 493)

12. Describe the information that can be obtained from a bone marrow biopsy, a complete blood count, a white blood cell differential, a bleeding time, a protime (PT), an activated partial thromboplastin time (APTT), and a reticulocyte count. (pp. 494-495)

Chapter 20 - Alterations of Hematologic Function

1. Define anemia. Describe the common clinical manifestations of anemia.

2. Classify the anemias in one of the following groups: macrocytic-normochromic, microcytic-hypochromic, and normocytic-normochromic. Describe the pathophysiology and any unique clinical manifestations of the following anemias: pernicious, folic acid deficiency, iron deficiency, sideroblastic, aplastic, posthemorrhagic, hemolytic, and anemia of chronic inflammation. (pp. 500-506)

3. Describe the types, causes, manifestations, and treatment of polycythemia. (pp. 506-508)

4. Describe terms and causes associated with high or low leukocyte counts: leukocytosis, leukopenia, granulocytosis (neutrophilia), neutropenia, eosinophilia, monocytosis, lymphocytosis, and lymphocytopenia. (pp. 508-510)

5. Describe the pathogenesis of infectious mononucleosis. (pp. 511-512)

6. Classify, contrast, and describe the manifestations of leukemia: acute lymphoblastic leukemia (ALL), chronic lymphocytic leukemia (CLL), acute myeloblastic leukemia (AML), chronic myelocytic leukemia (CML). (pp. 512-515)

7. Describe the pathophysiology and manifestations of multiple myeloma. (pp. 520-521)

8. Compare and contrast Hodgkin disease (lymphoma) to non-Hodgkin lymphoma. (pp. 516-520)

9. Describe the appropriate platelet levels and the clinical manifestations of thrombocytopenia. (pp. 523-524)

10. Describe the etiology of thrombocythemia. (pp. 525-526)

11. Describe the potential causes of abnormal platelet function. (p. 526)

12. Describe causes of impaired hemostasis including vitamin K deficiency and liver disease. (pp. 526-527)

13. Describe the pathophysiology and manifestations of disseminated intravascular coagulation (DIC). (pp. 527-530)

Chapter 21 - Alteration of Hematologic Function in Children

1. Compare and contrast the two major causes of hemolytic disease of the newborn. (pp. 536-539)

2. Describe the inheritance pattern, disease process, and clinical manifestations of sickle cell disease. (pp. 539-542)

3. Describe the inheritance pattern and clinical manifestations of the thalassemias. (pp. 542-543)

4. Identify the causes and clinical manifestations of hemophilia A (factor VIII deficiency) and hemophilia B (factor IX deficiency). (pp. 544-545)

Unit 3
Chapter 19
Structure and Function of the Hematologic System

Characteristics of Blood

- Composed of formed elements (45%) and plasma (55%)
  - Cells vs. formed elements
- Viscous (thick)
- Volume: 4-6 liters
- pH - 7.35-7.45
- 0.85-0.90% NaCl

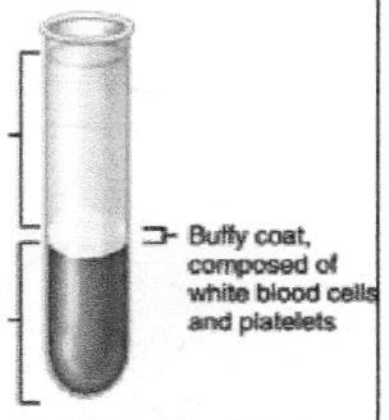

Plasma (55%)
Buffy coat, composed of white blood cells and platelets
Red blood cells (45%)

(a) Appearance of centrifuged blood

19-1

Blood Plasma

- Plasma is the straw-colored, **"liquid"** portion of unclotted blood
- Accounts for 55-60% of the blood volume
  - 92% water
  - 8% solutes
    - 7% plasma proteins
      - Albumins
      - Globulins
      - Fibrinogen
    - 1% other solutes
      - Electrolytes, nutrients, gases, hormones, wastes

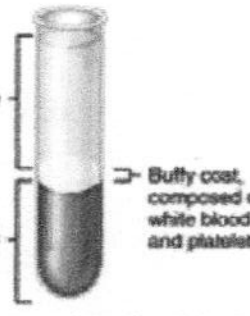

Plasma (55%)
Buffy coat, composed of white blood cells and platelets
Red blood cells (45%)

(a) Appearance of centrifuged blood

19-1

Plasma Proteins

- **Albumin**
  - A low-molecular-weight plasma protein synthesized in the liver
  - Contributes to blood viscosity and maintains blood pressure
    - Albumin does not diffuse freely across the vascular endothelium
  - Acts as an osmotically-active **carrier molecule**

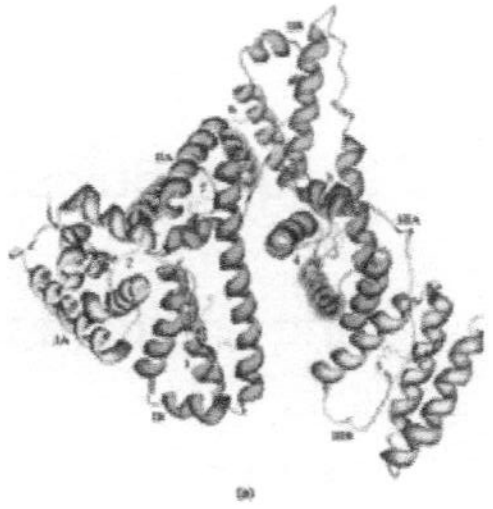

19-1

Plasma Proteins

- There are several types of globulins
  - Four main groups
    - Alpha$_1$ (α_1), alpha$_2$ (α_2), beta (β), and gamma (γ)
  - Function individually, as well as collectively
    - α - and β -globulins act individually as carrier molecules. Collectively, they control blood osmotic pressure.
    - γ -globulins (immunoglobulins or antibodies) are made by plasma cells (activated B lymphocytes)

19-1

Plasma Protein

- **Clotting Factors**
  - Soluble factors that are activated to produce a insoluble clot
  - Fibrinogen (factor I) is the most plentiful, but there are a number of others.
  - They promote clotting in a cascading fashion.
    - Much more on this later

19-1

Plasma vs. Serum

- Plasma and serum differ simply in the presence or absence of soluble clotting factors
- Serum is the liquid portion of clotted blood.
- Plasma is the liquid portion of unclotted blood.
- Patients in the ER who need extra blood volume are transfused with fresh frozen plasma **(FFP)**, not FFS

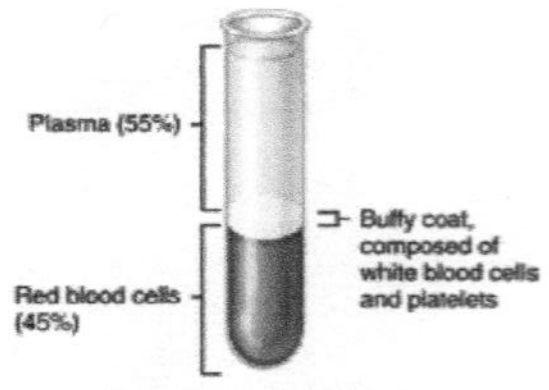
Plasma (55%)
Buffy coat, composed of white blood cells and platelets
Red blood cells (45%)
(a) Appearance of centrifuged blood

19-1

Other Plasma Components

- Electrolytes
- Lipids and lipoproteins
- Amino acids
- Gases
- Waste products
  - Urea, creatinine, uric acid, and bilirubin

19-1

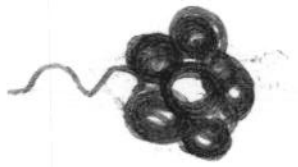

Formed Elements of Blood

		BLOOD CELL TYPE	DESCRIPTION	FUNCTION	LIFE SPAN
RED BLOOD CELLS		Erythrocyte	Flat disk with a central depression; no nucleus; contains hemoglobin.	Transports oxygen (O_2) and carbon dioxide (CO_2).	About 120 days.
WHITE BLOOD CELLS (LEUKOCYTES)	GRANULOCYTES	Neutrophil	Spherical; many-lobed nucleus; no hemoglobin; pink-purple staining cytoplasmic granules.	Cellular defense—phagocytosis of small microorganisms.	Hours to 3 days.
		Eosinophil	Spherical; two-lobed nucleus; no hemoglobin; orange-red staining cytoplasmic granules.	Cellular defense—phagocytosis of large microorganisms such as parasitic worms; releases anti-inflammatory substances in allergic reactions.	8 to 12 days.
		Basophil	Spherical; generally two-lobed nucleus; no hemoglobin; large purple staining cytoplasmic granules.	Inflammatory response—contains granules that rupture and release chemicals enhancing inflammatory response.	Hours to 3 days.
	AGRANULOCYTES	Monocyte	Spherical; single nucleus shaped like kidney bean; no cytoplasmic granules; cytoplasm often blue in color.	Converted to macrophages, which are large cells that entrap microorganisms and other foreign matter.	Days to months.
		B-lymphocyte	Spherical; round single nucleus; no cytoplasmic granules.	Immune system response and regulation; antibody production; sometimes causes allergic response.	Days to years.
		T-lymphocyte	Spherical; round single nucleus; no cytoplasmic granules.	Immune system response and regulation; cellular immune response.	Days to years.
PLATELETS		Platelets	Irregularly shaped fragments; very small pink staining cytoplasmic granules.	Control blood clotting or coagulation.	7 to 10 days.

Alters & Alters, Biology: Understanding Life, 1/e

19-1

Formed Elements of Blood

- **Red Blood Cells (RBCs)**
  - Erythrocytes
  - Lifespan 80-120 days
  - Function in gas transport
  - 1) High surface-to-volume ratio
    - Why would a biconcave disk be a better shape for a RBC than a sphere?
  - 2) Demonstrate reversible deformity

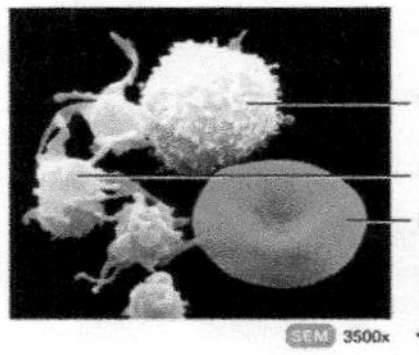
White blood cell
Platelet
Red blood cell
SEM 3500x

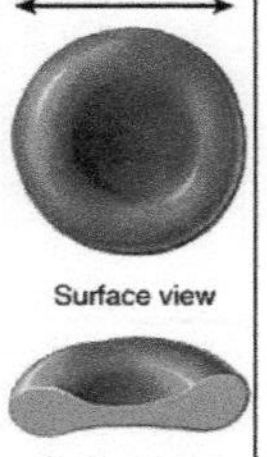
8μm
Surface view
Sectioned view

19-2 RBC shape

RBC Laboratory Values

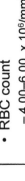

- Hematocrit (Hct)
  - % of whole blood volume occupied by red blood cells
  - 38-46% females, 40-54% for males
- Hemoglobin (Hgb)
  - Oxygen-carrying molecule
  - Heme (4) + 4 globin proteins
  - 14–16 g/dl
- RBC count
  - 4.00–6.00 x 10^6/mm^3

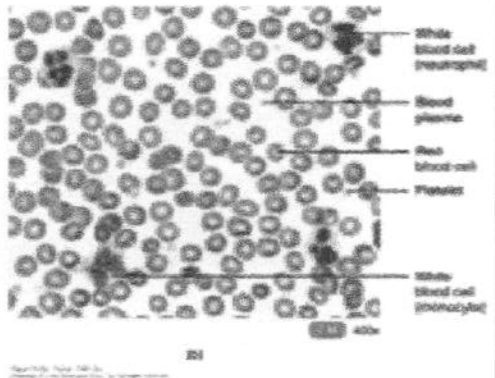

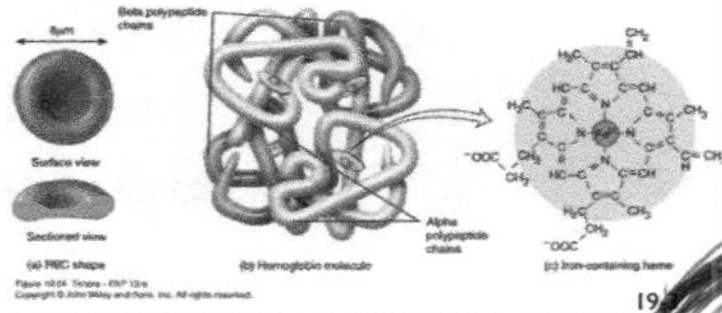

19

RBC Laboratory Values

- Mean Corpuscular (Cell) Volume **(MCV)**
  - Volume of an average RBC
    - 80-96 fL (femtoliters = 10^{-15} L)
- Mean Corpuscular (Cell) Hemoglobin **(MCH)**
  - Amount of hemoglobin in an average RBC
    - 20-32 pg (picograms = 10^{-12} g)
- Mean Corpuscular (Cell) Hemoglobin Concentration **(MCHC)**
  - Concentration of hemoglobin in an average RBC
    - 32-36 g/dl

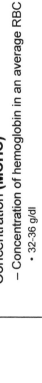

19-3

Leukocytes

- White Blood Cells (WBCs)
  - –5.0 – 10.0 x $10^3/mm^3$
  - –**Granulocytes**
    - Life spans of 0.5 – 9.0 days
    - Most die doing their job
  - –**Agranulocytes**
    - Lymphocytes live from days to decades
    - Monocytes live for several months
    - Phagocytes or immunocytes

19-4

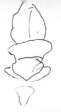

Leukocyte Terminology

- **Leukocytosis**
  - –WBC count > 10.0 x $10^3/mm^3$
    - Occurs in both viral and bacterial infections:
    - Normal physiological response to disease, up to a certain point
- **Leukopenia**
  - –WBC count < 5.0 x $10^3/mm^3$
    - Never a normal response

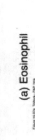

19-4

Granulocytes

- **Neutrophils**
  - –Pinkish cytoplasm
  - –Segmented nucleus
  - –Fight bacterial infections
  - –Phagocytic cells
  - –60-70% of circulating white cells
  - –Quickly respond to disease

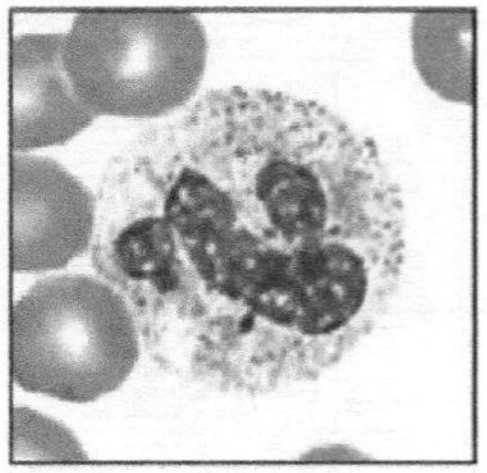

(c) Neutrophil

19-4

Granulocytes

- **Eosinophils**
  - –Large red granules
  - –Target antigen-antibody complexes
  - –Increased in
    - Allergies
    - Parasites
  - –1-4% of circulating WBCs

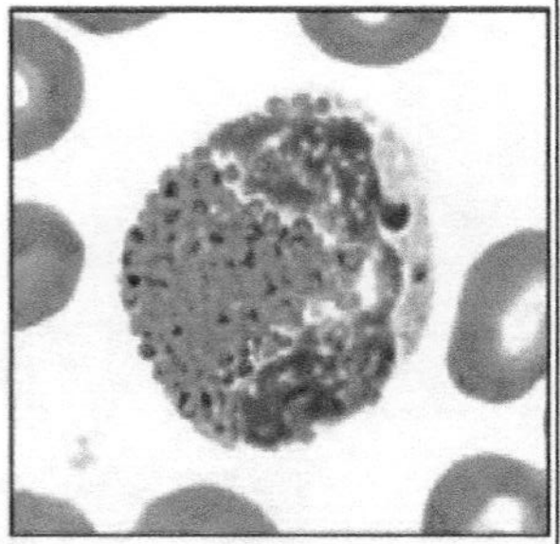

(a) Eosinophil

19-4

Granulocytes

- **Basophils**
  - Large dark blue granules
  - Participate in inflammatory responses
  - Release histamine and heparin
  - 0-1% of circulating WBCs
    - Minimal correlation with disease

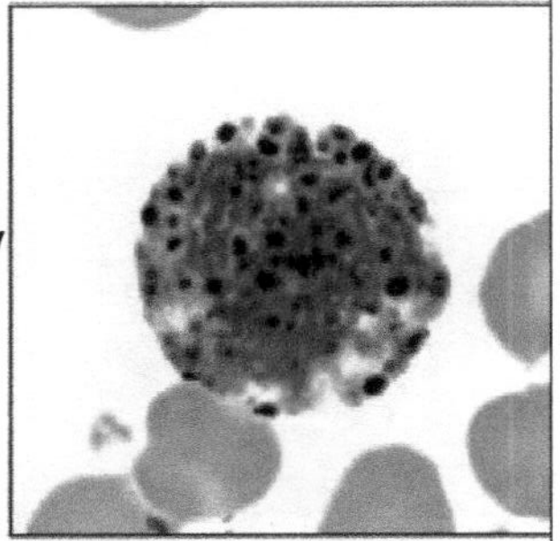

(b) Basophil

19-4

Agranulocytes

- **Monocytes/Macrophages**
  - Very powerful phagocytes
  - 3-8% of circulating white cells
  - Macrophages have different names depending on their location
    - Wandering macrophages
    - Fixed macrophages in tissue
      - Kupffer cells, histiocytes, microglial cells, alveolar macrophages, etc.

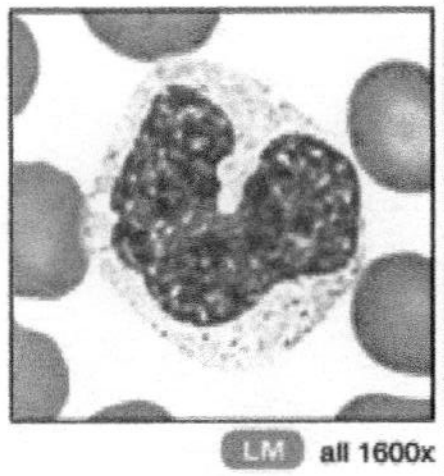
LM all 1600x

(e) Monocyte

19-4

Agranulocytes

- **Lymphocytes**
  - Most lymphocytes are contained within the lymph system
    - T and B cells
  - Fight viral infections and cancers
  - 20-30% of WBCs
  - Major role in adaptive immune response

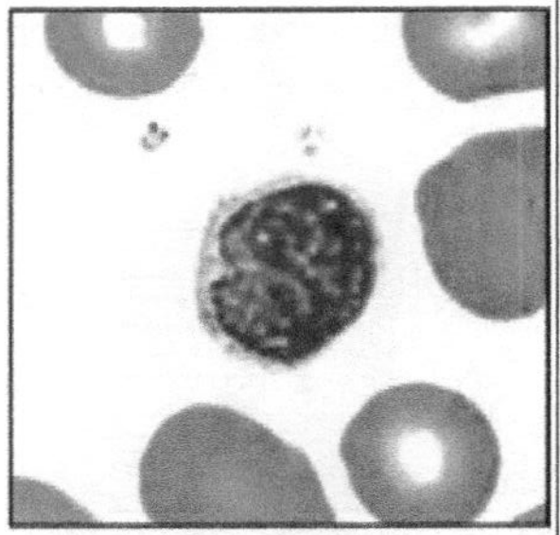

(d) Lymphocyte

19-4

Lymphatic System

- A system consisting of organs and **lymph vessels** through which **lymphatic fluid** passes.
- It functions to
  - Drain interstitial fluid
  - Transport dietary lipids absorbed by the GI tract to the blood
  - Facilitate an immune response

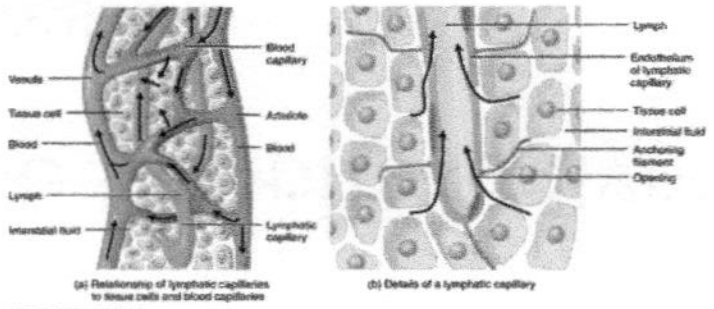

19-5

Lymphoid Organs

- **Primary** lymphoid organs
  - Thymus and bone marrow
- **Secondary** lymph organs
  - Spleen, lymph nodes, tonsils, and Peyer Patches of the small intestine
- Lymph organs link the hematologic and immune systems

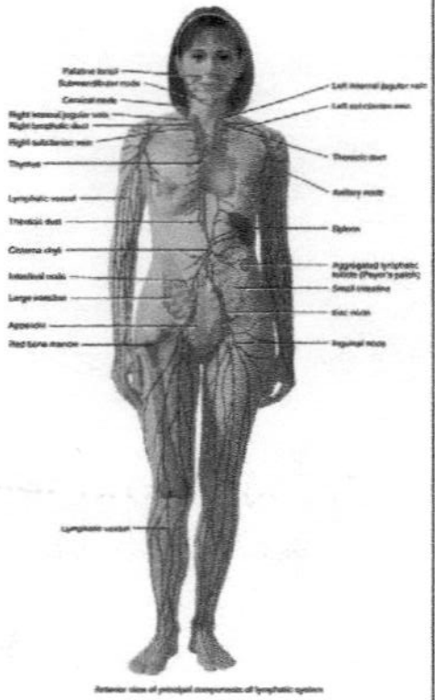

Figure 22.01 Tortora - PAP 12/e

19-5

The Lymphatic System

- Lymph Vessels
- Lymph Nodes
- Right and left lymphatic ducts
- Tonsils
- Spleen
- Thymus
- Bone marrow

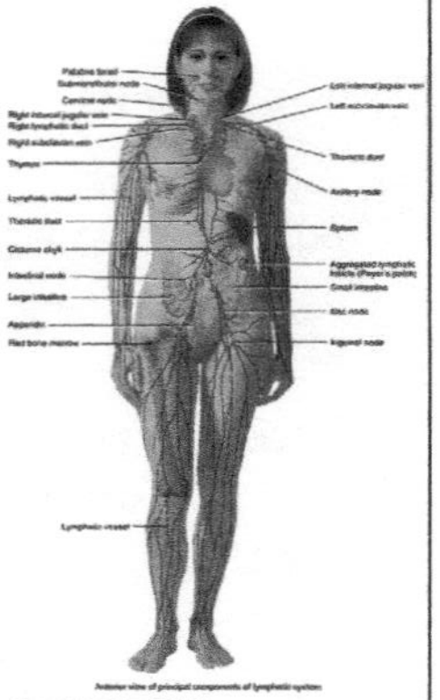

Figure 22.01 Tortora - PAP 12/e

19-5

The Spleen

- **Filters and cleanses** the blood
- Contains masses of lymphoid tissue (white pulp)
- Removes **old or damaged cells** from the blood.
- Storage area for extra blood that can be released by sympathetic stimulation.
- Storage of platelets, up to 1/3 of blood supply

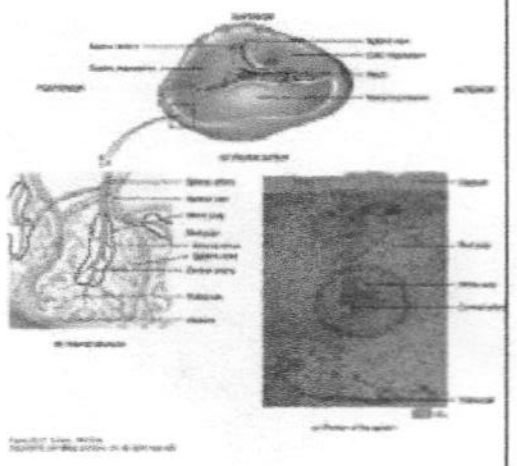

19-5

Lymph Nodes

- Lymph nodes serve as filters for lymph fluid.
- Foreign objects are trapped and destroyed.
- Important groups of lymph nodes
  - Submandibular, cervical, axillary, inguinal
- Lymph node enlargement may often indicate a pathological condition.

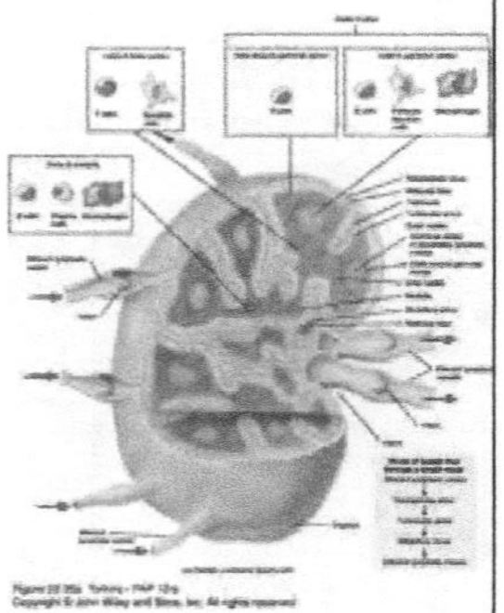

19-5

Hematopoiesis

- Formed element production
- Cells are formed in red bone marrow from **pluripotent stem cells** and mature in the bone marrow or lymphoid tissue (spleen, thymus, tonsils, lymph nodes).
- Active red bone marrow in adults
  - Pelvis, sternum, vertebrae

19-6

Hematopoiesis

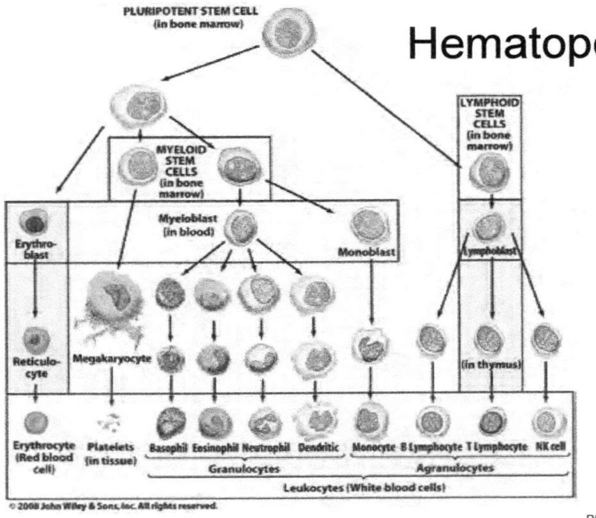

PLURIPOTENT STEM CELL (in bone marrow)
MYELOID STEM CELLS (in bone marrow)
LYMPHOID STEM CELLS (in bone marrow)
Erythro-blast
Myeloblast (in blood)
Monoblast
Lymphoblast
Reticulo-cyte
Megakaryocyte
(in thymus)
Erythrocyte (Red blood cell)
Platelets (in tissue)
Basophil
Eosinophil
Neutrophil
Dendritic
Monocyte
B Lymphocyte
T Lymphocyte
NK cell
Granulocytes
Agranulocytes
Leukocytes (White blood cells)
© 2008 John Wiley & Sons, Inc. All rights reserved.

19-6
Black, *Microbiology*, 7/e

Hematopoiesis

- **Medullary hematopoiesis** is cellular production in the bone marrow
- Disease conditions can cause **extramedullary hematopoiesis**
  - Production outside of the bone marrow
    - liver
    - spleen
    - other tissues less frequently

19-6

Erythropoiesis as Part of Hematopoiesis

- **Erythropoiesis**
  - The production of RBCs
  - Hypoxia (oxygen deficiency) stimulates the kidneys to release the hormone erythropoietin (EPO) which circulates to the red marrow and speeds up the maturation of immature RBCs
  - The **rate of erythropoiesis** is reflected in the **reticulocyte (retic)** count
    - A "retic" is a new, not yet fully mature red cell

19-6
19-12

Reticulocytes

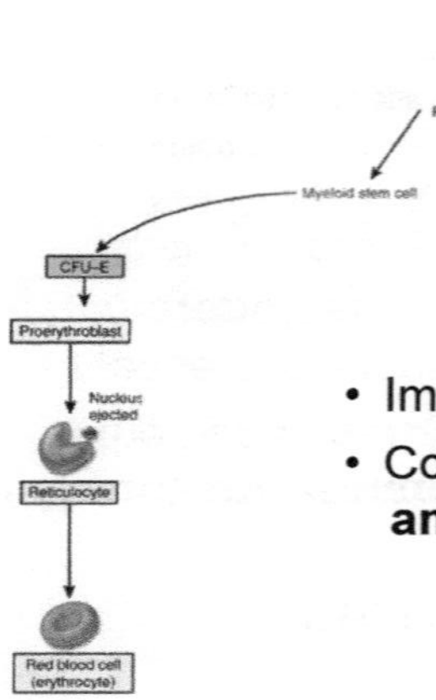
Pluripotent stem cell
Myeloid stem cell
CFU-E
Proerythroblast
Nucleus ejected
Reticulocyte
Red blood cell (erythrocyte)

- Immature RBCs
- Contains **hemoglobin**, **RNA**, **and mitochondrial remnants**

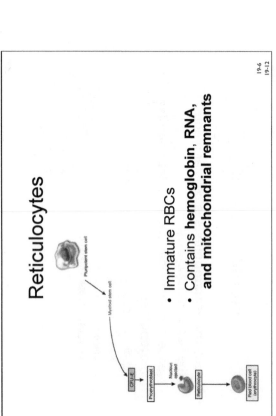

19-6
19-12

Hematopoiesis and Cytokines

- Hematopoietic cells will develop, proliferate, and differentiate if they are provided with specific **growth factors**
- Colony Stimulating Factors (CSF)
  - These **cytokines** act as hormones to stimulate the proliferation of progenitor (early) cells
  - Specific CSFs are necessary for growth of myeloid, erythroid, lymphoid, and megakaryocytic cells

19-7

Colony Stimulating Factors

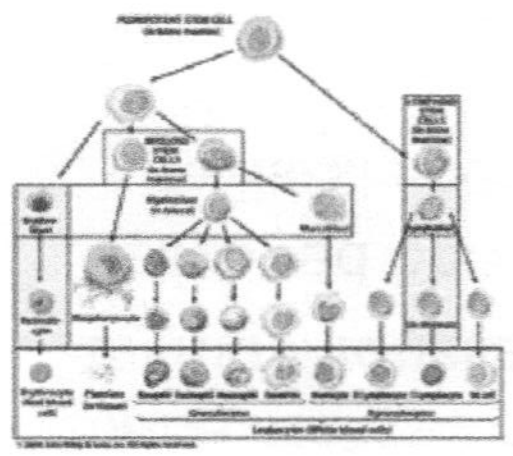

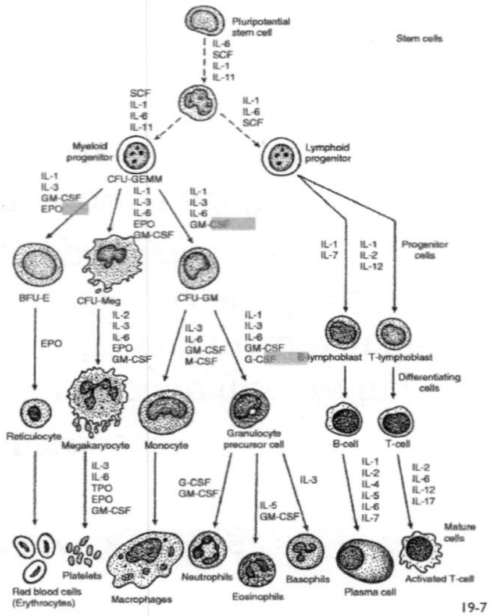
Pluripotential stem cell
Stem cells
Myeloid progenitor
CFU-GEMM
Lymphoid progenitor
Progenitor cells
BFU-E
CFU-Meg
CFU-GM
EPO
Reticulocyte
Megakaryocyte
Monocyte
Granulocyte precursor cell
B-lymphoblast
T-lymphoblast
Differentiating cells
B-cell
T-cell
Red blood cells (Erythrocytes)
Platelets
Macrophages
Neutrophils
Eosinophils
Basophils
Plasma cell
Activated T-cell
Mature cells

19-7

Colony Stimulating Factors

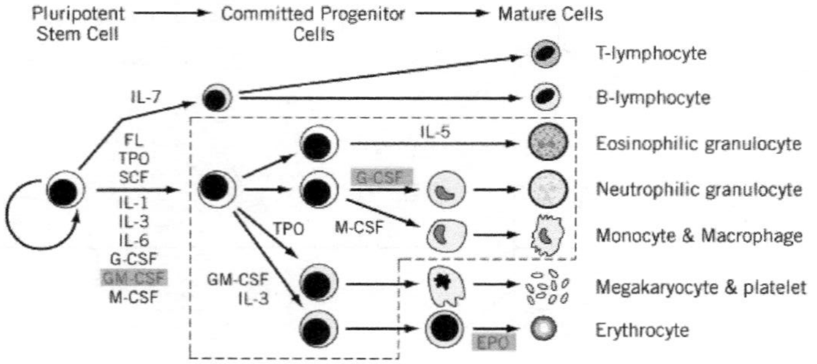
Pluripotent Stem Cell
Committed Progenitor Cells
Mature Cells
IL-7
FL
TPO
SCF
IL-1
IL-3
IL-6
G-CSF
GM-CSF
M-CSF
IL-5
G-CSF
TPO
M-CSF
GM-CSF
IL-3
EPO
T-lymphocyte
B-lymphocyte
Eosinophilic granulocyte
Neutrophilic granulocyte
Monocyte & Macrophage
Megakaryocyte & platelet
Erythrocyte

19-7

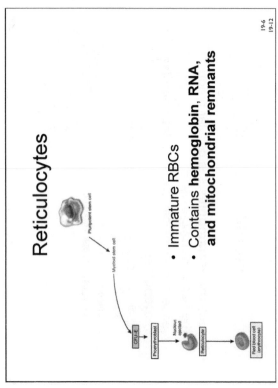

Hematopoiesis and Cytokines

- Colony Stimulating Factors originate from one cell to stimulate the proliferation of another

CSF	Cell Origin	Cell Stimulated
G-CSF	Macrophage, fibroblast	Granulocytes
GM-CSF	T cell	Neutrophil, Macrophage
Erythropoietin	Kidney cells and Kupffer cells	Erythrocytes

19-7

Thrombocytes (Platelets)

- Cell Fragments
  - 150–400 x $10^3/mm^3$
- Originate from megakaryocytes
- Aid in clotting by clumping (agglutination) and the release of biochemical mediators
- **Thrombocytopenia**
  - Low platelet count
- **Thrombocytosis**
  - Increased platelet count

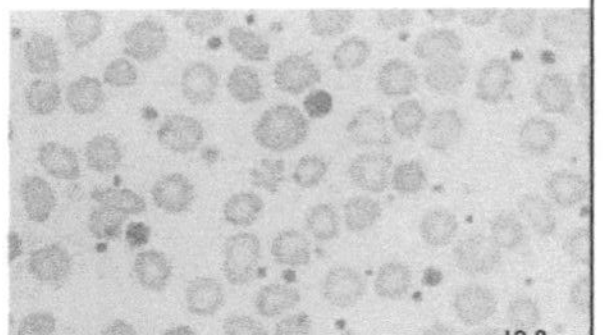

Bain BJ. *Blood Cells: A Practical Guide*, 4e, 2006.

19-8

Hemostasis

- There are three distinct steps in forming a blood clot:
  - 1) Vascular spasm
  - 2) Platelet plug formation
  - 3) Activation of the coagulation cascade

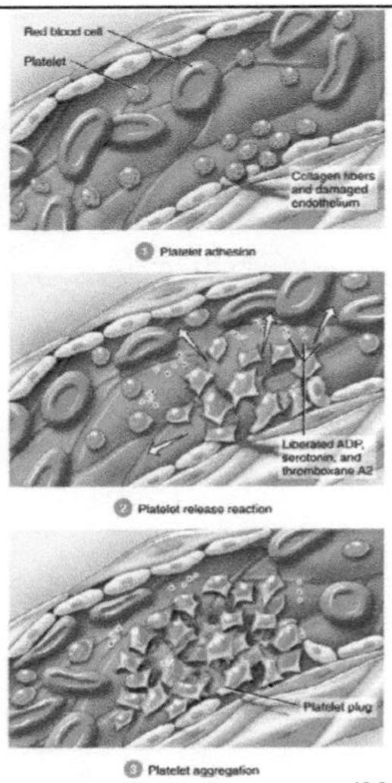
Red blood cell
Platelet
Collagen fibers and damaged endothelium
1 Platelet adhesion
Liberated ADP, serotonin, and thromboxane A2
2 Platelet release reaction
Platelet plug
3 Platelet aggregation

Figure 19.09 Tortora - PAP 12/e

19-9

The Clotting Cascade

- **Positive-feedback** system
- Begins with the activation of several **soluble**, **inactive** clotting factors stimulated in a cascading fashion
- There are two main pathways:
  - **Extrinsic pathway**
  - **Intrinsic pathway**
- Both systems or pathways **merge at** a common point, forming the **common pathway**
- Coagulation is usually fast and localized

19-9

Clotting Pathways

- **"Extrinsic" pathway**
  - Activated by tissue factor (tissue thromboplastin)
- **"Intrinsic" pathway**
  - Activated by contact with the injured vessel
    - Collagen and endothelium
- **"Common" pathway**
  - Converge at factor X
- **Ca^{++} plays a role in many steps of coagulation**

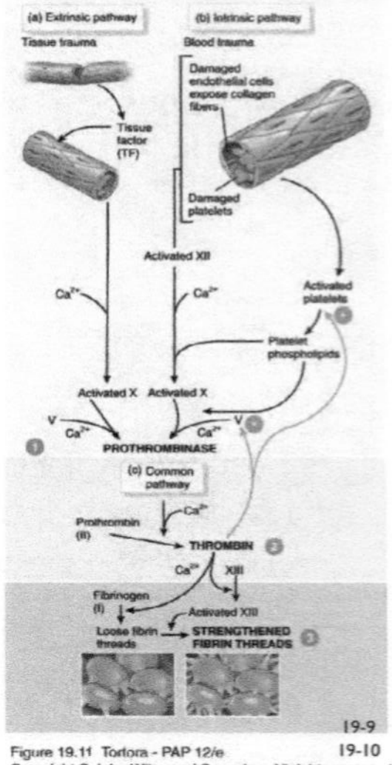

(a) Extrinsic pathway
(b) Intrinsic pathway
Tissue trauma
Blood trauma
Damaged endothelial cells expose collagen fibers
Tissue factor (TF)
Damaged platelets
Activated XII
Activated platelets
Platelet phospholipids
Activated X
Activated X
PROTHROMBINASE
(c) Common pathway
Prothrombin (II)
THROMBIN
Fibrinogen (I)
Activated XIII
Loose fibrin threads
STRENGTHENED FIBRIN THREADS

19-9

Figure 19.11 Tortora - PAP 12/e 19-10

Don't memorize these steps: just know there are two pathways that converge on a common pathway

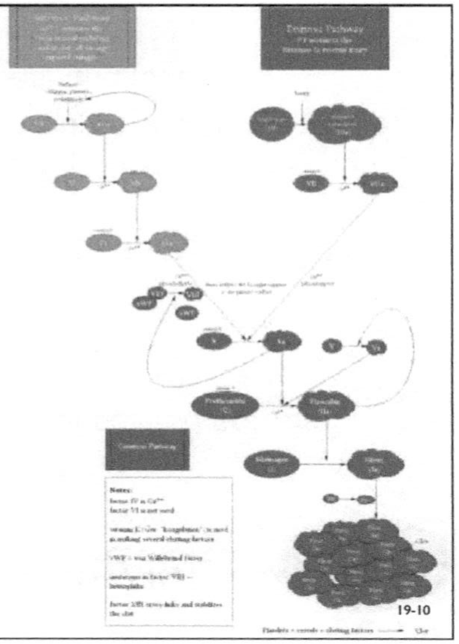

19-10

Stages of Coagulation

- Extrinsic and intrinsic activation
- The common pathway begins with the formation of prothrombinase (prothrombin activator)
- The prothrombin activator activates **prothrombin** to **thrombin**
- Thrombin induces the formation of **fibrin** from **fibrinogen**

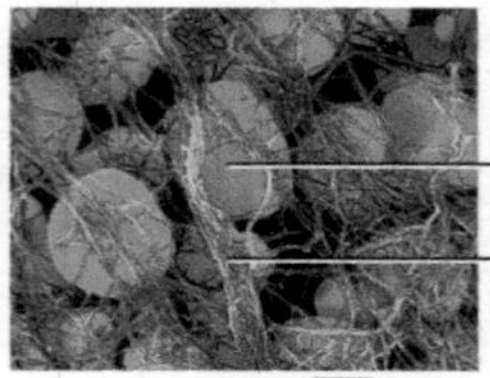

Red blood cell
Fibrin threads
SEM 1600x

(d) Red blood cells trapped in fibrin threads

19-10

Clot Retraction

- After 30-60 min, the platelets contract
  - Platelets contain actin and myosin proteins
  - This squeezes out the serum
- The clot becomes impacted and the edges of the blood vessel are brought closer together
- Healing is also beginning
  - Smooth muscle cells & fibroblasts are stimulated to divide
- Endothelial cells begin to restore endothelial lining of the vessel
- Now the clot has to be removed
  - **Fibrinolysis**

19-11

Fibrinolysis

- **Fibrinolytic System**
  - Large amounts of plasminogen (a plasma protein) are incorporated into clots
  - When endothelial cells produce **tissue plasminogen activator (TPA),** it causes the plasminogen to become **plasmin**
  - Factors within the coagulation cascade (factor XII and thrombin) also change plasminogen into its active form, **plasmin**
  - Either way, when plasmin is formed, it digests clots
    - TPA ("clot buster") is widely used in stroke/MI patients

19-11

Diagnostic Tests of Blood

Bone Marrow Biopsy

- Small amounts of bone marrow tissue are removed from the bone and observed microscopically.
- Usually collected from the posterior iliac crest
- Assists in the diagnosis of: anemias, leukemias, platelet disorders, immunoglobulin disorders, etc.

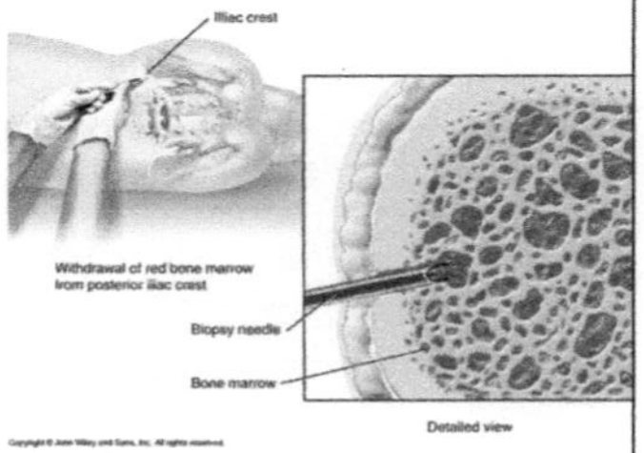

Iliac crest
Withdrawal of red bone marrow from posterior iliac crest
Biopsy needle
Bone marrow
Detailed view

19-12

Diagnostic Tests of Blood

Complete Blood Count

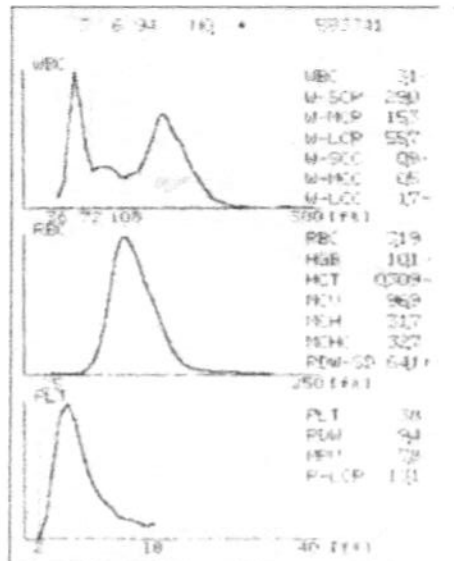

Fig. 2.10 Numerical printout and histograms of white blood cell (WBC), red blood cell (RBC) and platelet (PLT) volume produced by a Sysmex NE 5000 automated haematology analyser. White cells are classified into small cells (W-SC), which are mainly lymphocytes, intermediate sized cells (W-MC), which are mainly monocytes and large cells (W-LC), which are mainly neutrophils.

Bain BJ. *Blood Cells: A Practical Guide*, 4e, 2006.

- White blood cell (WBC) count
- White blood cell differential
- Red blood cell (RBC) count
- Hemoglobin
- Hematocrit
- Platelet count
- MCV
- MCH
- MCHC
- Red cell distribution width (RDW)

19-12

Diagnostic Tests of Blood

White Blood Cell Differential

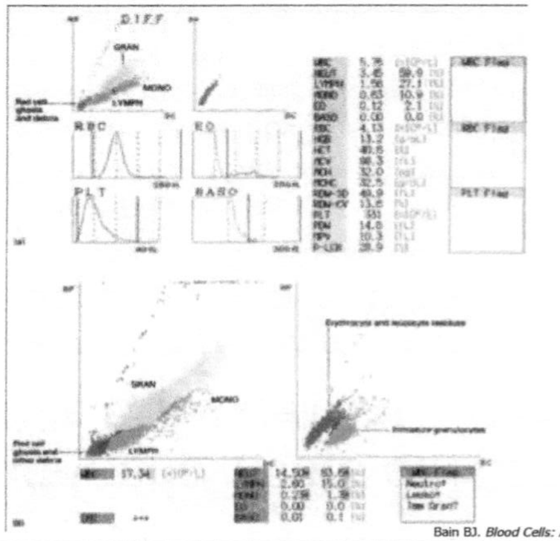

DIFF
GRAN
MONO
LYMPH
RBC
RO
PLT
BASO

19-12

Bain BJ. *Blood Cells: A Practical Guide*, 4e, 2006.

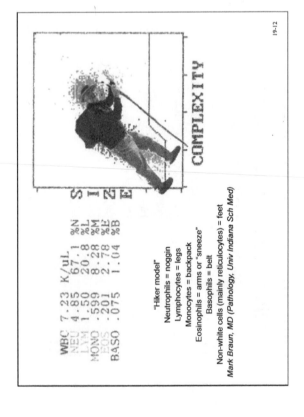

WBC	7.23	K/uL		
NEU	4.85		67.1	%N
LYM	1.50		20.8	%L
MONO	.599		8.28	%M
EOS	.201		2.78	%E
BASO	.075		1.04	%B

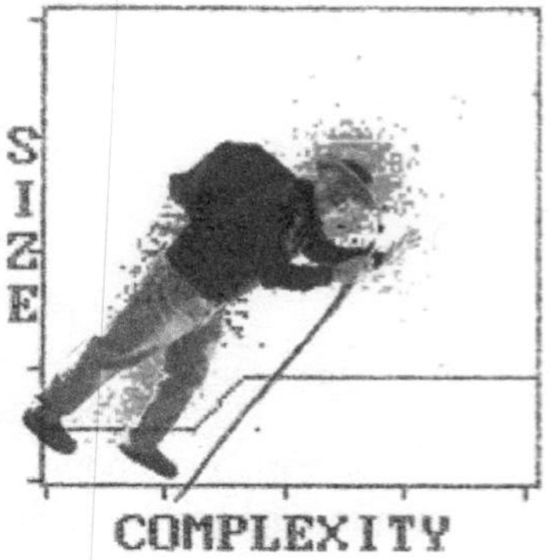
SIZE
COMPLEXITY

"Hiker model"
Neutrophils = noggin
Lymphocytes = legs
Monocytes = backpack
Eosinophils = arms or "sneeze"
Basophils = belt
Non-white cells (mainly reticulocytes) = feet
Mark Braun, MD (Pathology, Univ Indiana Sch Med)

19-12

Diagnostic Tests of Blood
White Blood Cell Differential

- Physicians use the percentage of the individual white blood cells in the blood to aid in the diagnosis of specific diseases.
  - Bacterial appendicitis
    - WBC = 15.0 x 10^3/mm^3 and 90% **neutrophils**
  - Infectious mono caused by Epstein-Barr virus
    - WBCs = 11.0 x 10^3/mm^3 and 80% **lymphocytes** (many activated or "atypical")
  - Chronic lymphocytic leukemia (CLL)
    - WBCs = 175.0 x 10^3 /mm^3 90% **lymphocytes**

19-12

Diagnostic Tests of Blood
Coagulation Tests

- Prothrombin Time / International Normalized Ratio **(PT/INR)**
  - Measures the **extrinsic** pathway
  - Usually to check status after anticoagulant administration
- Activated Partial Thromboplastin Time **(APTT)**
  - Measures the **intrinsic** pathway
- **Bleeding Time**
  - Measures **platelet function**, not platelet number
  - New instrumentation is replacing this test

19-12

Diagnostic Tests of Blood
Reticulocyte Count

- A low reticulocyte count (<0.5%) indicates a **low rate of erythropoiesis**.
- A high reticulocyte count (>1.5%) indicates a **high rate of erythropoiesis.**

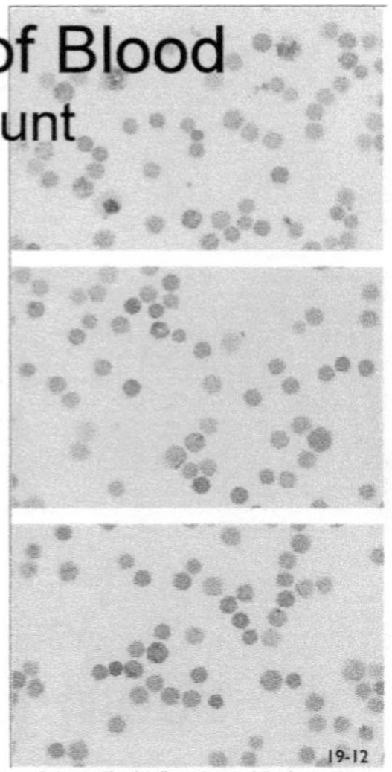

19-12

Bain BJ. *Blood Cells: A Practical Guide*, 4e, 2006.

Unit 3
Chapter 20
Alterations of Hematologic Function

Imbalances of Erythropoiesis
Anemia

- **Anemia**
  - Insufficient RBCs or a decrease in the quality or quantity of hemoglobin
    - Low iron intake, hemolysis, autoimmune disease, lack of production in the bone marrow
  - Typical symptoms: fatigue, weakness, dyspnea, and pallor

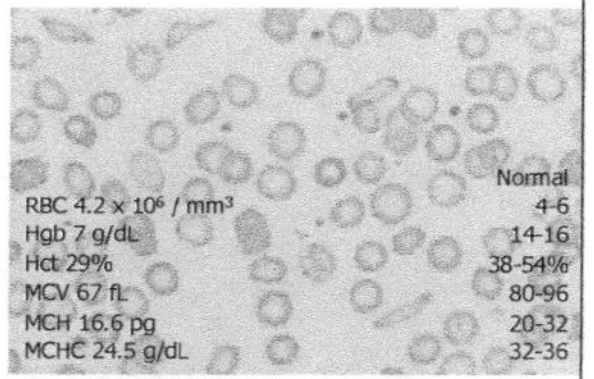

RBC 4.2 x 10⁶ / mm³
Hgb 7 g/dL
Hct 29%
MCV 67 fL
MCH 16.6 pg
MCHC 24.5 g/dL
Normal
4-6
14-16
38-54%
80-96
20-32
32-36

Bain BJ. *Blood Cells: A Practical Guide*, 4e, 2006.

20-I

Imbalances of Erythropoiesis

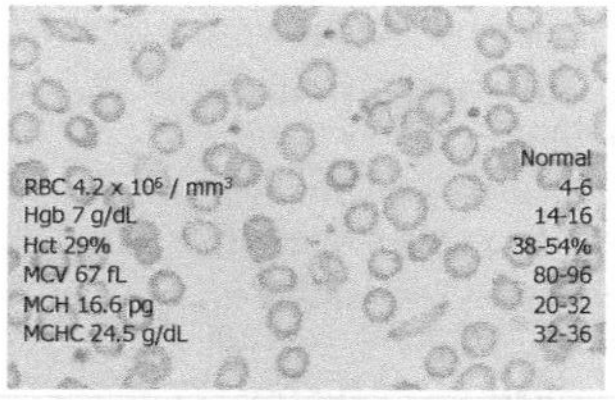

RBC 4.2 x 10⁶ / mm³
Hgb 7 g/dL
Hct 29%
MCV 67 fL
MCH 16.6 pg
MCHC 24.5 g/dL
Normal
4-6
14-16
38-54%
80-96
20-32
32-36

Anemia
- Insufficient RBCs or a decrease in the quality or quantity of hemoglobin
- i.e., a decrease in the oxygen carrying capacity of the blood

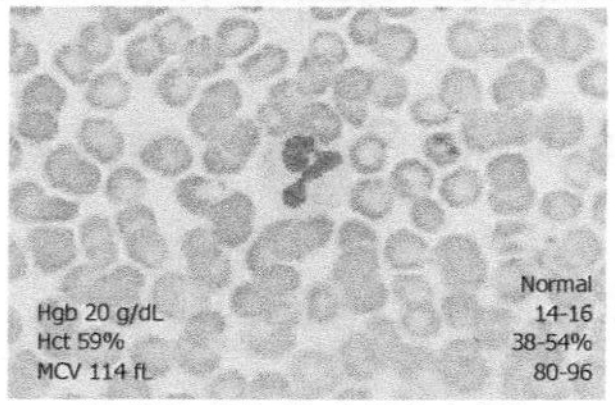

Hgb 20 g/dL
Hct 59%
MCV 114 fL
Normal
14-16
38-54%
80-96

Polycythemia
- Excess RBC formation
  - Develops in states of hypoxia, smoking, dehydration

Bain BJ. *Blood Cells: A Practical Guide*, 4e, 2006.

20-I
20-3

Anemias

Classified according to **etiology (origin)** and/or **morphology**

- **Etiologies**
  - Fe^{++} deficiency anemia
  - folate/B_{12} deficiency anemia
  - hemorrhagic anemia
  - anemia of chronic disease (ACD)
  - hemolytic anemia
- **Morphologies**
  - **Volume**
    - microcytic
    - macrocytic
    - normocytic
  - **Chromasia** (color)
    - hypochromic
    - normochromic

20-I
20-2

Anemias

- **Microcytic – Hypochromic Anemia**
  - Pale, small cells
  - Usually Fe^{++} deficiency anemia
- **Macrocytic – Normochromic Anemia**
  - Large cells
  - Usually folic acid or vitamin B_{12} deficiency anemia
- **Normocytic – Normochromic Anemia**
  - RBCs are normal size and hemoglobin content
  - Usually caused by hemorrhage or hemolysis

20-2

Anemias

- **Normocytic-Normochromic Anemia**
  - **Hemolytic anemia**
    - Anemia due to red cell lysis
    - Fragile cells, infections, drugs, autoimmunity, circulating antibodies
    - Symptoms: enlarged spleen and jaundice
  - **Hemorrhagic anemia**
    - Anemia due to blood loss
    - Surgery or trauma
    - Symptoms: shock and acidosis

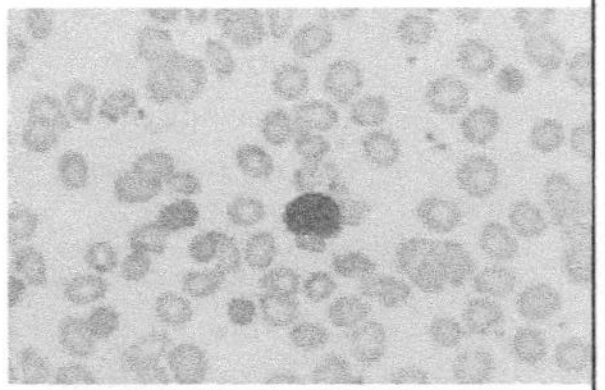

Bain BJ. *Blood Cells: A Practical Guide*, 4e, 2006.

20-2

Anemias

- **Normocytic-Normochromic Anemia**
  - **Anemia of Chronic Disease (ACD)**
    - Bacterial toxins, cytokines from WBCs, suppression of progenitor cells – usually mild
  - **Aplastic Anemia**
    - Bone marrow hypo- or aplasia
    - Causes: acquired due to drugs (chemotherapy), viruses, genetics, and neoplasia
    - Symptoms: petechiae, bleeding, infection, pancytopenia

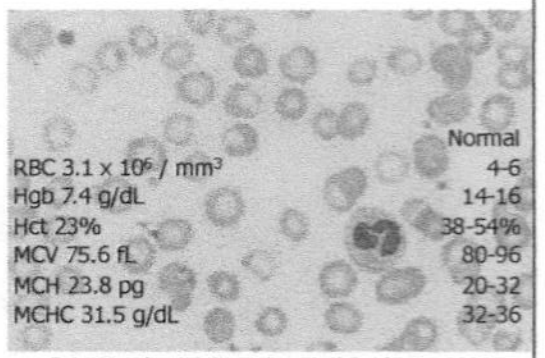
Normal
RBC 3.1 x 10⁶ / mm³ 4-6
Hgb 7.4 g/dL 14-16
Hct 23% 38-54%
MCV 75.6 fL 80-96
MCH 23.8 pg 20-32
MCHC 31.5 g/dL 32-36

Bain BJ. *Blood Cells: A Practical Guide*, 4e, 2006.

20-2

Anemias

- **Macrocytic-Normochromic Anemia**
  - **Pernicious Anemia**
    - Intrinsic factor (IF) deficiency leads to insufficient absorption of vitamin B_{12} which is necessary for developing RBCs.
    - Autoimmunity – autoantibody to gastric parietal cells
    - Symptoms: digestive symptoms, glossitis, peripheral neuropathy (demyelination)
    - Treatment: replace the B_{12}

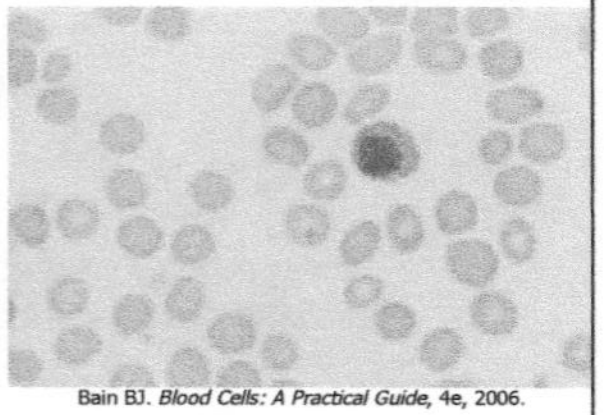

Bain BJ. *Blood Cells: A Practical Guide*, 4e, 2006.

20-2

Anemias

- **Macrocytic-Normochromic Anemia**
  - **Folic Acid Deficiency**
    - Dietary deficiency inhibits DNA synthesis
    - Alcoholics and the malnourished are at high risk
    - Symptoms similar to pernicious anemia, but no neurological symptoms
    - Treatment: replacement therapy

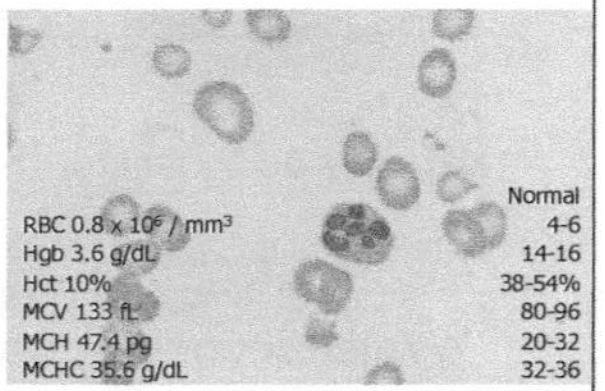
RBC 0.8 x 10^6 / mm^3
Hgb 3.6 g/dL
Hct 10%
MCV 133 fL
MCH 47.4 pg
MCHC 35.6 g/dL
Normal
4-6
14-16
38-54%
80-96
20-32
32-36

Bain BJ. *Blood Cells: A Practical Guide*, 4e, 2006.

20-2

Anemias

- **Microcytic-Hypochromic Anemia**
  - **Iron-Deficiency Anemia**
    - Most common cause is due to excessive bleeding and/or poor diet
    - High risk:
      - Pregnant women, adolescents, children, elderly, or anyone with chronic blood loss

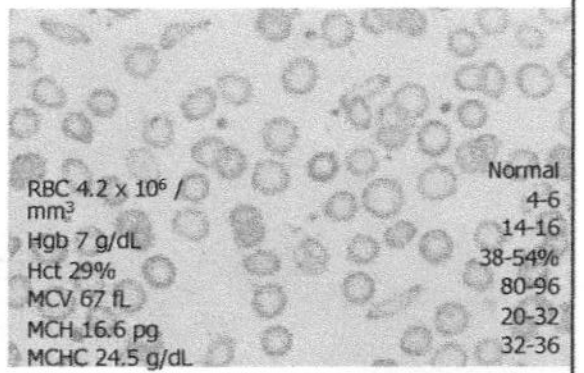
RBC 4.2 x 10^6 / mm^3
Hgb 7 g/dL
Hct 29%
MCV 67 fL
MCH 16.6 pg
MCHC 24.5 g/dL
Normal
4-6
14-16
38-54%
80-96
20-32
32-36

Bain BJ. *Blood Cells: A Practical Guide*, 4e, 2006.

20-2

Iron-Deficiency Anemia

- **Signs and Symptoms**
  - Fatigue, weakness, and shortness of breath
  - Pale earlobes, palms, and conjunctivae
  - Spoon-shaped nails, sore tongue, dryness of the epithelium in the corners of the mouth

Anemias

- **Microcytic-Hypochromic Anemia**
  - **Sideroblastic Anemia**
    - **Dysfunctional iron uptake** by erythroblasts producing sideroblasts and resulting in decreased synthesis of heme
    - Causes
      - lead
      - ethanol
      - other drugs
    - Symptoms
      - hepatosplenomegaly
      - hemochromatosis

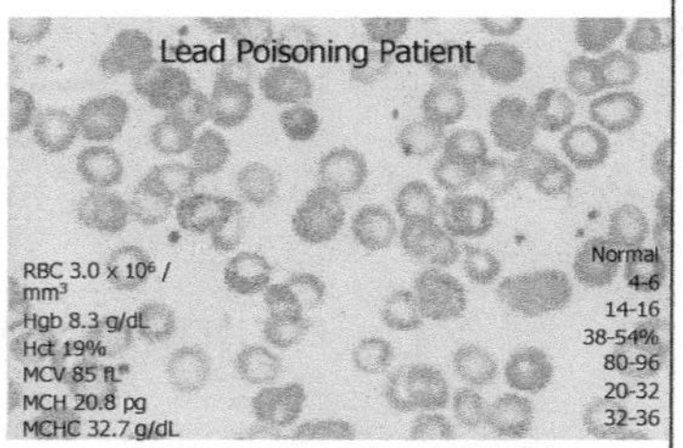
Lead Poisoning Patient
RBC 3.0 x 10^6 / mm^3
Hgb 8.3 g/dL
Hct 19%
MCV 85 fL
MCH 20.8 pg
MCHC 32.7 g/dL
Normal
4-6
14-16
38-54%
80-96
20-32
32-36

Bain BJ. *Blood Cells: A Practical Guide*, 4e, 2006.

Pb can occupy and block this site

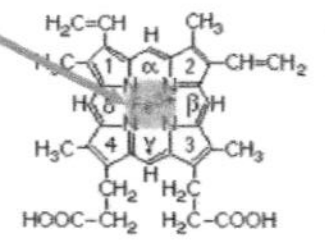

heme

20-2

Nutritional Requirements for the Development of RBCs

Nutrient	Role	Deficiency Consequence
Vitamin B_{12}	DNA synthesis	Macrocytic anemia
Folic Acid	DNA and RNA synthesis	Macrocytic anemia
Iron (Fe)	Hgb synthesis	Microcytic hypochromic anemia

20-2

Polycythemias

- Diseases/conditions that cause excessively large numbers of RBCs in the blood
- Two types, **relative and absolute**
  - **Relative** polycythemia
    - Simply an increase in RBCs due to a loss of plasma
  - **Absolute** polycythemia
    - Primary and secondary

20-3

Absolute Polycythemias

- **Polycythemia Vera (PCV)**
  - Is a primary polycythemia because it is not due to another diagnosis
  - It's a rare, **non-malignant** proliferative abnormality of the bone marrow…hence, it can also affect WBCs and platelets
  - Thought to be caused by hypersensitive bone marrow
  - Hct can be as high as 70-80%
  - It tends to occur in men between the ages of 40-60 of Jewish or European descent

20-3

Absolute Polycythemias

- **Secondary Polycythemia**
  - This is common because its a **physiologic response** to hypoxia
    - Hypoxic conditions
      - Chronic obstructive pulmonary disease (COPD)
      - High altitude
      - Smoking
      - Sleep apnea

20-3

Polycythemia

- **Pathological Effects:**
  - Increased blood viscosity promotes clotting (hypercoagulation) and poor oxygenation in distal tissues.
- **Symptoms**
  - Red color of the face, hands, feet, ears, and mucous membranes
  - High blood pressure, engorgement of retinal and sublingual veins, and hepatosplenomegaly

20-3

Treatment of Polycythemia

- Reduction of red cells and blood volume achieved by performing a therapeutic phlebotomy ("bloodletting"), which helps prevent the hyperviscosity and thrombus formation
- Treat the cause of the hypoxia and the number of red blood cells will decrease

20-3

Neutrophilia

- Granulocytosis or neutrophilia is evident in the first stages of an infection or inflammation.
- If the need for neutrophils increases beyond the supply, immature neutrophils **(band neutrophils, or just "bands")** are released into the blood.
- This premature release is detected in the manual WBC differential and is termed a **"shift-to-the-left"**.

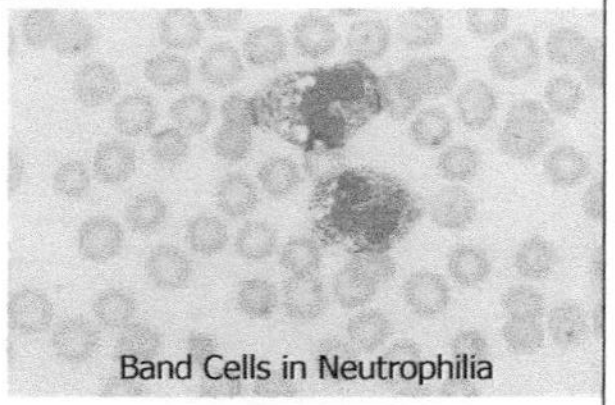
Band Cells in Neutrophilia

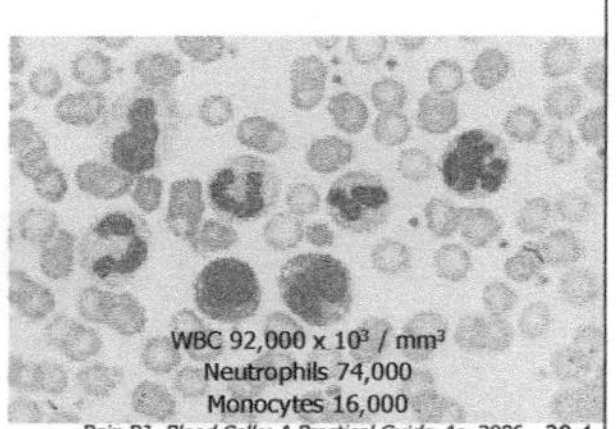
WBC 92,000 x 10³ / mm³
Neutrophils 74,000
Monocytes 16,000

Bain BJ. *Blood Cells: A Practical Guide*, 4e, 2006. 20-4

Neutropenia

- **All etiologies of neutropenia represent severe disease!**
  - Prolonged severe infection
    - Depletes cellular numbers
  - Decreased production
    - Starvation, aplastic bone marrow, **chemotherapy**
  - Reduced survival
    - Autoimmune diseases: lupus and rheumatoid arthritis

20-4

Alterations of Eosinophils

- **Eosinophilia**
  - –Increased in allergic disorders
    - Asthma, hay fever, drug reactions
  - –Increased in parasitic invasions

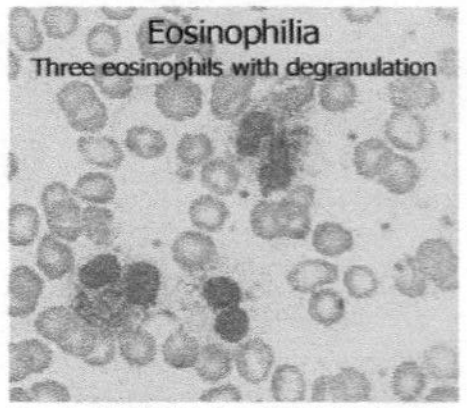
Eosinophilia
Three eosinophils with degranulation

Bain BJ. *Blood Cells: A Practical Guide*, 4e, 2006.

20-I
20-4

Alterations of Monocytes

- **Monocytosis**
  - –Monocytes are needed to phagocytose organisms and debris
  - –Measurement in blood has **poor correlation** with disease
  - –Usually occurs **with neutropenia** in later stages of infections

20-4

Alterations of Lymphocytes

- **Lymphocytosis**
  - –Acute viral infections
  - –Malignancies
    - Lymphocytic leukemias
- **Lymphocytopenia**
  - –Immune deficiencies, drug destruction, viral destruction (AIDS)

20-4

Infectious Mononucleosis

- Acute, self-limiting infection characterized by fever, sore throat, lymphadenopathy, and hepatosplenomegaly
- **Transmitted** by saliva through close personal contact
- Caused by the Epstein-Barr virus (EBV)
  - – Similar symptoms can be caused by other diseases
    - Cytomegalovirus (CMV) and Herpes viruses
- B cells have a **EBV receptor site** making them a primary site of the infection

20-4

Infectious Mononucleosis

- While the peak incidence occurs in 15-17 year-olds, the infection may occur at any age, most often between the ages of 10 and 35
- Lab findings
  - Leukocytosis
    - Lymphocytosis
- Diagnostic test: **Monospot** agglutination test for presence of **heterophilic antibodies**
- Symptomatic treatment

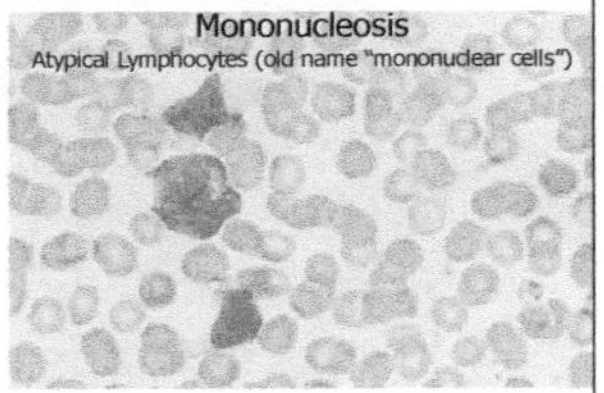
Mononucleosis
Atypical Lymphocytes (old name "mononuclear cells")

Bain BJ. *Blood Cells: A Practical Guide*, 4e, 2006.

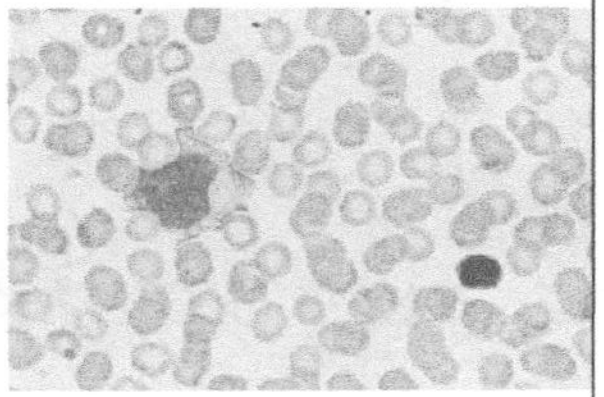

20-5

Leukemias

- Malignant disorder of the blood-forming cells, most commonly white blood cells and blood-forming organs
- **Uncontrolled** proliferation of white blood cells
- Classified by
  - Speed of onset
    - **acute**
    - **chronic**
  - Predominant cell type
    - **myeloid**
    - **lymphoid**

20-6

Leukemias

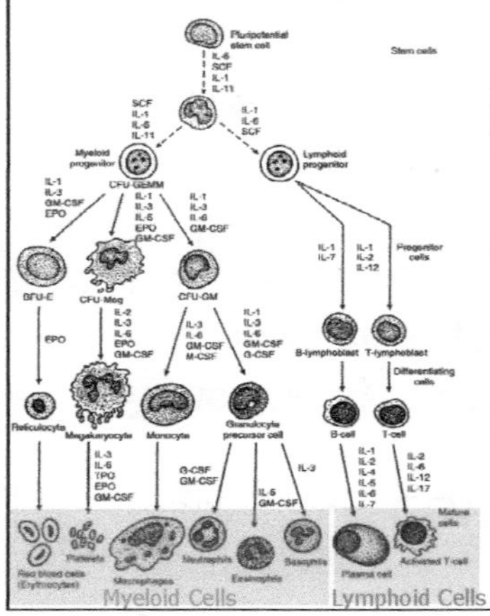
Myeloid Cells
Lymphoid Cells

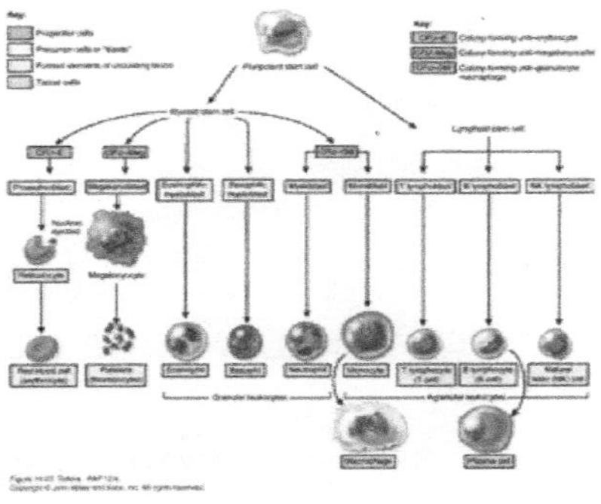

20-6

Leukemias

- **Acute Leukemia**
  - Undifferentiated or immature cells, usually "blasts"
  - Sudden onset of symptoms
  - Acute myeloid leukemia (AML) and acute lymphoid leukemia (ALL)
- **Chronic leukemia**
  - Predominant cells are **well-differentiated** and easily recognized… but they do not function normally
  - Gradual onset with longer survival times
  - Chronic myeloid leukemia (CML) and chronic lymphoid leukemia (CLL)

20-6

Leukemias

- Signs and symptoms are diverse
  - **Asymptomatic (19%)**
  - Splenomegaly
  - Infections
  - Night sweats
  - Fatigue
  - Weight loss
  - Anemia
  - Bleeding

20-6

Leukemias

- Leukemias occur with varying frequencies, depending mostly on age.
- **Adults**
  - Acute myeloblastic (myelocytic) **(AML)**
  - Chronic lymphocytic **(CLL)** most common
- **Children**
  - Acute lymphoblastic (lymphocytic) leukemia **(ALL)** is the most common

20-6

Leukemias of the Myeloid Line

AML

- Acute onset
- Myeloblasts
- Still has poor survival rate

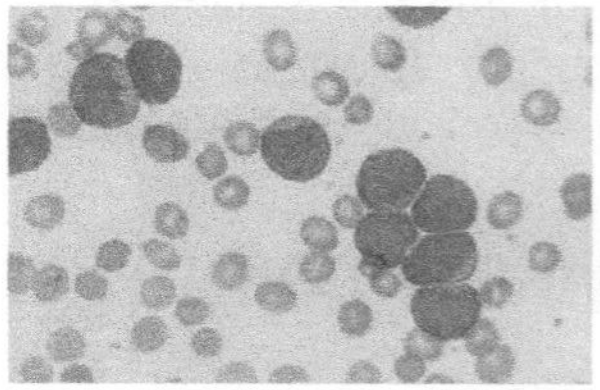

CML

- Gradual onset
- Most demonstrate the Philadelphia chromosome (t9:22)

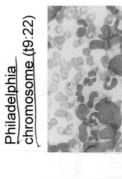

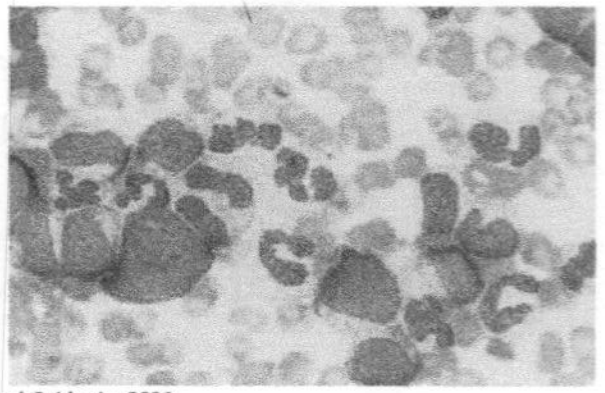

Bain BJ. *Blood Cells: A Practical Guide*, 4e, 2006.

20-6

Lymphoid Leukemias

ALL

- Acute
- B and T cells
- Lymphoblasts

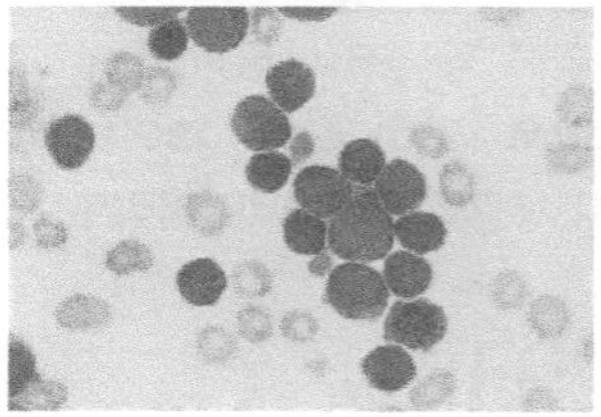

CLL

- Chronic with lengthy survival
- Primarily a diagnosis of the elderly
- Usually B cells

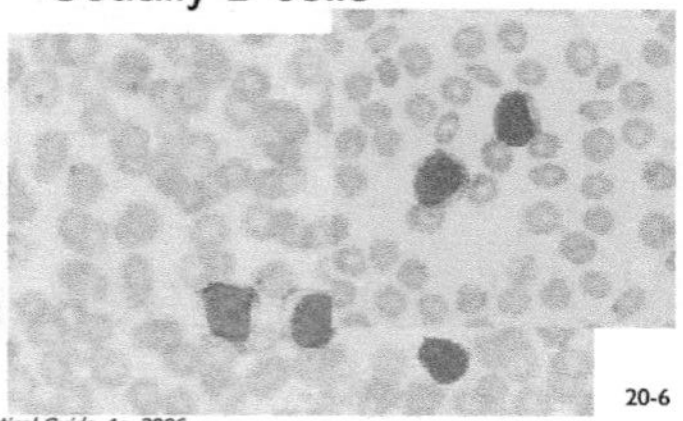

Bain BJ. *Blood Cells: A Practical Guide*, 4e, 2006.

20-6

Multiple Myeloma

- **Plasma cell (B lymphocyte) cancer of the bone marrow**
  - not a leukemia *per se*
- **Plasma cells** usually make up less than 1% of bone marrow cells
- In multiple myeloma, they proliferate to predominate in the marrow
- Usually occurs in people over 50 years old

20-7

Multiple Myeloma

- Characterized by:
  - Its involvement in the bone marrow and multiple other sites throughout the body
  - Destruction of bone
    - Myeloma cells can produce enzymes to infiltrate bone and stimulate **osteoclastic activity.**
  - Abnormal protein production
    - M-protein
    - Abnormal proteins in the urine
      - Bence-Jones proteins

20-7

Multiple Myeloma

- The malignant plasma cells produce abnormally large amounts of one class of immunoglobulin (antibody) or pieces of the immunoglobulin.
- The abnormal immunoglobulin is called the **M protein**
- The light chains of the immunoglobulins **(Bence Jones proteins)** can pass through the glomerulus and damage the renal tubular cells (50% of patients).
- The high plasma protein level causes hyperviscosity of the blood

20-7

Lymphomas

- Proliferation of lymphocytes and their precursors in **lymphoid tissues**
- The major types:
  - Hodgkin's disease (lymphoma)
  - Non-Hodgkin's lymphoma
    - Many diverse types

20-8

Hodgkin Disease

- Etiology remains inconclusive
  - Correlation with Epstein-Barr virus (targets B-cells)
- Bimodal age distribution (19-35 and >50)
- Characterized by the presence of **Reed-Sternberg cells** in the lymph nodes.
  - Usually localized
    - Arises in a **single** lymph node or chain of nodes, and tends to remain fairly localized

20-8

Hodgkin Disease

- Lymphadenopathy in the neck
- Mediastinal node involvement
- Signs
  - fever
  - weight loss
  - **night sweats**
  - pruritis (itching)
- Treatment with radiation and chemotherapy is very effective
  - tumor is localized and can be targeted

20-8

Non-Hodgkin Lymphomas

- Proliferation of lymphocytes in the lymphatic system
- No Reed-Sternberg cells
- Onset of disease is usually after 50
- **Disseminated**
  - Multiple node and organ involvement
- Because this disease is rarely localized, the prognosis for the patient is worse than Hodgkin lymphoma

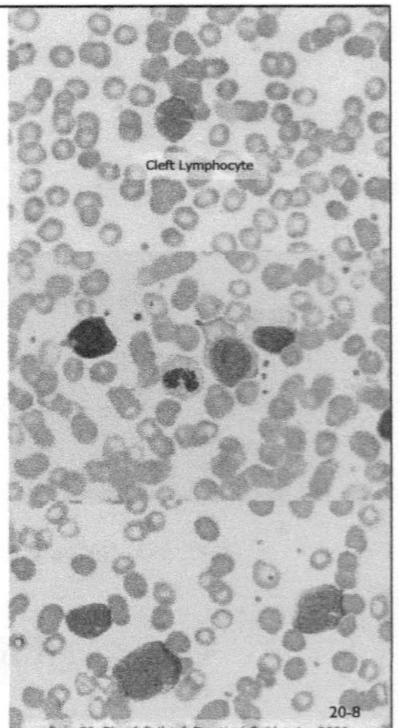
Cleft Lymphocyte
Bain BJ. Blood Cells: A Practical Guide, 4e, 2006.

20-8

Platelet Disorders

- Disorders of platelet **numbers**
  - Thrombocythemia
  - Thrombocytopenia
- Disorders of platelet **function**
  - Adhesion, aggregation, and secretion
- Alterations of platelets and soluble coagulation factors affect hemostasis
  - can prevent it from occurring

  or
  - can cause it to happen when it is not needed

20-9

Disorders of Platelet Numbers

- **Thrombocytopenia**
  - Platelet count < 100,000/mm^3
    - <50,000/mm^3 – hemorrhage from minor trauma
    - <15,000/mm^3 – spontaneous bleeding
    - <10,000/mm^3 – severe bleeding
  - Causes
    - hypersplenism
    - aplastic bone marrow
    - autoimmune disease
    - hypothermia
    - viral or bacterial infections that lead to **disseminated intravascular coagulation (DIC)**
      - more about DIC later

20-9

Disorders of Platelet Numbers

- **Essential** (Primary) **Thrombocythemia**
  - Thrombocythemia is characterized by platelet counts >600,000/mm^3
  - More common in middle age 50-60s
  - **Myeloproliferative disorder** of stem cells in which platelets are produced in excess
  - Risk of microvasculature thrombosis

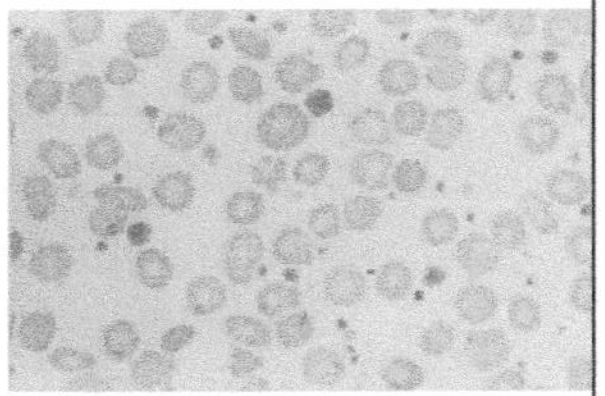

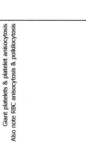

Thrombocytosis
Giant platelets & platelet anisocytosis
Also note RBC anisocytosis & poikilocytosis

20-10

Disorders in Platelet Function

- Platelet numbers can be normal, yet not function correctly.
- Demonstrated by a **normal platelet count**, but an **increased bleeding time (BT).**
- Symptoms: petechiae, mucosal bleeding, and gingival bleeding
- Two types
  - **Acquired** and **congenital**

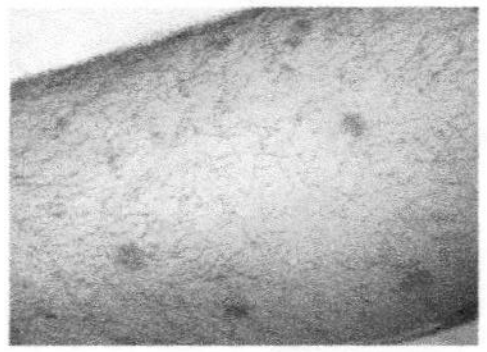

20-11

Disorders in Platelet Function

- **Acquired**
  - Drugs: aspirin and NSAIDs
  - Systemic conditions: renal failure and autoimmune diseases like thrombotic thromboycytopenic purpura (TTP)
  - Hematologic alterations: leukemias
- **Congenital**
  - Disorders of platelet adhesion, aggregation, secretion, and procoagulant activity

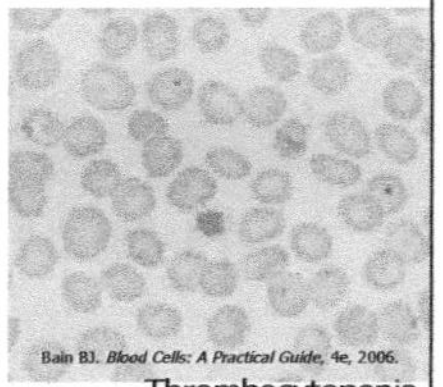
Bain BJ. *Blood Cells: A Practical Guide*, 4e, 2006.

Thrombocytopenia
Single giant platelet
Howell-Jolly bodies (DNA leftovers in RBCs)

20-11

Vitamin K and Clotting

- **Vitamin K** is named after its role in clotting
  - German: *koagulation*
  - vitamin K–dependent clotting factors
    - IX
    - VII
    - X
    - II

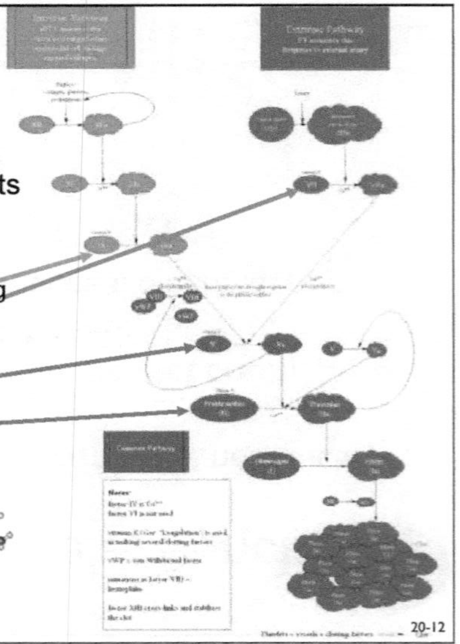

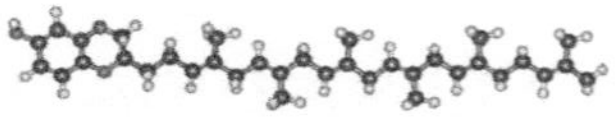

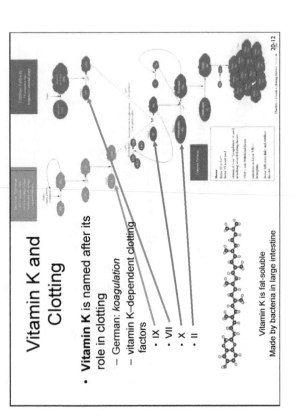

Vitamin K is fat-soluble
Made by bacteria in large intestine

20-12

Alterations of the Coagulation Cascade

- Administration of the drug Warfarin (coumadin) causes temporary, reversible **vitamin K deficiency**
  - Interferes with the synthesis of vitamin K–dependent clotting factors
    - II, VII, IX, and X

20-12

Platelet/Coagulation Disorders

- **Disseminated Intravascular Coagulation (DIC)**
  - Acquired, deadly and fairly common coagulation disorder
  - Excessive utilization of clotting factors
    - Caused by anything that can activate widespread coagulation
    - Infection, inflammation, damaged tissue
  - **DIC** is a disorder in which **clotting** and **hemorrhage** simultaneously occur

20-13

DIC

- Activation of **Intrinsic (Contact) Pathway**
  - Gram-negative sepsis, hypoxia, low blood flow rates
- Activation of **Extrinsic (Tissue) Pathway**
  - Gram-positive toxins, burn injuries, infarctions, surgeries, obstetric accidents, and malignancies
- Activation of **Common Pathway** (factor X)
  - Activated by substances that enter the bloodstream (enzymes, snake venom)

20-13

DIC

- The amount of activated thrombin exceeds the body's anti-thrombins, clotting ensues and **becomes systemic** (not localized)
- The wide-spread thromboses causes **widespread ischemia, infarction**, and organ **hypoperfusion**

20-13

DIC

- The **fibrinolytic system** is also **activated**
  - Plasmin breaks down fibrin and fibrinogen
  - This increases the patient's **fibrin degradation products (FDP)** levels
- The result is a **consumptive coagulopathy** with a high mortality rate
- Treatment is to try and **remove the stimulus**

20-13

Unit 3
Chapter 21
Alterations of Hematologic Function in Children

Hemolytic Disease of the Newborn

- HDN has two main causes:
  - ABO incompatibility – most common, but usually **mild**
  - Rh factor incompatibility – **life threatening**
- **ABO incompatibility**
  - In 20-19% of pregnancies, there is a difference in the fetal and maternal blood types.
  - Only 1 in 10 results in HDN
  - More mild because A and B antigens are poorly developed at birth, and A and B antibodies in plasma typically don't cross the placenta

21-1

Hemolytic Disease of the Newborn

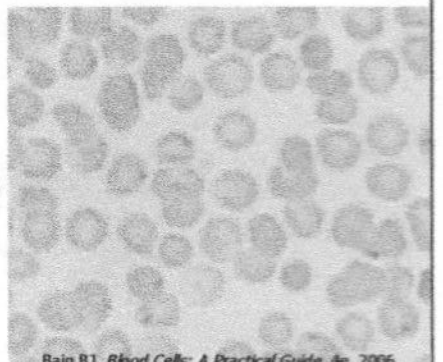

Bain BJ. *Blood Cells: A Practical Guide*, 4e, 2006.

- Rh factor incompatibility
  - The incompatibility occurs when maternal anti-Rh, IgG antibodies cross the placenta and attach to fetal erythrocytes
  - Antibody production occurs in Rh- mothers that have Rh+ babies, not the other way around
  - Rh incompatibility can lead to:
    - Severe anemia, edema, CNS damage, and fetal death
    - Other names: erythroblastosis fetalis and hydrops fetalis

21-1

Hemolytic Disease of the Newborn

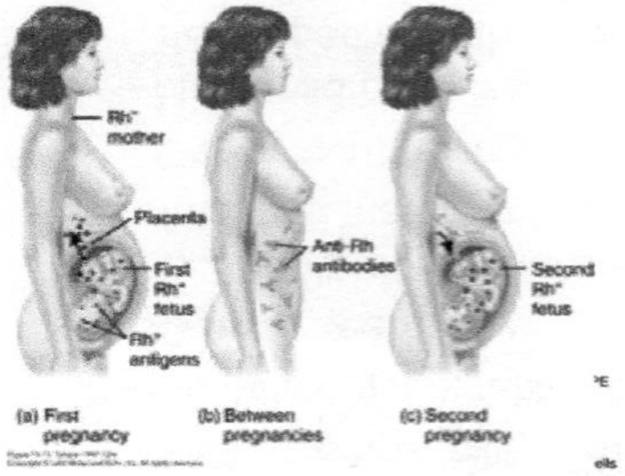

Placenta
First Rh⁺ fetus
Rh⁺ antigens
Anti-Rh antibodies
Second Rh⁺ fetus
(a) First pregnancy
(b) Between pregnancies
(c) Second pregnancy

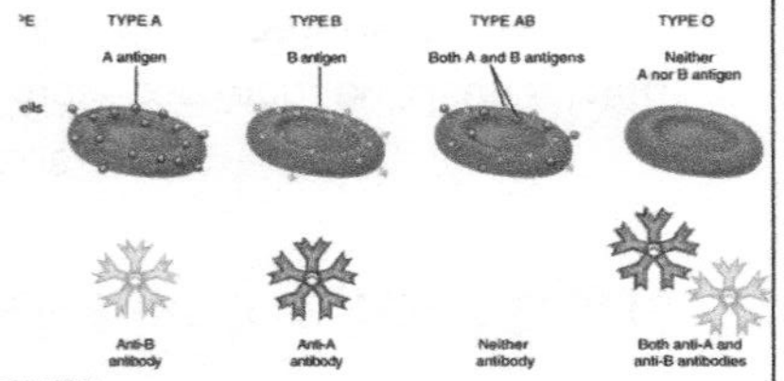

TYPE A
TYPE B
TYPE AB
TYPE O
A antigen
B antigen
Both A and B antigens
Neither A nor B antigen
Plasma
Anti-B antibody
Anti-A antibody
Neither antibody
Both anti-A and anti-B antibodies

21-1

Sickle Cell Anemia

- Autosomal recessive
- Characterized by the presence of an abnormal form of hemoglobin **(hemoglobin S, Hgb S)**
- Hgb S forms when valine replaces glutamic acid in the hemoglobin molecule
  - The side chain of valine is hydrophobic & uncharged
  - The side chain of glutamic acid is hydrophilic & acidic

21-2

Sickle Cell Anemia

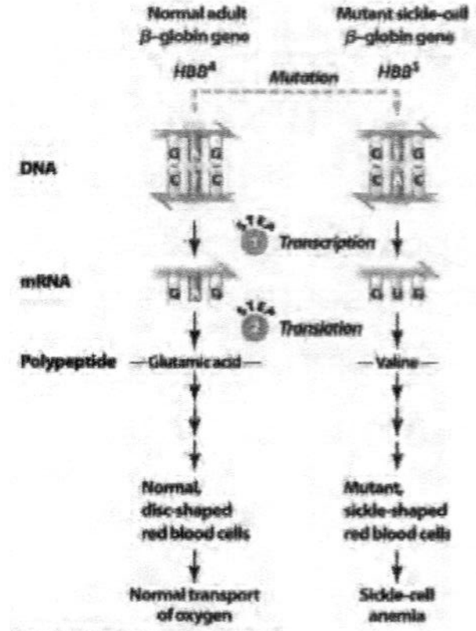

Normal adult β-globin gene
Mutant sickle-cell β-globin gene
Mutation
DNA
Transcription
mRNA
Translation
Polypeptide
Glutamic acid
Valine
Normal, disc-shaped red blood cells
Mutant, sickle-shaped red blood cells
Normal transport of oxygen
Sickle-cell anemia

Principles of Genetics, 5e, Snustad and Simmons

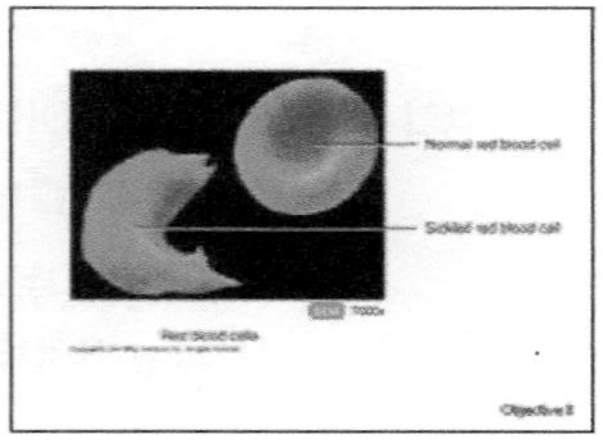

Normal red blood cell
Sickled red blood cell
Red blood cells

21-2

Sickle Cell Anemia

- During episodes of deoxygenation and dehydration, the erythrocyte can stretch and solidify into an elongated sickle shape
- This sickle-shaped cell is susceptible to splenic sequestration and can cause **vasoocclusive crisis (sickle cell crisis)**

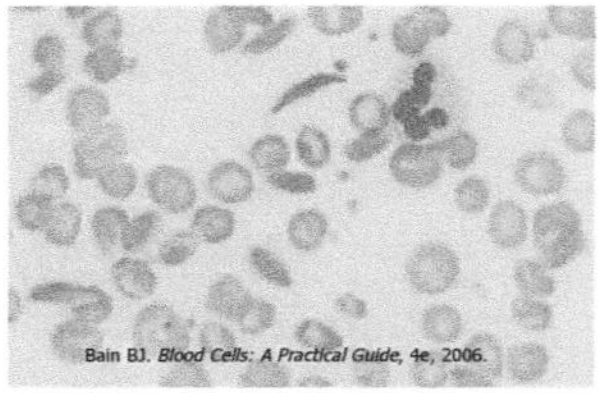

Bain BJ. *Blood Cells: A Practical Guide*, 4e, 2006.

21-2

Thalassemia

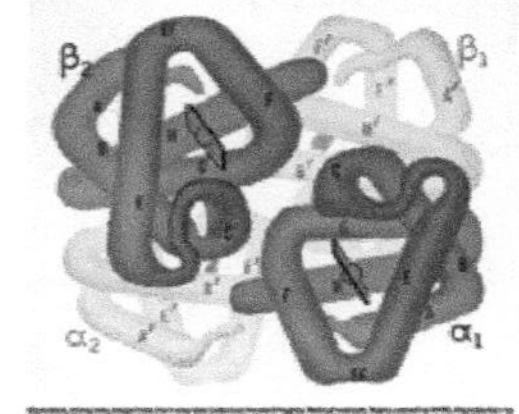

β_2
β_1
α_2
α_1

Karp, Cell and Molecular Biology

- The thalassemias are inherited **autosomal recessive** disorders that cause an impaired rate of synthesis of the alpha (α) or beta (β) hemoglobin chains
- Beta-thalassemia is the most common
  - Defect in β-chain formation
  - Results in too much α-chain
  - The α-chains become unstable and precipitate inside the cells
  - Bone marrow macrophages and the spleen sequester and destroy the cells

21-3

Thalassemias

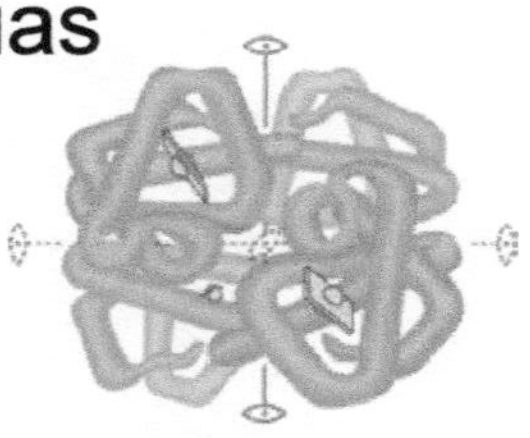

- Thalassemia minor
  - Heterozygous
  - Usually asymptomatic
    - Maybe an enlarged spleen and slightly smaller RBCs
- Thalassemia major
  - Homozygous
  - Severe anemia
  - Regular transfusions required

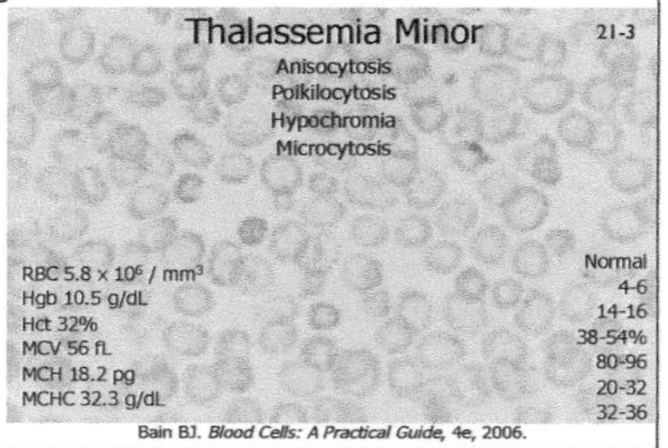

Thalassemia Minor
Anisocytosis
Poikilocytosis
Hypochromia
Microcytosis
RBC 5.8 x 10^6 / mm^3
Hgb 10.5 g/dL
Hct 32%
MCV 56 fL
MCH 18.2 pg
MCHC 32.3 g/dL
Normal
4-6
14-16
38-54%
80-96
20-32
32-36

Bain BJ. *Blood Cells: A Practical Guide*, 4e, 2006.

21-3

Congenital Alterations of the Coagulation Cascade

- The most common of the **inherited disorders** of the coagulation system are the X-linked hemophilias
  - **Hemophilia A**
    - Classical hemophilia
    - X-linked recessive deficiency of factor VIII
    - 1:5000-10,000 male births
  - **Hemophilia B**
    - X-linked recessive deficiency of factor IX
    - 1-30,000 male births

21-4

UNIT 4

Study Guide Objectives – Introductory Pathophysiology (HTHS 2230)

Unit 4

Chapter 5 - Innate Immunity: Inflammation and Wound Healing

1. Define and describe innate immunity (natural immunity). (p. 118)

2. Compare and contrast key components of the first, second, and third lines of defense. (pp. 118-119)

3. Describe the role of inflammation as a response to injury. (p. 121)

4. Identify and describe the local signs of acute inflammation. (pp. 121; 132)

5. Characterize the benefits of inflammation. (pp. 121-122)

6. Describe the following systemic manifestations of acute inflammation: fever, leukocytosis, and increased plasma protein synthesis. (pp. 132-133)

7. Identify and describe the plasma protein systems and their interactions in inflammation: complement system, coagulation system, and kinin system. (pp. 122-124)

8. Characterize the role of the cellular components of inflammation: cytokines, mast cells, and phagocytes. (pp. 125-132)

9. Describe the role of interleukins and interferons in inflammation. (pp. 126-127)

10. Indicate the causes of mast cell degranulation and the effects of the released preformed biomechanical mediators, histamine and neutrophil chemotactic factor. (p. 127)

11. Identify and state the effects of leukotrienes and prostaglandins synthesized by mast cells. (p. 128)

12. Describe the process of phagocyte migration and phagocytosis. (pp. 129-132)

13. Identify the role of neutrophils and macrophages in the inflammatory process. Describe how their functions differ. (pp. 129-130)

14. Characterize chronic inflammation and contrast it with acute inflammation. (pp. 133-134)

15. Define and differentiate between tissue regeneration and repair processes. (p. 134)

16. Identify the adverse factors that affect resolution and result in dysfunctional wound healing. (pp. 136-138)

Chapter 6 - Adaptive Immunity

1. Characterize the third line of defense, adaptive immunity. (pp.142-143)

2. Compare and contrast cell-mediated and antibody-mediated (humoral) immunity. (p. 143)

3. Contrast immunogen, antigen, hapten, allergen, and epitope. Identify criteria that can influence immunogenicity. (p. 144)

4. Describe and give examples of active and passive immunity. (pp. 143-144)

5. Identify and describe the structural components of an antibody. (pp. 146-148)

6. Identify the structure and an important role of each of the five classes of immunoglobulins (antibodies): IgG, IgM, IgE, IgA, and IgD. (p. 146)

7. Describe the actions of antibodies that provide protection against infections: opsonization, neutralization, agglutination, and precipitation. (pp. 149-150)

8. Characterize the secretory immune response. (p. 152)

9. Compare and contrast the titer and the class of immunoglobulin in the primary and secondary immune responses. (p.154)

10. Characterize fetal and neonatal immune function. (p. 162)

11. Describe the major histocompatability complex (MHC) and its influence on the immune response. (pp. 155-156; 198-199)

12. Describe the cluster of differentiation system (CD) for identifying cell-surface molecules. Identify cells that are CD4+ and CD8+.

13. Describe the role of antigen-presenting cells (APCs). (pp. 156-157)

14. Characterize the cellular interactions within the immune response: antigen-presenting cells (APC), T_h cells, T_c cells, T_{reg} cells, B cells, plasma cells, and memory cells. (pp. 156-160)

Chapter 7 - Infection and Defects in Mechanisms of Defense

1. Describe the dynamic relationship between humans and microorganisms. (pp. 165-166)

2. Define the following as they relate to pathologic infections: communicability, toxigenicity, infectivity, pathogenicity, and virulence. (p. 167)

3. Describe the mechanisms of infection and injury by bacteria, viruses, and fungi. (168-174)

4. Characterize examples of primary (congenital) immunodeficiencies: DiGeorge syndrome, Bruton agammaglobulinemia syndrome, Wiskott-Aldrich syndrome, and selective IgA deficiency. (p. 179-181)

5. Compare primary and secondary immunodeficiencies. Cite examples of acquired (secondary) immune deficiencies. (p. 181)

6. Describe the reasons a patient may develop graft-versus-host (GVH) disease. (p. 182)

7. Describe the immune deficiency disorder, AIDS: signs, symptoms, and pathophysiology (pp. 183-186)

8. Define hypersensitivity, allergy, autoimmunity, and alloimmunity. (pp.188-190)

9. Compare and contrast the four hypersensitivities (I, II, III, and IV). (pp. 189-196)

10. Characterize the origin of autoimmune disease. (p. 197)

11. Describe the pathophysiology of systemic lupus erythematosus (SLE): clinical signs and symptoms, and complications. (pp. 197-198)

12. Characterize alloimmune graft rejection and categorize a graft rejection as hyperacute, acute, or chronic based on the immune response. (pp. 199-200)

Unit 4
Chapter 5
Innate Immunity: Inflammation and Wound Healing

Body Defense Systems

- Innate (natural) immunity
  - Chemical and physical barriers
  - **Non-specific** mechanisms
  - **Non-adaptive** mechanisms
- Adaptive (acquired) immunity
  - Both **specific** and **adaptive**

5-1

The First Line of Defense

- First line of defense
  - **Physical** barriers
    - Skin, mucous membranes, vomiting, coughing, urination, defecation
  - **Biochemical** barriers
    - Mucus, perspiration, saliva, tears, cerumen, chemicals derived from normal flora, sebum

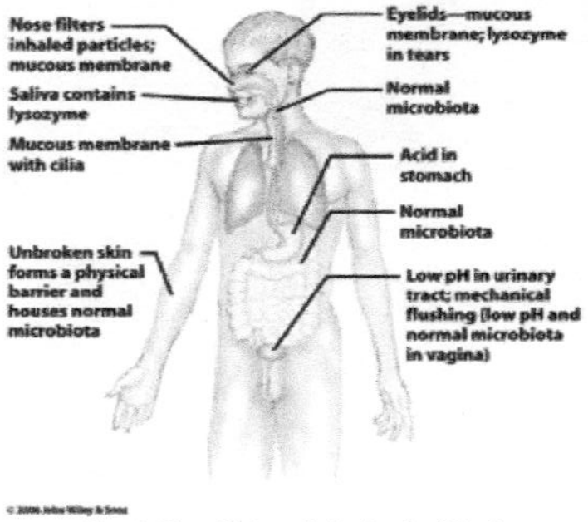
Nose filters inhaled particles; mucous membrane
Saliva contains lysozyme
Mucous membrane with cilia
Unbroken skin forms a physical barrier and houses normal microbiota
Eyelids—mucous membrane; lysozyme in tears
Normal microbiota
Acid in stomach
Normal microbiota
Low pH in urinary tract; mechanical flushing (low pH and normal microbiota in vagina)

Alters & Alters, *Biology: Understanding Life*, 1/e

5-2

Lines of Defense

- Second line of defense
  - Focus of this chapter
    - Inflammation
    - Phagocytosis
- Third line of defense
  - Adaptive, specific immunity
    - Cell-mediated
    - Antibody-mediated ("humoral")

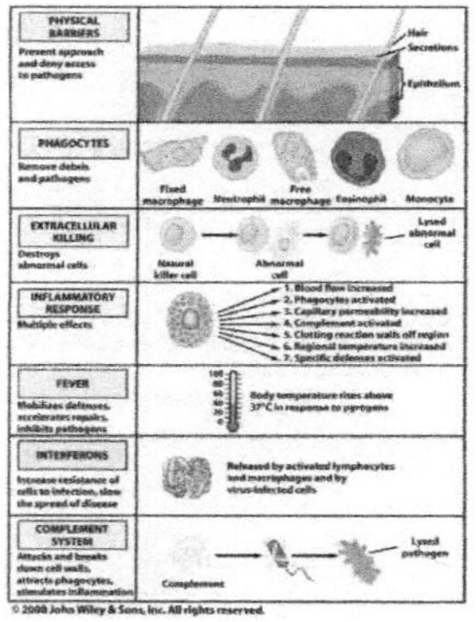
PHYSICAL BARRIERS
PHAGOCYTES
EXTRACELLULAR KILLING
INFLAMMATORY RESPONSE
FEVER
INTERFERONS
COMPLEMENT SYSTEM

5-2

Lines of Defense

- Second line of defense
  - Nonspecific mechanisms of immunity
    - Inflammation
  - Phagocytosis
  - Search and Destroy

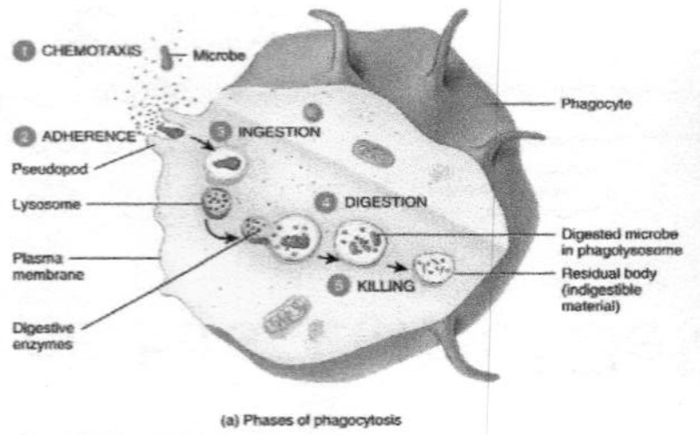

1 CHEMOTAXIS
Microbe
2 ADHERENCE
3 INGESTION
Pseudopod
Lysosome
4 DIGESTION
Plasma membrane
5 KILLING
Digestive enzymes
Phagocyte
Digested microbe in phagolysosome
Residual body (indigestible material)

(a) Phases of phagocytosis

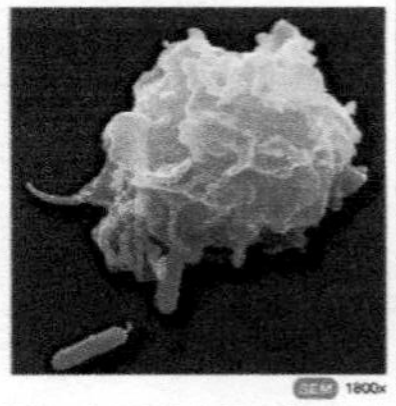

SEM 1800x

(b) Phagocyte (white blood cell) engulfing a microbe

Figure 22.09 Tortora - PAP 12/e

5-2

Innate defenses

Component	*Functions*
First Line of Defense: Skin and Mucous Membranes	
Physical Factors	
Epidermis of skin	Forms a physical barrier to the entrance of microbes.
Mucous membranes	Inhibit the entrance of many microbes, but not as well as intact skin.
Mucus	Traps microbes in respiratory and gastrointestinal tracts.
Hairs	Filter out microbes and dust in nose.
Cilia	Together with mucus, trap and remove microbes and dust from upper respiratory tract.
Lacrimal apparatus (tears)	Dilutes and washes away irritating substances and microbes.
Saliva	Washes microbes from surfaces of teeth and mucous membranes of mouth.
Urine	Washes microbes from urethra.
Defecation and vomiting	Expel microbes from body.
Chemical Factors	
Sebum	Forms a protective acidic film over the skin surface that inhibits growth of many microbes.
Lysozyme	Acts as antimicrobial substance in perspiration, tears, saliva, nasal secretions, and tissue fluids.
Gastric juice	Destroys bacteria and most toxins in stomach.
Vaginal secretions	Discourages bacterial growth by being slightly acidic; flushes microbes out of vagina.
Second Line of Defense: Internal Defenses	
Antimicrobial Proteins	
Interferons (IFNs)	Protect uninfected host cells from viral infection.
Complement system	Causes bursting of microbes, promotes phagocytosis, and contributes to inflammation.
Natural killer (NK) cells	Kill infected target cells by releasing granules that contain perforin. Phagocytes then kill the released microbes.
Phagocytes	Ingest foreign particulate matter.
Inflammation	Confines and destroys microbes and initiates tissue repair.
Fever	Intensifies the effects of interferons, inhibits growth of some microbes, and speeds up body reactions that aid repair.

Ireland, *Visualizing Human Biology*, 2/e

5-2

Inflammation

- Non-specific
- Non-adaptive
  - A secondary exposure to a stimulus will demonstrate the same response as the initial incident
- Immediate
- A universal response to injury occurring in vascular tissues of the body
- Mediated by chemicals found in the circulation
- Increases movement of plasma and blood cells into the tissues surrounding the injury
- Defends against infections
- Promotes tissue repair and healing
- Inflammation is necessary but can be painful and risky

5-3

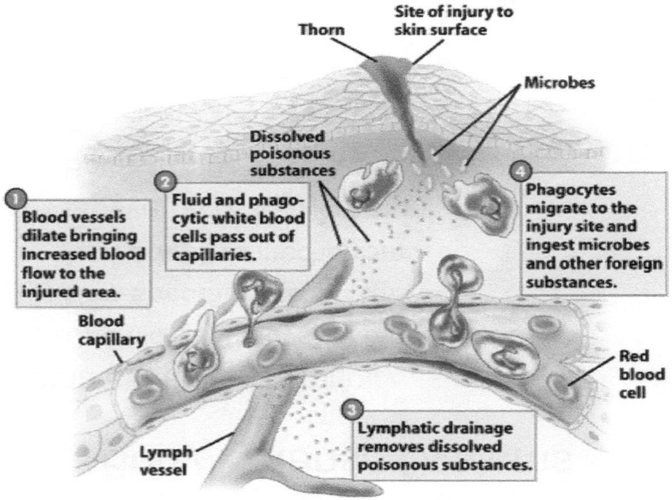

Thorn
Site of injury to skin surface
Microbes
Dissolved poisonous substances
1 Blood vessels dilate bringing increased blood flow to the injured area.
2 Fluid and phagocytic white blood cells pass out of capillaries.
3 Lymphatic drainage removes dissolved poisonous substances.
4 Phagocytes migrate to the injury site and ingest microbes and other foreign substances.
Blood capillary
Red blood cell
Lymph vessel

Alters & Alters, *Biology: Understanding Life*, 1/e

5-3

Local Manifestations of Inflammation

- Local symptoms
  - Changes in the microcirculation
    - Vasodilation
    - Increased capillary permeability
    - White cell migration from the capillaries to the site of inflammation
    - Inflammatory chemicals stimulate nociceptors
  - Observable characteristics
    1. **Heat**
    2. **Redness**
    3. **Swelling**
    4. **Pain**

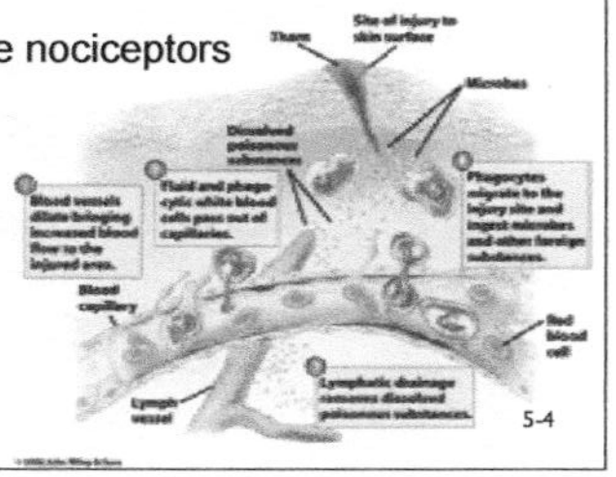

Site of injury to skin surface
Thorn
Microbes
Blood vessels dilate bringing increased blood flow to the injured area.
Fluid and phagocytic white blood cells pass out of capillaries.
Phagocytes migrate to the injury site and ingest microbes and other foreign substances.
Blood capillary
Red blood cell
Lymph vessel
Lymphatic drainage removes dissolved poisonous substances.

5-4

Local Manifestations of Inflammation

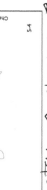

- **Vasodilation** to increase blood flow and decrease blood flow velocity
- Stimulation of endothelial cells to retract and become "leaky".
  - **Exudation** of plasma and blood cells ,clear – clots – pus
    - Serous, fibrinous, purulent, hemorrhagic – bloody
      - Dilutes toxins and toxic products
      - Brings in plasma proteins
      - Removes bacterial products and dead cells
  - **Migration** of immune cells

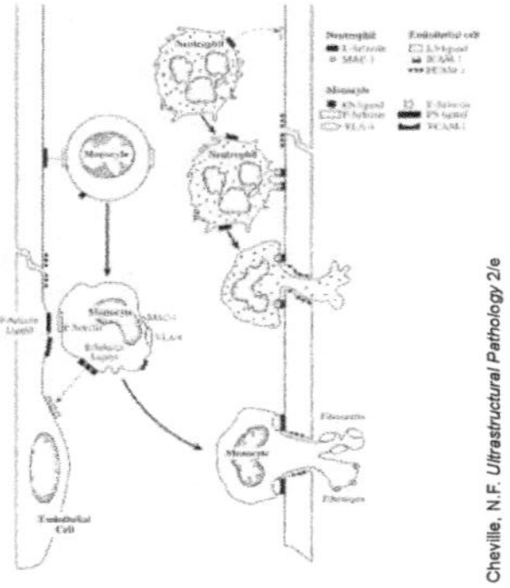

Cheville, N.F. *Ultrastructural Pathology 2/e*

5-4

Exudation – inflamatory – ↑ plasma, ↑ permeability.
Transudation – ↑ BHP blood hydrostatic pressure

2nd line (Inflammation) defense
stim 3rd line defense (adaptive)

Purposes and Benefits of Inflammation

- Destroy injurious agents
- Confine agents to limit their effects on the host
- Stimulate components of the adaptive immune system
- Promote regeneration and repair of tissue

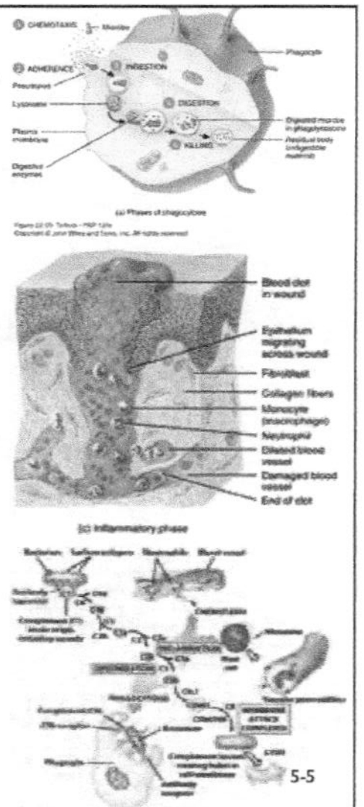

5-5

Systemic Manifestations of Inflammation

- **Fever** – change the thermostat – evidence systemic inflamation. ↑ WBC in blood.
  - Exogenous and endogenous chemical mediators act to reset the hypothalamic thermostat
- **Increase in both pro-inflammatory and anti-inflammatory plasma proteins produced by the liver**
  - Elevates so-called "**acute-phase reactants**" proteins of inflammation.
    - Erythrocyte sedimentation rate (ESR) sinking. mm/hr do RBC's settle
      - rate at which RBCs fall through plasma
      - reflects levels of fibrinogen and adhesion of RBCs
        - » ESR levels increase as acute-phase reactants increase
    - Blood levels of C-reactive protein (CRP) → helps enhance immune response.
      - liver produces this quickly after inflammation
- **Leukocytosis** – more things need to die. – ↑ inflammation
  - Increases circulating neutrophils
    - "Shift-to-the-left"
      - increase in immature granulocytes because of mature neutrophil depletion

5-6

makes RBC's group together + r heavier

hyperthermia – accumulate more heat but you don't want to.

– Rheumatoid arthritis ESR ↑ ~200 mm/hr

Events of Acute Inflammation

- **Activation of three plasma protein systems:**
  - –Complement System (lock + key)
    - Direct or indirect destruction of cells (esp. bacteria)
  - –Coagulation System
    - Isolates infections by trapping pathogens and prevents hemorrhage
  - –Kinin System
    - Interacts with the coagulation system
    - Pro-inflammatory

5-7

the c protein attach to phagocyte the number help it to target one certain thing. so a lab test could know why by the #.

Plasma Protein Systems

- **Complement System**
  - –A group of plasma proteins (C1-9)
  - –Participate at all levels of inflammation
    - Opsonization, chemotaxis, and anaphylaxis
  - –Three pathways
    - Classical
      - – Activated by antigen-antibody complexes
    - Alternative and Lectin
      - – Activated by biologic substances (bacteria, fungi, toxins)
      - – Non-antibody dependent

5-7

complement protein. break it & activate next step

WBCs follow chemical trail/gradient.

flagging for eating to know which ones to eat.

MAC - membrane attack complexes. (1-9) full complement attack cells.

Complement System

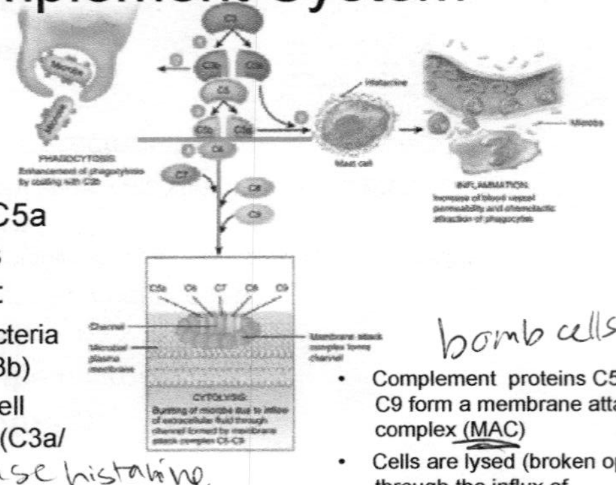

PHAGOCYTOSIS
INFLAMMATION
CYTOLYSIS

- C1 activates a cascade of C2-C5a which enhances inflammation by:
  - – **Opsonizing** bacteria (end product C3b) (flagging)
  - – Inducing mast cell **degranulation** (C3a/ C5a) (release histamine)
    - This, in turn, encourages neutrophil chemotaxis
- Complement proteins C5b-C9 form a membrane attack complex (MAC) (bomb cells.)
- Cells are lysed (broken open) through the influx of extracellular fluids

5-7

Complement System

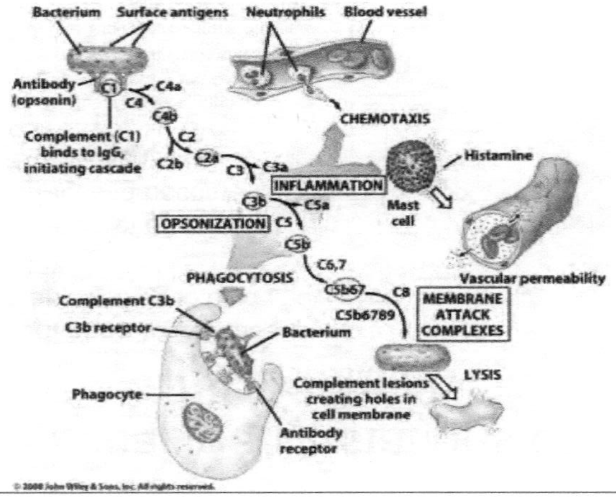

Bacterium
Surface antigens
Neutrophils
Blood vessel
Antibody (opsonin)
C1
C4a
C4
C4b
Complement (C1) binds to IgG, initiating cascade
C2
C2b
C2a
C3
C3a
CHEMOTAXIS
Histamine
INFLAMMATION
C3b
C5a
Mast cell
OPSONIZATION
C5
C5b
C6,7
PHAGOCYTOSIS
C5b67
C8
Vascular permeability
Complement C3b
C3b receptor
C5b6789
MEMBRANE ATTACK COMPLEXES
Bacterium
LYSIS
Phagocyte
Complement lesions creating holes in cell membrane
Antibody receptor

5-7

Plasma Protein Systems

- **Coagulation system**
  - Stops bleeding
  - Localizes microorganisms
  - Provides a meshwork for healing
- **The Kinin System**
  - Activated by the coagulation system (intrinsic pathway)
  - The primary kinin is bradykinin
  - Augments inflammation (pro-inflammatory): vascular permeability, vasodilation, smooth muscle contraction

ex) Erythropoitien from kidney cell to bone marrow cell.

Cellular Components of Inflammation

- **Cytokines** – chem signal from one cell to initiate response in another cell.
  - More than 100 different cytokines have been discovered.
  - Chemical signal from one cell that affects another
  - It's how cells talk!
  - Can be pro- or anti-inflammatory
  - Examples:
    - Interleukins, interferons, chemokines, etc.

Interleukins

communication btwn WBCs

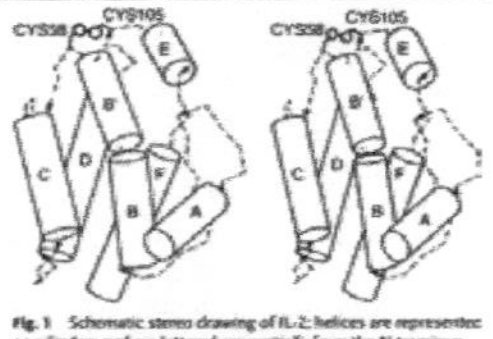
CYS58
CYS105
CYS58
CYS105
A
B
C
D
E
F

Fig. 1 Schematic stereo drawing of IL-2: helices are represented as cylinders and are lettered sequentially from the N-terminus. (Reprinted with permission from Brandhuber et al. (1987) Science 238, 1707. Copyright 1987 by American Association for the Advancement of Science.)

- Cytokines produced primarily by macrophages and lymphocytes in response to microorganisms and products of inflammation
  - Encourages cell adhesion molecule expression
  - Chemotaxis
  - Proliferation and maturation of white blood cells
  - Both pro- and anti-inflammatory

Interferons

- Proteins (IFN-α, IFN-β, IFN-γ) produced to protect against viral infections and encourage the immune system. encourage chemotaxis
  - Defense against viral infections
  - Made by leukocytes to help other cells defend against viruses

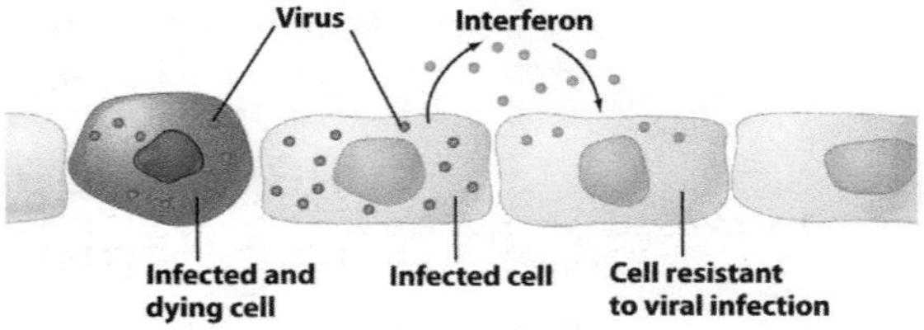
Virus
Interferon
Infected and dying cell
Infected cell
Cell resistant to viral infection

Ireland, *Visualizing Human Biology*, 2/e

try to control the spread to other cells

Mast Cells

huge bags chem

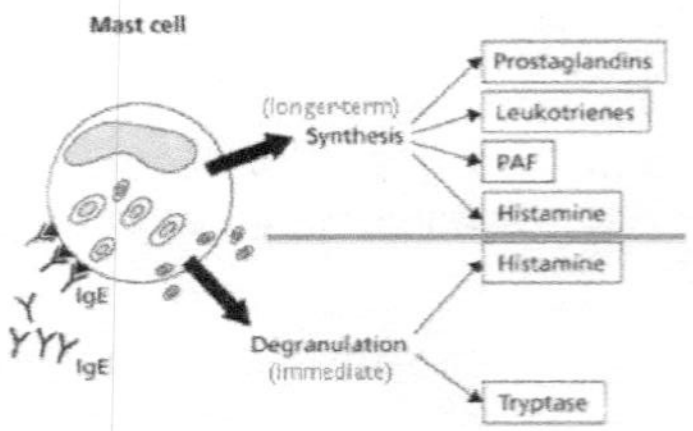

Mast cell
(longer-term)
Synthesis
Prostaglandins
Leukotrienes
PAF
Histamine
Histamine
IgE
IgE
Degranulation
(immediate)
Tryptase

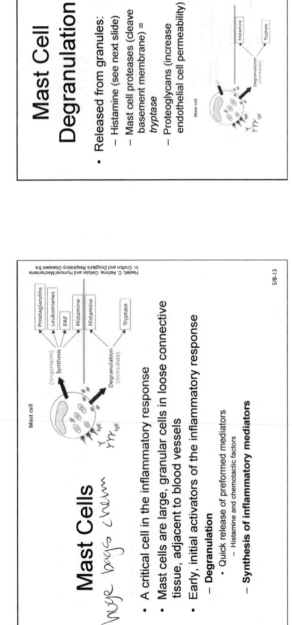

- A critical cell in the inflammatory response
- Mast cells are large, granular cells in loose connective tissue, adjacent to blood vessels
- Early, initial activators of the inflammatory response
  - **Degranulation**
    - Quick release of preformed mediators
      - Histamine and chemotactic factors
  - **Synthesis of inflammatory mediators**

Haslett, C. Asthma: Cellular and Humoral Mechanisms
In: *Crofton and Douglas's Respiratory Diseases 5/e*

5/8-13

Mast Cell Degranulation

- Released from granules:
  - Histamine (see next slide)
  - Mast cell proteases (cleave basement membrane) = *tryptase*
  - Proteoglycans (increase endothelial cell permeability)

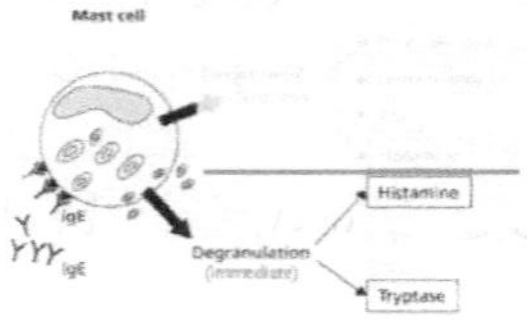

Mast cell
IgE
IgE
Histamine
Degranulation
Tryptase

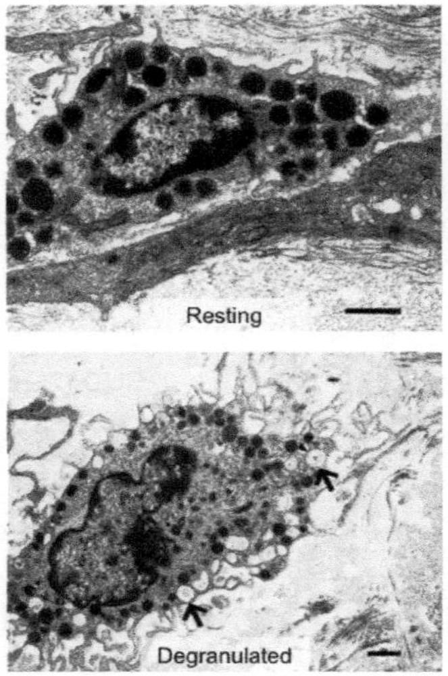

Resting
Degranulated

Bradding P and Cruse G. Mast Cells: Biological Properties and Role in Health and Allergic Diseases In: *Allergy and Allergic Diseases*

5/8-13

Effects of Histamine

- The effects of histamine relate to type of histamine receptors on the cells.
  - **Inflammation**
    - **Causes vasodilation of capillaries**
    - **Increases vascular permeability**
  - Contracts smooth muscle in the bronchi, GI tract, and uterus
  - Increases bronchial, intestinal, and salivary secretions
  - Dilation of cerebral blood vessels (headache)
  - Stimulates secretion of gastric juices
  - Stimulates nerve endings to cause pain and itching

asthma inhaler broncho dilator

5/8-13

Mast Cell Mediator Synthesis

- These are made by the mast cell when it is stimulated
- Lipid mediators
  - Prostaglandins
  - Leukotrienes
  - Platelet-activating factor (PAF)

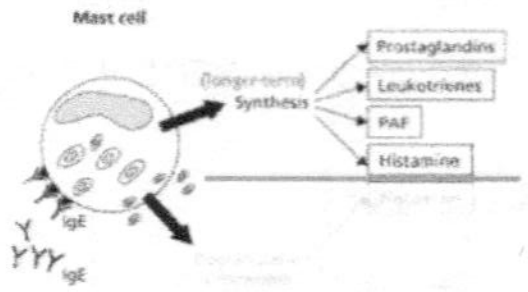

Mast cell
(longer-term)
Synthesis
Prostaglandins
Leukotrienes
PAF
Histamine
IgE
IgE

Haslett, C. Asthma: Cellular and Humoral Mechanisms
In: *Crofton and Douglas's Respiratory Diseases 5/e*

5/8-13

Leukotrienes

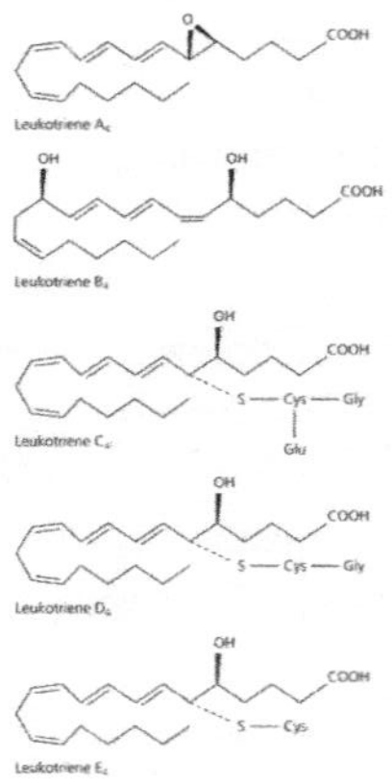

Leukotriene A4
Leukotriene B4
Leukotriene C4
Leukotriene D4
Leukotriene E4
COOH
OH

Allergy and Allergic Diseases, v. 1, 2/e

- Produce histamine-like effects
- Slower, more prolonged response
- Leukotrienes play an important role in the pathophysiology of asthma
- Leukotriene inhibitors used for more severe forms of asthma and also to prevent exercise-induced asthma; may be helpful in allergic rhinitis
  - Montelukast (Singulair™)
  - Zafirlukast (Accolate™)
  - Zileuton (Zyflo™)

5/8-13

Prostaglandins

- Encourage vascular permeability, chemotaxis, and pain
- Prostaglandins (PGs) are made by enzymes called cyclo-oxygenases (COX)
- Non-steroidal anti-inflammatory drugs (NSAIDs, such as aspirin) are COX inhibitors

5/8-13

Phagocytosis and Phagocyte Migration

- **Rolling**
  - Cells slowed by interaction with endothelium
- **Margination**
  - Increased stickiness by producing adhesion proteins on the cell
- **Diapedesis**
  - Emigration through the retracted endothelial junctions and basement membrane
- **Exudation**
- **Phagocytosis**

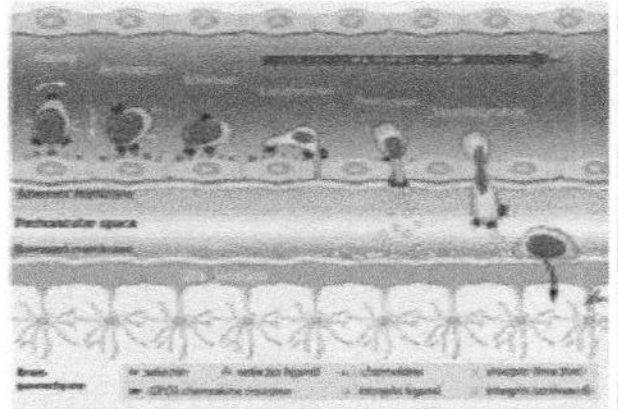

Perivascular space

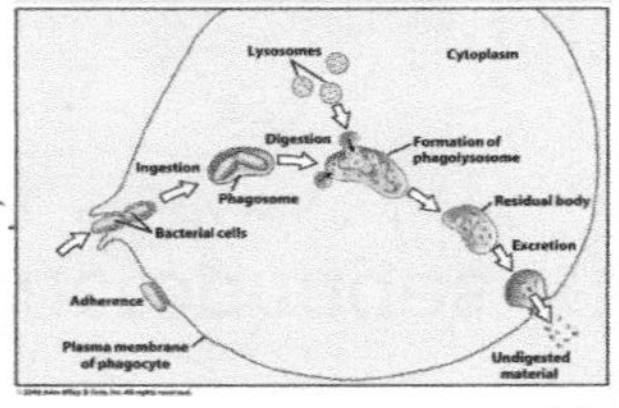

Lysosomes
Cytoplasm
Digestion
Formation of phagolysosome
Ingestion
Phagosome
Bacterial cells
Residual body
Excretion
Adherence
Plasma membrane of phagocyte
Undigested material

5/8-13

Neutrophils and Macrophages

- Neutrophils
  - 70% of WBCs, live 5 days on average (die by apoptosis)
  - "Dive into pus and die" (Linda Clayton)
  - Phagocytose invaders, then drop chemical bombs on them to kill them

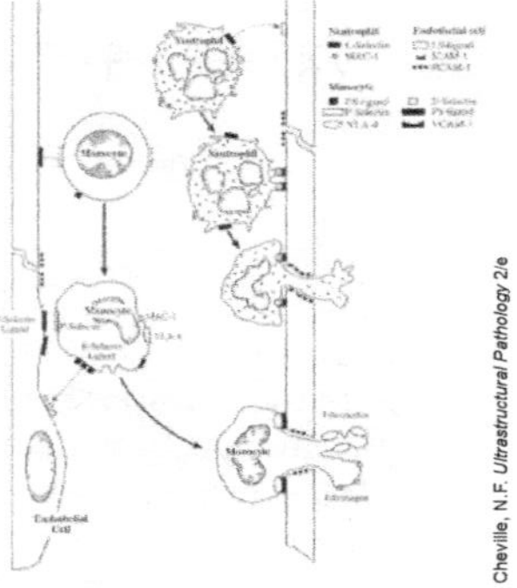

Cheville, N.F. Ultrastructural Pathology 2/e

5/8-13

Neutrophils and Macrophages

more chronic + cleanup tissue

- Macrophages
  - Migrate into tissues, where they lie in wait as macrophages
  - Enter the site after 24-hours to help replace the neutrophils
  - Survive longer than neutrophils
  - **Professional antigen-presenting cells** (more about this later)

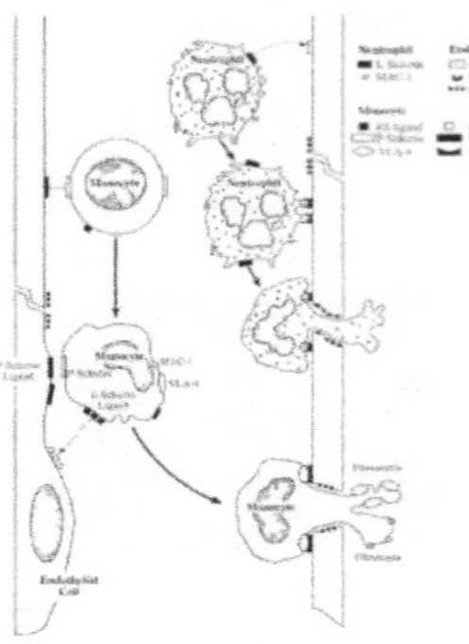

Cheville, N.F. *Ultrastructural Pathology 2/e*

5/8-13

Chronic Inflammation

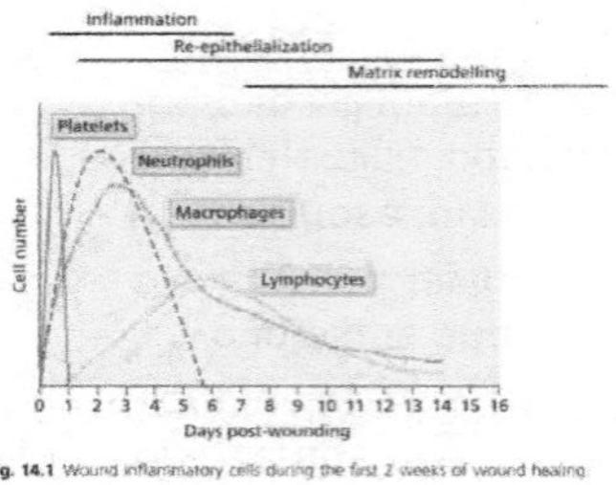

Inflammation
Re-epithelialization
Matrix remodelling
Platelets
Neutrophils
Macrophages
Lymphocytes
Cell number
0 1 2 3 4 5 6 7 8 9 10 11 12 13 14 15 16
Days post-wounding

Fig. 14.1 Wound inflammatory cells during the first 2 weeks of wound healing.

Rook's Textbook of Dermatology, Volume 1, Eighth Edition

- The difference between acute and chronic inflammation is simply **duration**; chronic inflammation lasts longer than 2 weeks
- Think about it: Chronic inflammation is often the result of unsuccessful acute inflammation.
- Chronic inflammation occurs when the body fails to remove the cause of the inflammation
  - Weak pathogens
  - Large, resistant or persistent pathogens
  - Weak immune response

5-14

Chronic Inflammation

- Histologically, acute and chronic inflammation are different
  - Chronic inflammation demonstrates a dense infiltration of lymphocytes and macrophages
    - If macrophages can't protect the tissue from damage, the body will protect itself by walling off the infected site, forming a **granuloma**
  - **Granulomas** are formed by macrophages which join together like bricks in a wall to encircle the offender

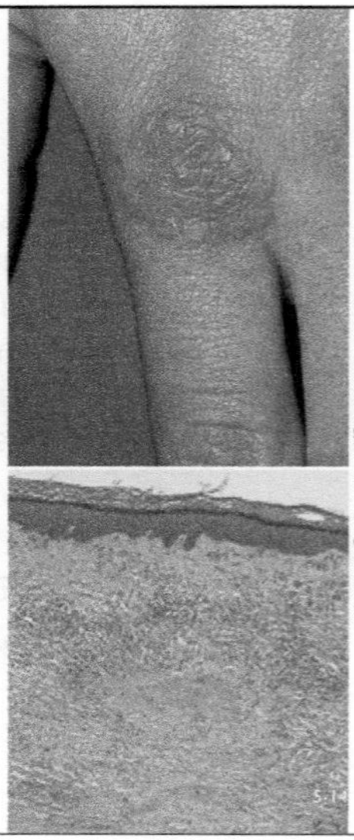

Rook's Textbook of Dermatology, Volume 1, Eighth Edition

Wound Healing

- The goal of healing in inflammation is the **regeneration** of the tissue
  - Regeneration results in the restoration of the structure, therefore function
- If a tissue isn't able to adequately regenerate because the wound is large, fibrin persists in the lesion, or if granulomas form, the wound will likely be **repaired,** not regenerated.
- **Repair** is the replacement of destroyed tissue with scar tissue
  - Scar tissue restores strength, but not function

5-15

Wound Healing

- The first step is to clean up the wound by phagocytizing particulate matter (fibrin, microorganisms, RBCs, and dead cells)
  - This cleanup process is called **debridement**
- Afterwards, healing continues by:
  - Filling in the wound
  - Covering/sealing the wound
  - Shrinking the wound

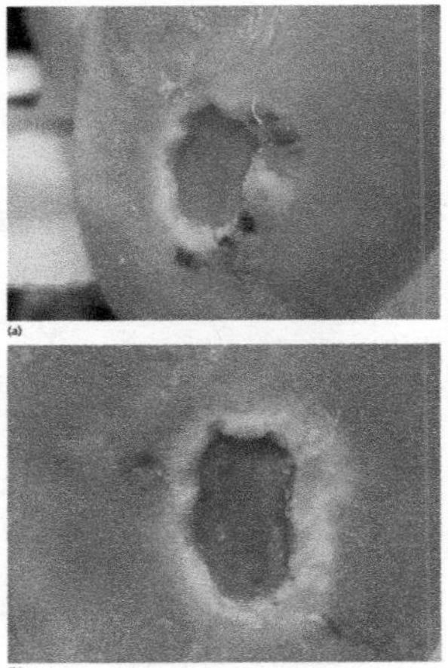

(a) (b)

Fig. 14.6 Neuropathic ulcer of the sole before (a) and after (b) debridement. (Courtesy of the Diabetic Foot Clinic, King's College Hospital, London.)

Rook's Textbook of Dermatology, Volume 1, Eighth Edition

5-15

Wound Healing

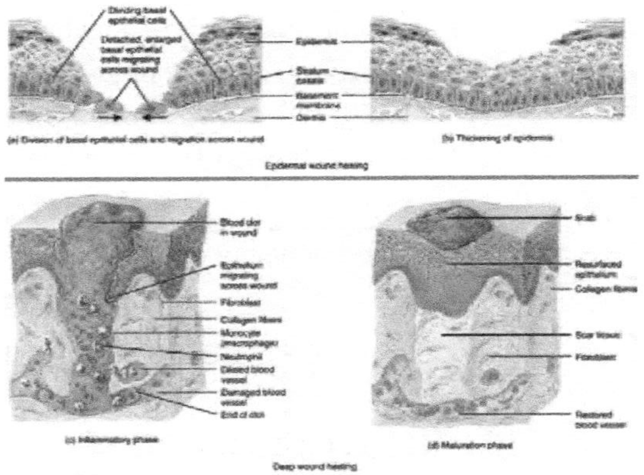

5-15

Wound Healing

- **Simple wounds** (minimal tissue loss) are regenerated and healed by **primary intention**
  - Examples: paper cut, incised wounds, sutured laceration
- Healing of a **open-wound** requires more tissue replacement and healing occurs through **secondary intention**
  - Examples: pressure sore, non-sutured laceration, burns

5-15

Regeneration and Repair Stages

- **Phase I: Inflammation**
  - Coagulation and infiltration of cells to facilitate healing
  - Debridement and angiogenesis
- **Phase II: Proliferation and New Tissue Formation**
  - Fibroblast proliferation, collagen synthesis, and epithelialization
- **Phase III: Remodeling and Maturation**
  - Cellular differentiation, scar tissue remodeling, capillaries removed from scar tissue

5-15

Dysfunctional Wound Healing

- Dysfunction during inflammatory phase
  - Hemorrhage
  - Infection
  - Chronic inflammation (excess granuloma formation)
- Affected by:
  - Diabetes, hypoxia, nutritional deficiency, reactivation of inflammatory responses, and anti-inflammatory medications

5-16

Dysfunctional Wound Healing

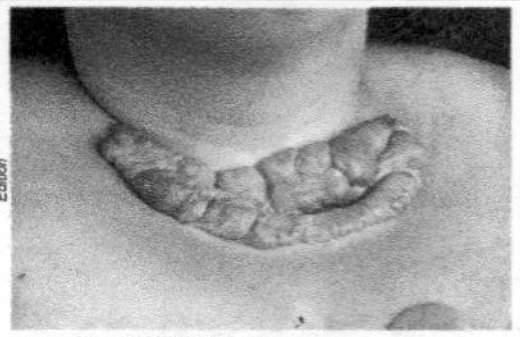

Rook's Textbook of Dermatology, Volume 1, Eighth Edition

Fig. 45.38 Spontaneous keloids of the neck.

- Impaired collagen synthesis from nutritional deficiency
  - Lack of vitamin C (scurvy), iron, calcium, and copper
- Excessive collagen synthesis
  - Adhesions, hypertropic and keloid scars
- Wound disruption
  - Reopening **(dehiscence)** due to collagen disruption
    - Wound healing by primary intention is now healing by secondary intention
- Excessive wound contraction
  - Vasoconstriction

5-16

Unit 4
Chapter 6
Adaptive Immunity

Acquired Immunity

- Third line of defense:
  - **Specific**
    - Responds to a unique pathogen
  - **Adaptive**
    - Variable response
  - Two components:
    - Cell-mediated
    - Antibody-mediated ("humoral")

6-1

Lymphocytes

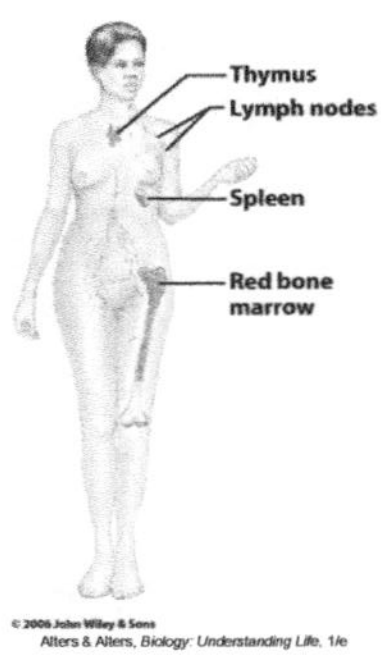

Thymus
Lymph nodes
Spleen
Red bone marrow
© 2006 John Wiley & Sons
Alters & Alters, Biology: Understanding Life, 1/e

- **Lymphocytes** are the most important cells of the **adaptive** immune response
  - They make up only 20-40% of the circulating WBCs, but there are many more in the secondary lymph organs
- Lymphocytes originate in the bone marrow as lymphocyte precursors or stem cells
- They mature either in the bone marrow or in the lymph system
  - Here, the precursor cells will differentiate into functional lymphocytes
    - T cells (in the thymus)
    - B cells (in the bone marrow)

B cells were originally named because they were discovered in the chicken Bursa of Fabricius. Luckily, bone marrow also starts with "B".

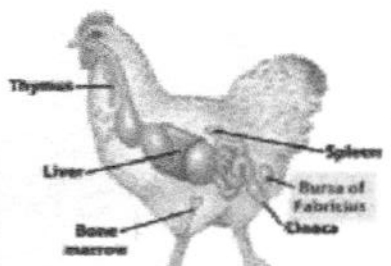

Thymus
Liver
Bone marrow
Spleen
Bursa of Fabricius
Cloaca

6-2

Black, Microbiology: Principles and Explorations, 7/e

Lymphatic System

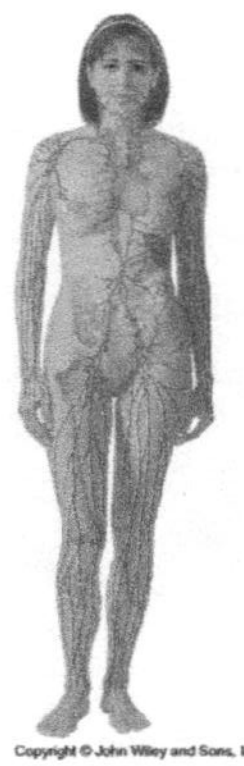

- Lymphocytes are very specific for certain antigens
- They must circulate in the lymphatic system to have the highest chance of coming in contact with their antigenic match
- The success of the immune system hinges on the cooperation and function of both **cell-mediated** and **antibody-mediated (humoral)** immunities

6-2

Activated B Lymphocytes Are Plasma Cells

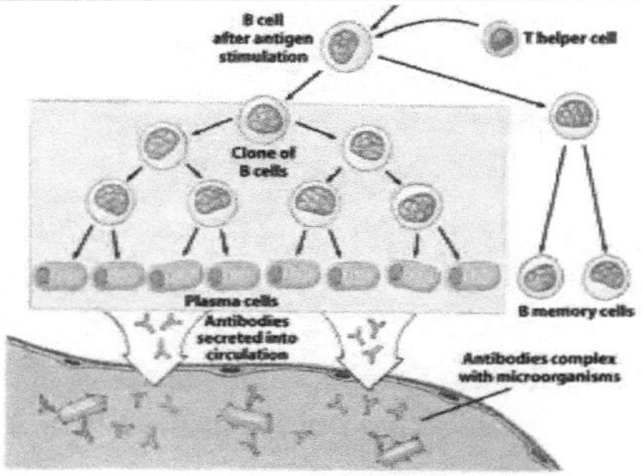

B cell after antigen stimulation
T helper cell
Clone of B cells
Plasma cells
Antibodies secreted into circulation
B memory cells
Antibodies complex with microorganisms

Black, Microbiology: Principles and Explorations, 7/e

- B lymphocytes
  - When stimulated, either directly or indirectly, B lymphocytes develop into **plasma cells**
  - The proteins released from plasma cells are antibodies
  - This is called **antibody-mediated (humoral)** immunity

6-2

T Lymphocytes Cooperate

- T lymphocytes
  - Recognize specific antigens
  - Can directly attack abnormal cells
  - Mediate adaptive immune responses
  - This is called **cell-mediated immunity**

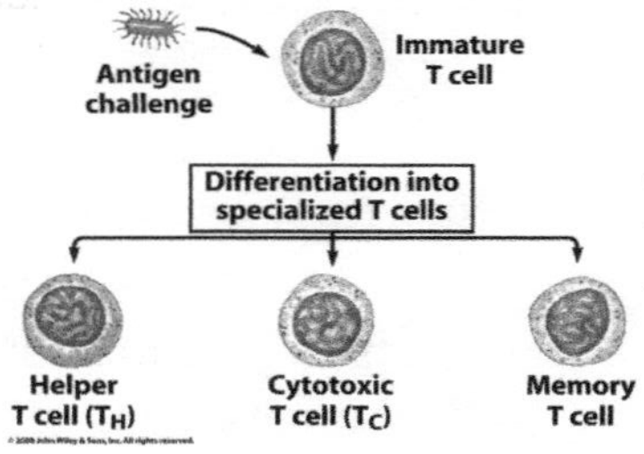

Antigen challenge
Immature T cell
Differentiation into specialized T cells
Helper T cell (T_H)
Cytotoxic T cell (T_C)
Memory T cell

Black, Microbiology: Principles and Explorations, 7/e

6-2

Immunogen versus Antigen

- Immunogen
  - Molecule that will induce an immune response
- Antigen
  - Molecule or molecular fragment that bind with products of the immune system (antibodies, T-cells, and B-cells)
    - Identifies the cell as self or non-self
    - Identifies the type of cell
    - Examples:
      - Viruses, bacteria, fungi, parasites, pollens, foods, drugs, cell markers, tumor cell markers

6-3

Antigen

- A **molecule** or **molecular fragment** is more immunogenic/antigenic if it is:
  - **Large** in size
    - 100 amino acids in a small protein would work
  - **Organic**
  - **Complex** in structure
  - **Foreign,** "non-self", or at least recognized as non-self

6-3

Haptens and Allergens

- A **hapten** is a molecule that is not large enough to react with the immune response by itself.
- It may trigger an immune response when bound to a larger molecule
  - Medications may act as haptens if they bind to something like a RBC surface protein and it could then become immunogenic
- An **allergen** is an antigen that induces an allergic response.

6-3

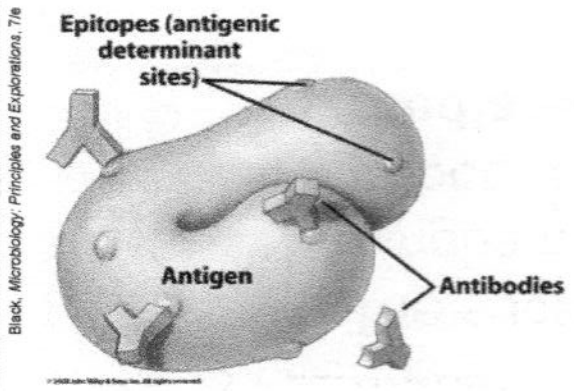

Black, Microbiology: Principles and Explorations, 7/e
Epitopes (antigenic determinant sites)
Antigen
Antibodies

Epitopes = Antigenic Determinants

- If an antigen is large and complex enough, there can be multiple immunogenic portions of the antigen
- These are called **antigenic determinants** or **epitopes**
  - If a patient has acute hepatitis B, they will produce at least three different antibodies to the virus
    - HBsAb, HBcAb, HBeAb
    - HBsAb is produced when a person is vaccinated for HBV

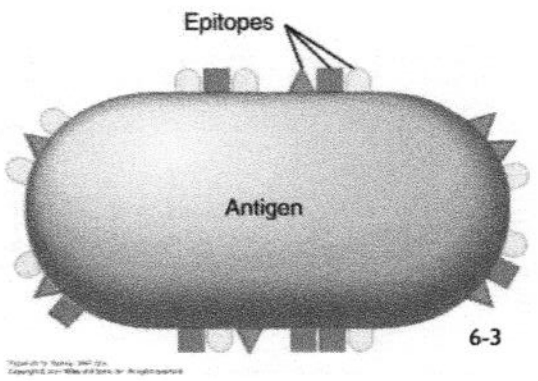

Epitopes
Antigen

6-3

Acquired Adaptive Immunity

- Natural Immunity
  - Immunity not gained through modern medicine
- Artificial Immunity
  - Immunity gained through artificial means
- Active Immunity
  - The body responds to a pathogen (antigen) to make antibodies (long-term immunity)
- Passive Immunity
  - The body simply receives antibodies with no effort of its own. (short-term immunity)
- Active immunity is long-term; passive is short-term.

6-4

Acquired Adaptive Immunity

- Examples
  - Natural active
    - Hepatitis A stimulates the production of anti-hepatitis A antibodies
  - Natural passive
    - A baby receives antibodies from its mother through the placenta and breast milk.
  - Artificial active
    - A person receives an injection of an attenuated (changed/weakened) pathogen that stimulates the body to form an antibody
  - Artificial passive
    - Injection of prepared antibody

6-4

Antigen and Antibody

- The adaptive immune system responds to antigens (antigens trigger adaptive immune responses)
- One of the results of this is production of an antibody
- An antibody is a protein molecule that can bind strongly to an antigen
  - binding is so strong, it's almost covalent (i.e., permanent)
  - antibodies are made in billions of different forms to bind any molecule the immune system may encounter

6-5

Immunoglobulins (Antibodies)

- Known by a few names: gamma globulins, immunoglobulins, and antibodies
- Immunoglobulins (Ig) are distinguished by a number of characteristics
  - Distinguished by structure, location, and function
    - **Classes: IgM, IgG, IgA, IgE, IgD**

6-5

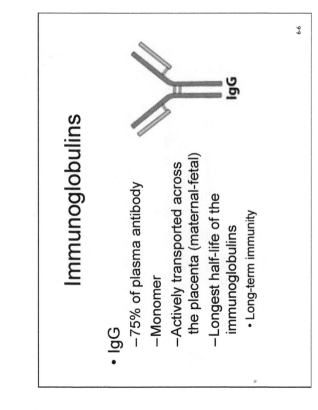

Immunoglobulin Structure

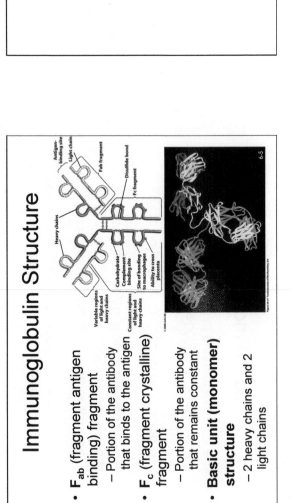

- F_{ab} (fragment antigen binding) fragment
  - Portion of the antibody that binds to the antigen
- F_c (fragment crystalline) fragment
  - Portion of the antibody that remains constant
- **Basic unit (monomer) structure**
  - 2 heavy chains and 2 light chains

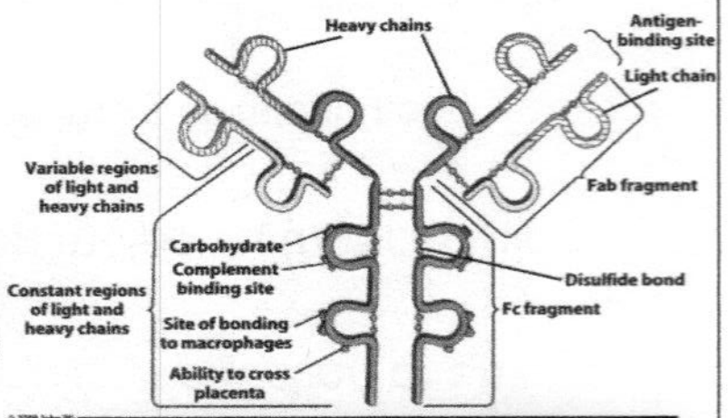

Heavy chains
Antigen-binding site
Light chain
Variable regions of light and heavy chains
Fab fragment
Carbohydrate
Complement binding site
Disulfide bond
Constant regions of light and heavy chains
Fc fragment
Site of bonding to macrophages
Ability to cross placenta

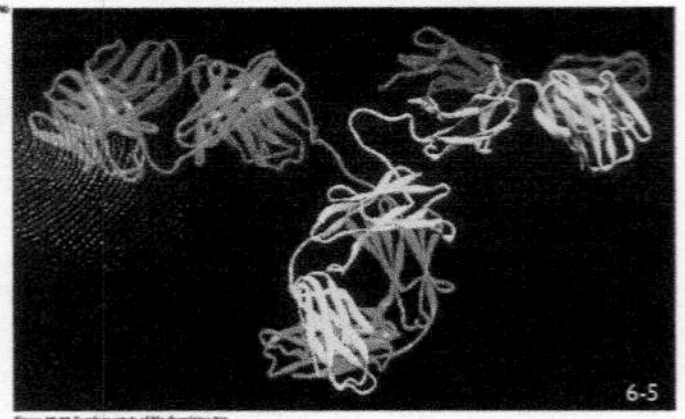

6-5

6-5

Antibody Classes

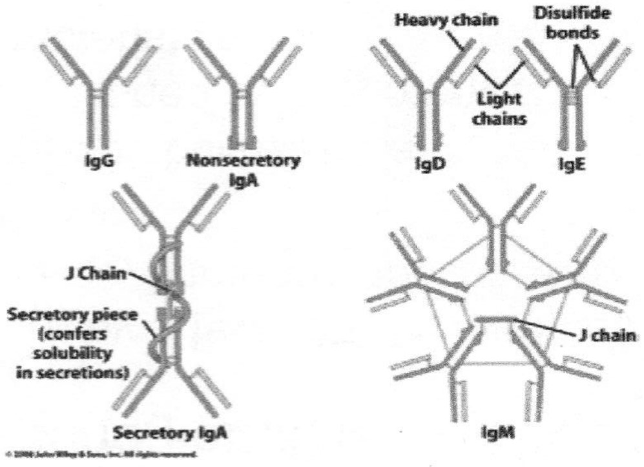

Heavy chain
Disulfide bonds
Light chains
IgG
Nonsecretory IgA
IgD
IgE
J Chain
Secretory piece (confers solubility in secretions)
Secretory IgA
J chain
IgM

6-6

Immunoglobulins

- IgM
  - 10% of total plasma antibody
  - Pentamer
  - 10 heavy & 10 light chains
  - **Very effective activator of the complement system**

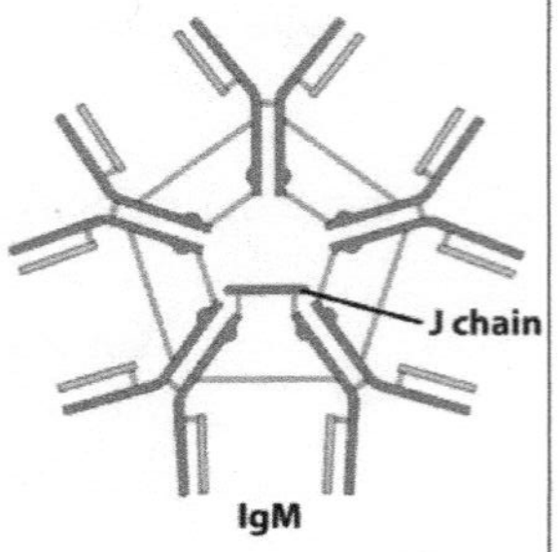

J chain
IgM

6-6

Immunoglobulins

- IgG
  - 75% of plasma antibody
  - Monomer
  - Actively transported across the placenta (maternal-fetal)
  - Longest half-life of the immunoglobulins
    - Long-term immunity

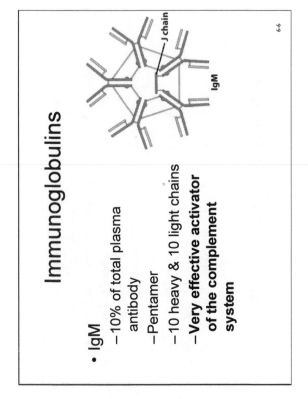

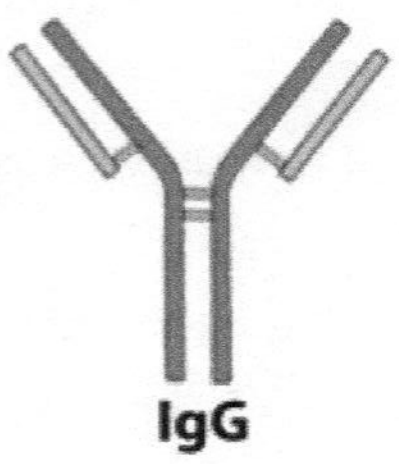

IgG

6-6

Immunoglobulins

- IgA
  - Located in the plasma and body secretions
  - sIgA - Contains a secretory component
    - Protects from enzymatic destruction
  - Lacrimal glands, salivary glands, and lymphoid tissues in the breasts, bronchi, intestines, and GI tract
  - Protects against pathogens that are inhaled, swallowed, or come in contact with external surfaces.

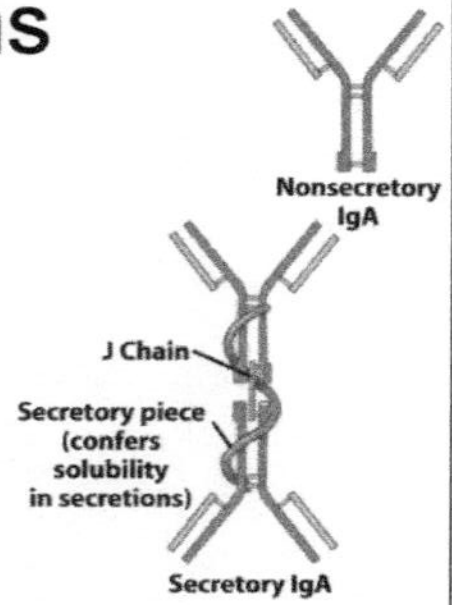
Nonsecretory IgA
J Chain
Secretory piece (confers solubility in secretions)
Secretory IgA

6-6

Immunoglobulins

- IgE
  - Low plasma concentration
  - Bound to eosinophils, basophils and mast cells
  - Triggers release of histamine from mast cells

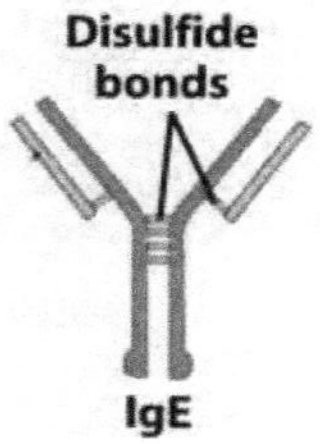
Disulfide bonds
IgE

6-6

How Antibodies Work

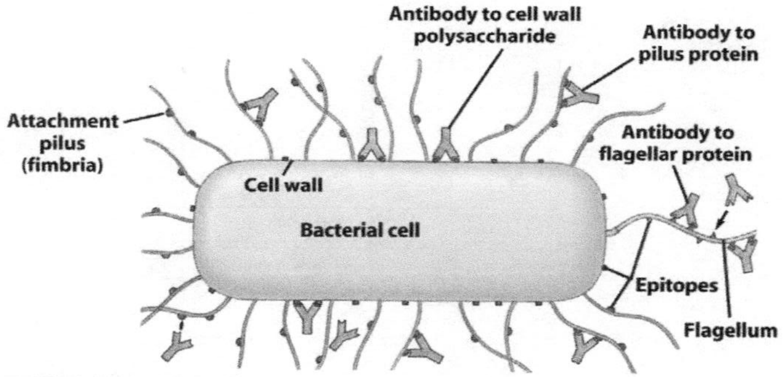
Antibody to cell wall polysaccharide
Antibody to pilus protein
Attachment pilus (fimbria)
Antibody to flagellar protein
Cell wall
Bacterial cell
Epitopes
Flagellum

6-7

Secretory Immune System

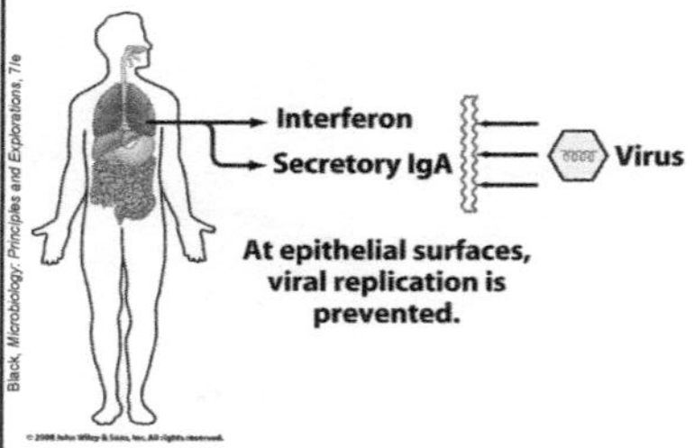
Interferon
Secretory IgA
Virus
At epithelial surfaces, viral replication is prevented.

Black, Microbiology: Principles and Explorations, 7/e

- IgA secreted in gut by **mucosal-associated lymphoid tissue (MALT)**
- These are similar to lymph nodes, but protrude into gut lumen
- **M cells** found in **Peyer's patches** within gut wall pass antigens from lumen to the MALT beneath
- There, B cells are stimulated to make IgAs
- Other epithelial surfaces use a similar system

6-8

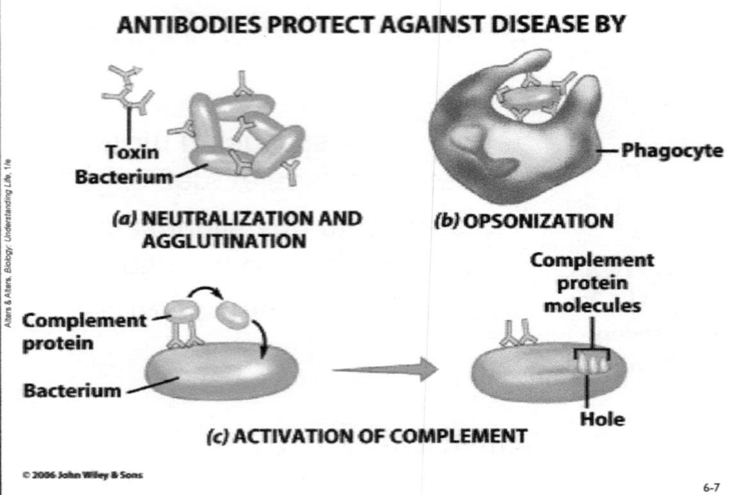
ANTIBODIES PROTECT AGAINST DISEASE BY
Toxin
Bacterium
(a) NEUTRALIZATION AND AGGLUTINATION
Phagocyte
(b) OPSONIZATION
Complement protein
Bacterium
Complement protein molecules
Hole
(c) ACTIVATION OF COMPLEMENT
Alters & Alters, Biology: Understanding Life, 1/e
© 2006 John Wiley & Sons

6-7

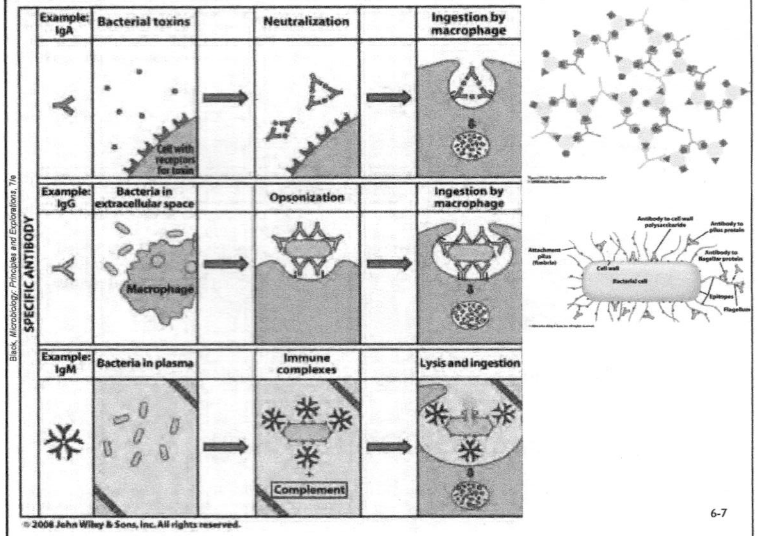
SPECIFIC ANTIBODY
Example: IgA
Bacterial toxins
Cell with receptors for toxin
Neutralization
Ingestion by macrophage
Example: IgG
Bacteria in extracellular space
Macrophage
Opsonization
Ingestion by macrophage
Example: IgM
Bacteria in plasma
Immune complexes
Complement
Lysis and ingestion
Black, Microbiology: Principles and Explorations, 7/e
© 2008 John Wiley & Sons, Inc. All rights reserved.

6-7

Primary vs Secondary Immune Responses

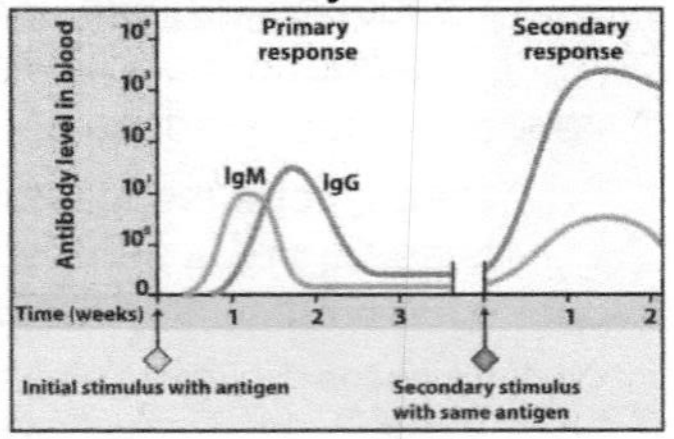
Antibody level in blood
Primary response
Secondary response
IgM
IgG
Time (weeks)
Initial stimulus with antigen
Secondary stimulus with same antigen

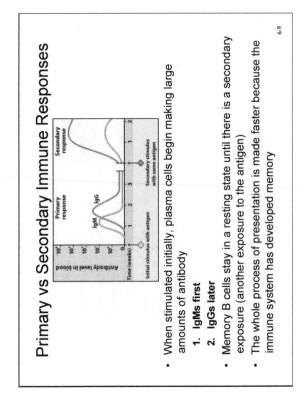

- When stimulated initially, plasma cells begin making large amounts of antibody
  1. **IgMs first**
  2. **IgGs later**
- Memory B cells stay in a resting state until there is a secondary exposure (another exposure to the antigen)
- The whole process of presentation is made faster because the immune system has developed memory

6-9

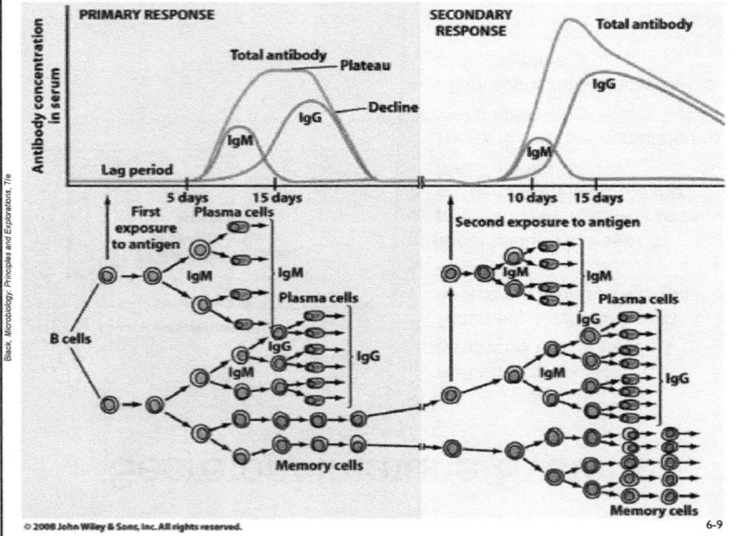
PRIMARY RESPONSE
SECONDARY RESPONSE
Antibody concentration in serum
Total antibody
Plateau
Decline
IgM
IgG
Lag period
5 days
15 days
10 days
First exposure to antigen
Second exposure to antigen
Plasma cells
B cells
Memory cells
Black, Microbiology: Principles and Explorations, 7/e
© 2008 John Wiley & Sons, Inc. All rights reserved.

6-9

Fetal and Neonatal Immunity

- Innate immunity is functioning (at reduced capacity) at birth
  - about half of newborns have rash (*erythema toxicum neonatorium*) as flora colonize skin, causing inflammation
  - IgG crosses the blood-placental barrier
    - At birth, baby's IgG levels are in equilibrium with mother's so baby has a natural passive immunity
    - Baby produces no IgG of his/her own at birth
  - IgM does not cross the blood-placental barrier
    - Must be made by newborn
    - Newborn levels 20% those of adult, and it takes about 2 years to reach adult levels
  - IgA levels very low at birth
    - Adult values of salivary IgA reached at about 2 months
    - Mother's breast milk provides passive natural immunity via her secreted IgA

6-10

Major Histocompatibility Complex (MHC Molecules and Human Leukocyte Antigens)

- The major histocompatibility complex is a group of genes on chromosome 6.
- MHC genes code for MHC proteins
- The MHC genes are grouped in classes (class I, class II, and class III)
- Because of their role in tissue transplants, the MHC molecules are also referred to as human leukocyte antigens (HLA).
  - A patient has a blood type, and they also have an HLA type.

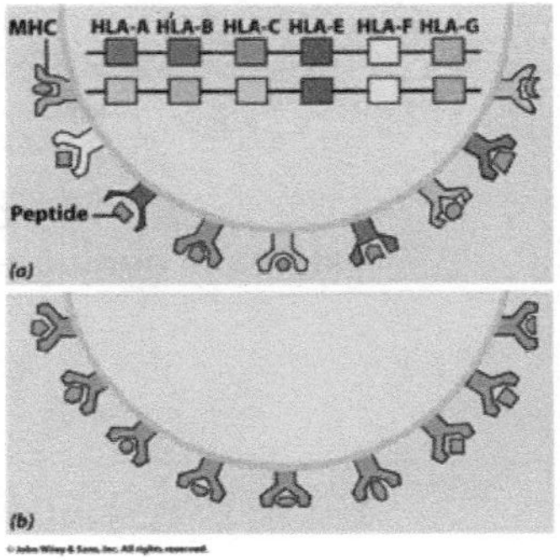

MHC
HLA-A HLA-B HLA-C HLA-E HLA-F HLA-G
Peptide
(a)
(b)

Karp, *Cell and Molecular Biology: Concepts and Experiments*, 6/e

6-11

Cell Surface Markers of Immune Cells Major Histocompatibility Complex (Human Leukocyte Antigens)

- MHC molecules are the "flags" that identify cells
  - who they belong to
  - what organ/tissue they belong to
- MHC molecules also play a role in the immune response by providing information about what the cell has encountered.
  - What the antigen-presenting cell "ate"
    - Exogenous antigen
  - Whether a cell is infected with a virus
    - Endogenous antigen

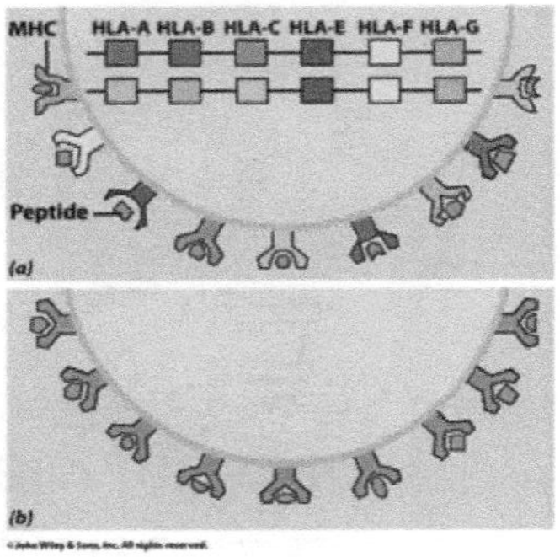

MHC
HLA-A HLA-B HLA-C HLA-E HLA-F HLA-G
Peptide
(a)
(b)

Karp, *Cell and Molecular Biology: Concepts and Experiments*, 6/e

6-11

Human Leukocyte Antigen Genes Code for Major Histocompatibility Complex Proteins

- **MHC (HLA) class I** molecules are located on all nucleated cells
  - Present endogenous antigen
- **MHC (HLA) class II** molecules are located on "professional" antigen presenting cells (APCs)
  - Macrophages, dendritic cells and some B lymphocytes
  - Present exogenous antigen

6-11

MHC Class I Molecules: "This Cell Is Virally Infected"

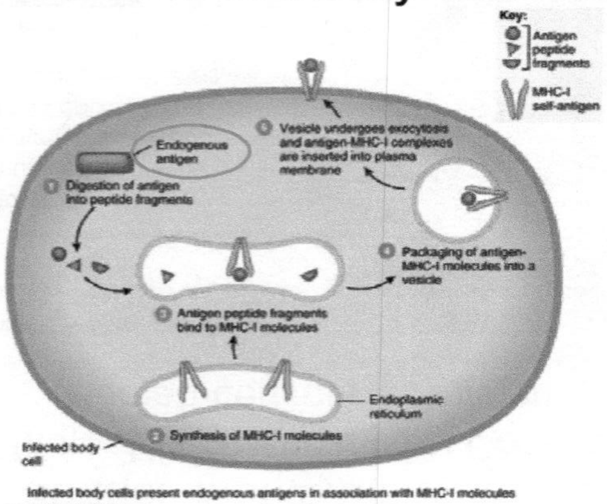
Key:
Antigen peptide fragments
MHC-I self-antigen
Endogenous antigen
1 Digestion of antigen into peptide fragments
2 Synthesis of MHC-I molecules
3 Antigen peptide fragments bind to MHC-I molecules
4 Packaging of antigen-MHC-I molecules into a vesicle
5 Vesicle undergoes exocytosis and antigen-MHC-I complexes are inserted into plasma membrane
Endoplasmic reticulum
Infected body cell

Infected body cells present endogenous antigens in association with MHC-I molecules

6-11

MHC Class II Molecules: "This Is an Invader"

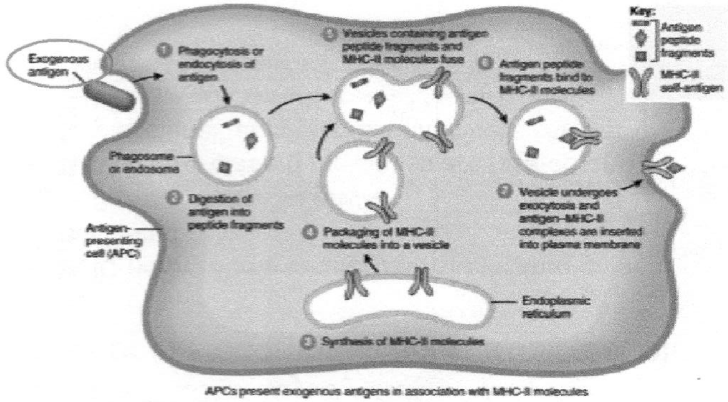
Key:
Antigen peptide fragments
MHC-II self-antigen
Exogenous antigen
1 Phagocytosis or endocytosis of antigen
Phagosome or endosome
2 Digestion of antigen into peptide fragments
Antigen-presenting cell (APC)
3 Synthesis of MHC-II molecules
4 Packaging of MHC-II molecules into a vesicle
5 Vesicles containing antigen peptide fragments and MHC-II molecules fuse
6 Antigen peptide fragments bind to MHC-II molecules
7 Vesicle undergoes exocytosis and antigen–MHC-II complexes are inserted into plasma membrane
Endoplasmic reticulum

APCs present exogenous antigens in association with MHC-II molecules

6-11

Cell Surface Markers

- Clusters of differentiation (CD) is another protocol for identification of cell surface markers.
  - These markers are not on a particular chromosome
  - Over 300 have been identified

Type of cell	CD markers
All leukocyte groups	CD45+
Granulocyte	CD45+,CD15+
Monocyte	CD45+,CD14+
T lymphocyte	CD45+,CD3+
T helper cell	CD45+,CD3+,CD4+
T Cytotoxic cell	CD45+,CD3+,CD8+
B lymphocyte	CD45+,CD19+

6-13

Links Between the Innate and Adaptive Immune Systems

- Innate immune system
  - Neutrophils
  - Monocytes/Macrophages
- **Linking innate and adaptive immune systems**
  - **Antigen-Presenting Cells (APCs)**
    - **Macrophages**
    - **Dendritic cells**
    - **Some B cells**
- Adaptive immune system
  - T cells (cell-mediated immunity)
  - B cells (antibody-mediated immunity)
  - Both B and T cells produce **memory** cells to speed responses

6-14

Antigen-Presenting Cells (APCs)

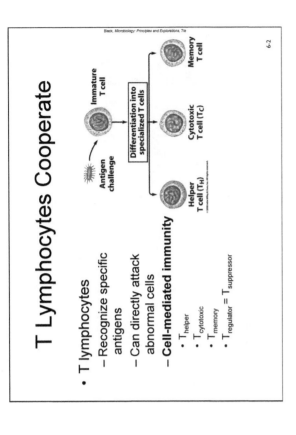

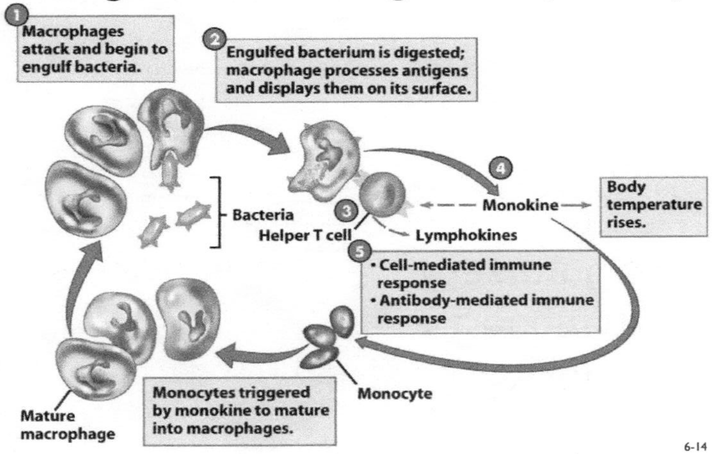
1
Macrophages attack and begin to engulf bacteria.
2
Engulfed bacterium is digested; macrophage processes antigens and displays them on its surface.
Bacteria
3
Helper T cell
4
Monokine
Body temperature rises.
Lymphokines
5
• Cell-mediated immune response
• Antibody-mediated immune response
Monocyte
Monocytes triggered by monokine to mature into macrophages.
Mature macrophage

6-14

Alters & Alters, *Biology: Understanding Life*, 1/e

T Lymphocytes Cooperate

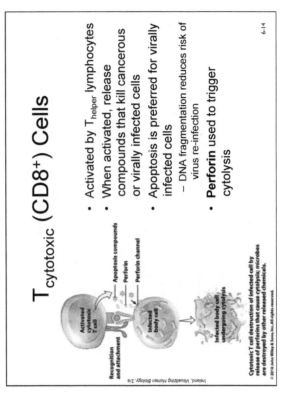

- T lymphocytes
  - Recognize specific antigens
  - Can directly attack abnormal cells
  - **Cell-mediated immunity**
    - T_{helper}
    - $T_{cytotoxic}$
    - T_{memory}
    - $T_{regulator} = T_{suppressor}$

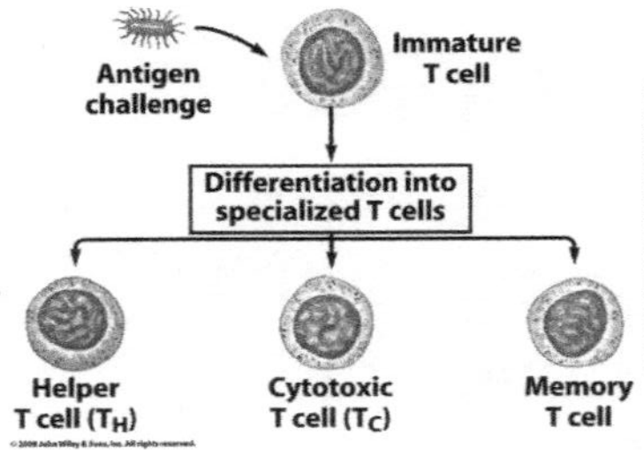
Antigen challenge
Immature T cell
Differentiation into specialized T cells
Helper T cell (TH)
Cytotoxic T cell (TC)
Memory T cell

Black, *Microbiology: Principles and Explorations*, 7/e

6-2

T_{helper} (CD4$^+$) Cells

- T_{helper} cells are "recruited" by "advertising" of antigens displayed by MHC II markers on the surface of APCs
- When found, they release cytokines and stimulate cell division by autocrine activation
- Divide to form:
  - T_{memory} cells
    → speed future responses
  - $T_{helper1}$ cells
    → cell-mediated immunity
  - $T_{helper2}$ cells
    → activate antibody-mediated immunity

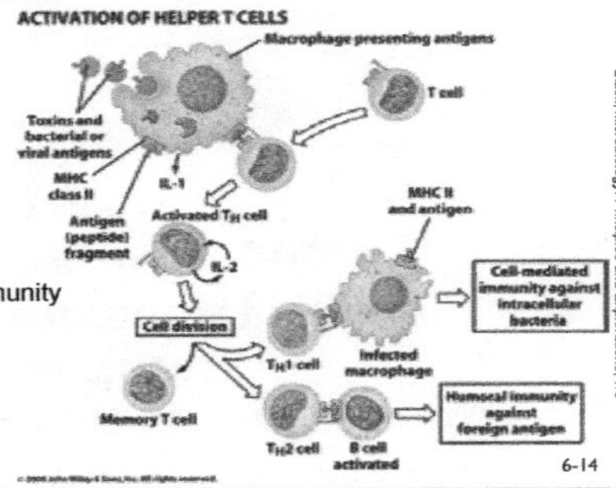
ACTIVATION OF HELPER T CELLS
Macrophage presenting antigens
T cell
Toxins and bacterial or viral antigens
MHC class II
IL-1
Activated TH cell
Antigen (peptide) fragment
IL-2
Cell division
MHC II and antigen
Infected macrophage
Cell-mediated immunity against intracellular bacteria
Humoral immunity against foreign antigen
TH1 cell
TH2 cell
B cell activated
Memory T cell

Black, *Microbiology: Principles and Explorations*, 7/e

6-14

$T_{cytotoxic}$ (CD8$^+$) Cells

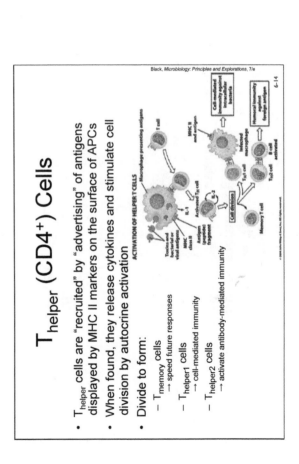

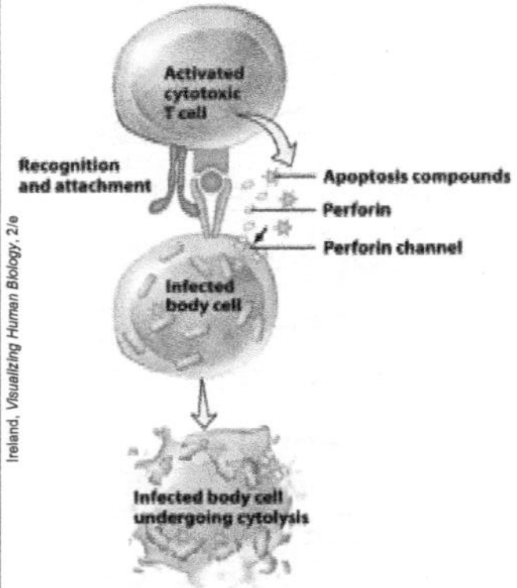
Activated cytotoxic T cell
Recognition and attachment
Apoptosis compounds
Perforin
Perforin channel
Infected body cell
Infected body cell undergoing cytolysis

Cytotoxic T cell destruction of infected cell by release of perforins that cause cytolysis; microbes are destroyed by other released chemicals.

Ireland, *Visualizing Human Biology*, 2/e

- Activated by T_{helper} lymphocytes
- When activated, release compounds that kill cancerous or virally infected cells
- Apoptosis is preferred for virally infected cells
  - DNA fragmentation reduces risk of virus re-infection
- **Perforin** used to trigger cytolysis

6-14

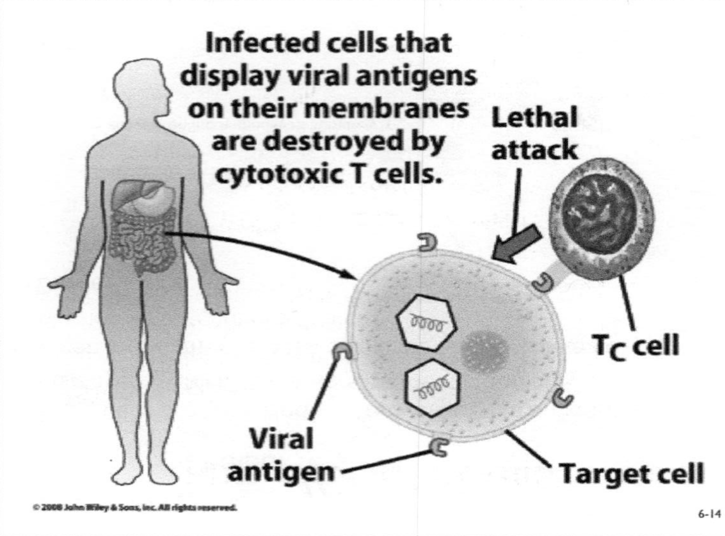
Infected cells that display viral antigens on their membranes are destroyed by cytotoxic T cells.
Lethal attack
Tc cell
Viral antigen
Target cell

Black, *Microbiology: Principles and Explorations*, 7/e

6-14

$T_{regulator}$ ($T_{suppressor}$) Cells

- Little known about these cells
  - Lack identified CD marker, making them harder to study
- Seem to down-regulate immune responses and save normal cells from destruction
- Over-active T_{reg} cells → cancer can get the upper hand (↓ immune surveillance)
- Under-active T_{reg} cells → autoimmune disease (↓ protection of normal cells)

6-14

B-Cells Becoming Plasma Cells

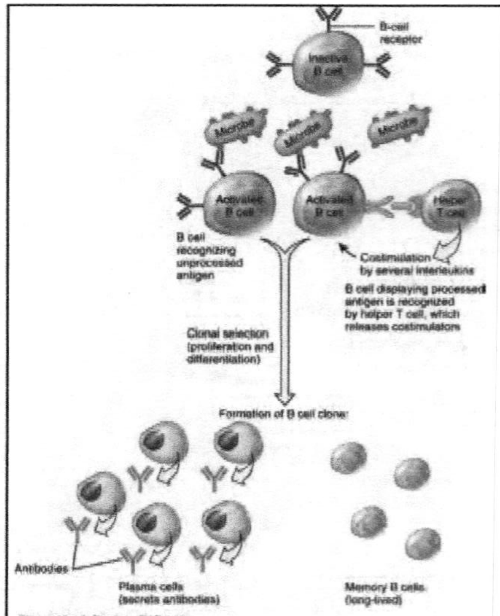
B-cell receptor
Inactive B cell
Microbe
Activated B cell
Helper T cell
B cell recognizing unprocessed antigen
Costimulation by several interleukins
B cell displaying processed antigen is recognized by helper T cell, which releases costimulators
Clonal selection (proliferation and differentiation)
Formation of B cell clone
Antibodies
Plasma cells (secrete antibodies)
Memory B cells (long-lived)

Figure 22.18 Tortora - PAP 12/e

6-14

Coordination of Innate and Adaptive Immunity

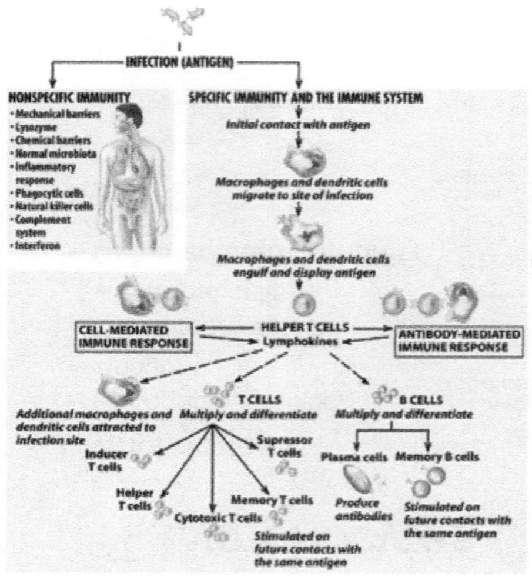
INFECTION (ANTIGEN)
NONSPECIFIC IMMUNITY
• Mechanical barriers
• Lysozyme
• Chemical barriers
• Normal microbiota
• Inflammatory response
• Phagocytic cells
• Natural killer cells
• Complement system
• Interferon
SPECIFIC IMMUNITY AND THE IMMUNE SYSTEM
Initial contact with antigen
Macrophages and dendritic cells migrate to site of infection
Macrophages and dendritic cells engulf and display antigen
CELL-MEDIATED IMMUNE RESPONSE
HELPER T CELLS
Lymphokines
ANTIBODY-MEDIATED IMMUNE RESPONSE
T CELLS
Multiply and differentiate
B CELLS
Multiply and differentiate
Additional macrophages and dendritic cells attracted to infection site
Inducer T cells
Supressor T cells
Helper T cells
Memory T cells
Cytotoxic T cells
Stimulated on future contacts with the same antigen
Plasma cells
Memory B cells
Produce antibodies
Stimulated on future contacts with the same antigen

Alters & Alters, *Biology: Understanding Life*, 1/e

6-14

Unit 4
Chapter 7
Infection and Defects in Mechanisms of Defense

Humans and Microorganisms

- Dynamic relationship
  - Mutualism
    - Both the host and the microorganism benefit
      - e.g. E. coli, a bacterium that lives in the large intestine
  - Commensalism
    - One organism benefits, the other is neutral
      - e.g. skin bacteria
  - Parasitism
    - One organism benefits, the other is harmed
      - e.g. tapeworm, round worms

7-1

Infectious Agents

- **Pathogenicity**
  - Ability of a pathogen to cause disease
  - Presence of enzymes, toxins, number (dosage), capsules, intracellular invasion
- **Virulence**
  - Ability of a pathogen to cause severe disease
  - Pathogens cause cellular injury because they circumvent defensive barriers
  - Pathogens directly damage cells, interfere with metabolism, and limit the functionality of the cell

7-2

Infectious Agents

- **Communicability**
  - Ability to spread from one individual to another and cause disease.
- **Infectivity**
  - Ability of a microorganism to invade and colonize within the host
  - Produce infection
- **Toxigenicity**
  - Ability to produce toxins and influence virulence

7-2

Bacteria

- Unicellular
- Classified as:
  - Aerobic
  - Anaerobic
- Bacteria can live as:
  - Opportunists, commensals, and intracellular and extracellular parasites
- Produce
  - Toxins: hemolysins, leukocidins, coagulases

7-3

Bacterial Shapes

- Bacteria are characterized by their shape and size.
- Before specific culture information is available, physicians use location and appearance characteristics to begin antibiotic therapy.

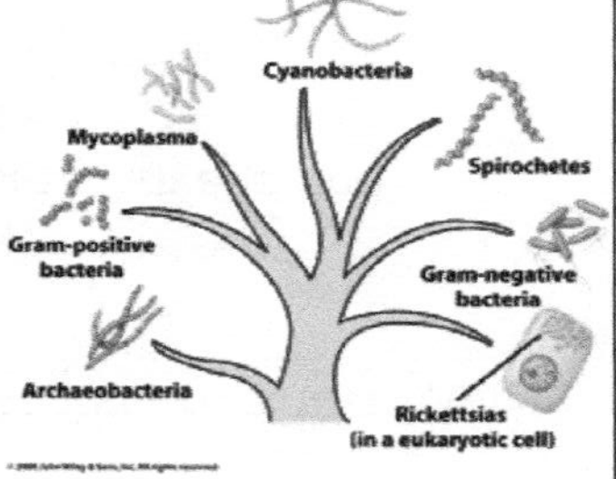
Cyanobacteria
Mycoplasma
Spirochetes
Gram-positive bacteria
Gram-negative bacteria
Archaeobacteria
Rickettsias (in a eukaryotic cell)

7-3

Bacterial Shapes

- Cocci
  - Spherical, non-motile bacteria
  - Subcategories
    - Diplo (pair)
    - Strepto (chain)
    - Staphylo (irregular cluster)

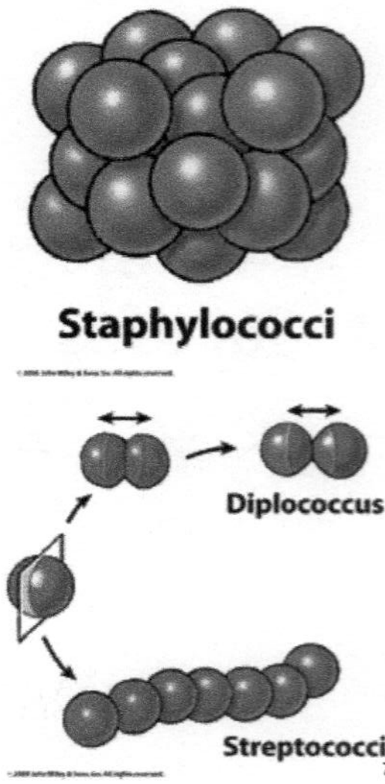
Staphylococci
Diplococcus
Streptococci

Black, Microbiology: Principles and Explorations 7e, Fig 4-2a,d

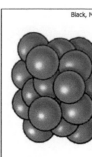

7-3

Bacterial Shapes

- Bacilli
  - Rod-shaped bacteria
- Spirillia
  - Rod-shaped, rigid, spiral organsims
- Spirochetes
  - Non-rigid, spiral rods
- Pleomorpic
  - Cells that do not fit in any of the above categories (i.e no defined shape)

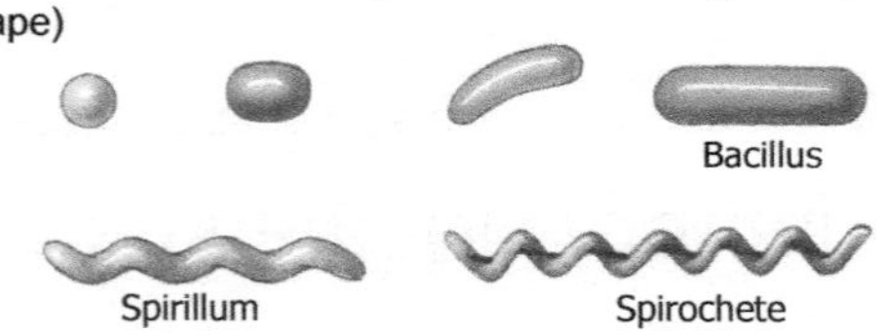
Bacillus
Spirillum
Spirochete

7-3

Bacterial Cell Wall

- The cell wall is composed of **peptidoglycan**
- Peptidoglycan is a large molecular network of glucose and amino acids
- Based on cell wall characteristics, bacteria are classified as **Gram +** or **Gram -**

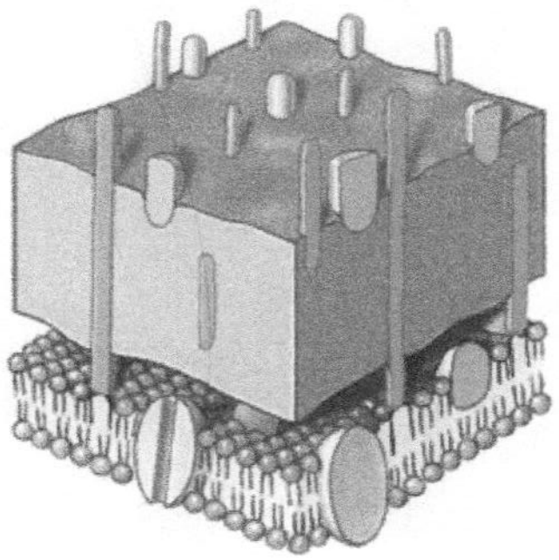

7-3

Putting It Together

- Spherical bacteria in clusters with a thick cell wall
  - Gram-positive staphylococci
- Spherical bacteria in pairs with a thin cell wall
  - Gram-negative diplococci
- Spherical bacteria in chains with a thick cell wall
  - Gram-positive streptococci
- “Kinda” spherical and “kinda” rod-shaped bacteria with a thin cell wall
  - Gram-negative coccobacilli

7-3

Bacterial Toxins

- **Gram + bacteria produce exotoxins**
  - Exotoxins are released during its life cycle
  - Exotoxins cause specific symptoms
  - Examples: botulism, tetanus, staph food poisoning, toxic shock syndrome
- **Gram – bacteria produce endotoxins**
  - Endotoxins are released during cell death
  - Produce generalized symptoms
  - Example: salmonella food poisoning

7-3

Sporulation

- **Sporulation** is the formation of endospores
- Produced when conditions are unfavorable
- Endopores help the chromosomal contents of the bacteria survive extreme temperatures, radiation, and harsh chemicals
- Once optimum conditions return, the spores will germinate

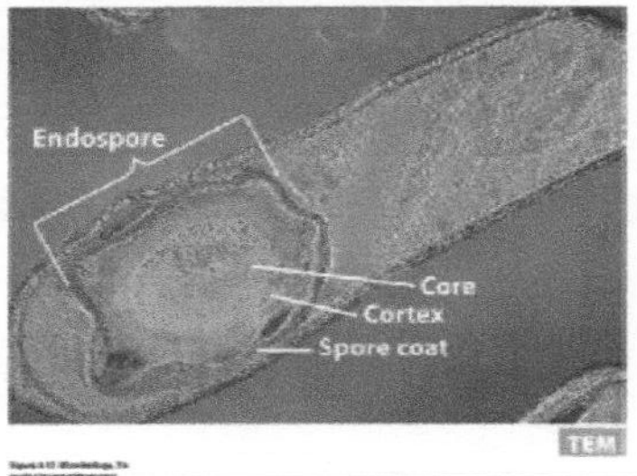
Endospore
Core
Cortex
Spore coat
TEM

7-3

Viruses

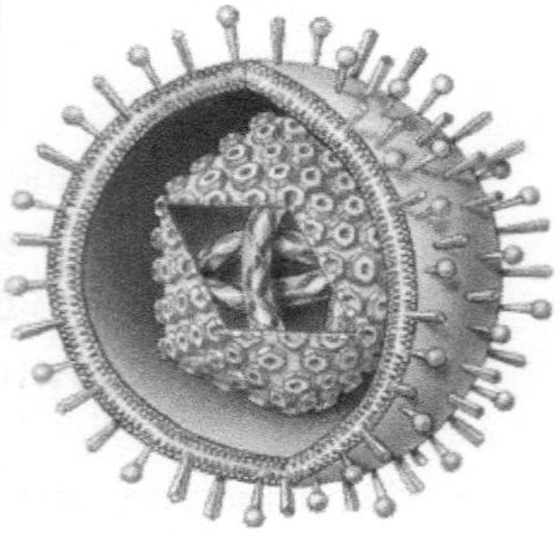

- A virus is not technically living
  - it has no metabolism
- **Obligate intracellular parasite**
- The virus provides the RNA and DNA to replicate, and the host cells provide the energy and resources.
- Components include nucleic acid, capsid, and an optional envelope

7-3

Viruses

- **Viral replication**
  - Depends on:
    - Absorption
    - Penetration
    - Uncoating
    - Replication
    - Assembly
    - Release new virions

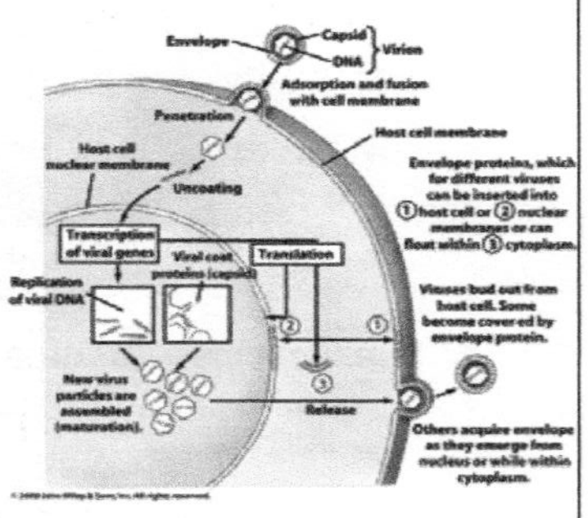

7-3

Fungi

- Fungi are important for the decomposition and recycling of organic material
- Fungi are divided into two groups, yeasts and molds
  - *Candida ablicans* (yeast infection)
  - *Tinea corporis* (ringworm)

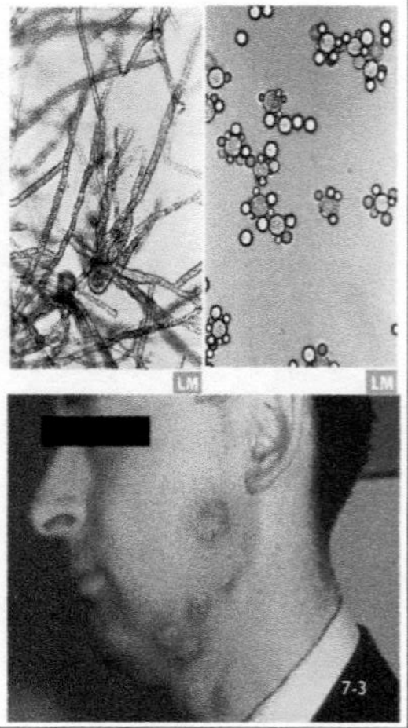

7-3

Fungi

- Fungi release mycotoxins and enzymes that damage connective tissues
- Diseases caused by fungi are called **mycoses**
- Fungi can caused **superficial** and **deep** infections
- Some fungi are part of the normal body flora and act as opportunists

7-3

Immunodeficiencies

- Usually manifested by the tendency to develop **unusual or recurrent infections**
- Immune deficiencies occur because of the impairment of one or more components of the immune or inflammatory response.
- Can be unsafe to administer vaccines
  - Why?

7-4

Immunodeficiencies

- Primary immunodeficiencies **(congenital)**
  - Occurs during leukocyte development in the fetus or embryo
  - Can affect one or more white cell lines
    - The number of cells affected dictates the degree of the deficiency
    - If the T and B cell lines are affected, the patient will have normal number of the other leukocytes, but they will have low number of lymphocytes, and diminished levels of antibodies.

7-4

Primary Immunodeficiencies

- **Di George Syndrome**
  - Partial or complete **lack of the thymus**
  - Patient demonstrates lymphopenia and **decreased T cell function**
- **Bruton's Agammaglobulinemia Syndrome**
  - **Failure of early B cells** to become mature B cells

7-4

Immunodeficiencies

- **Wiskott-Aldrich Syndrome**
  - X-linked recessive disorder
  - **IgM** production is depressed
- **Selective IgA deficiency**
  - Produce other types of antibody but not IgA
  - Can cause chronic intestinal candidiasis
  - Increased allergen uptake and more severe allergic responses

7-4

Immunodeficiencies

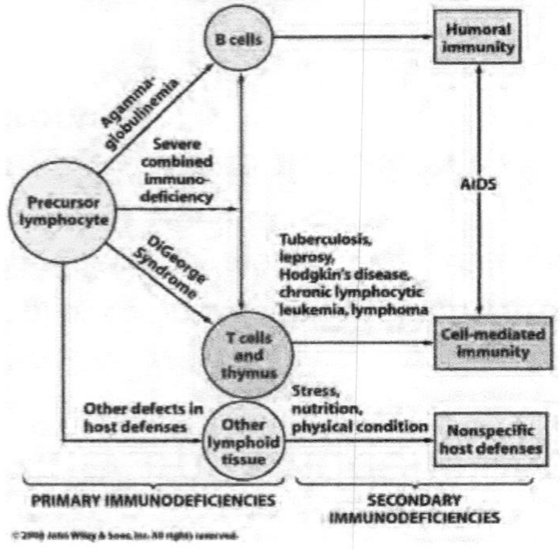

B cells
Humoral immunity
Agammaglobulinemia
Severe combined immunodeficiency
Precursor lymphocyte
AIDS
DiGeorge Syndrome
Tuberculosis, leprosy, Hodgkin's disease, chronic lymphocytic leukemia, lymphoma
T cells and thymus
Cell-mediated immunity
Stress, nutrition, physical condition
Other defects in host defenses
Other lymphoid tissue
Nonspecific host defenses
PRIMARY IMMUNODEFICIENCIES
SECONDARY IMMUNODEFICIENCIES

Black, Microbiology: Principles and Explorations, 7/e

7-4

Acquired Immune Deficiencies

- **Secondary immunodeficiencies**
  - –Nutritional deficits
  - –Chemotherapeutic agents
  - –Corticosteroids
  - –Burn victims
  - –Emotional stress
  - –Others: pregnancy, infancy, infections, malignancies, aging, diabetes, anemia

7-5

Graft-Versus-Host Disease (GVHD)

- Immunodeficiencies can put a patient at risk for graft-versus-host disease **(GVHD)**
  - –T-cells in transfused blood or bone marrow transplants can be immunologically active, therefore capable of cell-mediated immunity.
  - –Recipient's cells are not immunologically active, or they don't have any, so they can't fight back.

7-6

Human Immunodeficiency Virus

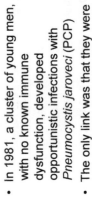

- In 1981, a cluster of young men, with no known immune dysfunction, developed opportunistic infections with *Pneumocystis jaroveci* (PCP)
- The only link was that they were homosexual
- In 1982, it was discovered in hemophiliacs
- The virus HIV-1 was identified in 1982
- HIV-2 was discovered in 1986

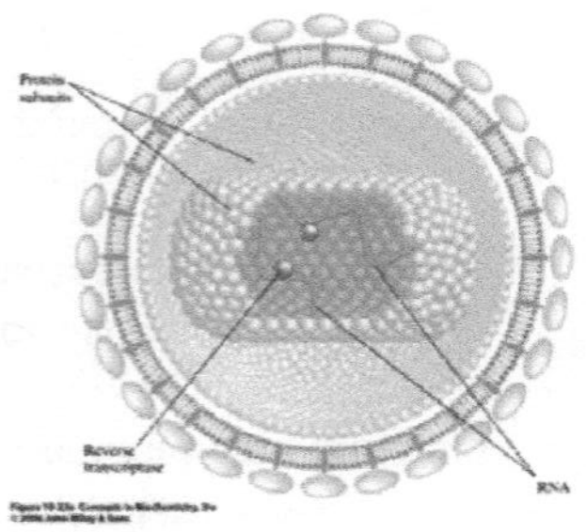

RNA

7-7

HIV

- HIV is a **retrovirus.**
- Retroviruses infect cells by binding to a surface receptor and inserting their RNA into the target cell.
- A viral enzyme, reverse transcriptase converts the RNA to DNA and inserts the viral genetic material into the target cell DNA.
- The genetic material can begin replicating immediately or remain latent for a period of time.

7-7

HIV

- HIV is spread primarily through contact with **blood** or **body fluids** containing the virus. It is also speculated that **lesions** from other sexually transmitted diseases provide opportunities for the virus to enter the host.
- Concentrations of HIV
  - High: blood and semen
  - Low: vaginal fluid, tears, sweat, breast milk
- Has also been transmitted through infected tissue transplants

7-7

AIDS Pathophysiology

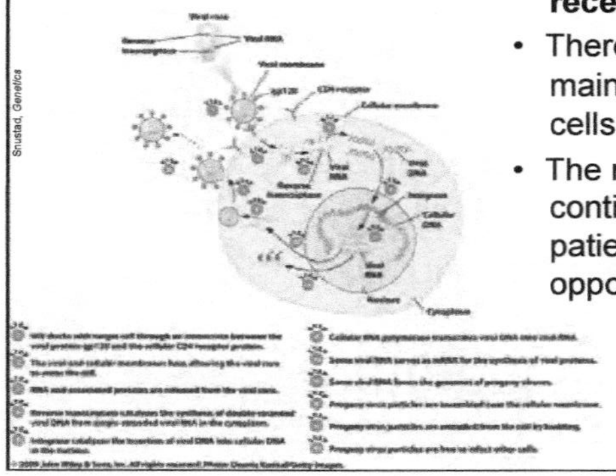

Snustad, Genetics

- Virus has a gp120 protein which binds the **CD4 receptor**
- Therefore, HIV infects mainly $CD4^+$ (helper T) cells
- The number of $CD4^+$ cells continues to diminish until patient is prone to opportunistic infections

7-7

Testing for HIV

- Window period
  - Lag time between infection and detection
  - Currently about 7 days
- Antigen and antibody tests for screening and confirmation
- Count $CD4^+$ cells

Black, *Microbiology: Principles and Explorations*, 7/e

7-7

Treatment for HIV

- Since 1996, Highly active antiretroviral therapy **(HAART):**
  - Three synergistic drugs
- Drugs can be:
  - Entry inhibitors
  - Reverse transcriptase inhibitors (NNRTIs)
  - Integrase inhibitors
  - Others
- HIV vaccine

7-7

Hypersensitivity

- Inappropriate immune response that results in damage to the host.
  - **Allergy**: hypersensitivity to antigen from environment
  - **Autoimmunity**: hypersensitivity to antigen from self
  - **Alloimmunity**: hypersensitivity to antigen from donor

7-8

Hypersensitivity

- Type I
  - IgE-mediated
- Type II
  - Tissue-specific
- Type III
  - Immune complex-mediated
- Type IV
  - T cell-mediated
- Almost all types will overlap to some degree

7-9

Type I
Immediate Hypersensitivity

- Mast cell-bound IgE antibody reacts with antigen and stimulates mast cell degranulation
- Some individuals have an inherited tendency to respond to allergens with continual production of IgE
  - 1 parent with allergy – 40%, 2 parents – 80%
- **Symptoms**: allergic rhinitis, asthma, urticaria, anaphylactic shock, diarrhea, and/or vomiting

7-9

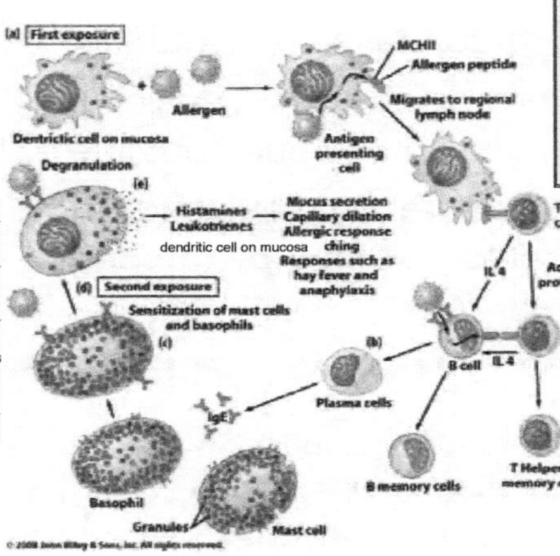

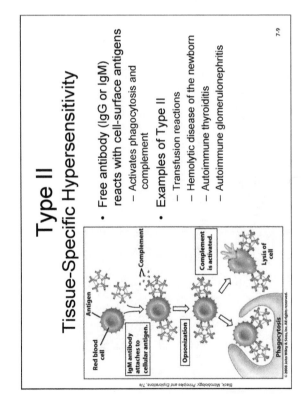

(a) First exposure
Allergen
Dentritic cell on mucosa
MCHII
Allergen peptide
Migrates to regional lymph node
Antigen presenting cell
Degranulation
(e)
Histamines
Leukotrienes
Mucus secretion
Capillary dilation
Allergic response
dendritic cell on mucosa
Responses such as hay fever and anaphylaxis
T Helper 2 cell
Activated proliferates
IL 4
(d) Second exposure
Sensitization of mast cells and basophils
(c)
(b)
B cell
IL 4
T Helper 2 cell
Plasma cells
IgE
Basophil
Granules
Mast cell
B memory cells
T Helper 2 memory cells
© 2008 John Wiley & Sons, Inc. All rights reserved.

- Choice of treatment depends on the severity of the response
  - Antihistamines (Benadryl)
  - Bronchodilators (Albuterol)
  - Corticosteriods
  - Epinephrine

Allergic Response

Black, Microbiology: Principles and Explorations, 7/e

7-9

Desensitization of Type I Hypersensitivity

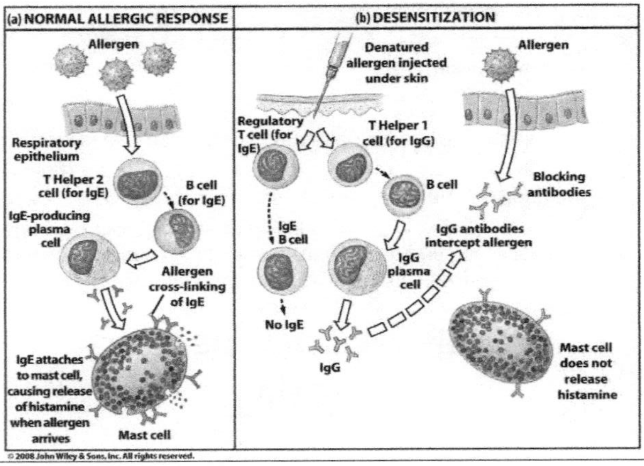

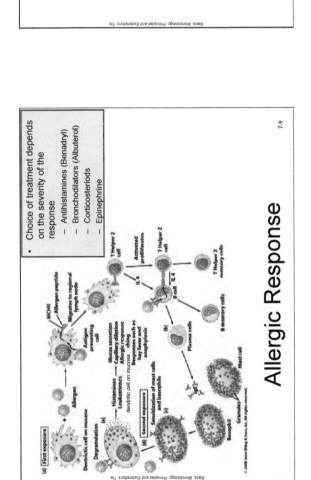

(a) NORMAL ALLERGIC RESPONSE
Allergen
Respiratory epithelium
T Helper 2 cell (for IgE)
B cell (for IgE)
IgE-producing plasma cell
Allergen cross-linking of IgE
IgE attaches to mast cell, causing release of histamine when allergen arrives
Mast cell
(b) DESENSITIZATION
Denatured allergen injected under skin
Allergen
Regulatory T cell (for IgE)
T Helper 1 cell (for IgG)
B cell
Blocking antibodies
IgE B cell
IgG antibodies intercept allergen
IgG plasma cell
No IgE
IgG
Mast cell does not release histamine
© 2008 John Wiley & Sons, Inc. All rights reserved.

Black, Microbiology: Principles and Explorations, 7/e

7-9

Type II
Tissue-Specific Hypersensitivity

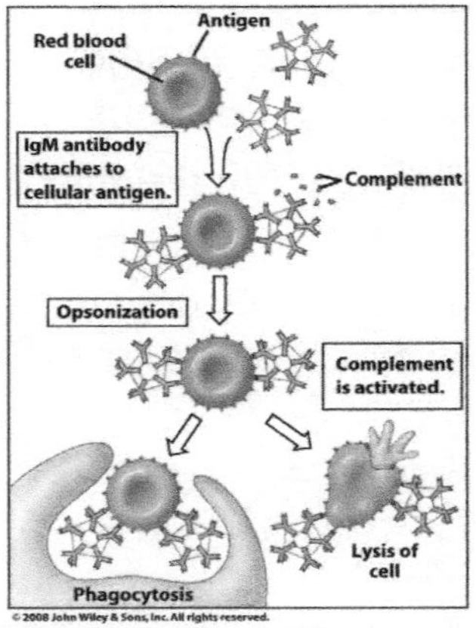

Red blood cell
Antigen
IgM antibody attaches to cellular antigen.
Complement
Opsonization
Complement is activated.
Phagocytosis
Lysis of cell
© 2008 John Wiley & Sons, Inc. All rights reserved.

- Free antibody (IgG or IgM) reacts with cell-surface antigens
  - Activates phagocytosis and complement
- Examples of Type II
  - Transfusion reactions
  - Hemolytic disease of the newborn
  - Autoimmune thyroiditis
  - Autoimmune glomerulonephritis

Black, Microbiology: Principles and Explorations, 7/e

7-9

Type II Hypersensitivity in Hemolytic Disease of the Newborn

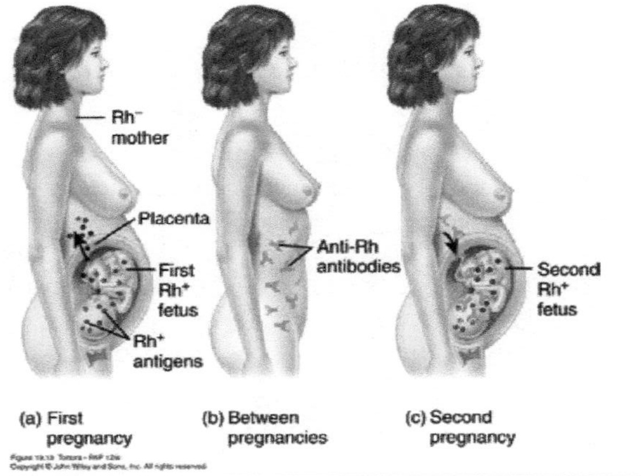

Rh⁻ mother
Placenta
First Rh⁺ fetus
Rh⁺ antigens
Anti-Rh antibodies
Second Rh⁺ fetus
(a) First pregnancy
(b) Between pregnancies
(c) Second pregnancy

7-9

Type III
Immune Complex Hypersensitivity

- Antibody reacts with free, soluble antigen to form complexes that precipitate in the tissues
- When soluble antigen combines with antibody, complexes precipitate out of the plasma and deposit in tissues, bind/ activate complement, and cause tissue damage

7-9

Type III

- Autoimmune diseases
  - Lupus
  - Rheumatoid arthritis
- "Farmer's lung"
  - Hypersensitivity to inhaled allergens in dairy farmers

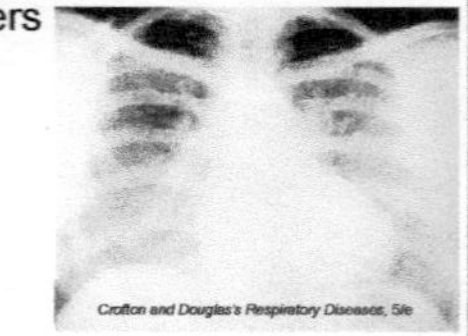

Crofton and Douglas's Respiratory Diseases, 5/e

- Glomerulonephritis
  - How can this be on the type II and type III list?

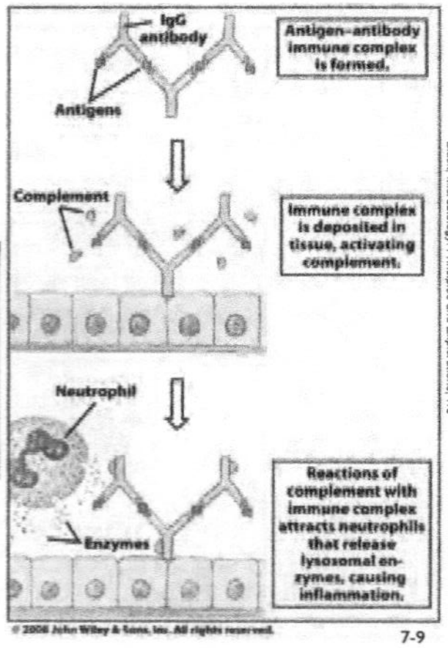
IgG antibody
Antigens
Antigen–antibody immune complex is formed.
Complement
Immune complex is deposited in tissue, activating complement.
Neutrophil
Enzymes
Reactions of complement with immune complex attracts neutrophils that release lysosomal enzymes, causing inflammation.

Black, Microbiology: Principles and Explorations, 7/e

7-9

Type IV
Delayed Hypersensitivity
Cell-Mediated Hypersensitivity
Contact Hypersensitivity

- **Sensitized cytotoxic T cells** attack tissues
- **Sensitized helper T cells** release lymphokines that recruit macrophages
- Antibody and complement not directly involved
- Symptoms delayed for 48-72 hours

7-9

Type IV
Delayed Hypersensitivity

- Poison ivy, poison oak, topical drugs, soaps, perfumes, sutures… really any chemical substance (many acting as haptens) including metals like nickel in cheap jewelry
- Process takes days but effects can last for years (blisters, peeling, weeping)
- TB skin test and acute transplant rejection are examples

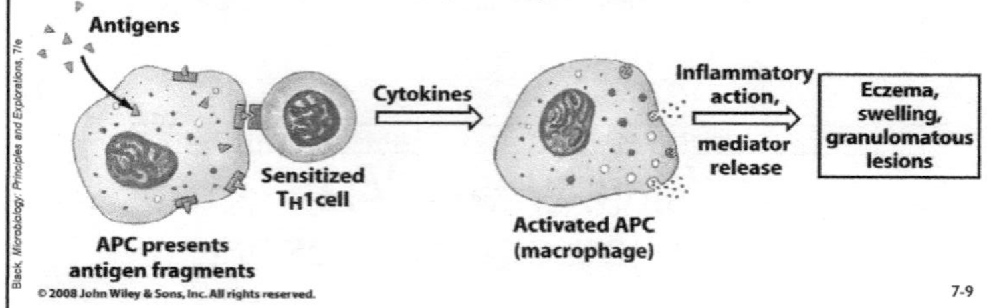
Antigens
Sensitized $T_H1$cell
Cytokines
Inflammatory action, mediator release
Eczema, swelling, granulomatous lesions
APC presents antigen fragments
Activated APC (macrophage)

Black, Microbiology: Principles and Explorations, 7/e

7-9

Type IV
Delayed Hypersensitivity Subtypes

Subtype	How long does it take?	Histology	Antigen
Contact	48-72 hr	lymphocytes → macrophages & edema	epidermal exposure to epidermal chemicals (poison ivy, heavy metals, etc.)
Tuberculin test	48-72 hr	lymphocytes, monocyte / macrophages	intradermal tuberculin
Granuloma	21-28 days	macrophages fusing to form giant cells, fibrosis	persistent antigen or foreign body (also tuberculosis)

Dr. Abdul Ghaffar, Univ South Carolina

7-9

Comparison of Hypersensitivity Types

Type	Ab	Source	Time	Appearance	Histology	Basis	Examples
I	IgE	exogenous	15-30 min	weals	basophils eosinophils	antibodies	allergies asthma hay fever
II	IgG, IgM	cell surfaces	mins-hrs	lysis necrosis	antibody complement	antibodies	hemolytic Dz newborn Goodpasture nephritis
III	IgG, IgM	soluble	3-8 hrs	erythema edema necrosis	complement neutrophils	antibodies	SLE Farmer's Lung Disease
IV	--	tissues & organs	48-72 hrs	erythema induration	monocytes lymphocytes	T cells	TB skin test poison ivy granuloma

Dr. Abdul Ghaffar, Univ South Carolina

7-9

Self vs Non-Self Recognition (Immune Tolerance)

- If billions of gene combinations are made, each capable of binding to its specific molecular shape, then it is critical to remove from the body those which bind to the body's own tissues
- This is called **self/non-self recognition** (or **tolerance**)
- T cells are tested in the thymus
  - 97% "fail" the test and die via apoptosis
  - 3% "pass" and are allowed into circulation
- B cells are tested in the bone marrow

7=10

Black, Microbiology: Principles and Explorations, 7/e

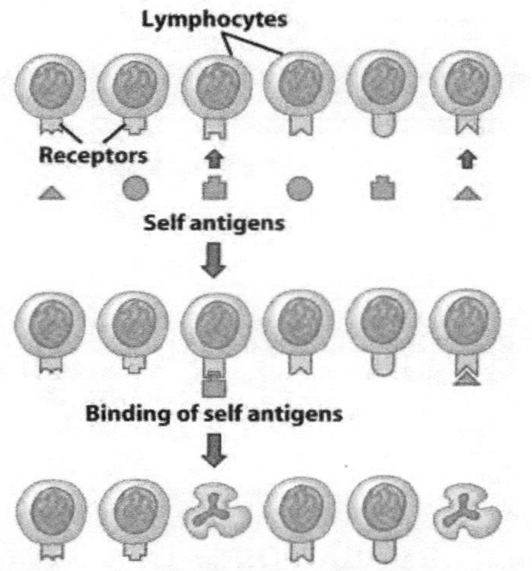

Lymphocytes
Receptors
Self antigens
Binding of self antigens

Clonal deletion of lymphocytes that have receptors for self

7-10

Autoimmunity

- Autoimmunity is a **breakdown of tolerance** in which the body's immune system begins to recognize self-antigens as foreign
- Common origin
  - Autoimmune diseases result from a genetic predisposition and a hypersensitivity to an environmental stimulus

7-10

MHC Types and Autoimmune Diseases

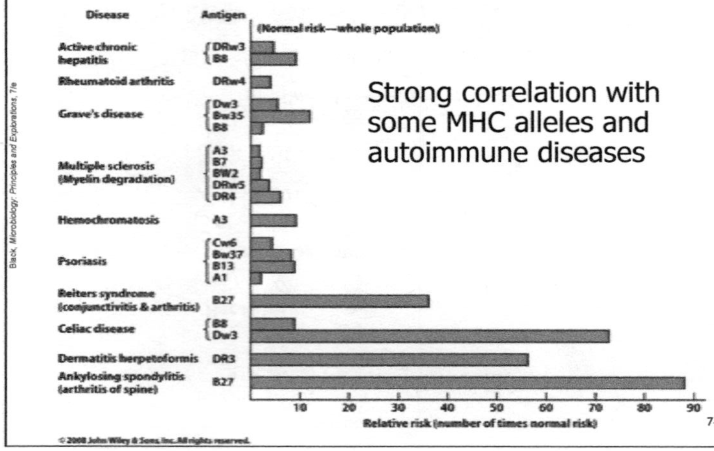
Black, Microbiology: Principles and Explorations, 7/e
Disease
Antigen
(Normal risk—whole population)
Active chronic hepatitis
DRw3
B8
Rheumatoid arthritis
DRw4
Grave's disease
Dw3
Bw35
B8
Multiple sclerosis (Myelin degradation)
A3
B7
BW2
DRw5
DR4
Hemochromatosis
A3
Psoriasis
Cw6
Bw37
B13
A1
Reiters syndrome (conjunctivitis & arthritis)
B27
Celiac disease
B8
Dw3
Dermatitis herpetoformis
DR3
Ankylosing spondylitis (arthritis of spine)
B27
10
20
30
40
50
60
70
80
90
Relative risk (number of times normal risk)
© 2008 John Wiley & Sons, Inc. All rights reserved.

Strong correlation with some MHC alleles and autoimmune diseases

7-10

Common Autoimmune Diseases

- There is one or more for every system of the body.
  - Graves' disease (thyroid)
  - Hashimoto thyroiditis
  - Type I (insulin-dependent) diabetes mellitus (pancreas)
  - Multiple sclerosis (myelin sheath in nervous system)
  - Rheumatoid arthritis (joints)
  - Myasthenia gravis (ACh receptors)
  - Goodpasture syndrome (kidney-glomerulus)
  - Autoimmune thrombocytopenia (platelets)
  - Pernicious anemia (parietal cells of stomach)

7-10

Autoimmunity

- **Systemic Lupus Erythematosus (SLE)**
  - Chronic, systemic inflammatory disease
  - Production of a variety of autoantibodies: nucleic acids (98% of patients), erythrocytes, phospholipids, and histone proteins
  - Positive anti-nuclear antibody (ANA) test
  - Circulating immune complexes deposit in tissue, especially the glomerular membrane.
  - "Lupus" (wolf-like), photo-sensitive "red" facial rash

7-11

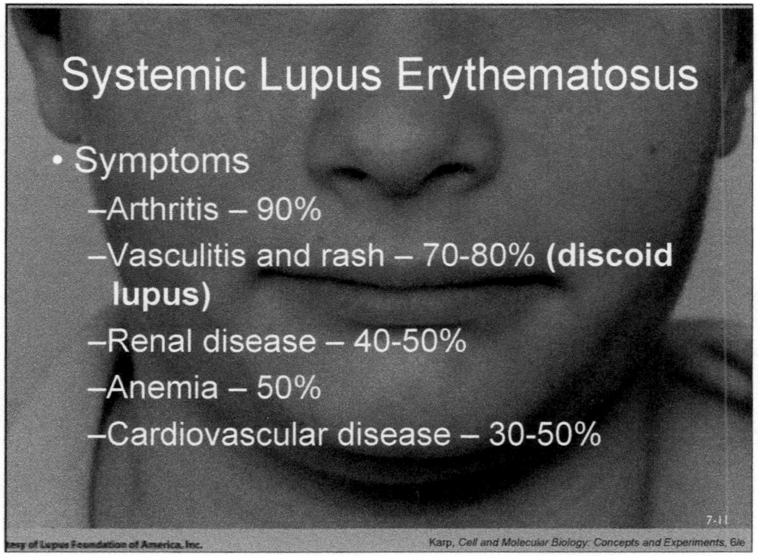
Systemic Lupus Erythematosus
• Symptoms
–Arthritis – 90%
–Vasculitis and rash – 70-80% (discoid lupus)
–Renal disease – 40-50%
–Anemia – 50%
–Cardiovascular disease – 30-50%
7-11
Karp, Cell and Molecular Biology: Concepts and Experiments, 6/e

Graft Rejection

- Alloimmunity occurs when an individual's immune system reacts against antigen of other members of **the same species**.
- Transplants are complicated by an alloimmune response to donor HLA antigens.
- Classified as **hyperacute**, **acute**, or **chronic** depending on activation time

7-12

Graft Rejection

- **Hyperacute**
  - –Patient has preexisting IgG or IgM antibody to the tissue
  - –Antibody binds to the tissue and activates an inflammatory response
    - Type II hypersensitivity
  - –This results in the cessation of blood flow to the graft – **"white graft".**
  - –Pre-transplant testing minimizes this risk.

7-12

Graft Rejection

- **Acute**
  - –The rejection is cell-mediated and occurs approximately 2 weeks after the transplant.
    - Type IV hypersensitivity
  - –Immunosuppressive drugs try to minimize this response.

7-12

Graft Rejection

- **Chronic**
  - –Can occur after months or years of normal function
  - –Reaction to minor HLA antigens
  - –No matter how much the immune response is suppressed, the tissue is still foreign.
  - –Signs and symptoms
    - Slow, progressive organ failure and damage to endothelial cells of the blood vessels.

7-12

UNIT 5

Study Guide Objectives – Introductory Pathophysiology (HTHS 2230)

Unit 5

Chapter 13 – Pain, Temperature Regulation, Sleep, and Sensory Function

1. Describe the gate control theory of pain. Describe systems that contribute to pain perception. Define pain threshold and tolerance. (pp. 325-326, 328-329)

2. Describe the neuroanatomy of pain to include pain transduction and pain transmission. Distinguish between sensory receptors and nerves that carry fast pain (Aδ) and slow pain (C). Define excitatory and inhibitory neuromodulators of pain. Explain how opiates act to relieve pain. (pp. 325-327)

3. Differentiate between acute and chronic pain. Characterize referred pain. Given a diagram, be able to state where pain from the appendix, kidneys, gall bladder, liver and heart are referred. (pp. 327-328)

4. Describe common chronic pain conditions to include hyperesthesias, hemiagnosia, fibromyalgia, and chronic fatigue syndrome. (pp. 328-329)

5. Describe symptoms of neuropathic pain. Give examples of peripheral and central neuropathic pain. (p. 328)

6. Explain how the hypothalamus regulates temperature. Describe how temperature regulation is altered in fever. Explain the pathophysiology of heat cramps, heat exhaustion, heat stroke, and malignant hyperthermia. State the signs and symptoms of accidental hypothermia, and explain why hypothermia is used as a therapy for some brain disorders. Describe how temperature regulation may be altered in infants and the elderly. (pp. 330-333)

7. Differentiate between REM and non-REM sleep. State the pathophysiology of the common dyssomnias: insomnia, obstructive sleep apnea syndrome, and narcolepsy. Define common parasomnias including somnambulism, night terrors, enuresis, and restless leg syndrome. (pp. 323-335)

8. Explain the pathophysiology of visual disorders: strabismus, amblyopia, nystagmus, cataract, glaucoma, macular degeneration, presbyopia, retinal detachment, myopia, hyperopia, astigmatism, alterations in color vision, and conjunctivitis. (pp. 335-338)

9. Explain the pathophysiology of auditory disorders: conductive hearing loss, sensorineural hearing loss, and ear infections. (pp. 338-341)

10. Explain the pathophysiology of vestibular disorders: vertigo and Ménière disease. (p. 340, 342)

Chapter 14 – Alterations in Cognitive Systems, Cerebral Hemodynamics, and Motor Function

1. Define consciousness. List CNS structures that contribute to consciousness. (p. 347)

2. Compare and contrast altered levels of consciousness to an unimpaired state. Describe causes of alterations in arousal including structural, metabolic, and psycogenic factors. Explain the clinical manifestations and evaluation of brain dysfunction. Differentiate between decorticate and decerebrate posture and describe the clinical significance of each. (pp. 347-351, 372).

3. List the three clinical tests used to determine level of consciousness for the Glasgow Coma Scale. Given a set of symptoms, demonstrate that you can use the Glasgow Coma Scale to "score" a patient. (no textbook reading)

4. Define criteria for brain death. Differentiate between total brain death, cerebral death (irreversible coma), persistent vegetative state, minimally conscious state, and locked-in syndrome. (351-353)

5. Differentiate between anterograde and retrograde amnesia. (p. 353)

6. Compare and contrast partial vs generalized seizure disorders. Define: seizure, epilepsy, epileptogenic focus, aura, prodroma, and tonic, clonic, and postictal phase. Explain why status epilepticus is a medical emergency. (pp. 354-356)

7. Describe the data processing deficits: agnosia, dysphasias, and dementia. (pp. 356-358)

8. Name the clinical features and pathophysiology of Alzheimer disease. (pp. 359-361)

9. Describe factors contributing to cerebral hemodynamics. Describe sources of increased intracranial pressure (ICP). Differentiate between stages of intracranial hypertension. Distinguish between supratentorial and infratentorial herniations. Explain the pathophysiology and clinical manifestations of hydrocephalus. (pp. 361-364)

10. Define terms associated with alterations in neuromotor function to include hypotonia, hypertonia, paresis, and paralysis. Compare and contrast upper motor neuron vs lower motor neuron disease. State which disease produces hyporeflexia and which produces hyperreflexia. Give an example of an abnormal reflex from upper motor neuron disease. (pp. 364-369)

11. Name the clinical features and pathophysiology of diseases of the basal nuclei: Parkinson disease and Huntington disease. (pp. 369-372)

Chapter 15 – Disorders of the Central and Peripheral Nervous Systems and the Neuromuscular Junction

1. Compare and contrast focal brain injuries from diffuse. Differentiate between closed (blunt) vs open brain trauma. Define coup versus contracoup injuries. (pp. 377-379)

2. Explain the location and pathophysiology of brain hematomas: extradural, subdural, subarachnoid, and intraparenchymal (intracerebral) hemorrhage. (pp. 379-380)

3. Name the key pathophysiologic features of diffuse brain injuries including concussions and diffuse axonal injury (DAI). (p. 381)

4. Name the major causes of spinal cord injury, and the symptoms that result from spinal cord injury. Define spinal shock and autonomic hyperreflexia. (pp. 382-387)

5. Describe the clinical manisfestations and pathophysiology of degenerative disc disease and herniated intervertebral disc. (pp. 387-388)

6. Classify and explain the cerebrovascular diseases. Differentiate between hemorrhagic vs ischemic stroke, and give the relative proportions of each. Describe the correlation between the blocked or leaky vessel and symptoms. Give examples of different types of brain aneurysm. State the features of arteriovenous malformations. Describe the significance of the ischemic penumbra. Differentiate between a transient ischemic attack and an ischemic stroke. (pp. 389-392)

7. Differentiate between migraine, cluster, and tension headaches. Describe the pathophysiology and epidemiology associated with each. (pp. 392-393).

8. Compare and contrast infectious diseases of the nervous system: bacterial vs viral meningitis; meningitis vs encephalitis. (pp. 393-396)

9. Classify and give the key features of: multiple sclerosis, amyotrophic lateral sclerosis, Guillain-Barré syndrome, and myasthenia gravis. (pp. 369, 397-400)

Unit 5
Chapter 13
Pain, Temperature, Sleep, and Sensory Function

Alterations in General and Special Senses
Pain, Temperature Regulation, Sleep Disorders, Dysfunctions of Special Senses

Pain

- Pain is a complex interaction between physical, cognitive, spiritual, emotional, and environmental factors.
- Cannot be characterized as only a response to injury.
- Pain is "whatever the experiencing person says it is, existing whenever he says it does."
  McCaffery, M. "Nursing practice theories related to cognition, bodily pain, and nonenvironment Interactions."
- Pain theories have evolved over time, attempting to explain the complex interactions contributing to the sensation of pain.

13-1

Gate Control Theory

- Proposed in 1965 by Melzack and Wall.
- If you hit your thumb with a hammer and then rub your thumb, does the pain decrease?
- Pain transmission is modulated by a balance of impulses conducted to the spinal cord.
- Cells in the gray matter of the dorsal spinal cord (substantia gelatinosa) act as a pain gate.
- A-delta and C fibers open the gate (neurons carrying pain).
- Other sensations may close the pain gate. For example, stimulating touch receptors on the skin, carried by large A-beta fibers close the gate, decreasing pain sensation.

13-1

Neuromatrix Theory

- Gate control theory does not explain all observeable pain.
- The neuromatix theory was proposed in 1999 by Melzack and Wall.
- Brain produces patterns of nerve impulses drawn from various inputs including genetic, psychologic, and cognitive experiences.
- Neuromatrix patterns are generally activated by sensory inputs.
- Other stimuli that do not produce pain may trigger pain patterns (as in phantom limb pain).

13-1

Pain Perception

- Conscious awareness of pain
- Pain perception is the result of the interaction of three systems:
  - **Sensory-discriminative: Somatosensory cortex** identifies presence, character, location, and intensity of pain.
  - **Affective-motivational:** Individual's emotional response to pain.
    - Mediated through reticular formation, limbic system, brain stem.
  - **Cognitive-evaluative:** Can modulate pain by overlying learned behavior.
    - Mediated through cerebral cortex.

13-1

Pain Threshold and Tolerance

- **Pain Threshold:** The lowest intensity of pain that a person can recognize.
  - Pain in one location may increase the threshold in another.
- **Pain Tolerance:** The greatest intensity of pain that a person can tolerate.
- Both influenced by genetics, gender, culture, expectations, and physical and mental health.

13-1

Neuroanatomy of Pain

- Three portions of the nervous system are responsible for the sensation and perception of pain:
  - Afferent pathways
    - Begin with pain receptors (nociceptors), travel to spinal gate in dorsal horn, then ascend to higher centers in CNS.
  - Interpretive centers
    - Located in brain stem, midbrain, diencephalon, and cerebral cortex.
  - Efferent pathways
    - Descend from CNS back to dorsal horn of spinal cord.

13-2

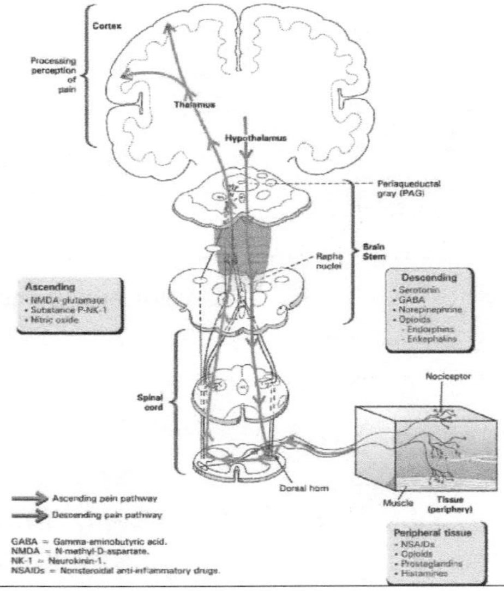
Cortex
Processing perception of pain
Thalamus
Hypothalamus
Periaqueductal gray (PAG)
Raphe nuclei
Brain Stem
Ascending
• NMDA-glutamate
• Substance P-NK-1
• Nitric oxide
Descending
• Serotonin
• GABA
• Norepinephrine
• Opioids
- Endorphins
- Enkephalins
Spinal cord
Nociceptor
Dorsal horn
Muscle
Tissue (periphery)
Ascending pain pathway
Descending pain pathway
GABA = Gamma-aminobutyric acid.
NMDA = N-methyl-D-aspartate.
NK-1 = Neurokinin-1.
NSAIDs = Nonsteroidal anti-inflammatory drugs.
Peripheral tissue
• NSAIDs
• Opioids
• Prostaglandins
• Histamines

13-2

Nociceptors

- Name means “receiving noxious information”, i.e. pain information
- Anatomically, appears as free nerve ending in skin
- Same anatomical type also receives temperature information
- **Axon** carries information to central nervous system (CNS)

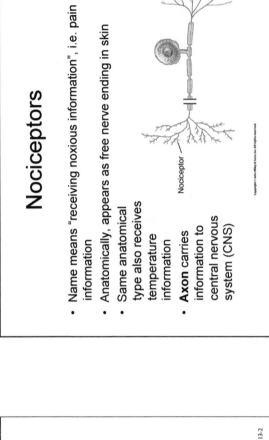

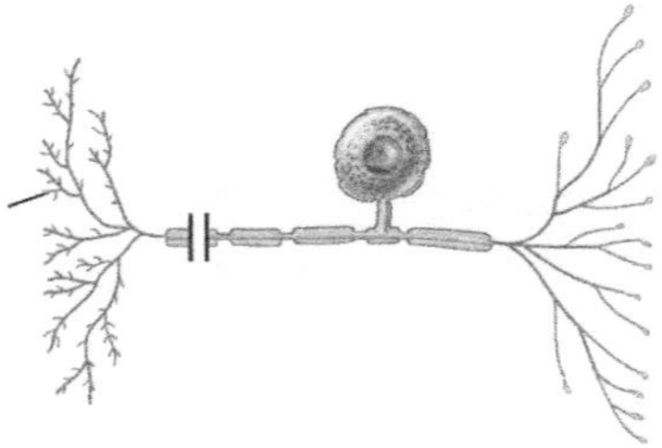
Nociceptor

13-2

Nociceptors

- Aα (biggest, fastest)
  - Carry information from muscles (proprioception)
- Aβ (intermediate size & speed)
  - Carry information from light touch and other skin sensations
- Aδ and C (smallest, slowest)
  - Aδ myelinated
  - C unmyelinated
  - Carry pain and temperature information
- Aδ = fast, “bright” pain
- C = slow, “dull” pain

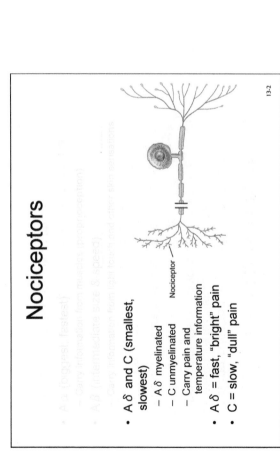

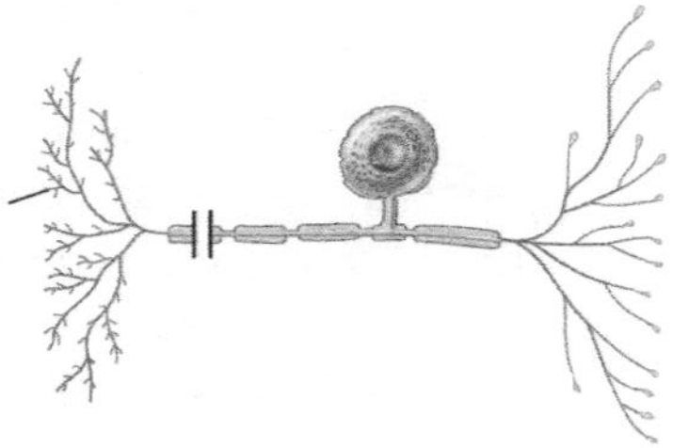
Nociceptor

13-2

Classification of Sensory Fibers

Name		Fiber diameter (μm)	Myelination	Receptor	Modality
Aα	Ia	17-20	Yes	Muscle spindle	Proprioception
	Ib	13-16	Yes	Golgi tendon organ	Proprioception
Aβ	II	6-12	Yes	Muscle spindle Meissner's Merkel's Pacinian Ruffini Hair follicle	Proprioception Light touch Light touch Vibration Vibration Touch, vibration
Aδ	III	1 – 5	Yes	Free nerve ending Free nerve ending	Pain sharp Temp (cool)
C	IV	0.2 – 1.5	No slow	Free nerve ending Free nerve ending Free nerve ending	Pain dull Temp (warm) Itch

13-2

Nociceptors: Chemistry of Pain

- **Pain transduction** begins when tissue is damaged by exposure to chemical, mechanical, or noxious stimuli stimulating nociceptors.
- **Nociceptors** are chemoreceptors
  - Detect chemicals released from damaged tissue
    - K^+, prostaglandins, leukotrienes
      - aspirin works as an analgesic (pain reducer) by blocking prostaglandin E2 synthesis
  - Detect blood products
    - serotonin from platelets, bradykinin from plasma
  - Detect products of inflammation
    - Histamine

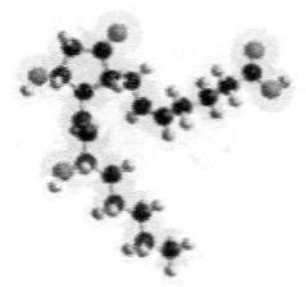

13-2

Pain Transmission

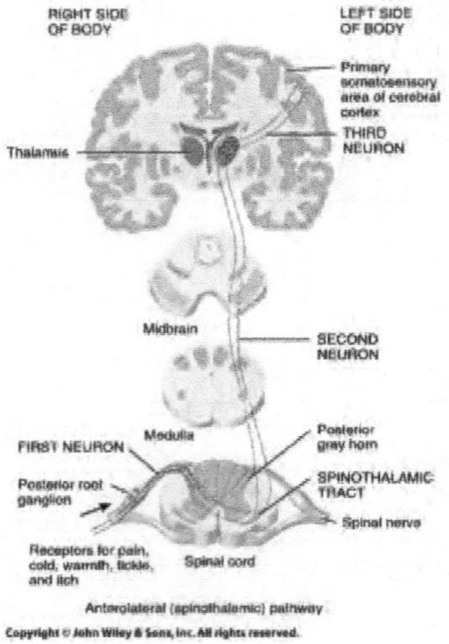
RIGHT SIDE OF BODY
LEFT SIDE OF BODY
Primary somatosensory area of cerebral cortex
Thalamus
THIRD NEURON
Midbrain
SECOND NEURON
Medulla
FIRST NEURON
Posterior gray horn
Posterior root ganglion
SPINOTHALAMIC TRACT
Spinal nerve
Receptors for pain, cold, warmth, tickle, and itch
Spinal cord
Anterolateral (spinothalamic) pathway

- **Pain transmission** is the conduction of pain impulses to the spinal cord
- Axons in spinal cord and brainstem on opposite side from where they entered
  - information on pain in left side of body carried in right **spinothalamic tract** and right brainstem
- Relayed in **thalamus**
- Information ends up in **somatosensory cortex (postcentral gyrus)**

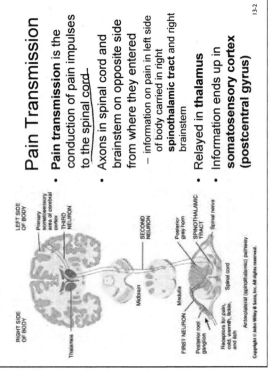

13-2

Transmitters of Ascending Pain Pathways

- Glutamate
- Substance P
  - remember “P is for pain”
- Nitric oxide (NO)

All of these are excitatory neuromodulators of pain

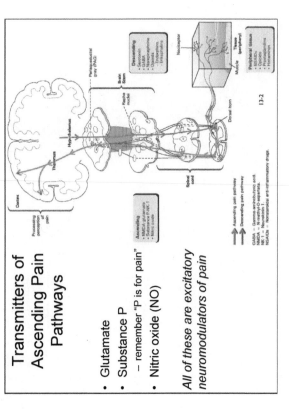

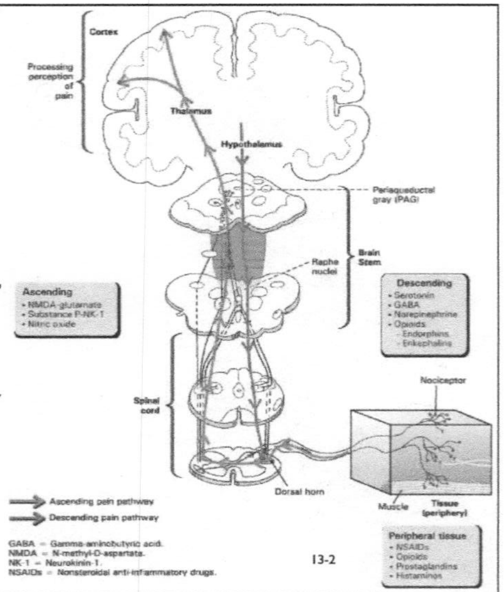
Cortex
Processing perception of pain
Thalamus
Hypothalamus
Periaqueductal gray (PAG)
Raphe nuclei
Brain Stem
Ascending
Descending
Spinal cord
Nociceptor
Dorsal horn
Muscle
Tissue (periphery)
Peripheral tissue
Ascending pain pathway
Descending pain pathway

13-2

Efferent Pathways

Neuromodulation of Pain

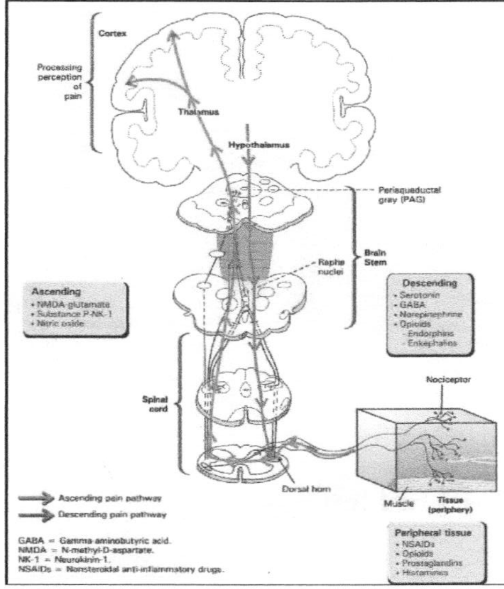
Cortex
Processing perception of pain
Thalamus
Hypothalamus
Periaqueductal gray (PAG)
Raphe nuclei
Brain Stem
Ascending
• NMDA-glutamate
• Substance P-NK-1
• Nitric oxide
Descending
• Serotonin
• GABA
• Norepinephrine
• Opioids
- Endorphins
- Enkephalins
Spinal cord
Nociceptor
Dorsal horn
Muscle
Tissue (periphery)
Peripheral tissue
• NSAIDs
• Opioids
• Prostaglandins
• Histamines
Ascending pain pathway
Descending pain pathway

GABA = Gamma-aminobutyric acid.
NMDA = N-methyl-D-aspartate.
NK-1 = Neurokinin-1.
NSAIDs = Nonsteroidal anti-inflammatory drugs.

Transmitters of Descending Pain Pathways

- Serotonin
- GABA
- Norepinephrine
- **Endogenous opioids**
  - **endorphin**
  - **enkephalin**
  - these act at the same receptors as opium, heroin, morphine, and related drugs

13-2

Endorphins and Enkephalins

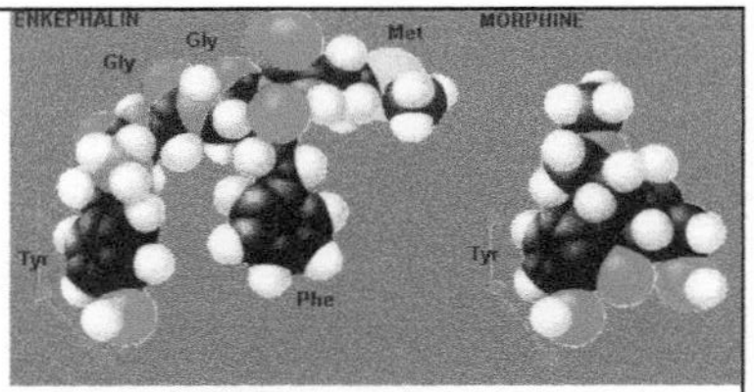
ENKEPHALIN
Tyr
Gly
Gly
Phe
Met
MORPHINE
Tyr

- Endorphins and enkephalins are peptide neurotransmitters made by the brainstem and released in the spinal cord
- All attach to opiate receptors
  - opiate receptor subtypes: mu (μ), kappa (κ), delta (δ)
- Stress, excessive physical exertion, acupuncture, and sexual intercourse all increase endorphin and enkephalin levels

13-3

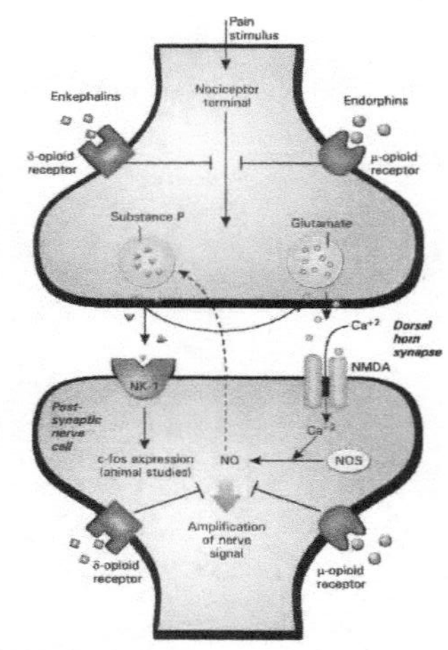
Pain stimulus
Nociceptor terminal
Enkephalins
Endorphins
δ-opioid receptor
μ-opioid receptor
Substance P
Glutamate
Dorsal horn synapse
NMDA
NK-1
Post-synaptic nerve cell
c-fos expression (animal studies)
NO
NOS
Amplification of nerve signal
δ-opioid receptor
μ-opioid receptor

Ca^{+2} = Calcium ion.
NK-1 = Neurokinin-1.
NMDA = N-methyl-D-aspartate.
NO = Nitric oxide.
NOS = Nitric oxide synthase.

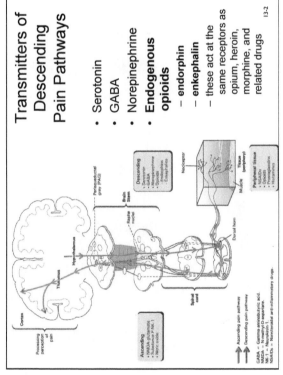

Action of Opioids

- Within the posterior (dorsal) horn, receptors for opioids shut off pain signal at synapses
- Reduce the release of pain transmitters
  - substance P
  - glutamate
- Reduce the response of postsynaptic cells
  - block nitric oxide (NO)

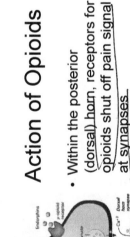

13-3

Clinical Descriptions of Pain

- Acute Pain
  - Protective mechanism against bodily harm
  - Transient, usually lasting seconds to days
  - Autonomic nervous system stimulated
    - Increased heart rate, hypertension, diaphoresis, dilated pupils
- Classified as:
  - Somatic. Superficial and well-localized pain.
    - Sharp, dull, aching, or throbbing.
  - Visceral. Pain in internal organs and linings of body cavities.
    - Poorly localized. Aching, gnawing, throbbing, cramping.
    - Pain often radiates from original site.

13-3

Dermatomes: Mapping the Skin Surface

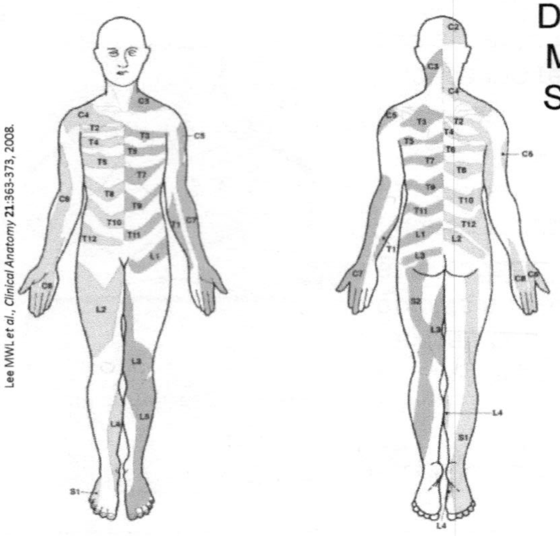

Lee MWL *et al.*, *Clinical Anatomy* 21:363-373, 2008.

13-3

Referred Pain: Mapping the Insides

- You have a map of your dermatomes
  - Touch something with your thumb, and the thumb region of somatosensory cortex is activated
  - This is "eye-hand" coordination
- No map of the internal organs exists
  - Can't touch something with your liver!
  - Pain must be "mapped" somewhere
  - Your mind constructs a rough map of where your body organs are
  - Depends on what nerve roots are shared with information coming in from both skin and organs

13-3

Referred Pain

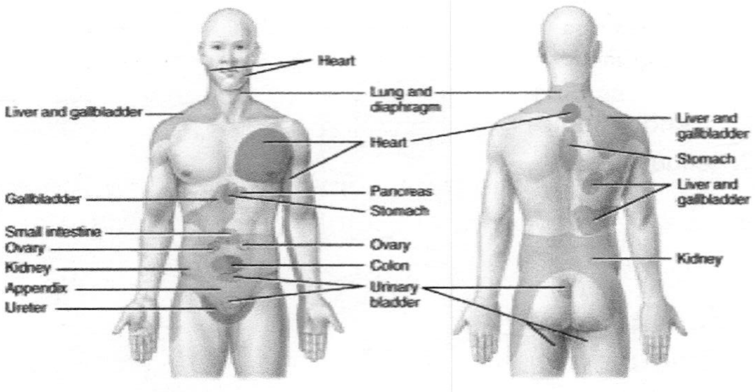
Heart
Liver and gallbladder
Lung and diaphragm
Heart
Gallbladder
Pancreas
Stomach
Small intestine
Ovary
Kidney
Appendix
Ureter
Ovary
Colon
Urinary bladder
Liver and gallbladder
Stomach
Liver and gallbladder
Kidney

(a) Anterior view

(b) Posterior view

13-3

Referred Pain

- Appendix
  - RLQ ("McBurney's point")
- Kidneys
  - flank on same side
- Gall bladder and liver
  - right flank, back, upper abdomen & shoulder
- Heart
  - usually left chest and arm
  - sometimes, neck or jaw

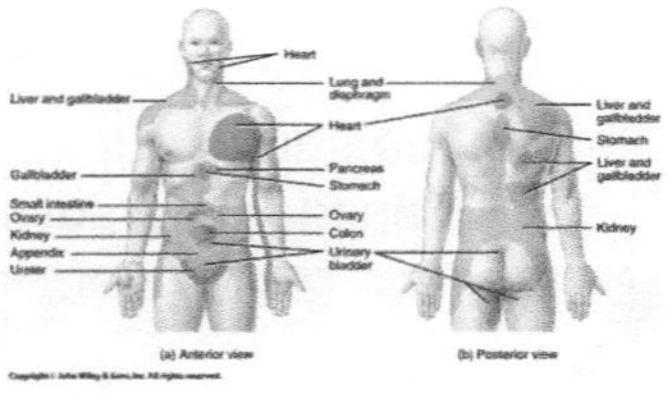

13-3

Chronic Pain

- Pain lasting 3-6 months or well beyond the expected normal healing time
  - Does not respond to usual therapy
  - Dysregulation of nociception and pain modulation
  - Neuroimaging studies have demonstrated brain atrophy leading to decreased ability to cope with pain

13-3

Common Chronic Pain Conditions

- Low Back Pain
- Postoperative Pain
- Cancer
- Hyperesthesias
  - Increased sensitivity and decreased pain threshold to tactile and painful stimuli
- Hemiagnosia
  - Loss of ability to identify source of pain on one side of body.
  - Associated with stroke

13-4

Chronic Pain
Myofascial Pain Syndrome
Fibromyalgia
Chronic Fatigue Syndrome

- These are interrelated chronic pain syndromes
- Borders between these diagnoses are not clear
- Compression of trigger points (shown) causes referred pain, movement disorders, and autonomic responses
- Little is known, and only effective treatment is antidepressants

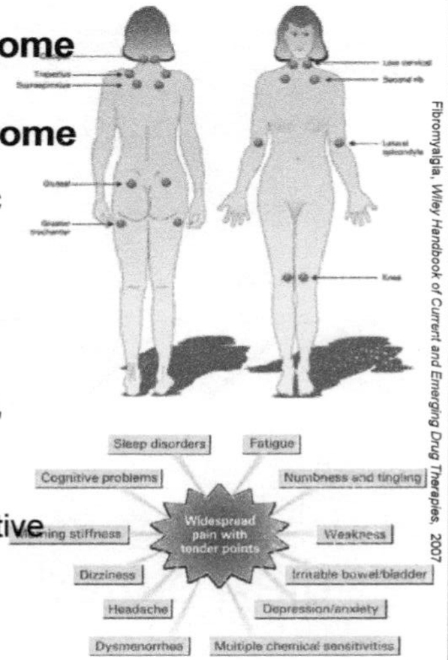

Sleep disorders
Fatigue
Cognitive problems
Numbness and tingling
Widespread pain with tender points
Weakness
Dizziness
Irritable bowel/bladder
Headache
Depression/anxiety
Dysmenorrhea
Multiple chemical sensitivities

Fibromyalgia, *Wiley Handbook of Current and Emerging Drug Therapies*, 2007

13-4

pressure on trigger point = spontaneous pain on unrelated spot in body

Δ way brain recieves pain signals

rest ∅ relive fatigue

Chronic Pain
Neuropathic Pain

- Caused by a primary lesion or dysfunction in the nervous system.
- Leads to long-term changes in pain pathway structure and abnormal processing of sensory function.
- Chronic pain characterized as burning, shooting, shock-like, or tingling.
  - Hyperalgesia: abnormally heightened sensitivity to pain.
  - Allodyina: pain from stimuli that are not normally painful.

13-5

Peripheral Neuropathic Pain

- Trauma or disease to one or more peripheral nerves
  - –Nerve entrapment
    - Nerves that are compressed or entrapped
    - Carpel Tunnel Syndrome is an example of nerve entrapment.

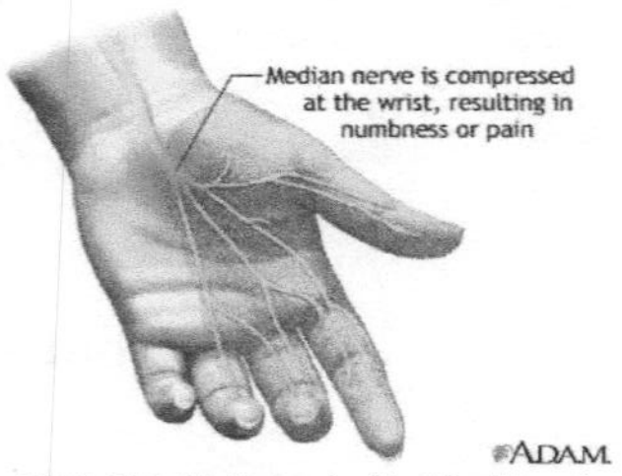
Median nerve is compressed at the wrist, resulting in numbness or pain
©ADAM.

A.D.A.M. Pub Med Health. A service of the National Library of Medicine. National Institute of Health.

13-5

Diabetic Neuropathy

- This is a type of **chronic** pain syndrome
- Pain in response to a stimulus happens, then it's over: this is **acute** pain
- In chronic pain, pain continues in absence of stimulus
- Lack of nutrition to nerve axons damages them
- Pain receptors activated and "always on"

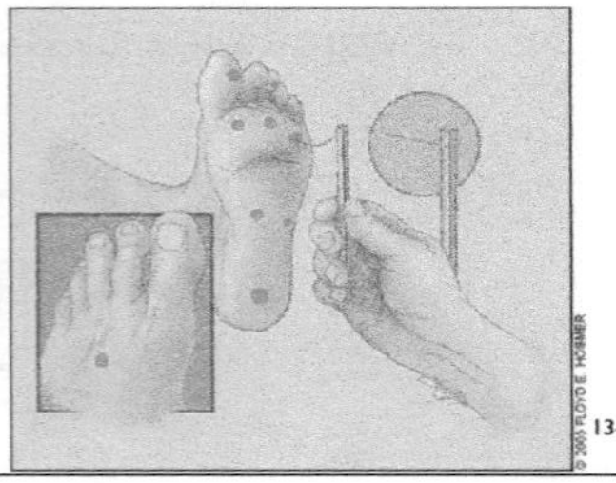

13-5

Central Neuropathic Pain

- **Phantom Pain**
  - –Brain perceives pain in amputated limb
  - –Obviously no receptors exist to trigger pain
  - –Recent studies suggest this is because of reorganization of the somatosensory cortex and "fight" for brain territory in remaining areas
    - e.g. right leg information tries to occupy space vacated by right arm after right arm amputation

13-5

Alterations in Temperature Regulation

Body Temperature

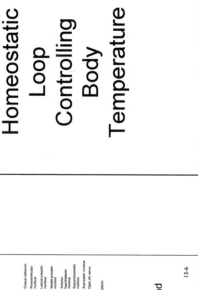

- Core temperature is carefully regulated: 37° C (98.6° F). Normal range (36.2° to 37.7° C).
- Body temperature warmer at the core (rectal) and cooler at the extremities(oral).

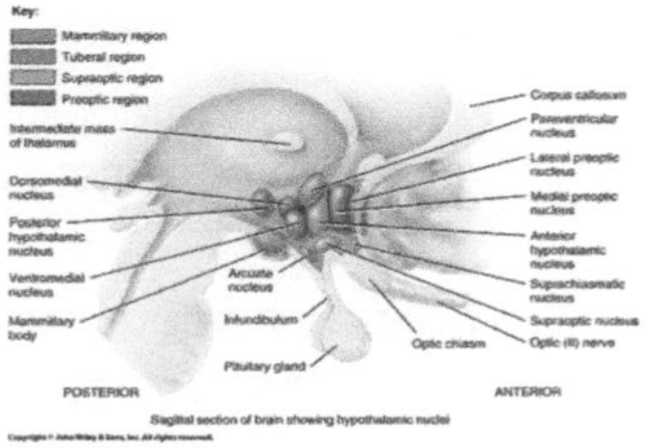

- The hypothalamus is the temperature control center

1. Hypothalamus dumps TSH-RH on pituitary →
2. Anterior pituitary releases TSH →
3. Thyroid releases **thyroxine** →
4. Thyroxin stimulates systemic release of **epinephrine** →
5. Epinephrine causes vasoconstriction in skin (heat conservation), and increases glycolysis and metabolism (heat production)

13-6

Homeostatic Loop Controlling Body Temperature

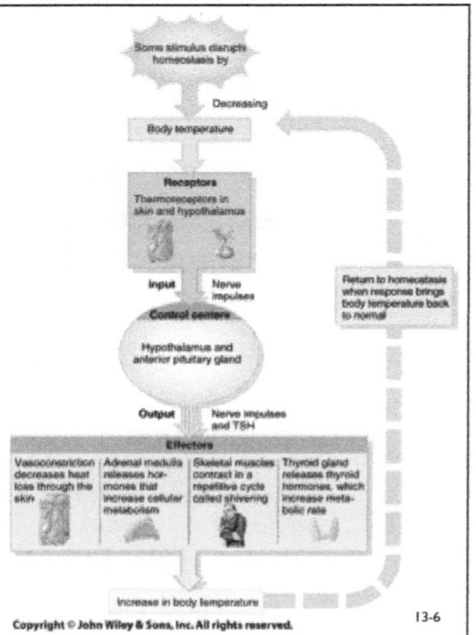

Decreasing
Body temperature
Receptors
Input
Nerve impulses
Control centers
Hypothalamus and anterior pituitary gland
Output
Nerve impulses and TSH
Effectors
Increase in body temperature

13-6

Temperature Regulation

- **Fever** is the resetting of the "hypothalamic thermostat" to a higher setting.
- Bacteria
  - **exogenous pyrogens**
  - are destroyed and absorbed by phagocytes
- Inflammation
  - **endogenous pyrogens** stimulate increased metabolism and body temperature
  - interleukin 1 (IL-1)
  - tumor necrosis factor alpha (TNF–α)
  - interferons

13-6

Temperature Regulation

- During fever, factors are released to help diminish the febrile response in a negative feedback loop
  - Endogenous cryogens released
    - arginine vasopressin
  - When the fever breaks, endogenous cryogens set the hypothalamic thermostat back to normal

13-6

Fever is Beneficial

- Increased body temperature kills some organisms directly, and affects the growth of others by sequestering needed nutrients (decreased levels of iron, copper and zinc in the serum).
- Increased temperature promotes lysosomal breakdown with autodestruction of cells to prevent viral replication in infected cells.
- Increased temperature increases lymphocyte transformation and phagocyte motility.

13-6

Hyperthermia

- Hyperthermia causes nerve damage, coagulation of cell proteins, and cell death
  - 41°C (105.8°) – produces convulsions
  - 43°C (109.4°) – causes death
  - Forms of accidental hyperthermia
    - **Heat cramps, heat exhaustion, and heat stroke**

13-6

Hyperthermia

- **Heat cramps**
  - Spasmodic cramps in the abdomen and limb musculature related to prolonged sweating and sodium loss.
  - Usually in people not accustomed to warm climates
  - May be accompanied by fever, rapid pulse, and increased blood pressure.
  - Administer dilute salt solutions.

13-6

Hyperthermia

- **Heat exhaustion**
  - Collapse due to prolonged high body core or environmental temperature.
  - Cause hypothalamic induction of large-scale vasodilation and profuse sweating.
  - Dehydration, hypovolemia, decreased cardiac output, hypotension, and tachycardia
  - Individual feels week, dizzy, nauseated, and faint.
  - Treat with warm fluids and replace fluid loss.

13-6

Hyperthermia

- **Heat Stroke**
  - The brain does not tolerate temperatures > 40°C (104°C)
  - Breakdown of thermoregulatory control
    - Sweating ceases
    - Skin becomes dry
    - Internal core temperature rises rapidly
  - Leads to vascular collapse
  - Causes degeneration of the CNS and muscles (**rhabdomyolysis**)
  - Death will result without gentle cooling
  - Treatment by rapid cooling is dangerous; causes peripheral vasoconstriction and prevents core cooling

13-6

Hypothermia

- **Hypothermia** causes depression of CNS and respiratory systems.
- Cognitive and muscular processes become sluggish.
- Slows down chemical reactions, **increases blood viscosity**, encourages **coagulation** and **vasoconstriction** and can lead to ischemic tissue damage.
- In severe hypothermia, ice crystals form on the inside of cells causing cell lysis and death.
- To overcome hypothermia, the hypothalamic center stimulates shivering to increase heat production.

13-6

Hypothermia

- Gradual re-warming of tissues is required
  - Superficial
  - Core rewarming
    - Warm IV fluids, gastric or peritoneal lavage, or inhalation of warmed gases
- FYI: Therapeutic hypothermia
  - Protects the brain by reduction in metabolic rate, ATP consumption, and reduces critical threshold for oxygen delivery
    - Can survive with core temps at 9°C (48.2°F)

13-6

Temperature Regulation Infants and the Elderly

- Infants and the elderly have difficulties with temperature regulation.
- Infants have little subcutaneous fat, greater ratio of body surface to body weight, inability to shiver to increase heat.
- Elderly have slow blood circulation, slowed activity levels, decreased shivering response, slowed metabolic rate, and decreased vasoconstrictor response and ability to sweat.

13-6

Alterations in Sleep

Sleep Stages and Terminology

- Sleep has stages (one night's sleep shown below)
- Rapid Eye Movement (REM) sleep (20-25% of sleep)
  - Occurs about every 90 minutes
  - roughly equivalent to dream sleep
  - body is paralyzed, eyes move
- Non-REM sleep
  - stages numbers 1 (light sleep) through 4 (deep sleep)

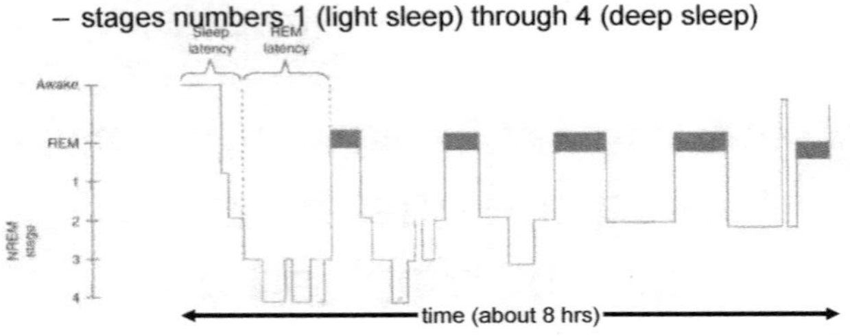

Sleep latency
REM latency
Awake
REM
1
2
3
4
NREM stage
time (about 8 hrs)

Erman M & Ancoli-Israel SA. *Psychiatry*, 3/e

13-7

Dysomnias

- Disorders of initiating and maintaining sleep and disorders of excessive sleepiness.
- Insomnia: Inability to fall or stay asleep
  - Long term insomnia may be associated with drug or alcohol abuse, chronic pain disorders, chronic depression, use of certain drugs, obesity, and aging.

13-7

Sleep Apnea

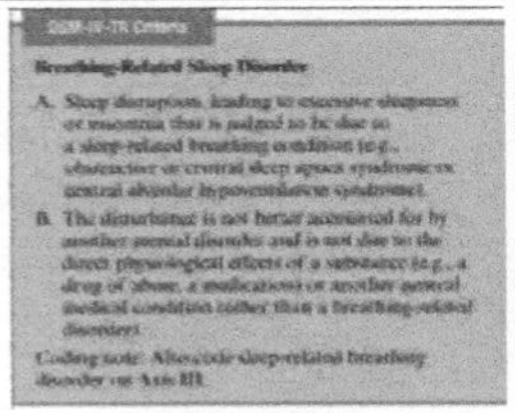

Erman M & Ancoli-Israel SA. *Psychiatry*, 3/e

- Lack of breathing during sleep (at least 10 seconds between breaths)
- Can be **central apnea, obstructive apnea**, or a combination of both
- Produces low O_2 saturation, pulmonary hypertension, polycythemia, cyanosis, edema, and right-sided heart failure (cor pulmonale)
- Treatments include: weight loss, O_2 therapy (CPAP), respiratory stimulant, surgery (relieve the obstruction)

13-7

Narcolepsy

- Narcolepsy symptoms:
  - Periods of extreme drowsiness for about 15 minutes every 3 to 4 hours during the day
  - Dream-like hallucinations during the transition from sleep to wakefulness
  - Inability to move at both sleeping and waking transitions
  - Often includes **cataplexy**: loss of muscle tone while awake
    - can be triggered by emotional excitement
  - http://bit.ly/CIZSn

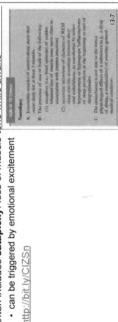

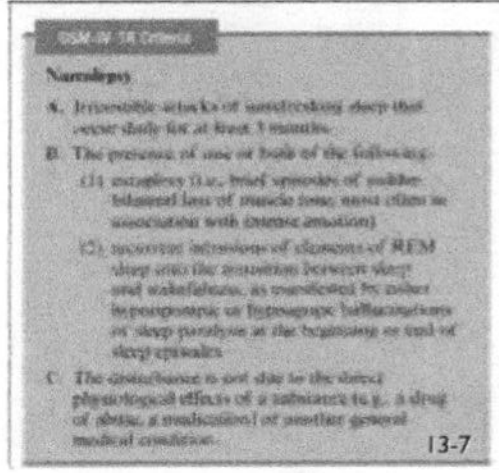

13-7

Erman M & Ancoli-Israel SA. *Psychiatry*, 3/e

Parasomnias
Unusual Behaviors Occurring During Sleep
Somnambulism

- **Somnambulism** (sleep-walking)
  - Individual functions at a very low level of arousal with no memory of the event
  - Individuals can end up in dangerous situations
  - Usually occurs in children during the first third of the night and resolves over time

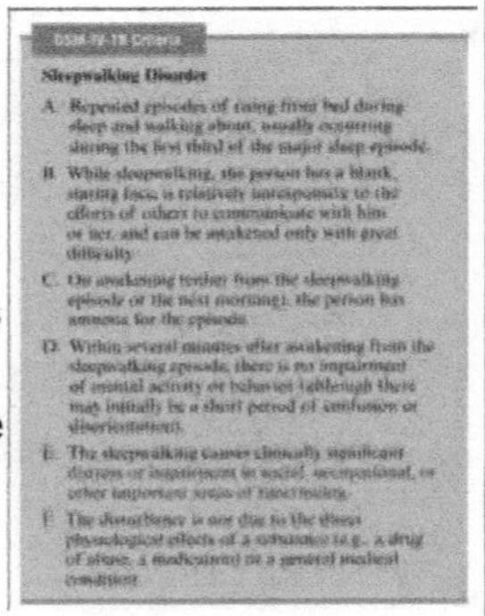

Erman M & Ancoli-Israel SA. *Psychiatry*, 3/e

13-7

Parasomnias
Night Terrors

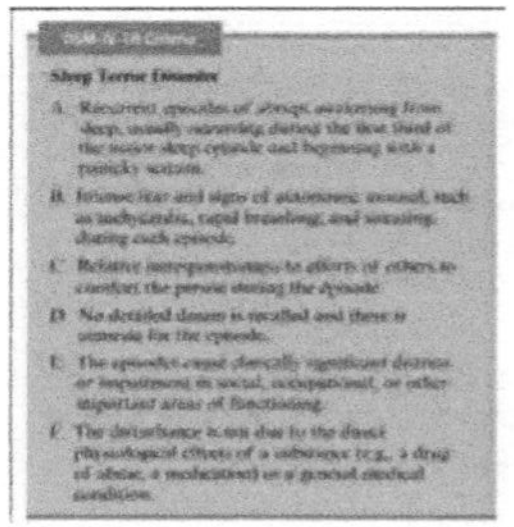

Erman M & Ancoli-Israel SA. *Psychiatry*, 3/e

- **Night terrors** are characterized by extreme terror and a temporary inability to regain full consciousness
- Patient awakens abruptly gasping, moaning, or screaming.
- No memory of the episode
  - true nightmares usually can be recalled
- Calm the person and convince them to "go back to sleep" (although they are already in stage 4 sleep)

13-7

Parasomnias
Enuresis

- **Enuresis**
  - "Bed-wetting"
  - Occurs when a child is difficult to arouse
  - Developmental delay, and is usually outgrown
  - Thought to have a hereditary component
  - Rule out medical causes: child is evaluated for infections, obstructions, neurogenic bladder, and decreased nocturnal antidiuretic hormone

13-7

Restless Leg Syndrome

- A strange name for a serious illness
- Prevalence about 3%
  - twice as many women as men
- One of the oldest neurological illnesses described (Willis 1683)
- About three-quarters of patients have **periodic limb movements in sleep (PLMS)**
- Diagnostic criteria based on symptoms, not signs
  1. An urge to move the legs, with an accompanying uncomfortable sensation
  2. Worse during rest or inactivity
  3. Relieved by movement
  4. Worse at night
- Iron deficiency in substantia nigra appears to be main cause (related to Parkinson Disease)

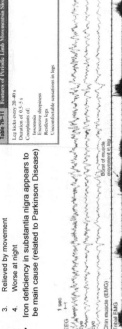

Table 79–11	Features of Periodic Limb Movementsin Sleep
Leg kicks every 20–40 s	
Duration of 0.5–5 s	
Complaints of:	
Insomnia	
Excessive sleepiness	
Restless legs	
Uncomfortable sensations in legs	

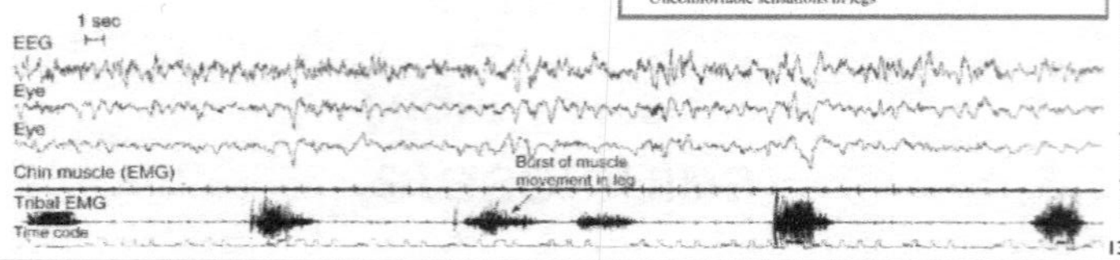
1 sec
EEG
Eye
Eye
Chin muscle (EMG)
Burst of muscle movement in leg
Tibial EMG
Time code

Erman M & Ancoli-Israel SA. *Psychiatry*, 3/e

13-7

Disorders of Special Senses

Vision

Disorders of Vision

Strabismus

- **Strabismus**
  - **Deviation** of one eye from the other when looking directly at a specific object
  - Usually caused by a weak muscle in one of the eyes
- Strabismus may often, but not always, lead to amblyopia
- Treatment: injections of botulinum toxin (Botox) to partially paralyze stronger muscle of the pair

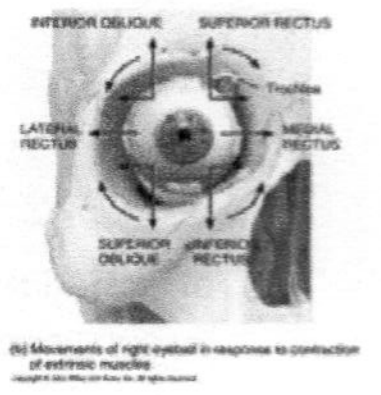
INFERIOR OBLIQUE
SUPERIOR RECTUS
LATERAL RECTUS
MEDIAL RECTUS
SUPERIOR OBLIQUE
INFERIOR RECTUS

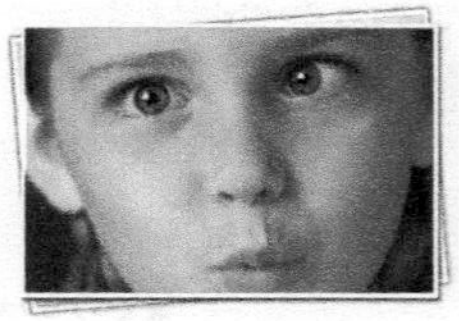

13-8

Disorders of Vision

Amblyopia

- Visual pathways develop during a **critical period**
- Not certain of critical period in humans, but thought to be birth to 6 years of age
- During this period, visual cortex constructs binocular image using input from both eyes
- If one eye does not focus or produces what the brain decides is an unreliable image, then the information is discarded and only one eye is “wired into” the brain
- Treatment is to alternately patch each eye

13-8

Nystagmus

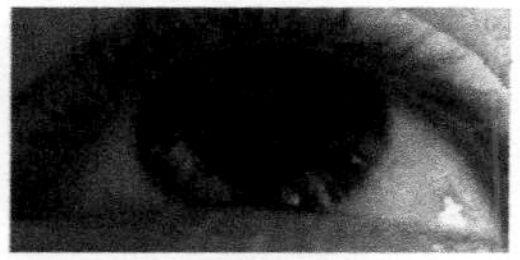

- Involuntary unilateral or bilateral rhythmic movement of the eyes.
- May be caused by an imbalanced reflex activity of the inner ear.
  - Inner ear sends a signal in the absence of movement.
  - Eyes move as if the head is rotating.
- Nystagmus may also be caused by drugs, retinal disease, and disease involving the cervical spinal cord.

13-8

Cataract

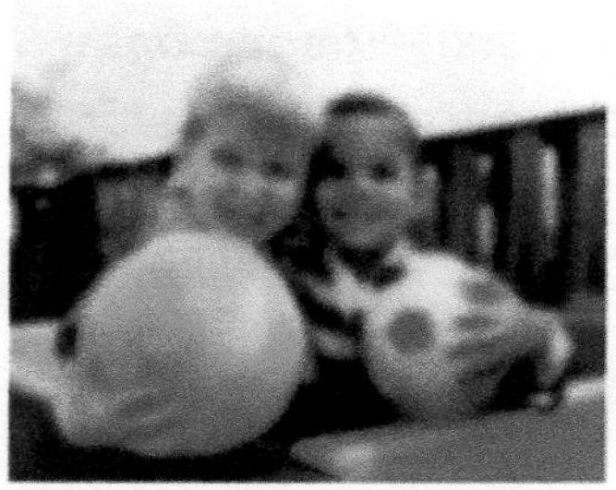

A scene as it might be viewed by a person with a cataract.

- Clouding of the lens
  - caused by UV light exposure, diabetes, infections, trauma, drugs
- Lens is liquified inside its capsule (**phakoemulsification**) and intraocular lens is implanted in its place

13-8

Glaucoma

- **Glaucoma** is an abnormal pressure in the **anterior chamber**
  - space between cornea and lens/iris
- Measure **intraocular pressure** with **tonometer**
- Increased pressure can reduce blood supply to retina and cause permanent vision loss

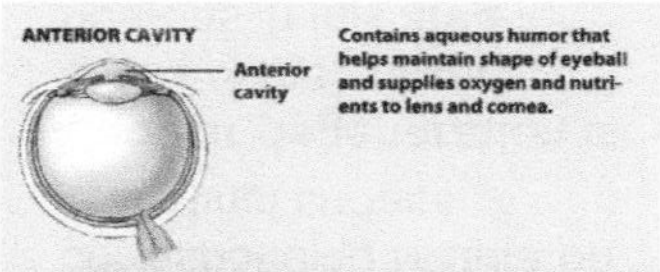
ANTERIOR CAVITY
Anterior cavity
Contains aqueous humor that helps maintain shape of eyeball and supplies oxygen and nutrients to lens and cornea.

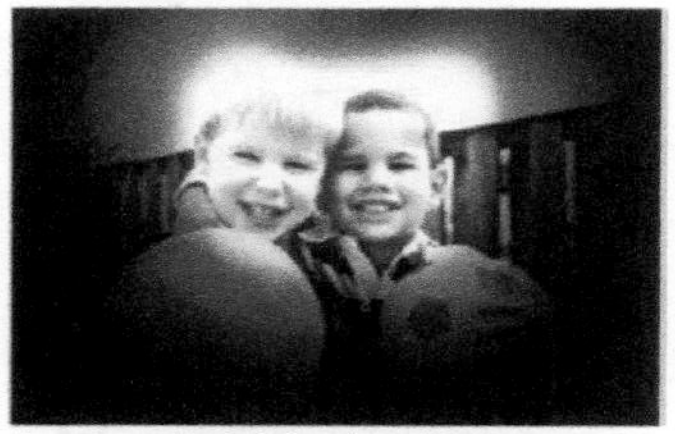

A scene as it might be viewed by a person with glaucoma.

13-8

Glaucoma

- Aqueous humor made by ciliary processes, then circulates along posterior surface of iris to pass out of the pupil
- Then, fills anterior chamber and is drained via the scleral venous sinus (canal of Schlemm)

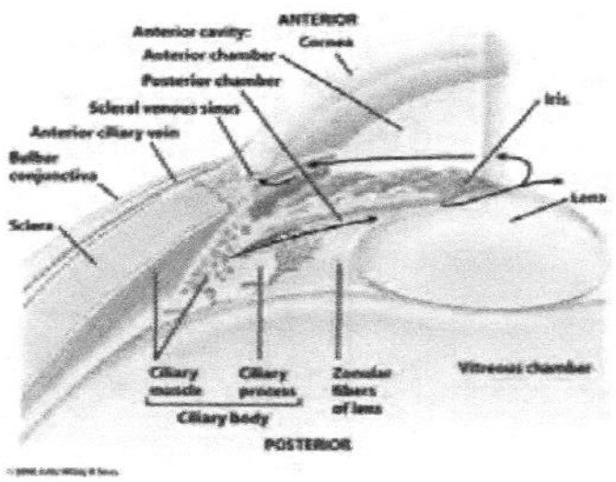
ANTERIOR
Cornea
Anterior cavity:
Anterior chamber
Posterior chamber
Scleral venous sinus
Anterior ciliary vein
Bulbar conjunctiva
Sclera
Iris
Lens
Ciliary muscle
Ciliary process
Ciliary body
Zonular fibers of lens
Vitreous chamber
POSTERIOR

- Glaucoma can result from:
  - overproduction by ciliary processes
  - obstruction in flow
  - obstruction in scleral venous sinus (most common)
- Drugs which cause pupil dilation (sympathetic nervous system stimulants) tend to close the sinus and make glaucoma worse

13-8

Macular Degeneration

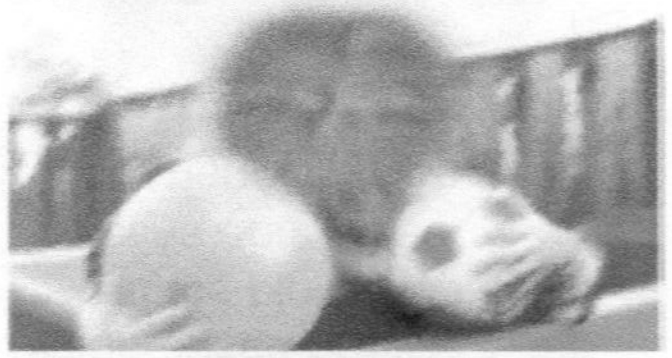
A scene as it might be viewed by a person with age-related macular degeneration.

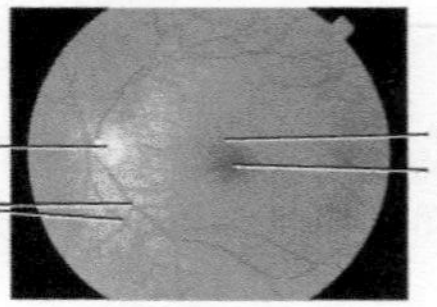
NASAL SIDE
TEMPORAL SIDE
Optic disc
Retinal blood vessels
Macula lutea
Fovea centralis
Left eye

- Almost all vision is carried out in a small, 1 mm diameter region of retina called the **fovea**
- The **macula** ("spot") is the corresponding feature on the retinal surface
- **Macular degeneration** is a loss of the critical neurons in this area for unknown reasons

13-8

Presbyopia

- As we age, lens loses its elasticity
- This prevents it from taking on a round shape when relaxed
- Round shape needed to focus on near objects
- After age 40, reading glasses needed to focus on near objects

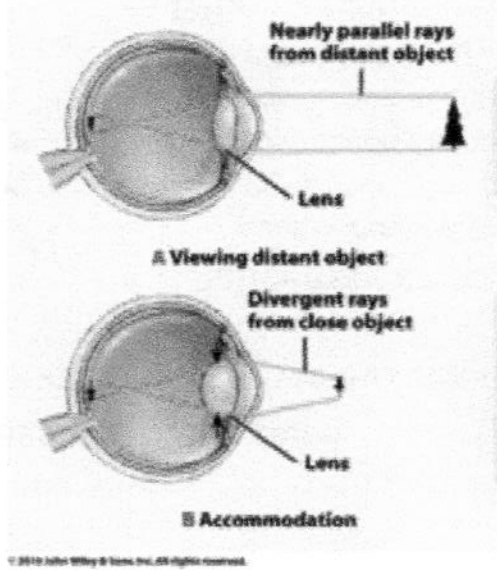
Nearly parallel rays from distant object
Lens
A Viewing distant object
Divergent rays from close object
Lens
B Accommodation

lens is flattened by pulling action of zonule fibers

when zonule fibers relax, elasticity of lens "snaps it back" into round shape

13-8
Ireland, Visualizing Human Biology, 2/e

Retinal Detachment

- Retina is one of several layers in the eye
- The inner retina receives blood supply and nutrition from the surface blood vessels
- The outer retina (including photoreceptors) receives nutrition from the retinal pigment epithelium (RPE, between retina and choroid)
- The retina is not attached to the RPE and can easily come loose
- Neurons of the retina lose their nutritional support and die
- Nerve tissue cannot repair; treatment is to limit spread of damage by "spot welding" retina to the sclera with either cold or heat

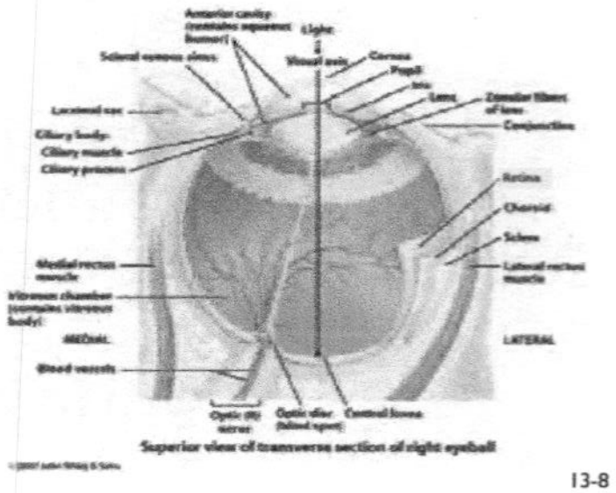
Superior view of transverse section of right eyeball

13-8

Disorders of Vision

- **Emmetropia** – normal vision
- **Myopia** – near-sighted, eyeball too long
- **Hypermetropia** – far-sighted, eyeball too short
- **Astigmatism** – unequal curvature of the cornea or lens

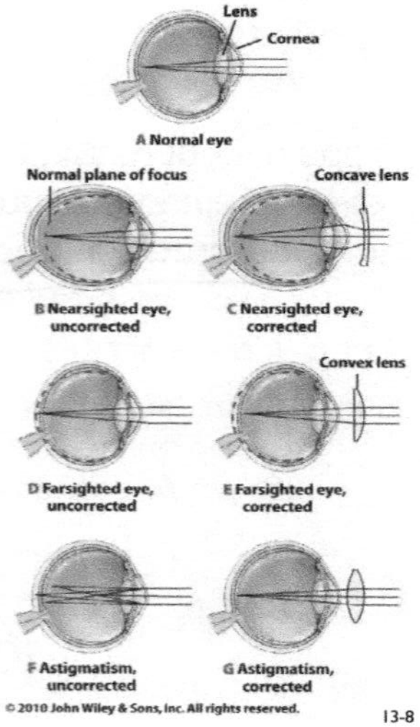
Lens
Cornea
A Normal eye
Normal plane of focus
Concave lens
B Nearsighted eye, uncorrected
C Nearsighted eye, corrected
Convex lens
D Farsighted eye, uncorrected
E Farsighted eye, corrected
F Astigmatism, uncorrected
G Astigmatism, corrected

13-8

Color Vision

- Can you trace a path between the Xs in the left figure? What about the right?
- About 5% of men are unable to perform this task

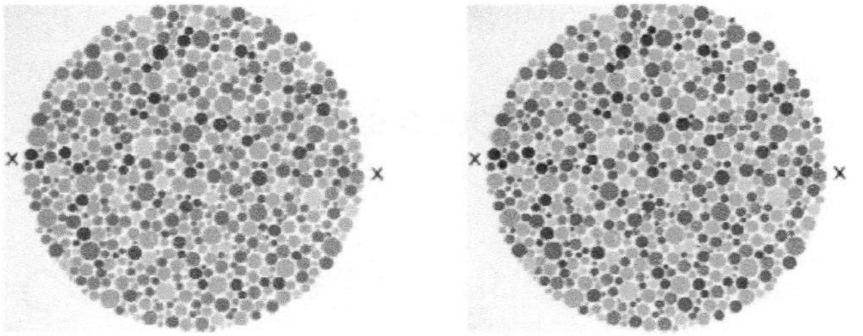

X
X
X
X

Alters, Biology: Understanding Life, 1/e
http://vischeck.com

13-8

Alterations in Color Vision

- There are three types of cone photoreceptor
  - each is most sensitive to a different wavelength of light (blue, green, red)
  - each has a different pigment protein
  - the genes coding for the red pigment and green pigment are on the X chromosome
  - mutations in the green pigment gene most common

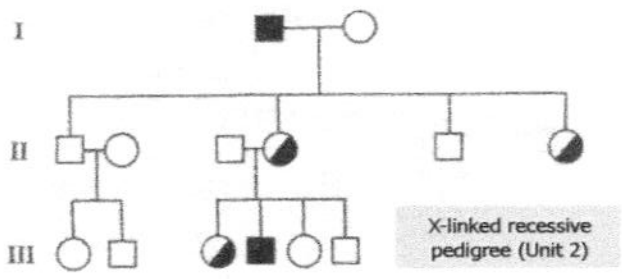

I
II
III

X-linked recessive pedigree (Unit 2)

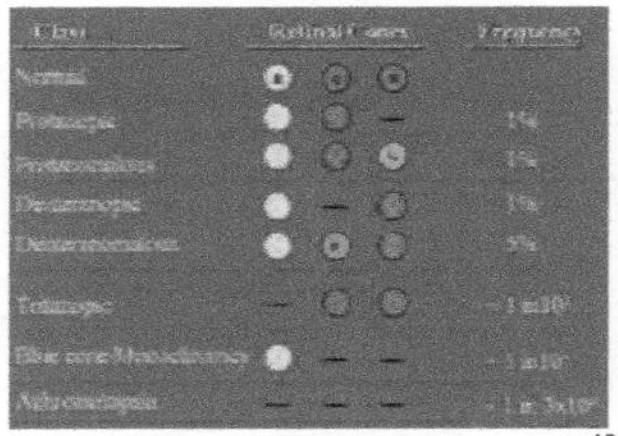

Deeb SS & Motulsky AG. Red-Green Color Vision Defects, www.ncbi.nlm.nih.gov

13-8

Alterations in Color Vision

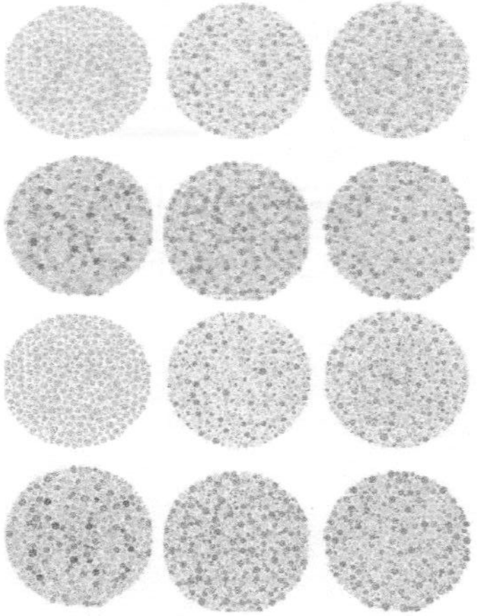

Deeb SS & Motulsky AG. Red-Green Color Vision Defects, www.ncbi.nlm.nih.gov
www.vischeck.com

- Top set of six circles: **Ishihara color vision test**
- Bottom set: same image processed through `vischeck.com`, which simulates alterations in color vision
- Note that "color blindness" is a bad term — this is color confusion
- Also note that dogs and deer have the same color vision defect, which is why hunter's orange works

13-8

Conjunctivitis

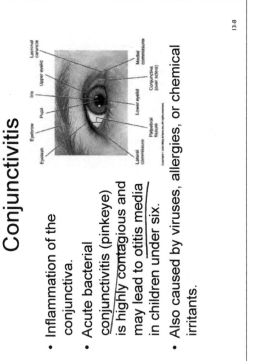

- Inflammation of the conjunctiva.
- Acute bacterial conjunctivitis (pinkeye) is highly contagious and may lead to otitis media in children under six.
- Also caused by viruses, allergies, or chemical irritants.

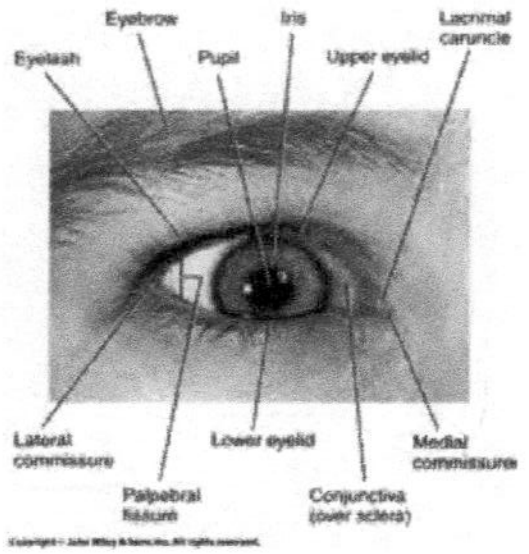

Eyebrow
Iris
Lacrimal caruncle
Eyelash
Pupil
Upper eyelid
Lateral commissure
Lower eyelid
Medial commissure
Palpebral fissure
Conjunctiva (over sclera)

13-8

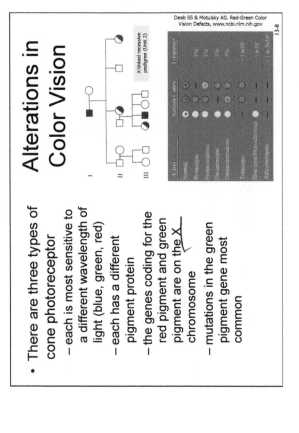

Disorders of Special Senses
Inner Ear: Hearing and Balance

Disorders of Hearing

- Hearing loss is divided into two broad catergories
  - **Conductive** hearing loss
    - Involves the external ear and middle ear structures
  - **Sensorineural** hearing loss
    - Involves the inner ear structures and cranial nerve VIII

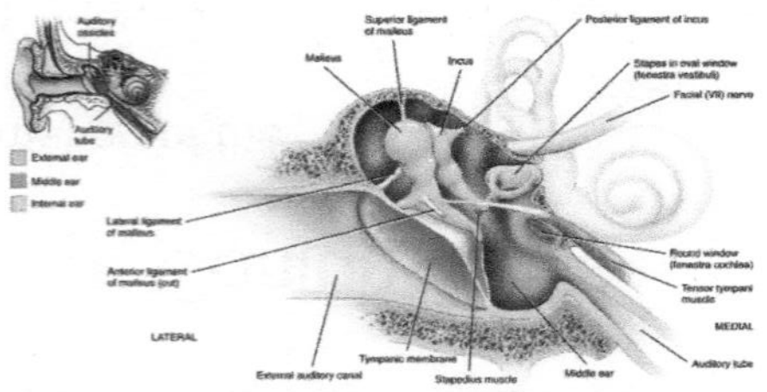

13-9

Conductive Hearing Disorders

- Occurs when a change in the outer and/or middle ear impairs conduction of sound waves
  - Foreign bodies, cerumen impaction, neoplasms of the external or inner ear, auditory tube (Eustachian tube) dysfucntion
  - Infections:
    - Acute otitis media **(AOM)**
    - Especially in children from 6 months to 5 years old

13-9

Sensorineural Hearing Loss

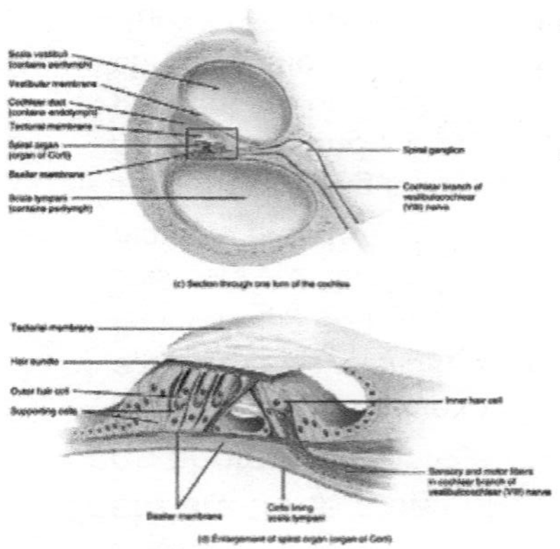
Figure 12.21(d) Tortora - PAP 12/e

- Anything affecting the **organ of Corti** or **cranial nerve VIII**
- Due to congenital, hereditary, or environmental factors
  - streptomycin and related antibiotics
  - loud noises
  - aspirin at toxic levels

13-9

Vertigo

- Sensation of spinning that is caused by inflammation or other disorders (e.g. cancer) of the **semicircular canals.**
- Vertigo is very different than dizziness or “lightheadedness” where someone feels “faint”
- Vertigo causes loss of balance, disorientation, nausea, and severe sensations that the room is spinning

13-9

Ménière Disease

- A not uncommon vestibular disorder of unknown etiology
  - Disturbance in the ionic composition of endolymph
- Results in a loss of proprioception, inability to walk or drive a car (affects gait and vision by causing vertigo) and persistent ringing in the ears

13-9

Unit 5
Chapter 14
Alterations in Cognitive Systems, Cerebral Hemodynamics, and Motor Function

Consciousness

Sources of Consciousness

Sleep

Coma

Consciousness

- **Consciousness = activity in cerebral cortex**
- All consciousness of sensory events is from cortex
- All conscious movement (motor activity) originates in cortex
- All conscious internal thoughts occur because of cortical activity (mostly in frontal cortex)

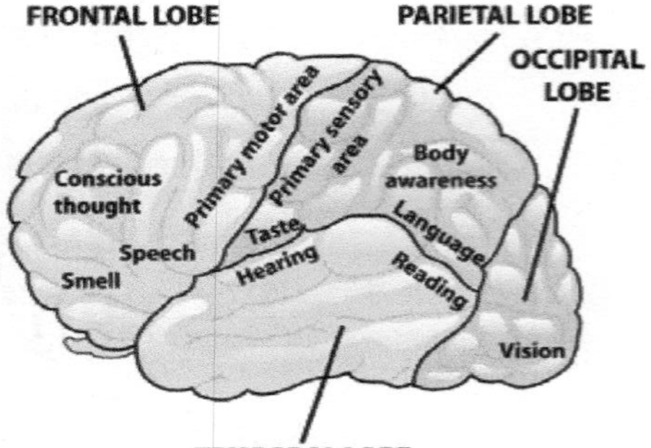
FRONTAL LOBE
PARIETAL LOBE
OCCIPITAL LOBE
Conscious thought
Primary motor area
Primary sensory area
Body awareness
Speech
Smell
Taste
Hearing
Language
Reading
Vision
TEMPORAL LOBE

Alters, Biology: Understanding Life, 1/e

14-I

Levels of Consciousness

- **Consciousness** is a function of **arousal** and **content of thought**
  - **Arousal** is the responsibility of the **reticular activating system** (RAS)
  - **Content of thought** is the responsibility of:
    - **cerebral cortex** (in general, rational thought)
    - **limbic system** (in general, emotional thought)

14-I

Limbic System Structures Controlling Memory and Consciousness

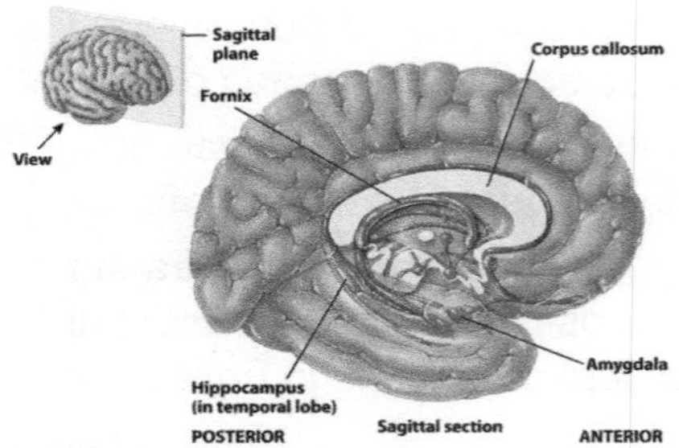
Sagittal plane
View
Fornix
Corpus callosum
Amygdala
Hippocampus (in temporal lobe)
POSTERIOR
Sagittal section
ANTERIOR

Ireland, Visualizing Human Biology, 2/e

- It's what's inside that counts
- Not just cortical activity on surface — remember internal cortical structures of **limbic lobe**
- These control and regulate memory and emotional states

14-I

Reticular Activating System (RAS)

- Not a defined area, just a bunch of neurons in the same general location with the same function

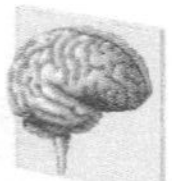

- These neurons control state of arousal
  - awake
  - asleep
  - somewhere in between
- RAS projects to all areas of cortex

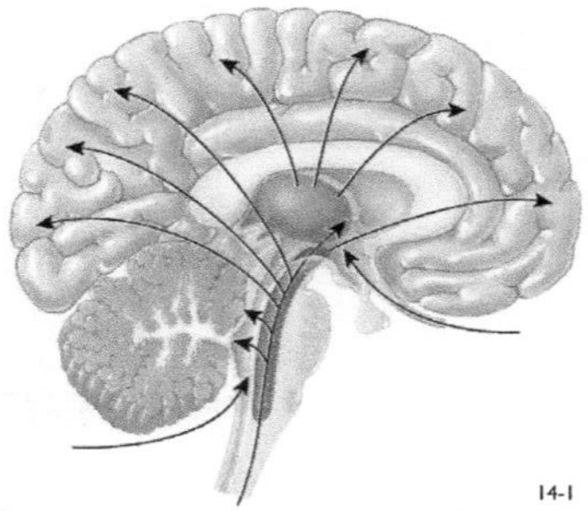

14-I

Reticular Activating System

- Inputs to RAS from sensory systems
- Outputs of RAS to cerebral cortex, regulating arousal

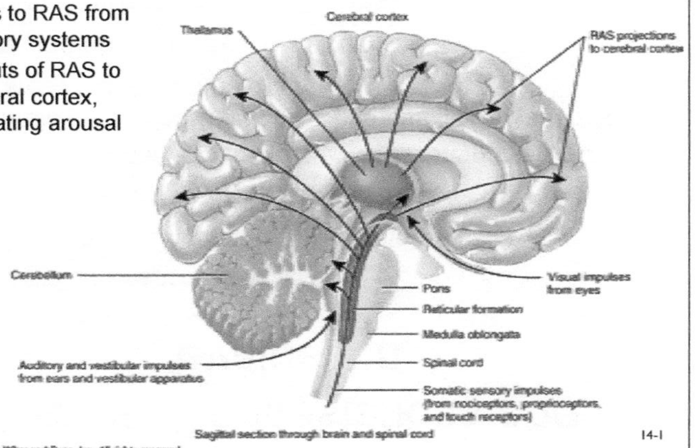

Thalamus
Cerebral cortex
RAS projections to cerebral cortex
Cerebellum
Visual impulses from eyes
Pons
Reticular formation
Medulla oblongata
Auditory and vestibular impulses from ears and vestibular apparatus
Spinal cord
Somatic sensory impulses (from nociceptors, proprioceptors, and touch receptors)

Sagittal section through brain and spinal cord

14-1

Alterations in Arousal

Levels of Consciousness

- We are said to be **unimpaired** (**fully functional**) when we are **alert** and we are oriented to person, place, and time
- **"Oriented X 3"**
  - *I know who I am*
  - *I know where I am (generally: city or "in a hospital")*
  - *I know what time it is (generally: year, day, who is President)*
- Normal speech, voluntary movement, oculomotor activity, respirations, and pupillary responses

14-2

Alterations in Arousal

- **Structural:** infections, vascular, neoplastic, traumatic, congenital, degenerative.
- **Metabolic:** hypoxia, electrolyte disturbances, hypoglycemia, drugs, and toxins.
- **Psychogenic** (unresponsiveness): may signal a general psychiatric disorder. Patient may appear unconscious but is physiologically awake.

14-2

Clinical Manifestations and Evaluation

Alterations in Arousal

Levels of Altered Consciousness

- Confusion
  - Loss of ability to think rapidly and clearly
- Disorientation
  - Disorientation to time, and then to place (usually orientation to person is preserved)
- Lethargy
  - Limited spontaneous movement; easily aroused; not oriented X 3
- Obtundation
  - Mild to moderate reduction in arousal. Falls asleep if not continuously stimulated. Single-syllable answers to questions.
- Stupor
  - Can only be aroused with vigorous and continuous stimulation
- Light Coma
  - Purposeful movement on stimulation
- Coma
  - Nonpurposeful movement, only if stimulated
- Deep Coma
  - No response

15-2

Clinical Manifestations and Evaluation

- Level of consciousness
- Pattern of breathing
  - Rate, rhythm, and pattern evaluated
- Size and reactivity of pupils
  - Indicate presence and level of brain stem dysfunction
  - Brain stem areas that control arousal are adjacent to areas that control pupils
- Eye position and eye reflexes
- Skeletal muscle motor responses
  - Purposeful, inappropriate, or not present

15-2

Skeletal Muscle Decorticate Posture

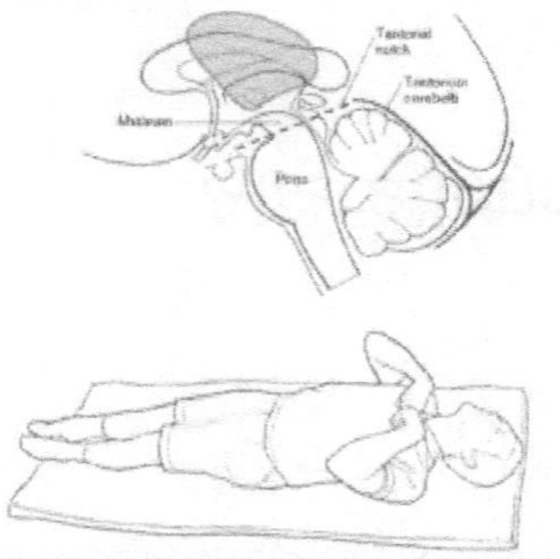
Decorticate rigidity

Decorticate = "no cortex"

- Upper extremities flexed at the elbows and held close to the body
- Lower extremities extended (toes pointed)
- Loss of connections between cortex and spinal cord/muscles

15-2

Skeletal Muscle Decerebrate Posture

- Upper extremity now extended
  - Thought to involve loss of inputs to arm muscles from the *red nucleus* in the midbrain
- Lower extremity the same
- Seen in extensive brain stem damage
- Death is imminent

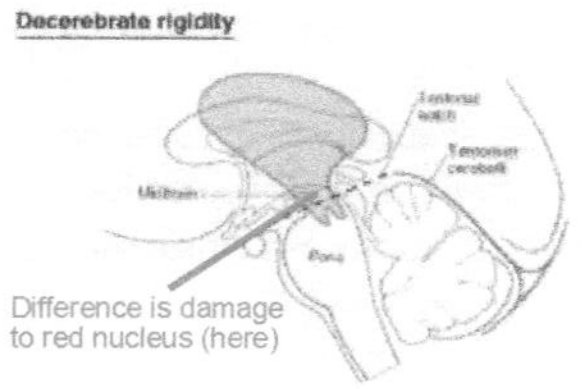
Decerebrate rigidity
Midbrain
Pons
Difference is damage to red nucleus (here)

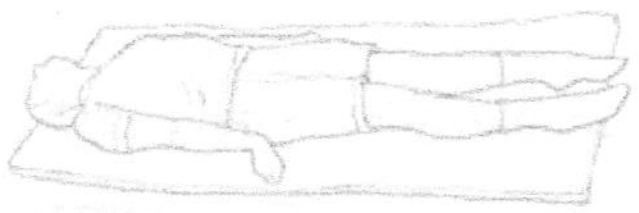

Decerebrate = "no brain"

15-2

Glasgow Coma Scale

Best eye response (E)	Spontaneous—open with blinking at baseline	4
	Opens to verbal command, speech, or shout	3
	Opens to pain, not applied to face	2
	None	1
Best verbal response (V)	Oriented	5
	Confused conversation, but able to answer questions	4
	Inappropriate responses, words discernible	3
	Incomprehensible speech	2
	None	1
Best motor response (M)	Obeys commands for movement	6
	Purposeful movement to painful stimulus	5
	Withdraws from pain	4
	Abnormal (spastic) flexion, decorticate posture	3
	Extensor (rigid) response, decerebrate posture	2
	None	1

15-3

Using the Glasgow Coma Scale

- Score of 3-15 possible
- Expressed as individual scores (E4, V4, M4) and sum (12)
- If it's just expressed as a sum ("12") then how can we tell if one is getting better while another one is getting worse (E4, V5, M3)?
- Brain injury defined as:
  - severe (GCS 3-8)
  - moderate (GCS 9-12)
  - minor (GCS 13-15)

15-3

Outcomes of Alterations in Arousal

- Outcomes fall into two categories: extent of disability (morbidity) and mortality.
- Outcomes range from full recovery to permanent disability or death.
- Brain death (total brain death)
  - Irreversible cessation of function of entire brain including the brain stem and cerebellum.
  - Flat EEG 6-12 hours
- Cerebral death (irreversible coma)
  - Death of cerebral hemispheres exclusive of the brain stem and cerebellum.
  - Brain stem may respond but individual is unable to respond to environment.

15-4

Outcomes of Alterations in Arousal

- Persistent Vegetative State
  - Complete unawareness of self or environment with complete loss of cognitive function
  - Brain stem reflexes intact
  - Recovery unlikely if state persists more than 12 months
- Minimally Conscious State
  - Individuals may follow simple commands, have intelligible speech, may blink or smile.
- Locked-in Syndrome
  - Complete paralysis of voluntary muscles except eye muscles.
  - Content of thought and level of arousal are intact but efferent pathways are blocked.

15-4

Alterations in Memory

Amnesias

- **Memory:** ability of brain to store and retrieve information
- **Anterograde amnesia**
  - Inability to form new memories
  - Usually damage to hippocampus
- **Retrograde amnesia**
  - Inability to recall memories from before traumatic event
  - May be a few seconds (e.g. motor vehicle collision) or years
    - Problem with memory storage system being "overwhelmed"
  - May be years
    - Damage to brain structures where memories stored
    - More distant events stored more strongly or in more locations and less likely to be lost
    - For example, name rarely lost

14-5

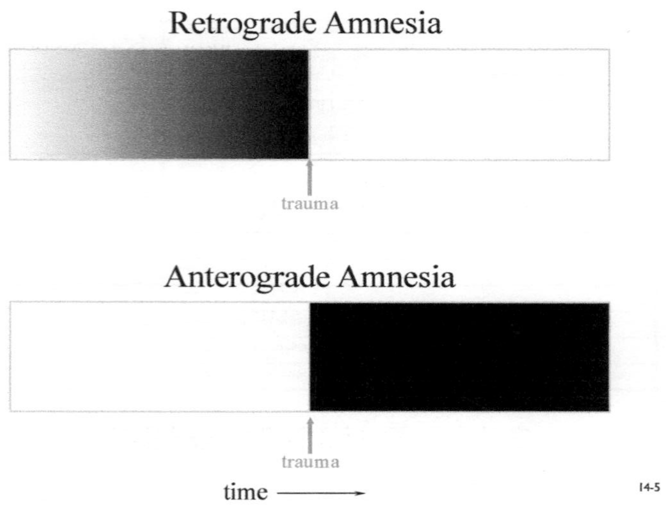

Retrograde Amnesia
trauma
Anterograde Amnesia
trauma
time

14-5

Seizures

Seizure Disorders

- **Seizure**: abnormal electrical activity in the brain
- Approximately 10% of the population will have a single seizure during their lifetime
  - Berg AT & Shinnar S. *Neurology* **41**:965, 1991
- Only about half of these people have another seizure, and only about one-third of these will be diagnosed with epilepsy
- About 3% of the population has **epilepsy**
- **Epilepsy =** "a transient occurrence of signs and/or symptoms as a result of abnormal excessive or enhanced synchronous neuronal activity in the brain"
  - Sathasivam S & Nicolson A. *Int J Clin Pract* **62**:1920, 2008.

14-6

Seizure Disorders

- Generalized seizures
  - Abnormal activity over a wide area of the brain
  - Consciousness always impaired or lost
  - Most common type: **absence seizures** ("spacing out")
- Partial seizures = focal seizures, unilateral
  - Specific area affected
  - For example, movement of hand
  - May progress to generalized seizures
    - movement of right hand → movement of right arm → movement of right side of body → movement of entire body
    - This pattern is called a **Jacksonian march**
    - Seizures involving abnormal activity over entire motor area of brain are called **generalized tonic-clonic seizures**

14-6

Seizure Disorders

- **Prodroma** (symptom): early clinical manifestation a few days or hours preceding a seizure
  - Maliase, headache, depression
- **Aura** (symptom): partial seizure, feeling that "something is about to happen"
  - Gustatory, visual, auditory, dizziness, numbness, funny feeling
- **Tonic phase** (sign): contraction of muscle(s)
- **Clonic phase** (sign): alternating contraction and partial relaxation of muscles
- **Ictus**: time that seizure is occurring (Latin *icere*, "whammo"
- **Postictal state**: Period immediately following end of seizure activity

14-6

Status Epilepticus

- Metabolic needs of neurons increase with increased firing rate
  - remember that sodium/potassium pump (ATPase) maintains the normal concentration of ions while each action potential degrades it a little bit
  - this increases the brain's need for glucose and oxygen
- Status epilepticus is a life-threatening emergency
  - Patient has a "string" of seizures with no respite
  - Usually caused by discontinuation of prescribed seizure medications

14-6

Data Processing Defects

Agnosia

Dysphasia

Dementias

Data Processing Defects

- Agnosia: defect of pattern recognition
  - Generally only one sense is affected
    - Tactile, visual, auditory
    - For example, an individual may be able to identify an object by touch but cannot name it by site.
- Dysphasia: Impairment of production or comprehension of language.
- Aphasia: More severe form of dysphasia and ability to communicate.

14-7

Language Disorders

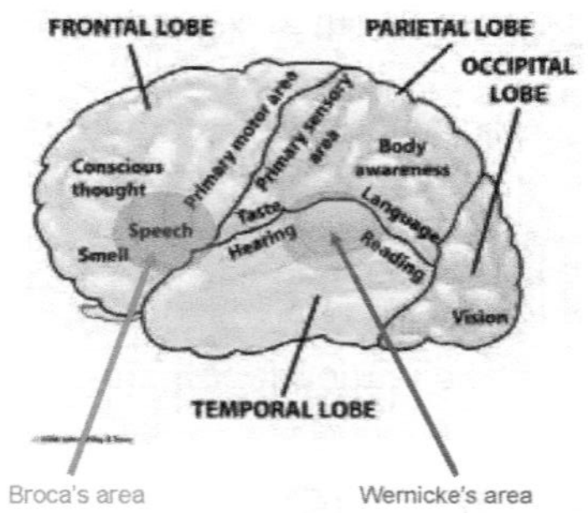
FRONTAL LOBE
PARIETAL LOBE
OCCIPITAL LOBE
TEMPORAL LOBE
Conscious thought
Primary motor area
Primary sensory area
Body awareness
Speech
Smell
Taste
Hearing
Language
Reading
Vision
Broca's area
Wernicke's area

- **Wernicke's area** (between hearing and language areas)
  - damage here produces **Wernicke's aphasia**
- **Broca's area** (near face area of primary motor cortex)
  - damage here produces **Broca's aphasia**

14-7

Broca Aphasia

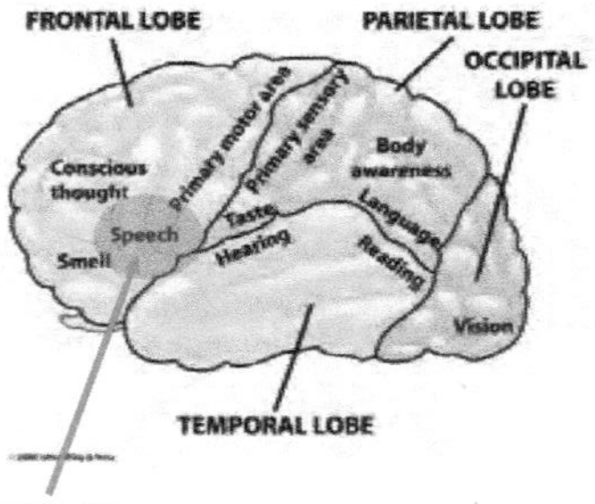
FRONTAL LOBE
PARIETAL LOBE
OCCIPITAL LOBE
Conscious thought
Primary motor area
Primary sensory area
Body awareness
Speech
Smell
Taste
Hearing
Language
Reading
Vision
TEMPORAL LOBE
Broca's area

- Also called "non-fluent aphasia"
  - Patient is unable to produce written or oral speech
  - Patient may have one syllable that he uses for all speech: "ma" or "fa" or "ba"
  - Patient appears frustrated or angry
  - Video: http://bit.ly/lwKdj
    - check out that groovy suit!

14-7

Wernicke Aphasia

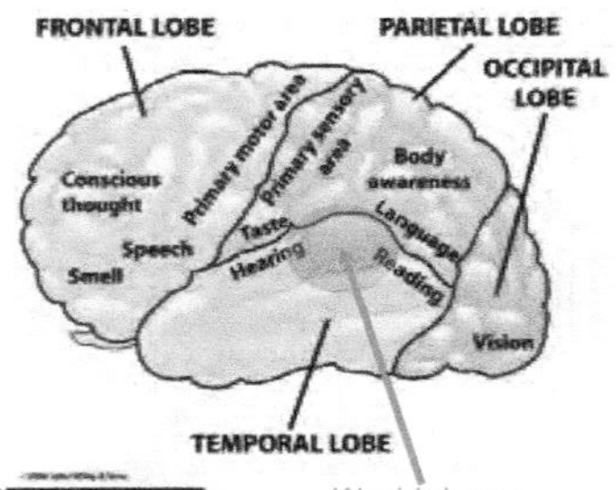
FRONTAL LOBE
PARIETAL LOBE
OCCIPITAL LOBE
Conscious thought
Primary motor area
Primary sensory area
Body awareness
Speech
Smell
Taste
Hearing
Language
Reading
Vision
TEMPORAL LOBE
Wernicke's area

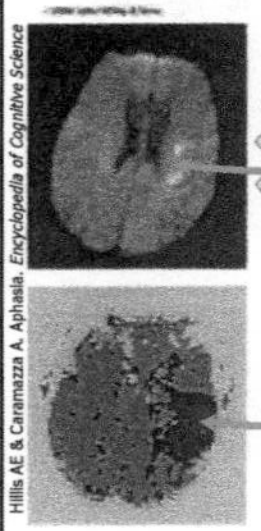
White area on diffusion-weighted imaging shows loss of blood supply to Wernicke's area
Dark area on perfusion-weighted imaging shows loss of blood supply to Wernicke's area

Hillis AE & Caramazza A. Aphasia. *Encyclopedia of Cognitive Science*

- Also called "fluent aphasia"
- Patients can speak, but language makes no sense and lacks grammatical structure
- Video: http://bit.ly/2iseGN

14-7

Testing for Aphasia and Other Brain Disorders

- Test for comprehension
  - top picture, *What is happening?*
    - "word salad": **Wernicke aphasia**
    - inability to speak: **Broca aphasia**
    - ignores left side of picture: **contralateral (left) hemineglect**
- Test for naming ability
  - bottom picture, *Name these objects.*
    - Does patient need prompting?
    - Are names correct?
    - Are answers slow or vague?

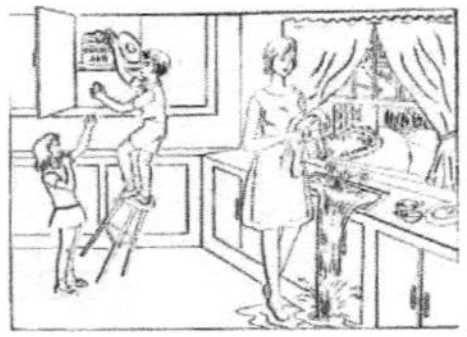

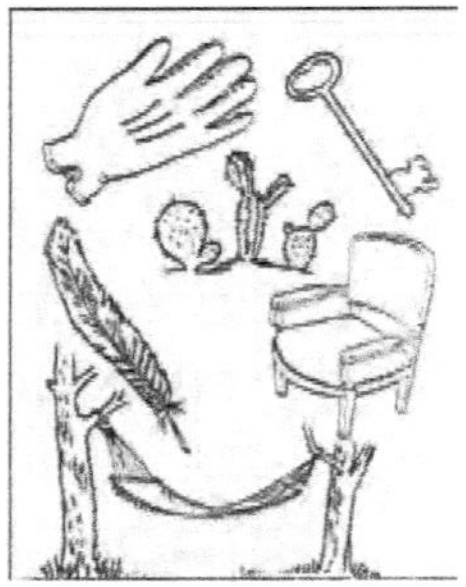

Ortiz GA & Sacco RL. National Institutes of Health Stroke Scale, in: *Wiley Encyclopedia of Clinical Trials*, 2008. Images courtesy National Institutes of Health

14-7

Dementia

- Progressive failure of many cerebral functions.
- Patient loses orientation to person, place and/or time; also memory loss.
- Decline in intellectual ability leads to alterations in behavior.

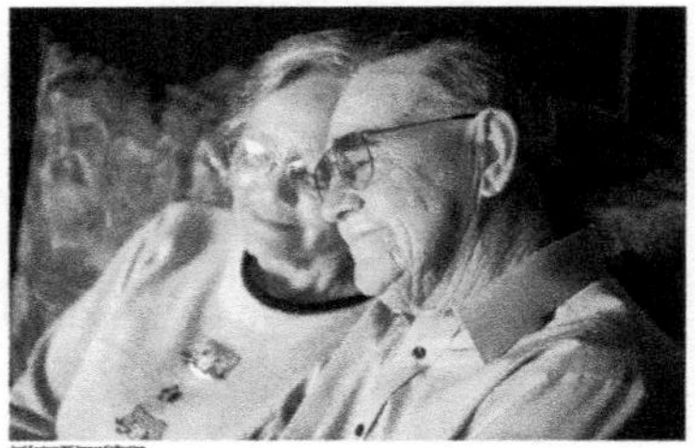

John Wiley & Sons Inc., 2011

14-7

Major Causes of Dementia

- Alzhemimer disease (>50% of cases)
- Alcoholism
- Parkinson disease
- Neoplasms of the CNS
- Neurosyphilis
- Prion disease (Creutzfeld-Jacob)
- Chronic meningitis

14-7

Alzheimer Disease

- Leading cause of dementia
- 4 million Americans affected
- 50% of people age 85 or greater have been diagnosed with Alzheimer Disease
- Declarative memory most severely affected
- Neuropsychological testing suggests diagnosis, but only definitive diagnosis is post-mortem examination of brain
- This is unsatisfying for everyone, especially for the patient

14-8

Neurpathological Changes in Alzheimer Brain

- **Tau** is a microtubule-associated protein
- **Amyloid precursor protein** is a normal protein of unknown function
  - APP is processed into β–amyloid, which is insoluble
- Both accumulate in abnormal intracellular structures in neurons
  - tau forms tangles
  - β–amyloid forms plaques
- Neurons die in larger numbers than normal

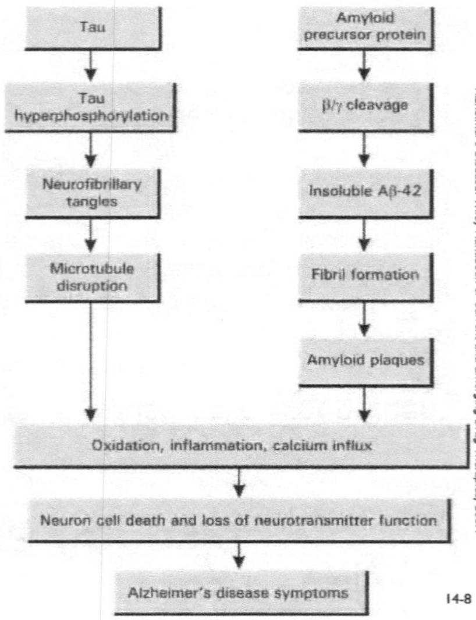

Tau
Tau hyperphosphorylation
Neurofibrillary tangles
Microtubule disruption
Amyloid precursor protein
β/γ cleavage
Insoluble Aβ-42
Fibril formation
Amyloid plaques
Oxidation, inflammation, calcium influx
Neuron cell death and loss of neurotransmitter function
Alzheimer's disease symptoms

Alzheimer's Disease. *Wiley Handbook of Current and Emerging Drug Therapies*, 2007.

14-8

Tau Forms Tangles Amyloid Forms Plaques

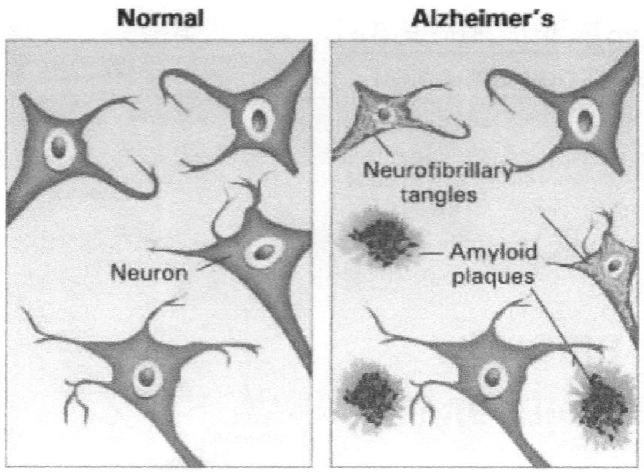

Normal
Alzheimer's
Neuron
Neurofibrillary tangles
Amyloid plaques

Alzheimer's Disease. *Wiley Handbook of Current and Emerging Drug Therapies*, 2007.

14-8

Alzheimer Brain

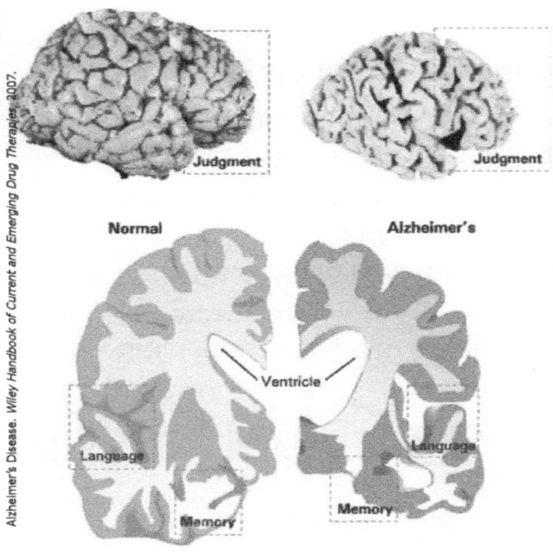
Judgment
Judgment
Normal
Alzheimer's
Ventricle
Language
Language
Memory
Memory

- As neurons die, brain shrinkage occurs
- Memory, language and judgment areas most affected
- Using imaging, it is difficult to distinguish between normal aging and Alzheimer

Sources: Oklahoma University Health Sciences Center.

Alzheimer's Disease. Wiley Handbook of Current and Emerging Drug Therapies, 2007.

14-8

Alzheimer Therapy

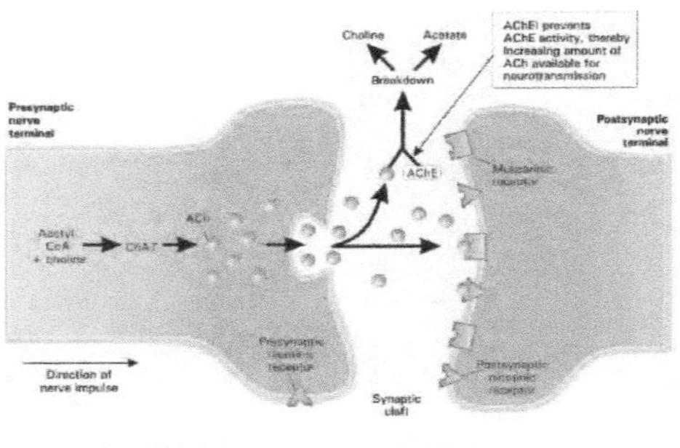
Choline
Acetate
Breakdown
AChEI prevents AChE activity, thereby increasing amount of ACh available for neurotransmission
Presynaptic nerve terminal
Postsynaptic nerve terminal
AChE
ACh
ChAT
Direction of nerve impulse
Synaptic cleft

Acetyl-CoA = Acetyl-coenzyme A; ACh = Acetylcholine; AChE = Acetylcholinesterase; AChEI = Acetylcholinesterase inhibitor; ChAT = Choline acetyltransferase.

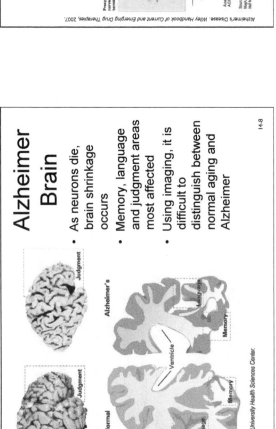

- Currently available therapies use acetylcholinesterase inhibitors (AChEIs) which make more acetylcholine available at the remaining synapses
- These therapies mostly ineffective, 10+ year disease course shifted by perhaps 3 months

Alzheimer's Disease. Wiley Handbook of Current and Emerging Drug Therapies, 2007.

14-8

Alterations in Cerebral Hemodynamics

Cerebral Hemodynamics

- Injuries to the brain may induce alterations in cerebral blood flow, intracranial pressure, and oxygen delivery.
- Increases in intracranial pressure (ICP) may cause a decrease in blood perfusion.

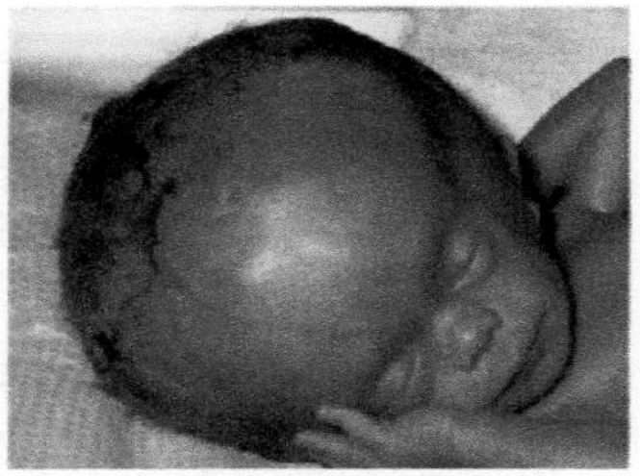

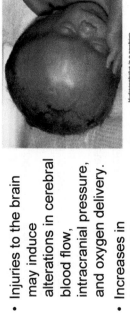

Hydrocephalus in a newborn

John Wiley & Sons, 2011

14-9

Sources of Intracranial Pressure

- Space-occupying lesion
  - hematomas
  - brain tumors
- Hydrocephalus
  - overproduction of CSF
  - under-absorption of CSF
  - blockage in circulation of CSF
- Brain edema

14-9

Increased ICP

- Stage 1: Vasoconstriction and external compression of venous system to decrease ICP.
  - Few symptoms. ICP may not change due to compensation.
- Stage 2: Continued expansion of intracranial content.
  - Systemic arterial vasoconstriction in an attempt to overcome increased ICP.
  - Patient may be confused, restless, drowsy, and may have slight pupillary and breathing changes.

14-9

Increased ICP

- Stage 3: ICP begins to approach arterial pressure.
  - Brain tissues begin to experience hypoxia and hypercapnia.
  - Patient's condition rapidly deteriorates.
  - Decreasing levels of arousal, widened pulse pressure, bradycardia, and small, sluggish pupils.
  - Dramatic rises in ICP when compensatory mechanisms exhausted.
- Stage 4: Brain tissue herniates.

14-9

Supratentorial vs Infratentorial

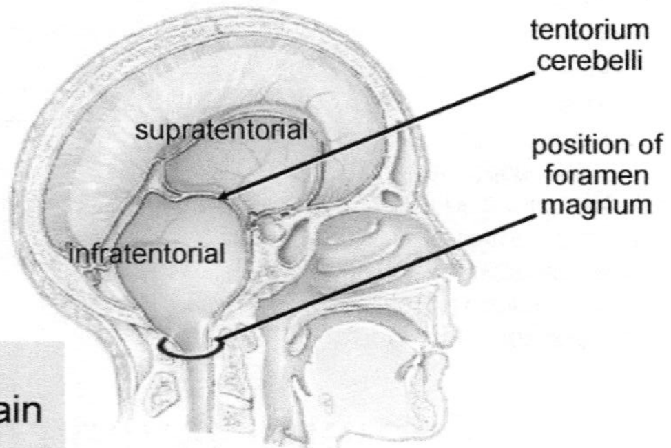
supratentorial
infratentorial
tentorium cerebelli
position of foramen magnum

The tentorium defines two brain compartments

14-9

Uncal Herniation

- When there is more pressure in the supratentorial compartment than the infratentorial compartment, the brain tries to "leave" (**herniates**) past the tentorium cerebelli
  - e.g., bleeding from skull fracture; tumor
- A part of the brain called the uncus is in the way
- This is called an **uncal herniation**
- Underneath the uncus are structures controlling **declarative memory**, memories of facts, dates and events
  - **"Orientation X 3"** depends on these structures

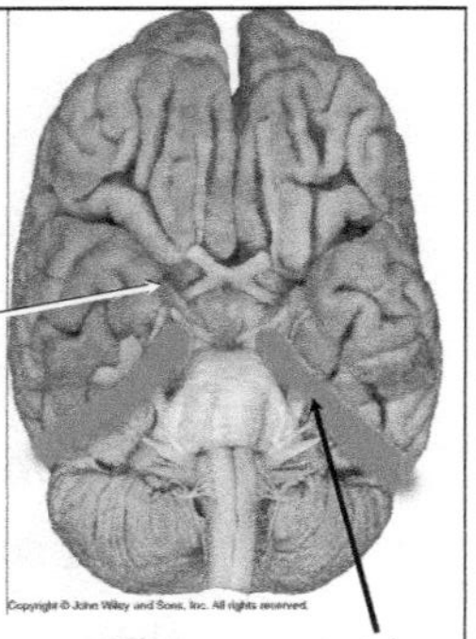
uncus
tentorium cerebelli

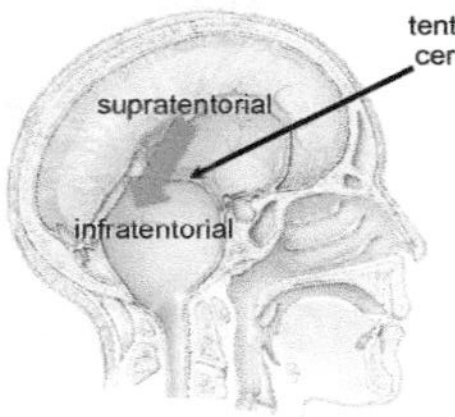
supratentorial
infratentorial

14-9

Tonsillar Herniation

- Death can result:
  - If supratentorial pressure continues
  - Or if pressure begins in infratentorial compartment
- Part of the cerebellum (**cerebellar tonsils**) and **medulla** try to "leave" skull at same time through same exit: the **foramen magnum**
- This part of the medulla controls heartbeat and respiration

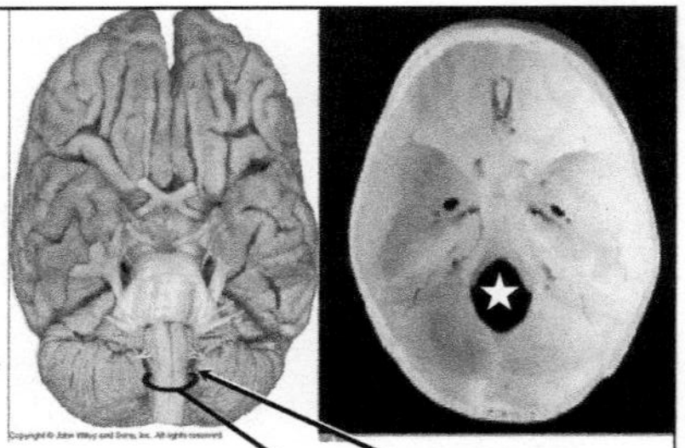
medulla
cerebellar tonsils

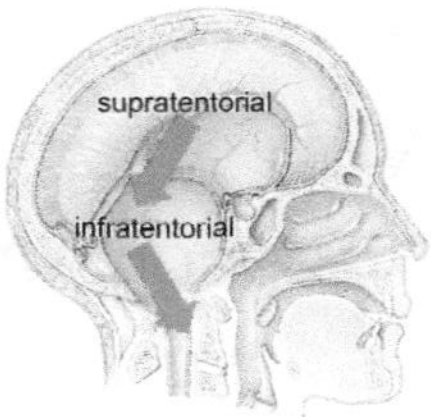
supratentorial
infratentorial

14-9

Motor (Muscle) Function

The Spinal Cord

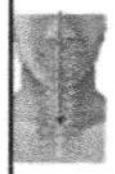

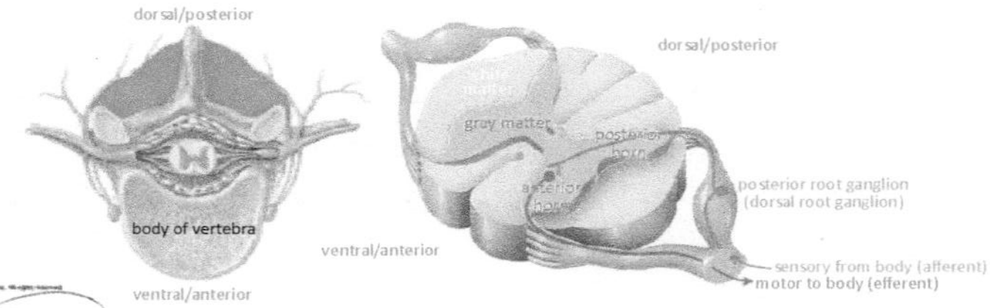
dorsal/posterior
body of vertebra
ventral/anterior
dorsal/posterior
gray matter
posterior root ganglion
(dorsal root ganglion)
ventral/anterior
sensory from body (afferent)
motor to body (efferent)

- White matter contains ascending (sensory) and descending (motor) tracts
- Gray matter is where neural information (including reflex) is processed
  - Posterior horn (also called dorsal horn) processes sensory information
    - cell body in posterior root ganglion (blue dot)
  - Anterior horn (also called ventral horn) contains cell bodies of neurons which control the voluntary muscles
    - motor neuron cell body is a red dot in this schematic

14-10

Motor Pathway
Lateral Corticospinal Tract

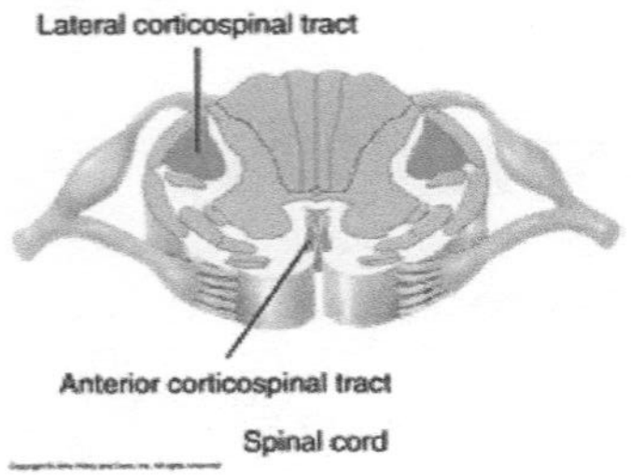
Lateral corticospinal tract
Anterior corticospinal tract
Spinal cord

- Axons from motor cortex
- Cross at pyramidal decussation (level of foramen magnum)
- In spinal cord, motor fibers are on same side as the muscles they will eventually innervate

14-10

Motor Pathways

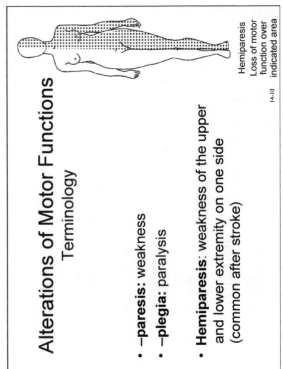

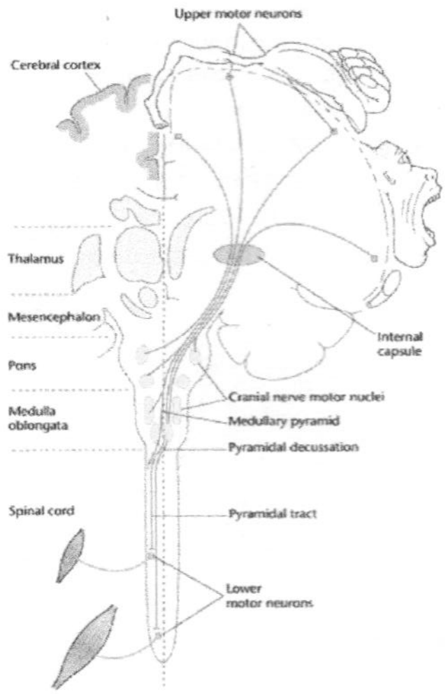
Upper motor neurons
Cerebral cortex
Thalamus
Mesencephalon
Pons
Medulla oblongata
Spinal cord
Internal capsule
Cranial nerve motor nuclei
Medullary pyramid
Pyramidal decussation
Pyramidal tract
Lower motor neurons

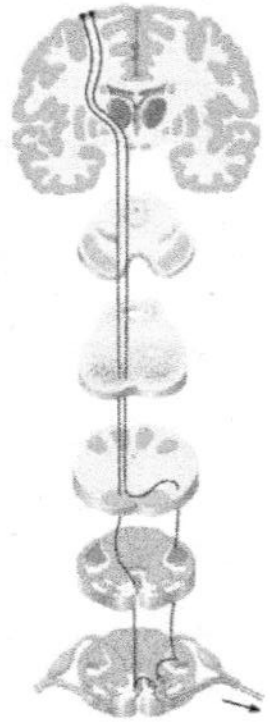

14-10

Alterations of Motor Functions
Terminology

- **Hypotonia**: decreased muscle tone
  - caused by decreased neuronal activity
- **Hypertonia**: increased muscle tone
- **Hyperkinesia**: excessive movement
- **Dyskinesia**: abnormal involuntary movements
- **Hypokinesia**: decreased movement

14-10

Alterations of Motor Functions
Terminology

- **–paresis:** weakness
- **–plegia:** paralysis

- **Hemiparesis**: weakness of the upper and lower extremity on one side (common after stroke)

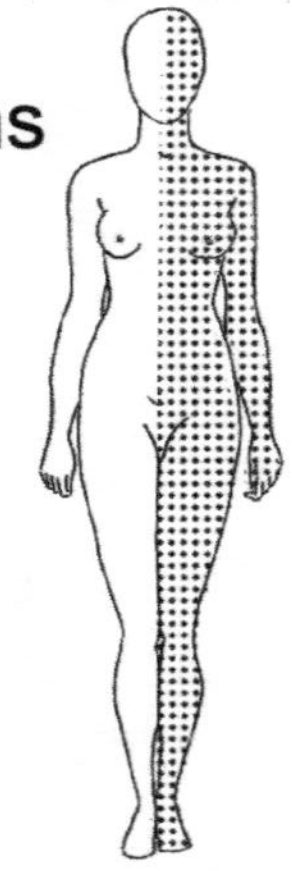

Hemiparesis
Loss of motor function over indicated area

14-10

Alterations of Motor Functions

Terminology

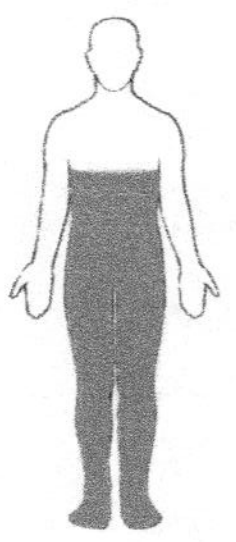

Paraplegia
Loss of motor function over indicated area
Damage to spinal cord at T4 (sensory and motor "level" at nipple line)

- **Diplegia**
  - Paralysis affecting both arms or both legs due to brain damage
    - e.g. cerebral palsy at birth
- **Paraplegia**
  - partial or total paralysis in the lower extremities
- **Tetraplegia**
  - partial or total paralysis in all four extremities due to spinal cord damage
    - the condition is also termed **quadriplegia**

14-10

Upper Motor Neuron vs Lower Motor Neuron

- All neurons which cause or regulate movement are called "motor neurons"
- *Lower motor neurons* are those in spinal cord that directly innervate skeletal muscle
- All others (including motor cortex neurons) are *upper motor neurons*

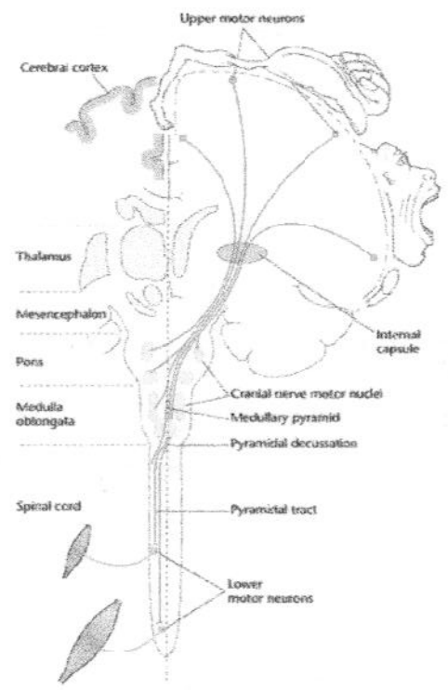
Upper motor neurons
Cerebral cortex
Thalamus
Mesencephalon
Pons
Medulla oblongata
Spinal cord
Internal capsule
Cranial nerve motor nuclei
Medullary pyramid
Pyramidal decussation
Pyramidal tract
Lower motor neurons

14-10

Reflexes in Lower Motor Neuron Disease

- Loss of lower motor neuron: there is no way to "drive" muscle
- This is called a **flaccid paralysis**
- Effect on reflexes is **hyporeflexia**

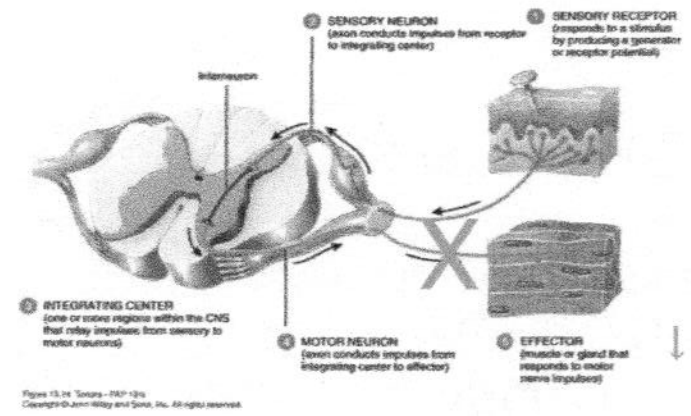
SENSORY NEURON
SENSORY RECEPTOR
Interneuron
INTEGRATING CENTER
MOTOR NEURON
EFFECTOR

↓ muscle tone

- Reflexes described clinically on 0–5 scale
- 2/5 or 3/5 is normal
- Flaccid paralysis is 0/5 or 1/5

14-10

Reflexes in Upper Motor Neuron Disease

- Loss of upper motor neuron thought to remove inhibition on reflexes, so patient exhibits **hyperreflexia**
- Some forms called **spastic paralysis** or **rigidity**

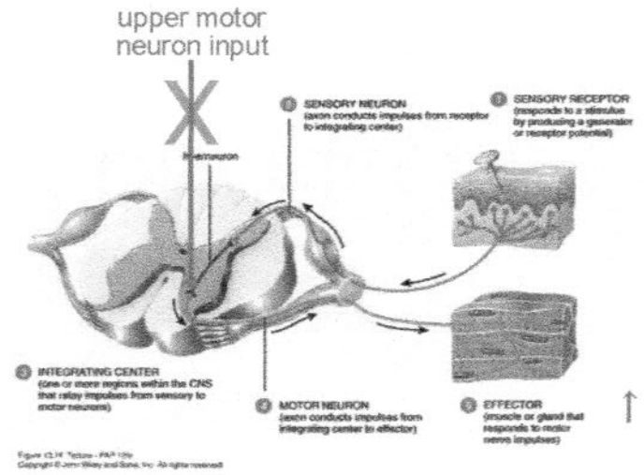
upper motor neuron input
SENSORY NEURON
SENSORY RECEPTOR
INTEGRATING CENTER
MOTOR NEURON
EFFECTOR

↑ muscle tone

- Reflexes described clinically on 0–5 scale
- 2/5 or 3/5 is normal
- Hyperreflexia and spastic paralysis are 4/5 or 5/5

14-10

Upper Motor Neuron Lesion

- Loss of control from brain means reflexes operate without modification
- Example: "the Babinski sign"
- Stroke the metal end of the reflex hammer along the sole of the foot
- In normal adults, response is plantar flexor: toes curl down, toward sole of foot
- In spinal cord damage, brain damage or in babies less than 1 yr old, response is plantar extensor: toes splay up, away from sole of foot

- How to elicit a Babinski: http://www.youtube.com/watch?v=kOq5Np0eZ6A
- A Babinski sign: http://www.youtube.com/watch?v=ZQh6zVxtYGc

14-10

Disorders of the Basal Nuclei (Basal Ganglia)

Parkinson Disease
Huntington disease

Neurotransmitters in the Basal Nuclei

- Basal nuclei control smooth movement
- Motor cortex signal is processed through this system
- Interactions between motor inhibiting neurotransmitters (GABA, Dopamine) and excitatory neurotransmitters (Acetylcholine) control movement.
- http://bit.ly/KO3fkZ

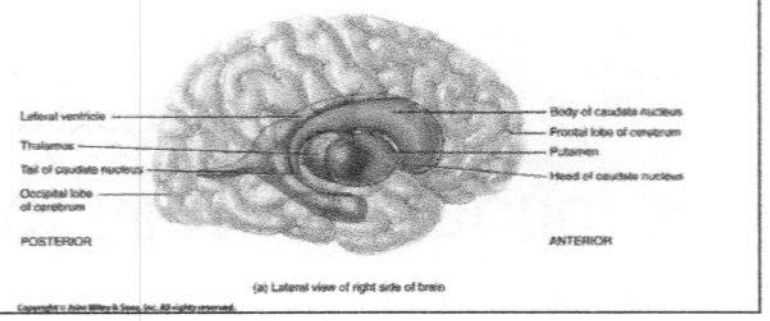
POSTERIOR
ANTERIOR

14-11

Parkinson Disease and the Substantia Nigra

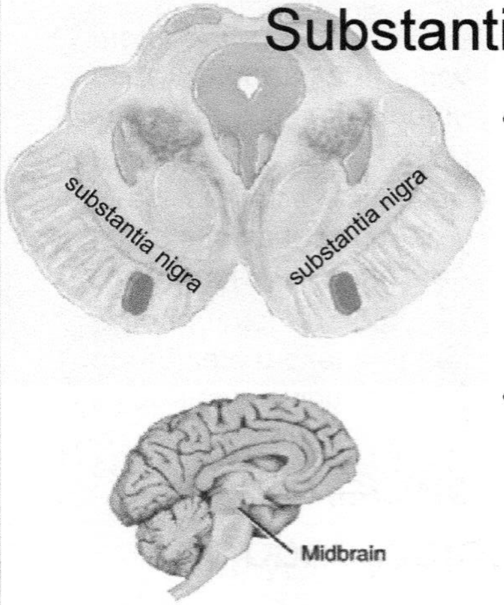
substantia nigra
substantia nigra
Midbrain

- Neurons in the substantia nigra make dopamine and send axons to the basal nuclei, where dopamine is released
- In Parkinson Disease, these neurons die for unknown reasons

14-11

Parkinson Disease Symptoms

- Symptoms:
  - “pill-rolling” tremor at rest (disappears with movement)
  - slow movement (**bradykinesia**)
  - stooped posture
  - characteristic gait
    - trouble getting through doorways
  - about 40% have dementia

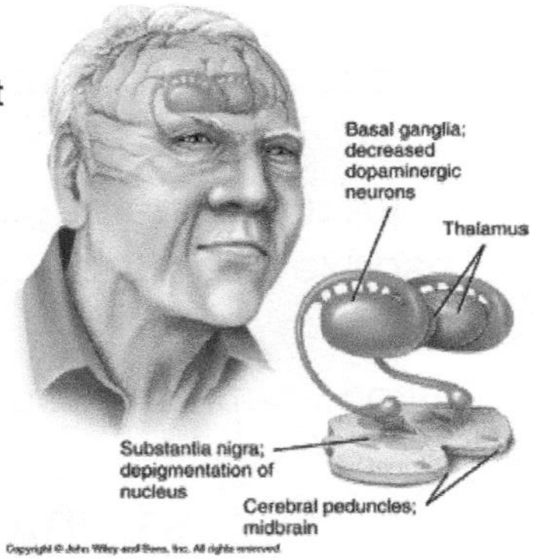

Basal ganglia; decreased dopaminergic neurons
Thalamus
Substantia nigra; depigmentation of nucleus
Cerebral peduncles; midbrain

14-11

Huntington Disease

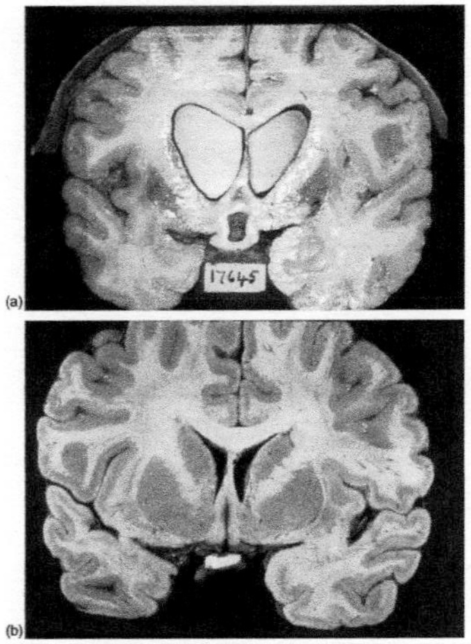

(a)
17645
(b)

- Disease with variable age of onset causing dementia and chorea (writhing, dance-like movements)
- Gene for protein huntington on chromosome 4
- Degeneration of basal nuclei with degeneration of GABA producing neurons (inhibitory) leads to hyperkinesia.
  - top: Huntington Disease
  - bottom: normal

14-11

Huntington Disease

- **Trinucleotide repeat disease**
  - non-Mendelian inheritance but resembles autosomal dominant
  - unaffected patients have 10-29 repeats of CAG in the huntington gene
  - diseased persons have 40 or more repeats
    - CAG is codon for glutamine
  - more repeats means more severe disease and earlier onset

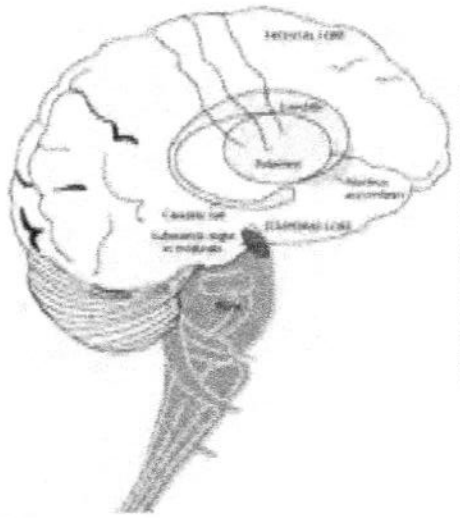

Encyclopedia of Cognitive Science

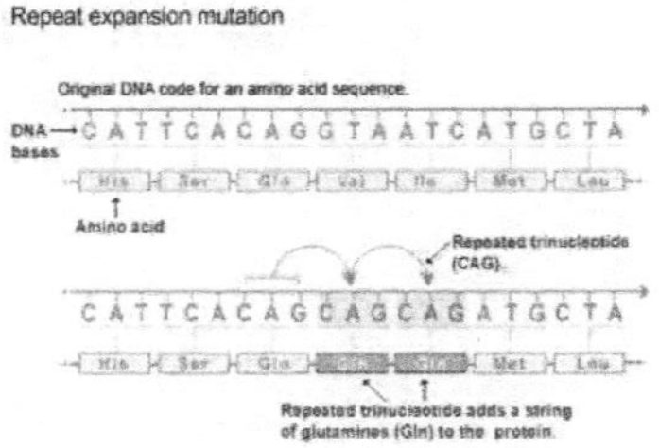

Repeat expansion mutation
Original DNA code for an amino acid sequence.
DNA bases
C A T T C A C A G G T A A T C A T G C T A
His Ser Gln Val Ile Met Leu
Amino acid
Repeated trinucleotide (CAG).
C A T T C A C A G C A G C A G A T G C T A
His Ser Gln Gln Gln Met Leu
Repeated trinucleotide adds a string of glutamines (Gln) to the protein.

U.S. National Library of Medicine

14-11

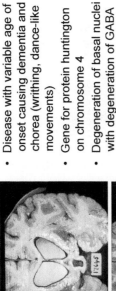

Unit 5
Chapter 15
Disorders of the Central and Peripheral Nervous Systems and the Neuromuscular Junction

Traumatic Brain Injury
Focal Brain Injury

Traumatic Brain Injury

- 1.4 million per year
  - 80% mild (GCS 13-15), 10% moderate (GCS 9-12), 10% severe (GCS 3-8)
  - 28% falls, 20% motor vehicle crashes, 19% something hits you or you hit something, 11% assaults
- **Open trauma**
  - Penetration of the skull by a missile, usually a bullet
- **Blunt trauma**
  - Brain is not exposed

15-1

Brain Injuries

- **Penetrating** or **open** head injuries occur from missile trauma
- These injuries break the dura and expose the cranial contents to the environment (infection; loss of CSF)
- Penetrating head traumas produce **focal** injuries which are **observable** by radiological examination

15-1

Blunt Trauma

- Focal injury
  - Epidural (extradural) hematoma
  - Subdural hematoma
  - Intracerebral hematoma
  - Contusion
- Diffuse injury
  - Concussion
    - mild (grade I-III)
    - severe, classic (grade IV)
  - Diffuse axonal injury (DAI)

15-1
15-3

Focal Brain Injury

- These type of closed-head injuries usually present as **coup-contrecoup** contusions
  - coup (French, "strike") is the direct impact between the brain and skull
  - contrecoup is directly opposite the coup injury, from the brain "bouncing" and impacting the opposite side of the skull
  - example: head hits windshield in motor vehicle collision
    - coup: frontal cortex
    - contrecoup: occipital cortex
- Coup-contrecoup injuries are commonly seen in **shaken baby syndrome**

15-1

Epidural vs Subdural Bleeding

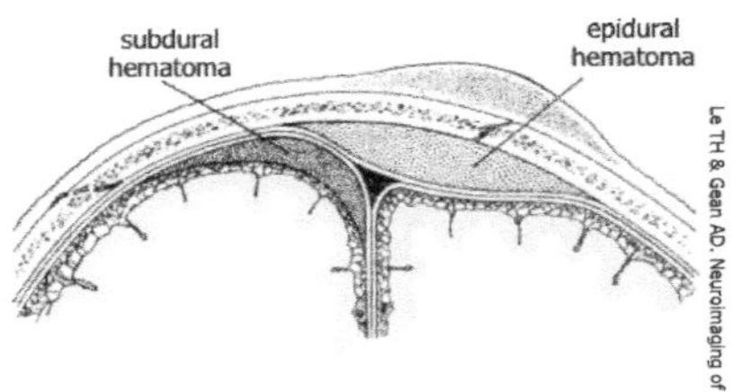
subdural hematoma
epidural hematoma

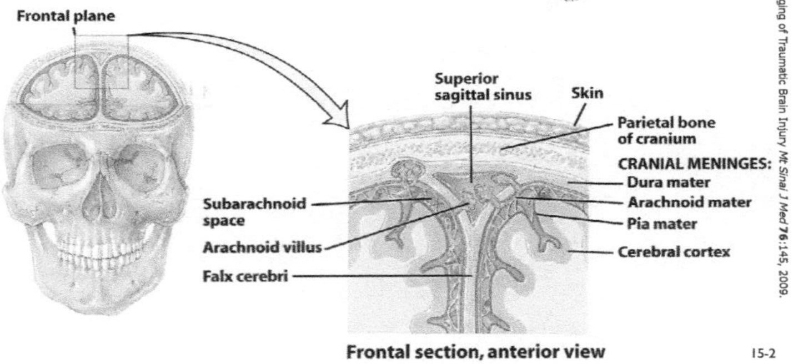
Frontal plane
Superior sagittal sinus
Skin
Parietal bone of cranium
CRANIAL MENINGES:
Dura mater
Arachnoid mater
Pia mater
Cerebral cortex
Subarachnoid space
Arachnoid villus
Falx cerebri
Frontal section, anterior view

© 2006 John Wiley & Sons

Le TH & Gean AD. Neuroimaging of Traumatic Brain Injury *Mt Sinai J Med* **76**:145, 2009.

15-2

Focal Brain Injury
Epidural Hematoma

- Epidural hematoma (extradural hematoma)
- Bleeding usually arterial
- Bleeding between skull and dura mater
- Can be insidious (slow onset)
- Usually show lens shape on CT or MRI
  - blood between bone and toucgh membrane
- Symptoms
  - Headache of increasing severity, vomiting, drowsiness, confusion, and seizure
  - Can produce paralysis on opposite side of body
  - May also cause brain herniation

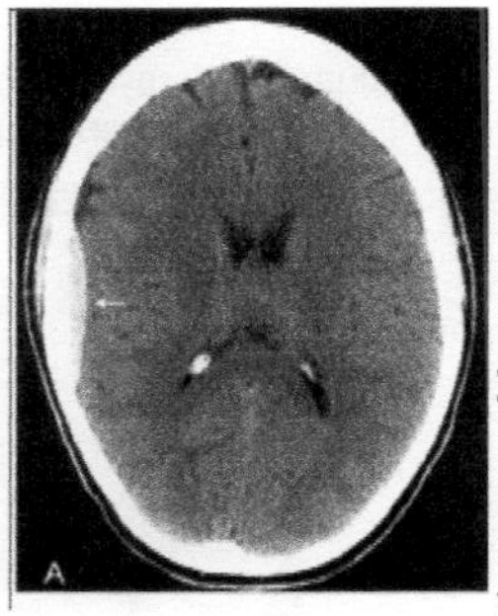
A

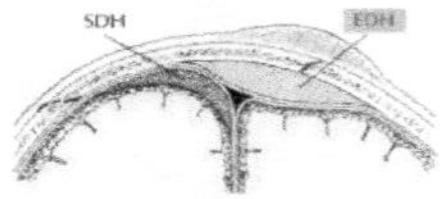
SDH
EDH

Le TH & Gean AD. Neuroimaging of Traumatic Brain Injury *Mt Sinai J Med* **76**:145, 2009.

15-2

Focal Brain Injury
Subdural Hematoma

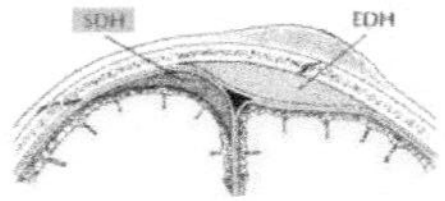
SDH
EDH

- **Subdural** hematomas
  - More difficult to see on CT or MRI
  - Symptoms usually more insidious and chronic: headache, drowsiness, slowed cognition, and confusion
  - Arrows show collections of blood putting pressure on brain

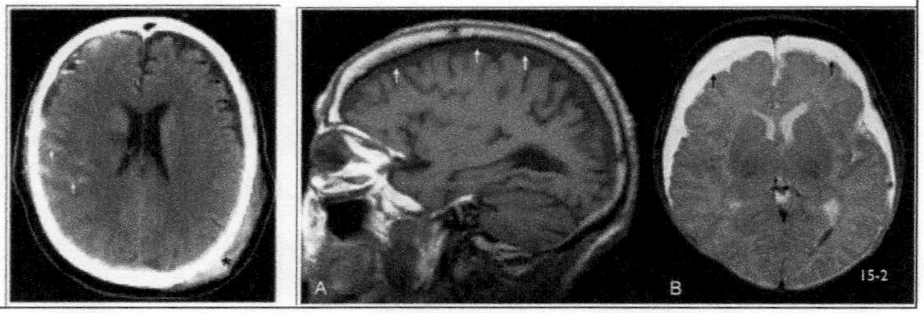
A
B

Le TH & Gean AD. Neuroimaging of Traumatic Brain Injury *Mt Sinai J Med* **76**:145, 2009.

15-2

Focal Brain Injury
Subdural Hematoma

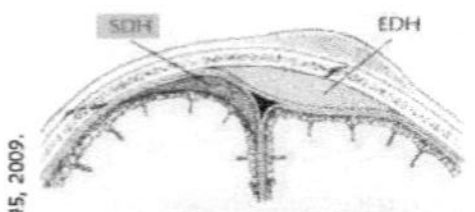
SDH
EDH

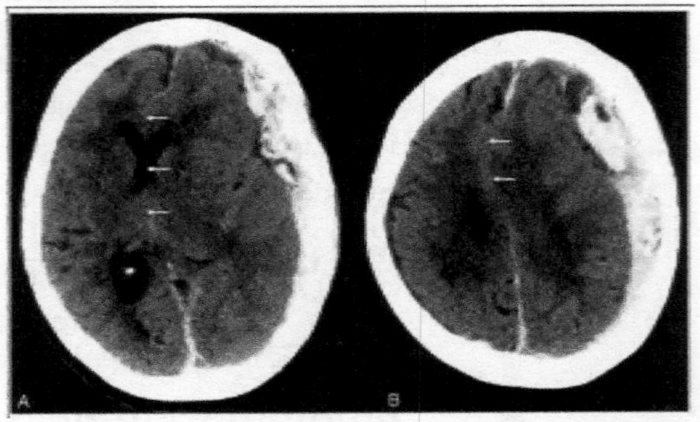
A
B

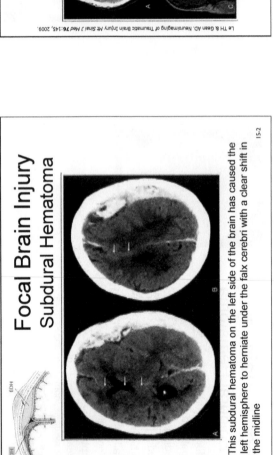

- This subdural hematoma on the left side of the brain has caused the left hemisphere to herniate under the falx cerebri with a clear shift in the midline

Le TH & Gean AD. Neuroimaging of Traumatic Brain Injury *Mt Sinai J Med* **76**:145, 2009.

15-2

Focal Brain Injury
Intracerebral Hematoma

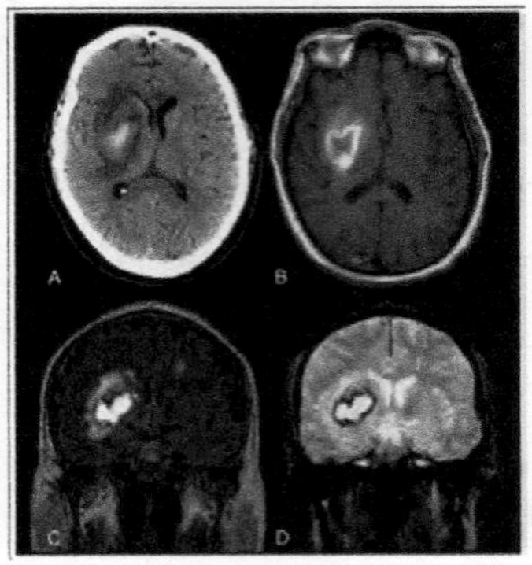
A
B
C
D

- Usually seen in falls and motor vehicle collisions
- Shearing forces tear blood vessels inside the brain
- May cause weakness or paralysis
- May progress to herniation

Le TH & Gean AD. Neuroimaging of Traumatic Brain Injury *Mt Sinai J Med* **76**:145, 2009.

15-2

Focal Brain Injury
Cortical Contusion

- Like a brain bruise
- Edema because of brain injury
- Can be very difficult to see on CT or MRI
- See evidence of edema (white shading) at arrows

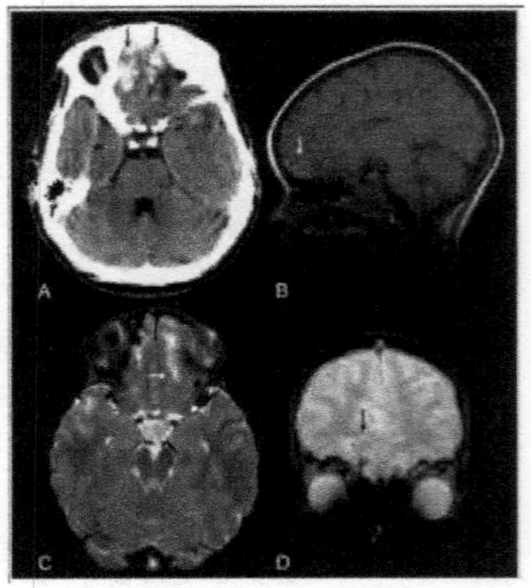
A
B
C
D

Le TH & Gean AD. Neuroimaging of Traumatic Brain Injury *Mt Sinai J Med* **76**:145, 2009.

15-2

Traumatic Brain Injury
Diffuse Brain Injury

Diffuse Brain Injury
Concussions

- Mild (Grades I-III)
  - **Temporary** axonal disturbances causing attention and memory deficits but no loss of consciousness
- Classic Concussion (Grade IV)
  - Disconnection of cerebral systems and the brain stem reticular activating system causing loss of arousal
  - Physiologic and neurologic dysfunction with no anatomic disruption.
  - Loss of consciousness (<6 hours)
  - Anterograde and retrograde amnesia

15-3

Diffuse Brain Injury
Diffuse Axonal Injury

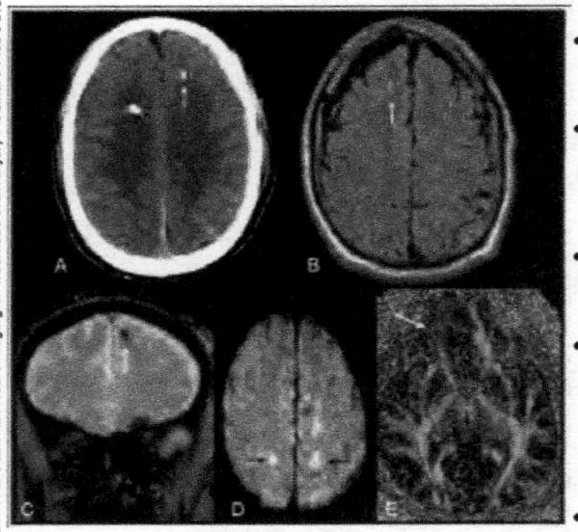
A
B
C
D
E

Le TH & Gean AD. Neuroimaging of Traumatic Brain Injury *Mt Sinai J Med* **76**:145, 2009.

- Result from shear injuries to brain
- Soft gray matter shifts against firmer white matter and axons get torn
- Difficult to see on conventional imaging
- New technique (fractional anisotropy, color) makes DAI easier to visualize (yellow arrow)
- Range from mild to severe.
  - 64% survival rate in severe cases with physical, cognitive, social, and psychologic/behavior consequences.

15-3

Spinal Cord Injuries

Hyperextension and Hyperflexion Injuries of Spinal Cord

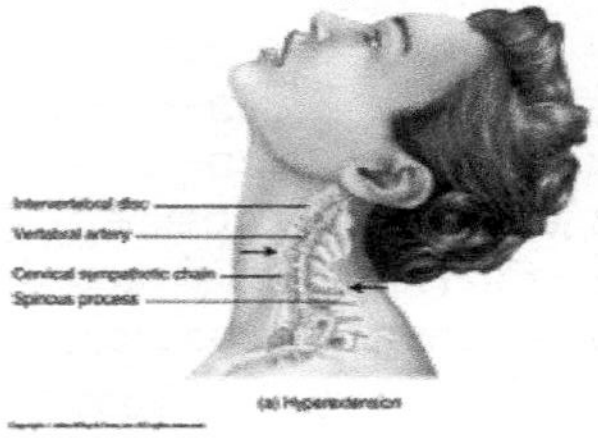
Intervertebral disc
Vertebral artery
Cervical sympathetic chain
Spinous process
(a) Hyperextension

- Commonly seen in motor vehicle collisions (**whiplash**)
- Hyperextension
- Hyperflexion

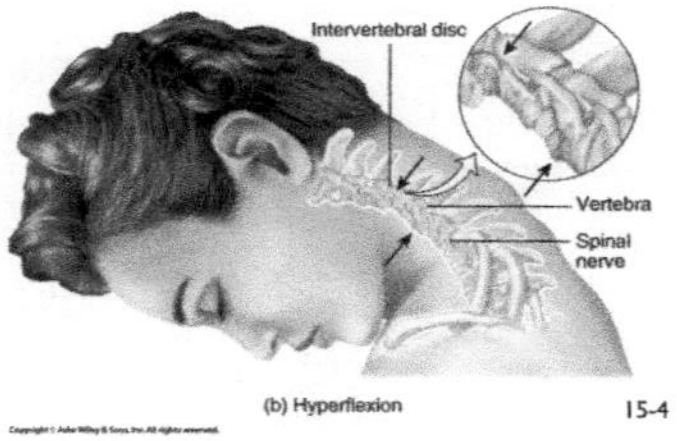
Intervertebral disc
Vertebra
Spinal nerve
(b) Hyperflexion

15-4

Spinal Cord Injury

- The cord is usually injured from broken fragments of injured vertebrae
- 12K new cases each year
- 260K Americans alive today
- 81% are men; average age is 34
- **Trauma**:
  - 44% motor vehicle collisions
  - 27% falls
  - 15% violence
  - 8% sports
    - diving injuries are 1/3 of sports injuries

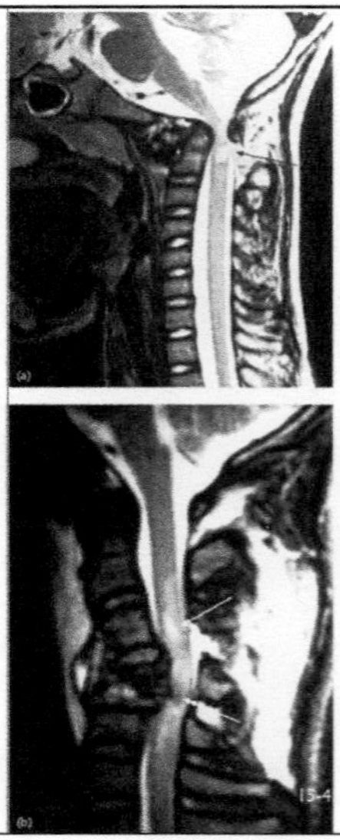
(a)
(b)

Stys PK. Traumatic Central Nervous System Injury, *Encyclopedia of Life Sciences*, 2001.

15-4

Spinal Cord Injuries

- Most common injury is vertebral bone fragments damaging spinal cord
- Most common location is where cord is relatively large and tightly packed in the vertebral canal:
  - **C1–C2**
  - **C4–C7**
  - **T12–L2**

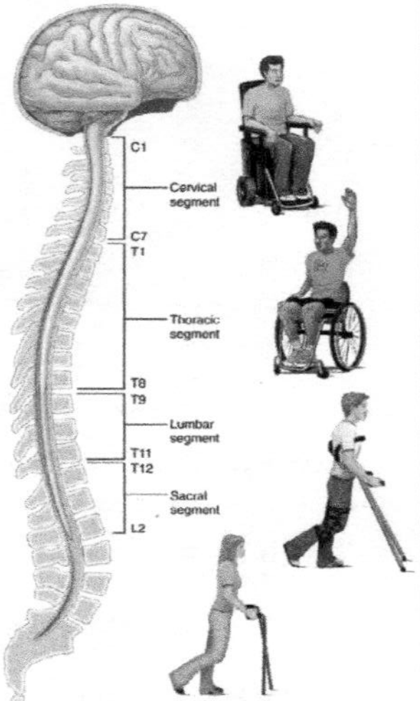
C1
Cervical segment
C7
T1
Thoracic segment
T8
T9
Lumbar segment
T11
T12
Sacral segment
L2

15-4

Alterations of Motor Functions

- **Spinal Shock**
  - Temporary cessation of cord function below a spinal lesion
  - Causes flaccid paralysis, areflexia or hyporeflexia (absent or diminished reflexes) and bowel/bladder dysfunction
  - If spinal cord is not permanently damaged, spinal shock is followed (in about 10-14 days) by a return of cord function, increased reflexes, and possibly autonomic **hyperreflexia** (hyperactivity)

15-4

Autonomic Hyperreflexia

- Massive, uncompensated cardiovascular response to stimulation of the sympathetic nervous system.
- Stimulated by visceral distention of bowel, bladder, or abdomen.
- Sensory afferent neurons stimulate reflex of major sympathetic outflow.
- Body tries to compensate sympathetic stimulation by activating parasympathetic system.
- Parasympathetic response above the lesion but not below.
- BP (up to 300 mm Hg, systolic), pounding headache, blurred vision, sweating above the level of the lesion, flushed skin, bradycardia.

15-4

Spinal Cord Injuries

- Diagnosis of spinal cord injuries
  - By physical examination (loss of reflexes) or by radiological examination:CT and/or MRI scans
- Treatment
  - Immobilization, surgery, administration of corticosteroids to reduce secondary cord swelling, and symptomatic treatment of autonomic hyperreflexia

15-4

Spinal Disc Disease

- **Degenerative Disc Disease**
  - Dehydration and loss of disc structure.
- **Herniated Disc**
  - Herniation of nucleus pulposus can lead to nerve impingement.

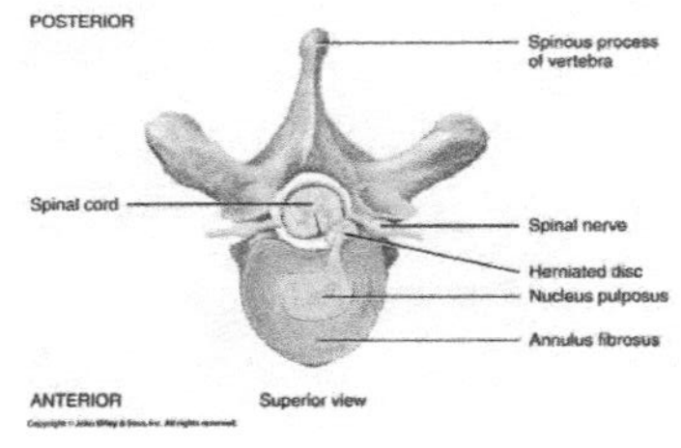

POSTERIOR
Spinous process of vertebra
Spinal cord
Spinal nerve
Herniated disc
Nucleus pulposus
Annulus fibrosus
ANTERIOR
Superior view

15-5

Cerebrovascular Disease

Ischemic Stroke

Hemorrhagic Stroke

Aneurysms

Transient Ischemic Attack (TIA)

Cerebrovascular Accident (CVA) Two Kinds of Stroke

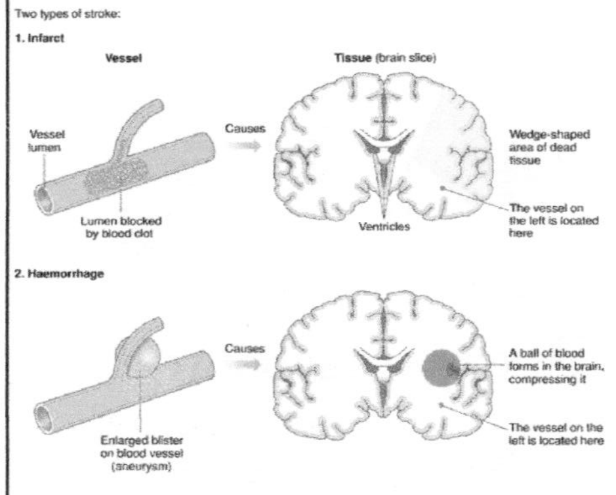

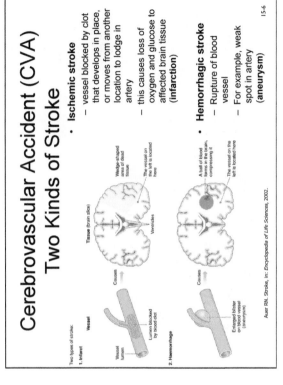

Two types of stroke:
1. Infarct
Vessel
Tissue (brain slice)
Vessel lumen
Causes
Wedge-shaped area of dead tissue
Lumen blocked by blood clot
Ventricles
The vessel on the left is located here
2. Haemorrhage
Causes
A ball of blood forms in the brain, compressing it
Enlarged blister on blood vessel (aneurysm)
The vessel on the left is located here

Auer RN. Stroke, in: *Encyclopedia of Life Sciences*, 2002.

- **Ischemic stroke**
  - vessel blocked by clot that develops in place, or moves from another location to lodge in artery
  - this causes loss of oxygen and glucose to affected brain tissue **(infarction)**
- **Hemorrhagic stroke**
  - Rupture of blood vessel
  - For example, weak spot in artery **(aneurysm)**

15-6

Stroke Classification

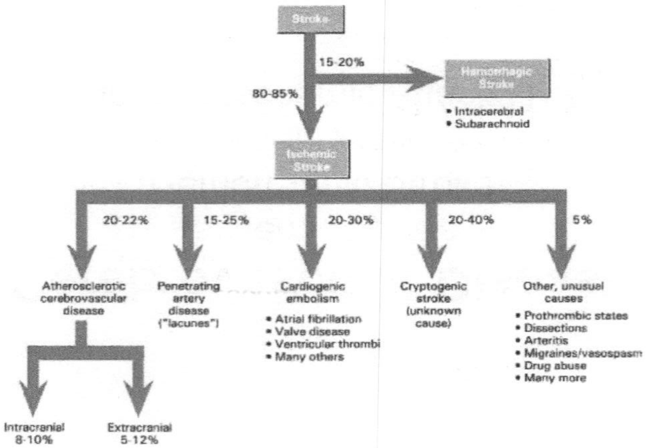

Stroke
15-20%
80-85%
Hemorrhagic Stroke
• Intracerebral
• Subarachnoid
Ischemic Stroke
20-22%
15-25%
20-30%
20-40%
5%
Atherosclerotic cerebrovascular disease
Penetrating artery disease ("lacunes")
Cardiogenic embolism
• Atrial fibrillation
• Valve disease
• Ventricular thrombi
• Many others
Cryptogenic stroke (unknown cause)
Other, unusual causes
• Prothrombic states
• Dissections
• Arteritis
• Migraines/vasospasm
• Drug abuse
• Many more
Intracranial 8-10%
Extracranial 5-12%

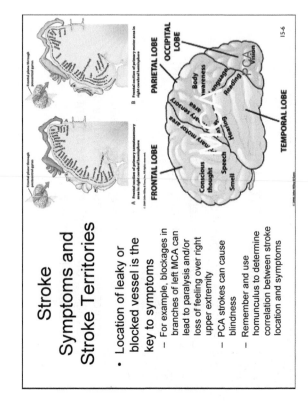

Meisel A et al. Pathophysiology of Stroke, in: *Encyclopedia of Molecular Cell Biology and Molecular Medicine*, 2005.

15-6

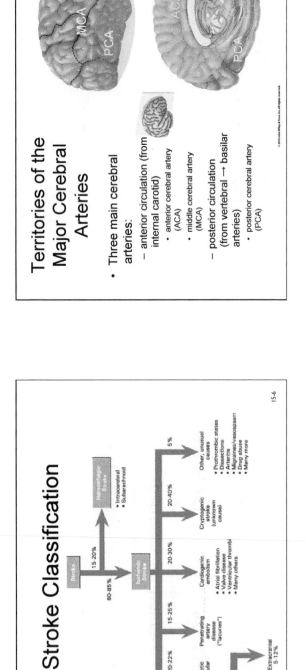

Territories of the Major Cerebral Arteries

- Three main cerebral arteries:
  - anterior circulation (from internal carotid)
    - anterior cerebral artery (ACA)
    - middle cerebral artery (MCA)
  - posterior circulation (from vertebral → basilar arteries)
    - posterior cerebral artery (PCA)

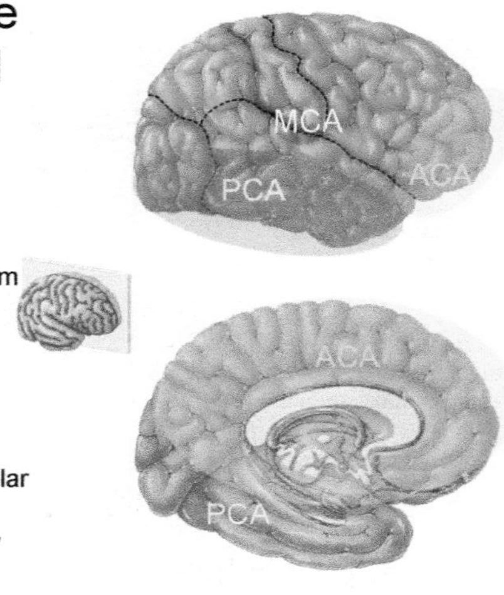

MCA
PCA
ACA
ACA
PCA

17-6

Stroke Symptoms and Stroke Territories

- Location of leaky or blocked vessel is the key to symptoms
  - For example, blockages in branches of left MCA can lead to paralysis and/or loss of feeling over right upper extremity
  - PCA strokes can cause blindness
  - Remember and use homunculus to determine correlation between stroke location and symptoms

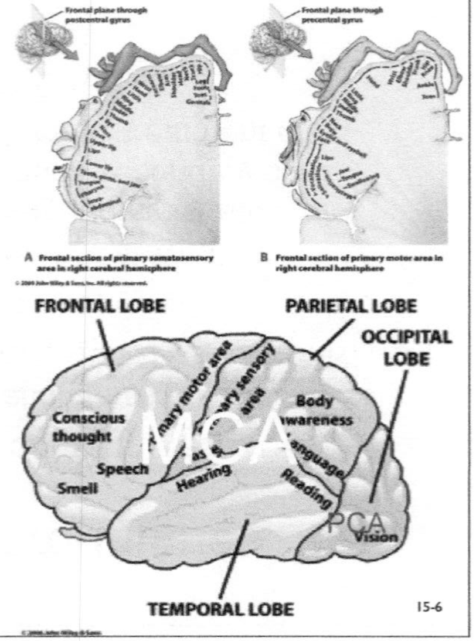

A Frontal section of primary somatosensory area in right cerebral hemisphere
B Frontal section of primary motor area in right cerebral hemisphere
FRONTAL LOBE
PARIETAL LOBE
OCCIPITAL LOBE
TEMPORAL LOBE
Conscious thought
Speech
Smell
Hearing
Body awareness
Language
Reading
Vision
MCA
PCA

15-6

Aneurysm

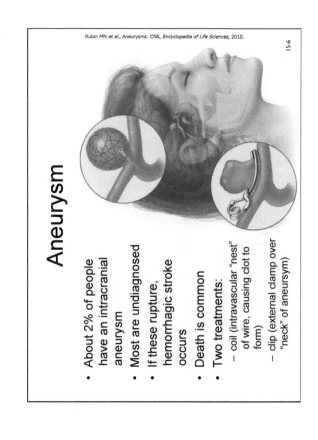

- About 2% of people have an intracranial aneurysm
- Most are undiagnosed
- If these rupture, hemorrhagic stroke occurs
- Death is common
- Two treatments:
  - coil (intravascular "nest" of wire, causing clot to form)
  - clip (external clamp over "neck" of aneursym)

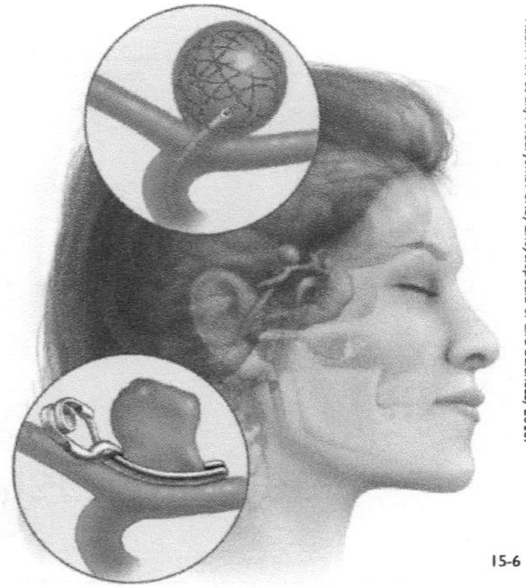

Rubin MN *et al.*, Aneurysms: CNS, *Encyclopedia of Life Sciences*, 2010.

15-6

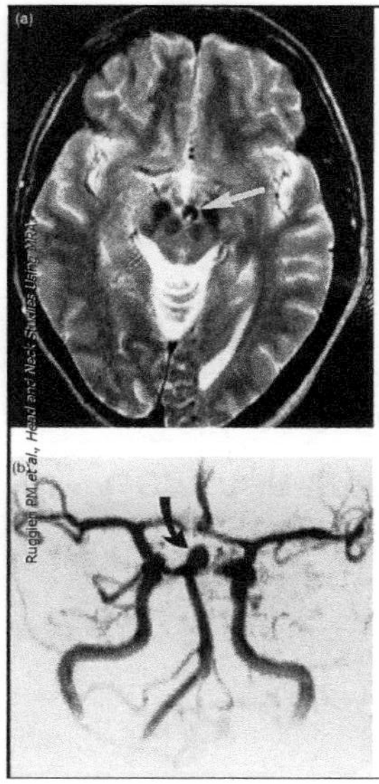
(a)
(b)
Ruggieri PM, et al., Head and Neck Studies Using MRA

Aneurysm

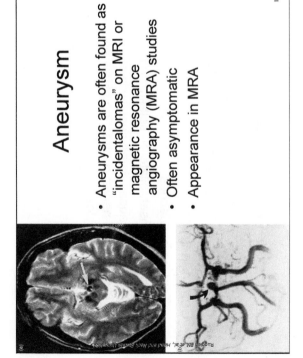

- Aneurysms are often found as "incidentalomas" on MRI or magnetic resonance angiography (MRA) studies
- Often asymptomatic
- Appearance in MRA

15-6

Arteriovenous Malformation

- Nest-like structure with anastomosing arteries and veins
- May appear as holes in CT or MRI scans
- Difficult to treat, frequently prone to rupture and hemorrhagic stroke

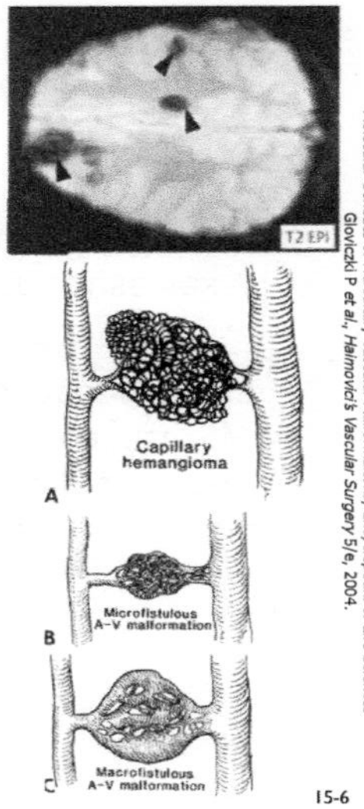
T2 EPI
A
Capillary hemangioma
B
Microfistulous A-V malformation
C
Macrofistulous A-V malformation

Molecular Genetics of Hereditary Vascular Malformaitons, *Encyclopedia of Life Sciences*
Gloviczki P *et al.*, *Haimovici's Vascular Surgery* 5/e, 2004.

15-6

The Ischemic Penumbra

- When a stroke occurs, there is an area of direct and immediate damage
- No one can save this tissue
  - infarction → cell death
- Surrounding the infarction is an area called the **ischemic penumbra**
- In the penumbra, tissue can be saved if we do the right thing, or will be killed if we do the wrong thing

15-6

The Ischemic Penumbra

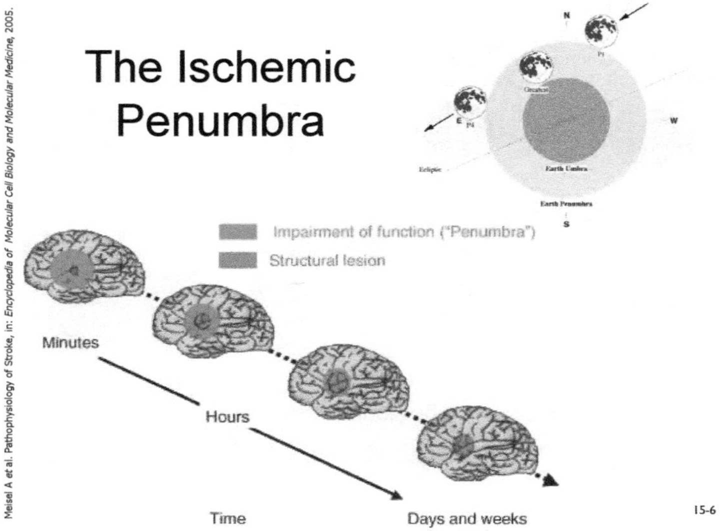
N
W
S
Impairment of function ("Penumbra")
Structural lesion
Minutes
Hours
Time
Days and weeks

Meisel A et al. Pathophysiology of Stroke, in: *Encyclopedia of Molecular Cell Biology and Molecular Medicine*, 2005.

15-6

Transient Ischemic Attack

"All Penumbra, No Infarction"

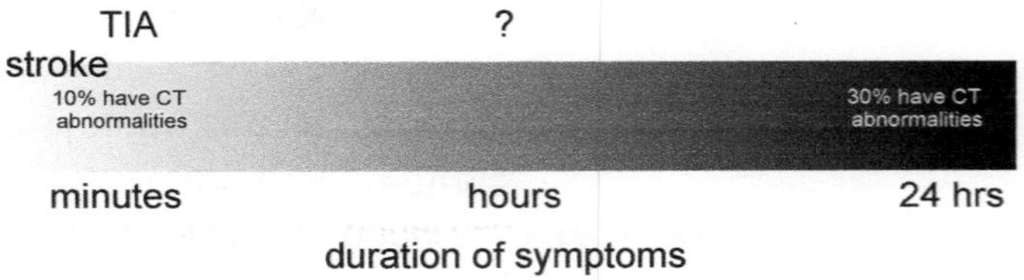
TIA
?
stroke
10% have CT abnormalities
30% have CT abnormalities
minutes
hours
24 hrs
duration of symptoms

15-6

Symptoms of a TIA

Percent of patients reporting each symptom

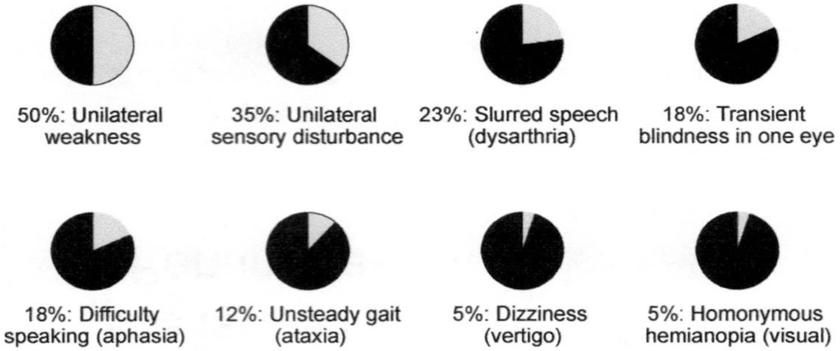
50%: Unilateral weakness
35%: Unilateral sensory disturbance
23%: Slurred speech (dysarthria)
18%: Transient blindness in one eye
18%: Difficulty speaking (aphasia)
12%: Unsteady gait (ataxia)
5%: Dizziness (vertigo)
5%: Homonymous hemianopia (visual)

15-6

Headache

- One of the most common neurological disorders, yet the least understood
- Common types:
  - –Tension headaches
    - gradual onset, bilateral, self-limiting
    - possible causes: hypersensitivity of trigeminal nerve; contraction of jaw and neck muscles

15-7

Headache

–Migraine headaches

- 5,4,3,2,1 criteria: 5 or more attacks, 4 hours to 3 days duration, 2 of: unilateral, pulsating, moderate to severe pain, aggravation by physical activity, 1 of: nausea/vomiting, photophobia, phonophobia
- vascular origin (blood vessel dilation)
  - –may be relieved by drugs which cause vessel constriction (caffeine, serotonin receptor agonists)
- 2x as common in ♀
- triggers (stress, hunger, foods, weather, hormonal changes in ♀) usually involved

15-7

Headache

–Cluster headaches

- occur in groups (several in one day for several days) then remit for a time
- 5x more common in ♂ (typical age 20-50)
- severe, unilateral stabbing pain behind eyes (retro-orbital) with eye watering and nausea

15-7

Infections of the Brain

Meningitis

Encephalitis

Meningitis

- Inflammation of the pia and arachnoid
- Caused by anything that can trigger inflammation
  - Usually infectious agents like viruses, bacteria, fungi, parasites
  - *Chemical meningitis* when drugs, toxins, or radiation trigger inflammation
- All types of meningitis exhibit an increased intracranial pressure
  - Increased production or
  - Impaired circulation or
  - Impaired resorption

  of cerebrospinal fluid

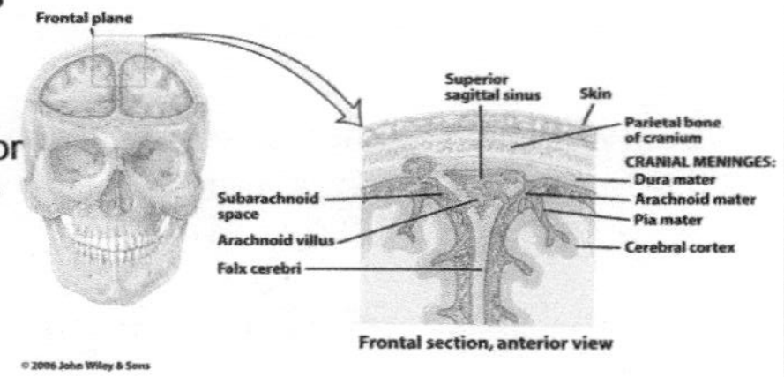

Frontal plane
Superior sagittal sinus
Skin
Parietal bone of cranium
CRANIAL MENINGES:
Dura mater
Arachnoid mater
Pia mater
Cerebral cortex
Subarachnoid space
Arachnoid villus
Falx cerebri
Frontal section, anterior view

15-8

Viral Meningitis

- Sometimes called "aseptic" or non-purulent meningitis
- Usually develops more gradually and is less severe, requiring only supportive care
- Visible examination of the cerebrospinal fluid (CSF) will show it to be clear
- Lumbar puncture with Gram stain of CSF may show some lymphocytes, *but no bacteria*
- Microscopic examination of a drop of CSF may also show the presence of a few lymphocytes

15-8

Viral Meningitis

- Chemistry analysis of the CSF may show a mildly elevated protein, but glucose levels usually remain within normal limits
- The white blood count (WBC) is usually just slightly elevated (10-12,000/mm^3) but the differential will show an elevation of lymphocytes to perhaps 40-50%
- Pathogens: Enteroviruses, HSV (type I), and others
- Signs and symptoms are similar to those of bacterial meningitis, but more mild and self-limiting

15-8

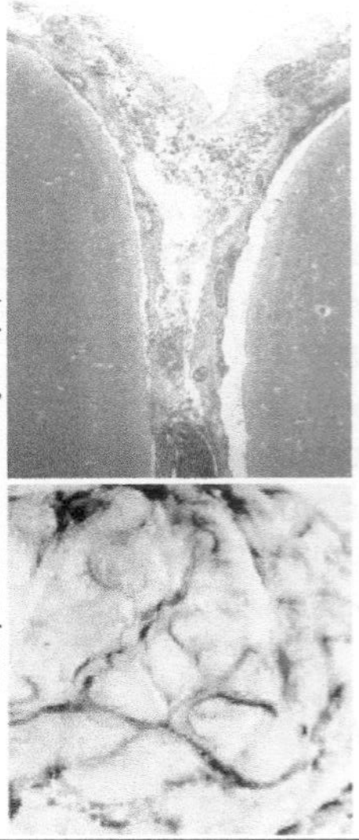

Helmsley C & Crook D. Bacterial Meningitis. *Encyclopedia of Life Sciences.*

Bacterial Meningitis

- Extends beyond the meninges to involve the cerebrospinal fluid in the subarachnoid space and ventricular system
- Usually more severe – can be life-threatening within hours if the infectious agent is *Neisseria meningitidis*
- The CSF will be visibly cloudy
- A gram stain of CSF will demonstrate bacteria
- Chemistry analysis of the CSF will show a markedly elevated protein, and a markedly decreased glucose.

15-8

Bacterial Meningitis

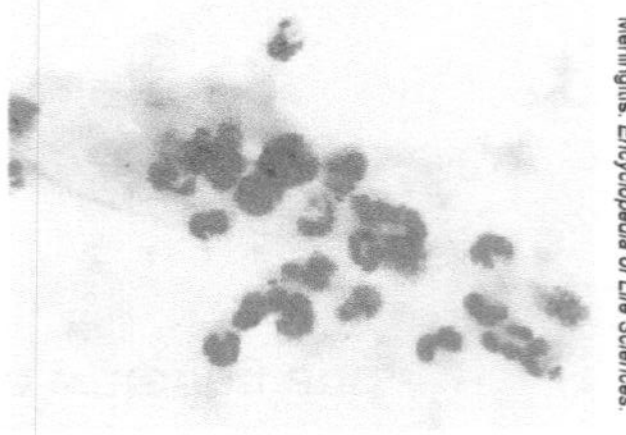

Helmsley C & Crook D. Bacterial Meningitis. *Encyclopedia of Life Sciences.*

- Microscopic examination of a drop of CSF from a lumbar puncture will show it to be full of neutrophils and monocytes
- The white blood count (WBC) will be significantly elevated (12-20,000/mm^3) with a definite left shift
- Pathogens: *N. meningitidis* (meningococcus), *S. pneumoniae*, *H. influenzae*
- Symptoms: throbbing headache, nausea/vomiting, nuchal rigidity (neck stiffness), a petechial rash on the palms of the hands, progressing to an altered mental status

15-8

Encephalitis

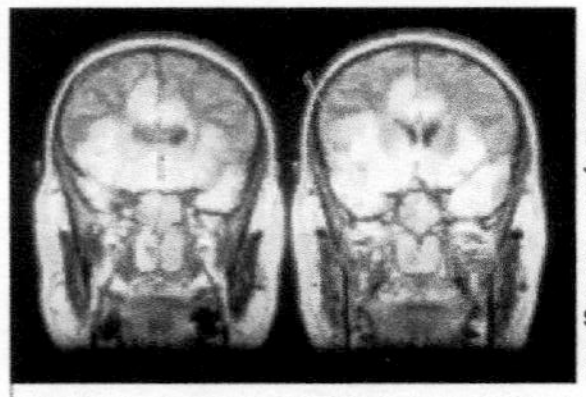

Howard R & Manji H. Infection in the Nervous System. *Neurology* 2009

- Acute inflammation of the brain matter; usually viral
- Caused by arthropod-born viruses and HSV-1
- Can occur due to systemic viral diseases
- Cause widespread nerve cell degeneration
- Increased intracranial pressure may progress to herniation
- Symptoms: fever, delirium, dementia, seizures, palsies, and paralysis

15-8

Degenerative Motor and Autoimmune Diseases of the Brain

Multiple Sclerosis

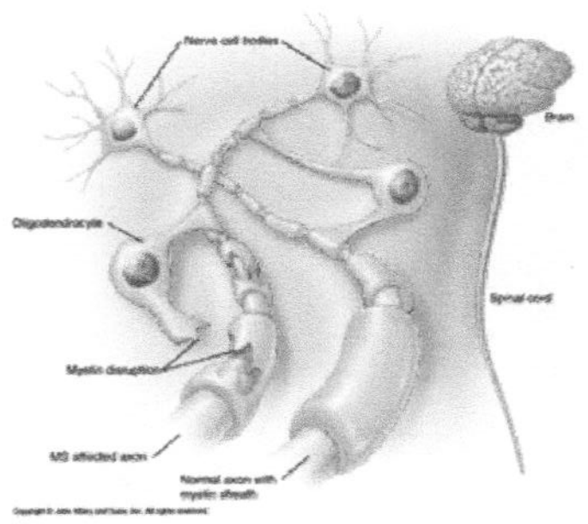
Nerve cell bodies
Brain
Oligodendrocyte
Spinal cord
Myelin disruption
MS affected axon
Normal axon with myelin sheath

- Autoimmune disease where the patient's immune system directs an attack on the myelin sheaths surrounding nerve axons
- As myelin sheaths are destroyed, more antigen is released into the body and problem gets worse (**exacerbation**)
- Immune attack diminishes and nervous system repairs as best it can (**remission**)
- Because demyelination can occur anywhere in nervous system, it can mimic almost any other neurological problem

15-9

Multiple sclerosis is a disease where myelin sheaths are destroyed

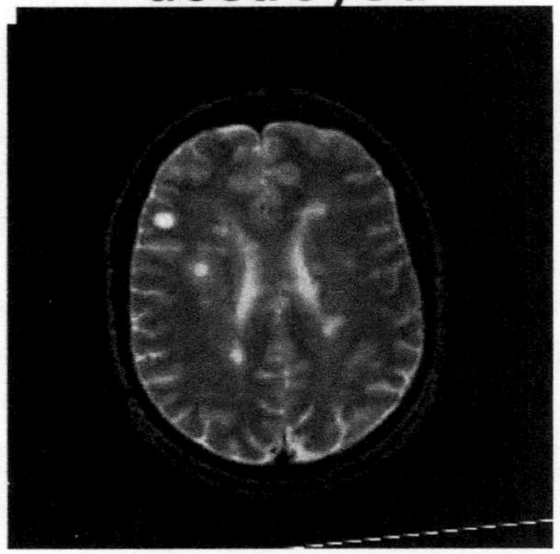

032.mpg

Whole Brain Atlas 15-9

Amyotropic Lateral Sclerosis

- Amyotrophic lateral sclerosis (ALS, Lou Gehrig's disease) affects upper and lower motor neurons
  - corticospinal tracts and anterior horn alpha motor neurons
- The disease leads to progressive weakness beginning in a single muscle group, muscle wasting, and death
- Patients have normal intellectual and sensory function until death
  - may be rapidly progressing, causing death from respiratory paralysis in less than a year

15-9

Guillain-Barré Syndrome

- Guillain-Barré Syndrome is an acute inflammatory demyelinating disorder of the peripheral nerves
- Signs:
  - rapid onset of weakness
  - paralysis of legs or arms or face muscles
  - paralysis of the respiratory muscles is possible
- The most common cause of rapidly acquired paralysis in the U.S.
  - affects about 2/100,000
  - about 5000 new cases each year
  - any person, any age

15-9

Myasthenia Gravis

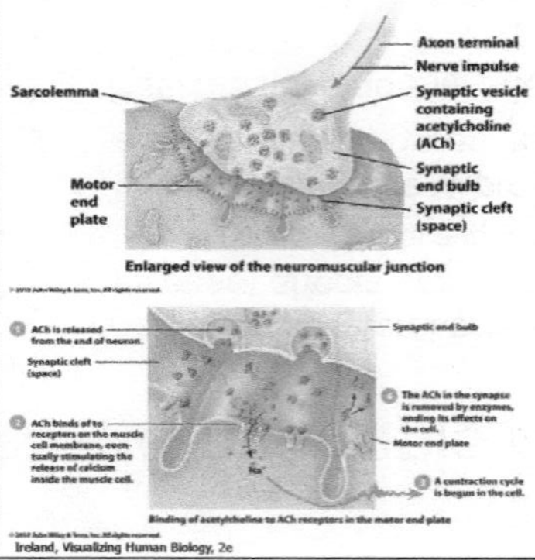

Sarcolemma
Motor end plate
Axon terminal
Nerve impulse
Synaptic vesicle containing acetylcholine (ACh)
Synaptic end bulb
Synaptic cleft (space)
Enlarged view of the neuromuscular junction

Ireland, Visualizing Human Biology, 2e

- Autoimmune disease
  - 70-80% of patients have pathologic changes in the thymus
- An IgG antibody is produced against the ACh receptor (#2 in the diagram)
  - Muscles innervated by cranial nerves affected earliest, later progresses to upper body and diaphragm
  - Weakness and fatigue affect the muscles of the eyes and the throat causing diplopia, difficulty chewing, talking and swallowing

15-9

UNIT 6

Study Guide Objectives – Introductory Pathophysiology (HTHS 2230)

Unit 6

Chapter 18 - Alterations of Hormonal Regulation

1. Identify common mechanisms leading to hyper- and hypo-secretion of hormones. (pp. 447-448).
2. Describe the two common diseases of the posterior pituitary gland, syndrome of inappropriate ADH secretion (SIADH) and central diabetes insipidus (DI). Compare and contrast the causes of central diabetes insipidus to nephrogenic diabetes insipidus. (pp. 448-450)
3. Describe the disorders of the anterior pituitary gland that result in abnormalities of growth: hypopituitarism and hyperpituitarism. Contrast hypersecretion of growth hormone during infancy with the disorder acromegaly. (pp. 450-453)
4. Characterize the causes and manifestations of hypothyroidism and hyperthyroidism Define goiter, and discuss the relationship of thyroid enlargement in both hyper- and hypothyroid states. (pp. 453-457)
5. Describe the disorders of hyperthyroidism: Graves' disease and thyrotoxic crisis (pp. 454-455).
6. Differentiate between primary and secondary causes of hypothyroidism. Define the term myxedema as it relates to the severity of a hypothyroid state. Describe congenital hypothyroidism (cretinism). (pp. 456-457)
7. Distinguish between hyperparathyroidism and hypoparathyroidism, and name their most common causes and clinical manifestations. (pp 458-459)

Compare and contrast insulin-dependent (type I) and non-insulin-dependent (type II) diabetes mellitus. (pp. 459-468)

8. Identify and describe the acute complications of diabetes mellitus: hypoglycemia (insulin shock), diabetic ketoacidosis (DKA), and hyperosmolar hyperglycemic nonketotic syndrome (HHNKS). (p. 465)

9. Discuss the chronic microvascular complications of diabetes mellitus: diabetic retinopathy, diabetic nephropathy, and diabetic neuropathy. Compare and contrast these complications with the macrovascular and infectious complications of diabetes mellitus. (pp. 468-468)

10. Describe the etiology, pathogenesis, and manifestations of hyperfunction and hypofunction of the adrenal cortex: Cushing disease/syndrome, Conn disease (primary hyperaldosteronism), Addison disease, and feminization and virilization syndromes. (pp. 469-472).

11. Define pheochromocytoma and describe the clinical manifestations that accompany excessive production of catecholamines from the adrenal medulla. (p. 472)

Chapter 8 - Stress and Disease

1. Define stress, and compare eustress and distress. Describe the interaction between stressors and the stress response. (pp. 204-205)

2. Describe Selye's historic general adaptation syndrome and clarify the salient features of each of its stages (pp. 204-205).

3. Summarize the major interactions of the nervous, endocrine, and immune systems in the stress response. (pp. 209-216)

Chapter 23 - Alterations of Cardiovascular Function

1. Distinguish between a thrombus and an embolus. List types of emboli. Name potential threats to the circulation of arterial and venous thrombi. (pp. 592-593)

2. Describe diseases of the veins to include varicose veins, chronic venous insufficiency, and deep vein thrombosis. (pp. 585-586)

3. Distinguish between primary, secondary, and complicated hypertension. Define orthostatic (postural) hypotension. (pp. 587-591)

4. Define aneurysm and list the various types (pp.591-592).

5. Describe the development, clinical presentation, and consequences of atherosclerosis. (pp. 594 – 597)

6. Compare and contrast the clinical presentation, and the underlying pathology of the two peripheral vascular diseases (PVD): thromboangiitis obliterans (Buerger disease) and Raynaud disease and phenomenon (pp.593-594).

7. Characterize coronary artery disease (CAD). List major and modifiable risk factors.
4. Specify the sequence of events leading to myocardial ischemia. Differentiate between angina and myocardial infarction. List common complications of a myocardial infarction. (pp. 597-609)

8. Characterize the conditions associated with pericardial disease: acute pericarditis, constrictive pericarditis, and pericardial effusion (including cardiac tamponade). (pp.609-611).

9. Compare the cardiomyopathies: dilated, hypertrophied, and restrictive. (pp.611-612)

10. Identify the causes and manifestations of valvular dysfunction: aortic stenosis, mitral stenosis, aortic regurgitation, mitral regurgitation, tricuspid regurgitation, and mitral valve prolapse syndrome. (pp. 612-616)

11. Distinguish between rheumatic heart disease and infective endocarditis. (pp. 616-619)

12. Characterize dysrhythmias of the heart. (pp. 619-622)

13. Compare the pathophysiology and manifestations of right (cor pulmonale) and left (congestive) heart failure. (pp. 623-626).

14. Define shock. Classify the different types of shock: cardiogenic, hypovolemic, neurogenic, anaphylactic, and septic. (pp. 627-634)

15. Define multiple organ dysfunction syndrome (MODS) to include triggers, pathophysiology, and clinical manifestations. (pp. 634-637).

Chapter 24 - Alterations of Cardiovascular Function in Children

1. Describe the congenital heart defects contributing to an increased pulmonary blood flow: patent ductus arteriosus, atrial septal defect (ASD), and ventricular septal defect (VSD). (pp. 643-644, 647-648)

2. Describe the following congenital heart defects and their clinical manifestations: tetralogy of Fallot, coarctation of aorta, and transposition of the great vessels. (pp. 644-645, 649-652).

Unit 6
Chapter 18
Alterations of Hormonal Regulation

Hormones

- Hormones are mediator molecules that are secreted directly into the blood by endocrine glands
- Hormone receptors are located on the plasma membrane or in the intracellular compartment of a target cell
- Hormones operate by **negative** or **positive** feedback

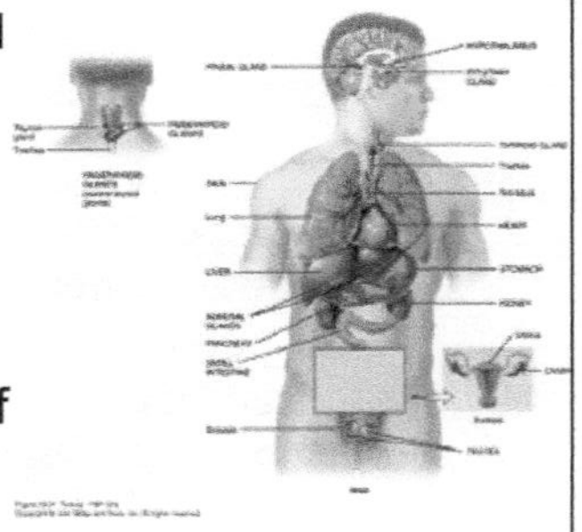

The Endocrine System

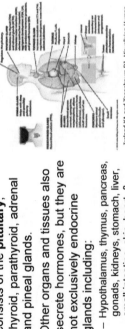

- The **endocrine system proper** consists of the **pituitary**, thyroid, parathyroid, adrenal and pineal glands.
- Other organs and tissues also secrete hormones, but they are not exclusively endocrine glands including:
  - Hypothalamus, thymus, pancreas, gonads, kidneys, stomach, liver, small intestine, skin, heart. & placenta

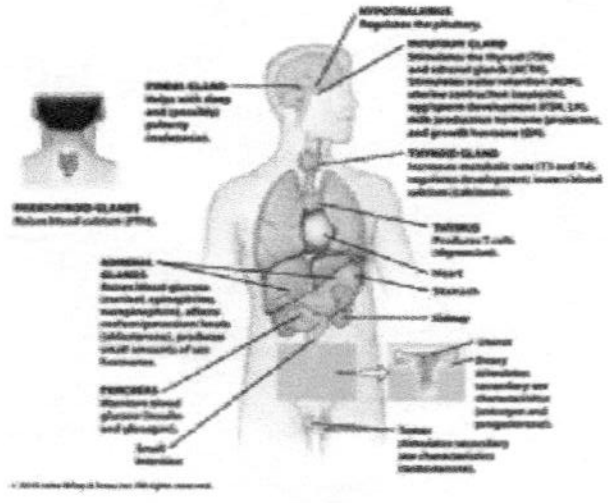

Ireland KA and Tenenbaum DJ. *Visualizing Human Biology*

Action of Hormones

- Control of the composition and the volume of the **internal environment**
- Emergency control during physical and mental **stress**
- Integration of **growth** and development
- **Reproductive** control
- Regulate **metabolism** and energy balance
  - –Glucose availability and metabolic rates

Action of Hormones

- If hormones are secreted into the blood and circulate through the body, **why aren't there widespread effects from the hormone?**
- There are, but only at specific target cells (tissue)
- They bind to specific protein or glycoprotein receptors on their target cells
  - For example, thyroid stimulating hormone (TSH), only affects the thyroid gland
- Target cells have the ability to up- or down-regulate receptors

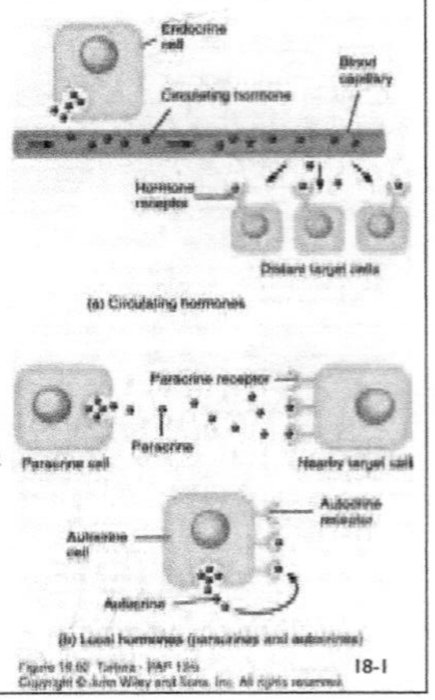

18-I

Alterations of Endocrine Function

- Inappropriate amounts of hormone delivered to target cell
- Inappropriate response by target cell
- **Hypersecretion**
  - Glandular neoplasms
  - Ectopic hormone release - hormone released from wrong area of body!
  - Antibody mimicking hormone - anti hormone antibodies.
- **Hyposecretion**
  - Receptor disorders
  - Inadequate hormone synthesis
  - Degraded or inactivated hormones
  - Blocking antibodies

18-I

The Pituitary and Hypothalamus

- The hypothalamus is the major link **between** the **nervous system** and endocrine system. It receives input from several regions in the brain: limbic, RAS, thalamus

reticular activating system: sleep wake cycle

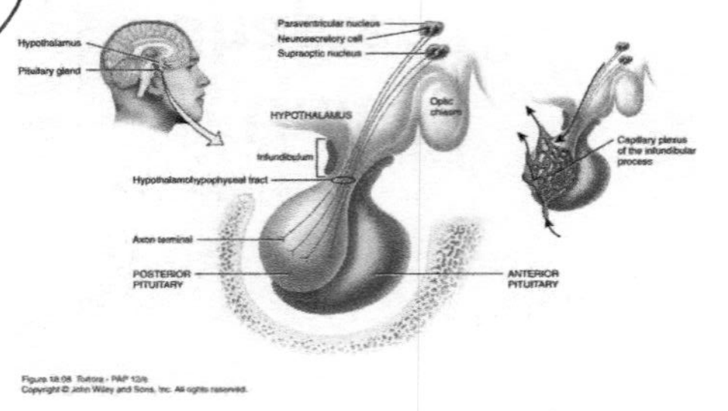

The Pituitary and Hypothalamus

- The anterior lobe of the pituitary (**adenohypophysis**) is anatomically and functionally connected to the hypothalamus by blood vessels
- The posterior lobe of the pituitary (**neurohypophysis**) is anatomically and functionally connected to the hypothalamus by neurosecretory neurons

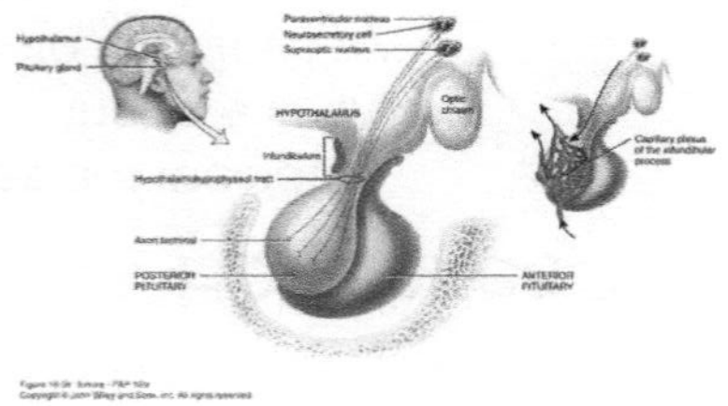

The Posterior Pituitary

- Oxytocin (OT) and antidiuretic hormone (ADH) are **produced** by the cell bodies of the neurosecretory neurons in the hypothalamus
- **Transported** down cell axons to the posterior pituitary
- The hormones are then secreted in respor to nerve impulses from the neurosecretory neurons
- Childbirth, suckling, and coitus stimulate oxytocin release
- Dehydration stimulates ADH release
- **Diseases of the posterior pituitary are rare** and are usually related to abnormal ADH secretion

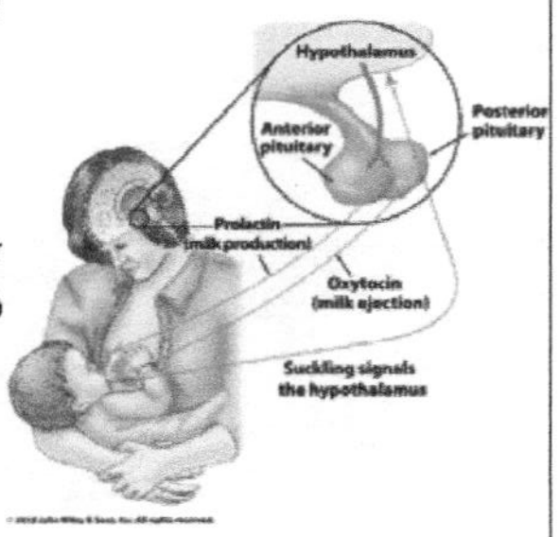

Hypothalamus
Anterior pituitary
Posterior pituitary
Prolactin (milk production)
Oxytocin (milk ejection)
Suckling signals the hypothalamus

18-2

Pituitary Disorders

- Antidiuretic hormone (ADH)
  - –ADH controls cells at the distal collecting tubule (DCT) of the kidney to prevent secretion of water
    - Increases aquaporin (water channel) production by DCT cells
  - –ADH thereby **decreases** the **plasma osmolality**

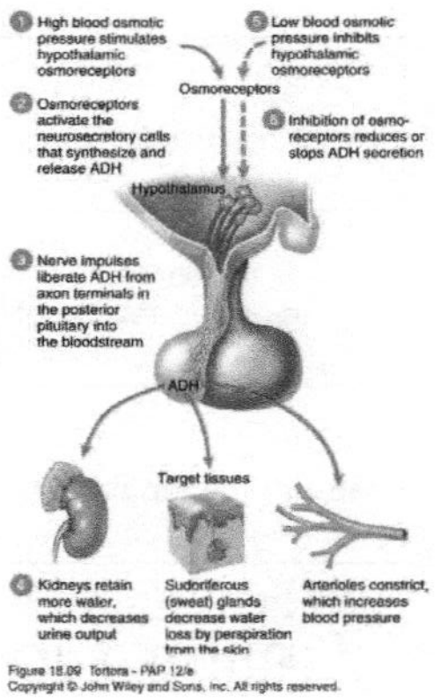

High blood osmotic pressure stimulates hypothalamic osmoreceptors
Low blood osmotic pressure inhibits hypothalamic osmoreceptors
Osmoreceptors
Osmoreceptors activate the neurosecretory cells that synthesize and release ADH
Inhibition of osmoreceptors reduces or stops ADH secretion
Hypothalamus
Nerve impulses liberate ADH from axon terminals in the posterior pituitary into the bloodstream
ADH
Target tissues
Kidneys retain more water, which decreases urine output
Sudoriferous (sweat) glands decrease water loss by perspiration from the skin
Arterioles constrict, which increases blood pressure

Figure 18.09 Tortora - PAP 12/e
Copyright © John Wiley and Sons, Inc. All rights reserved.

18-2

ADH

- Antidiuretic hormone controls cells at the distal collecting tubule (DCT), causing an increases expression of aquaporin channels
  - this facilitates reabsorption of water and decreases the plasma osmolality
  - it also decreases urine output (UOP)

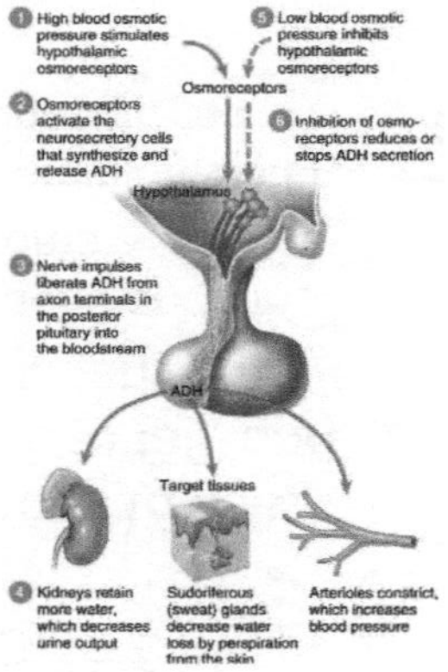

High blood osmotic pressure stimulates hypothalamic osmoreceptors
Low blood osmotic pressure inhibits hypothalamic osmoreceptors
Osmoreceptors
Osmoreceptors activate the neurosecretory cells that synthesize and release ADH
Inhibition of osmoreceptors reduces or stops ADH secretion
Hypothalamus
Nerve impulses liberate ADH from axon terminals in the posterior pituitary into the bloodstream
ADH
Target tissues
Kidneys retain more water, which decreases urine output
Sudoriferous (sweat) glands decrease water loss by perspiration from the skin
Arterioles constrict, which increases blood pressure

18-2

Syndrome of Inappropriate ADH (SIADH)

- In states of dehydration, releasing ADH is the right thing to do
- SIADH occurs when ADH is secreted despite normal or even elevated levels of body water, and without the absence of normal physiologic stimuli as in thirst.
  - This results in an inability to excrete excess water in the urine, and reabsorption of water to the point of causing hypervolemia and hyponatremia

18-2

too much ADH = swelling

when Ø thirsty

SIADH

- As excess body water continues to rise, serum sodium levels continue to fall, and more water is shifted intracellularly
  - Cellular edema leads to headache and other neurological signs and symptoms
  - At the same time the body is retaining water, the urine is inappropriately concentrated

18-2

too little ADH = pruning.

when very thirsty.

Diabetes Insipidus

- The disease of ***Diabetes Insipidus*** is the opposite of SIADH: DI is caused by the insufficient release of ADH despite dehydration
- With insufficient ADH secretion free water continues to be eliminated in the urine, even though it is needed in the body
  - normal urinary ouput is 1 – 1.5 L/day
  - with Diabetes Insipidus, urinary output is > 2.5 L/day lots of peeing
    - 50% of patients: 4-8 L/day
    - 25% of patients: 8-12 L/day

18-2

Diabetes Insipidus

- There are two types of DI
  - Neurogenic (most common), results from a lesion in the hypothalamus, pituitary, or infundibulum resulting in decreased ADH secretion
  - Nephrogenic is a state of insensitivity of the renal tubules to ADH

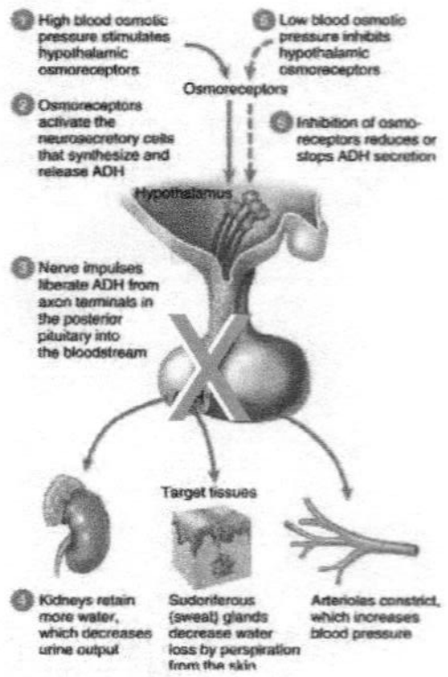
High blood osmotic pressure stimulates hypothalamic osmoreceptors
Low blood osmotic pressure inhibits hypothalamic osmoreceptors
Osmoreceptors
Osmoreceptors activate the neurosecretory cells that synthesize and release ADH
Inhibition of osmo-receptors reduces or stops ADH secretion
Hypothalamus
Nerve impulses liberate ADH from axon terminals in the posterior pituitary into the bloodstream
Target tissues
Kidneys retain more water, which decreases urine output
Sudoriferous (sweat) glands decrease water loss by perspiration from the skin
Arterioles constrict, which increases blood pressure

18-2

Hormones of the Anterior Pituitary

Hypothalamic Hormone	Hormone Released from Anterior Pituitary	Major Function/ Target
Growth Hormone Releasing Hormone (GHRH)	Human Growth Hormone (HGH)	Stimulates growth of body cells
Thyrotropin Releasing Hormone (TRH)	Thyroid Stimulating Hormone (TSH)	Stimulates thyroid gland
Corticotropin Releasing Hormone (CRH)	Adrenocorticotropic hormone (ACTH)	Stimulates adrenal cortex

Hormones of the Anterior Pituitary

Hypothalamic Hormone	Hormone Released from Anterior Pituitary	Major Function/ Target
Gonadotropic Releasing Hormone (GnRH)	Follicle Stimulating Hormone (FSH)	Ova/Sperm development and production
Gonadotropic Releasing Hormone (GnRH)	Lutenizing Hormone (LH)	Maturation of uterine lining, testosterone production, and ovulation
Prolactin Releasing Hormone (PRH)	Prolactin (PRL)	Lactation of mammary glands

Hormones of the Anterior Pituitary

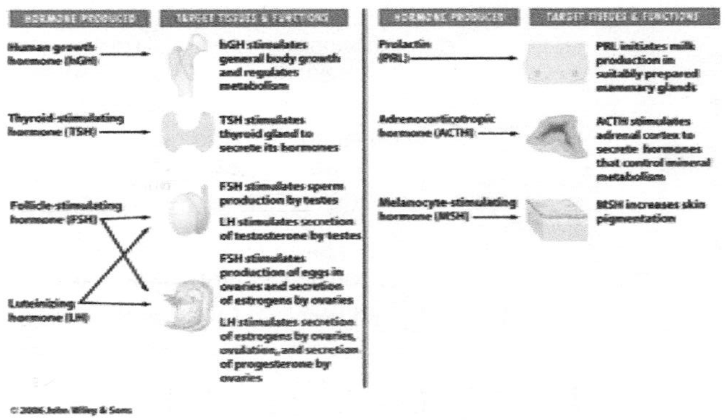

Pruitt NL & Underwood LS. *BioInquiry: Making Connections in Biology,* 3e

Anterior Pituitary Disorders

- Hypopituitarism
  - –Infarction of the gland
  - –Removal/ destruction of the pituitary
  - –Space-occupying pituitary adenomas
  - –Aneurysms that cause compression.
- Absence of all hormones is called
- **panhypopituitarism**
  - –Treatment may consist of replacing HGH, ACTH, TSH, and sex hormones

18-3

Disorder of HGH Secretion

- **Hypopituitarism**
  - – Depends on the affected hormone
  - – **Pituitary dwarfism** results from insufficient HGH release during an individual's growth phase.
    - Patient has normal face and intelligence, with **normal body proportions**
  - – *Compare to Achondroplasia-disorder of bone or cartilage development*
    - *Bone-growth disorder responsible for 70% of dwarfism.*
    - *Limbs are proportionately shorter than trunk with a larger head than average and characteristic facial features.*

18-3

Disorder of HGH Secretion

- The most common cause of excess secretion of hormones of the adenohypophysis is a pituitary adenoma
  - Giantism results from excess HGH during an individual's growth phase
    - this is now a fairly rare disorder because of early detection of adenomas

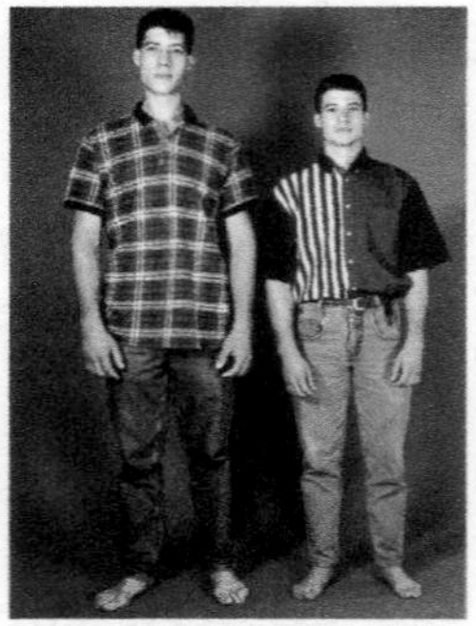

(a) A 22-year old man with pituitary giantism shown beside his identical twin

18-3

Disorders of HGH Secretion

- **Acromegaly**
  - Occurs as a result of excess HGH during adulthood
  - Acromegaly is marked by the enlargement and elongation of the bones of the face, jaw, cheeks, and hands
  - The long bones of the extremities are unaffected because the growth plates are closed

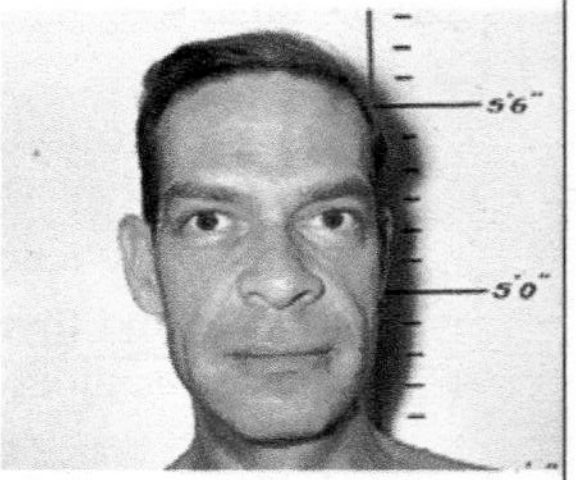
5'6"
5'0"

(b) Acromegaly (excess hGH during adulthood)

18-3

Disorders of HGH Secretion

- **Acromegaly**
  - With bony and soft tissue overgrowth, nerves can be entrapped
    - The patient may demonstrate muscle weakness, foot drop, and sensory changes
    - There is also an increase in the size and function of sebaceous and sweat glands (leading to acne and increased body odor)

18-3

The Thyroid Gland

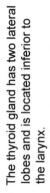

- The thyroid gland has two lateral lobes and is located inferior to the larynx.
- The gland stores a 100 day supply of hormones in sacs (thyroid follicles) that make up most of the gland.
  - Two hormones are secreted: Thyroxine (T_4) and Triiodothyronine (T_3)

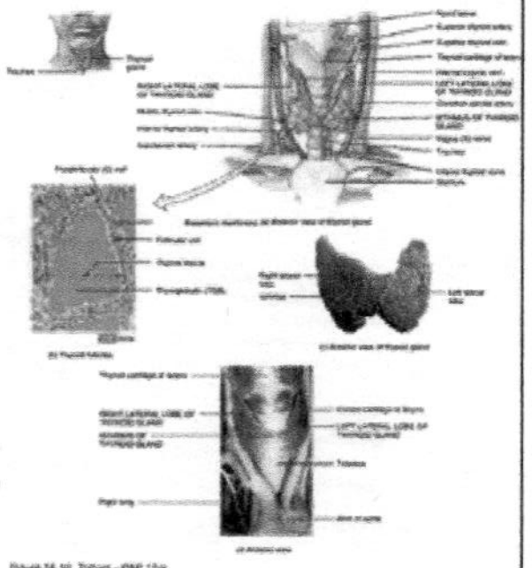

18-4

Thyroid Hormones

- Thyroid hormones
  - Regulate oxygen use
  - Increase the basal metabolic rate (BMR)
  - Increase cellular carbohydrate and protein catabolism
  - Increase reactivity of the nervous system
  - Along with HGH, controls tissue growth and development

18-4

Thyroid Hormones

Characteristics	Hypothyroidism	Hyperthyroidism
BMR	Decreased	Increased
Sympathetic response	Decreased	Increased
Weight	Gain	Loss
Temperature tolerance	Cold intolerance Decreased sweating	Heat intolerance Increased sweating

18-4

Thyroid Hormones

Characteristics	Hypothyroidism	Hyperthyroidism
GI Function	Constipation Decreased appetite	Diarrhea
Cardiac Function	Low output Bradycardia	Increased output tachycardia
Respiratory function	Hypoventilation	Dyspnea
Muscle/tone reflexes	Decreased	Increased

18-4

Thyroid Hormones

Characteristic	Hypothyroidism	Hyperthyroidism
Appearance	Myxedematous	Enlarged thyroid Decreased blinking
General Behavior	Mental retardation (infant) Mental and physical sluggishness	Restlessness, irritable, anxiety, wakefulness

18-4

Thyroid Hormone Release is Controlled By a Homeostatic Loop

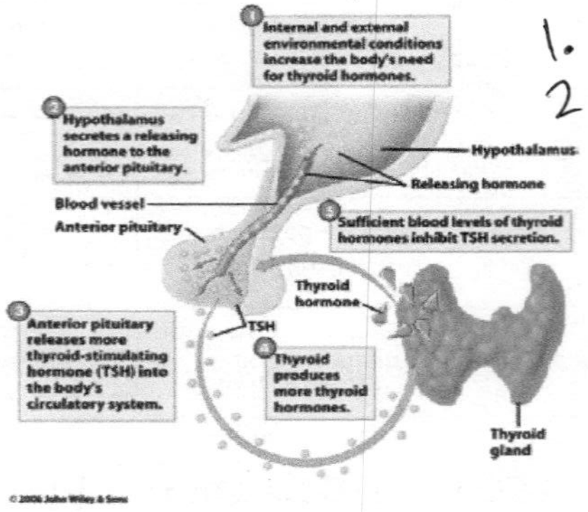

Internal and external environmental conditions increase the body's need for thyroid hormones.
Hypothalamus secretes a releasing hormone to the anterior pituitary.
Hypothalamus
Releasing hormone
Blood vessel
Anterior pituitary
Sufficient blood levels of thyroid hormones inhibit TSH secretion.
Thyroid hormone
TSH
Anterior pituitary releases more thyroid-stimulating hormone (TSH) into the body's circulatory system.
Thyroid produces more thyroid hormones.
Thyroid gland
© 2006 John Wiley & Sons

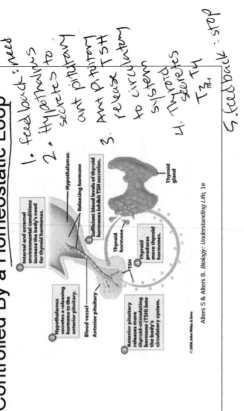

Alters S & Alters B. *Biology: Understanding Life*, 1e

18-4

1. feedback: need
2. Hypothalmus secretes to ant pituitary
3. Ant Pituitary release TSH to circulatory system
4. Thyroid secretes T_3 T_4
5. feedback: stop

Thyroid Disorders

- A ***goiter*** is an enlarged thyroid gland due to increase demand for thyroid hormones, or anything that causes an increase of TSH
  - Goiters can occur in states of euthyroid, hypothyroidism, and hyperthyroidism
    - common causes include I_2 deficiency, viral or genetic disease, puberty, and pregnancy

normal

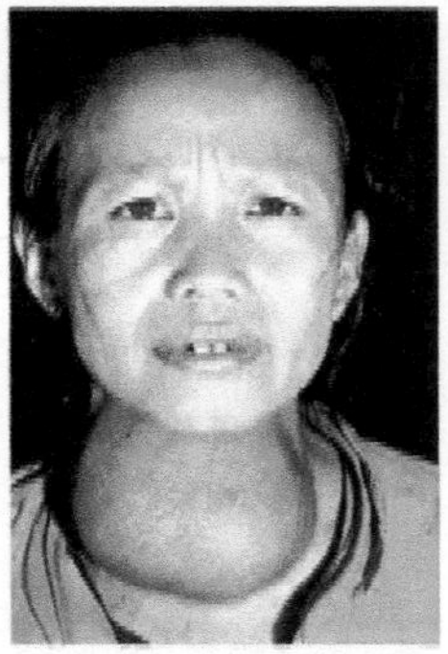

(c) Goiter (enlargement of thyroid gland)

18-4

euthyroid sick syndrome - adaptation or Ø feedback loop due to no food, bad water, etc, etc.

Graves Disease

- A **autoimmune** disorder where antibodies are made against TSH receptors of thyroid cells
  - the antibodies act as TSH receptor agonists (i.e., they turn on the production of thyroxin)
- Excess thyroxin secretion leads to thyrotoxicosis (*symptomatic hyperthyroidism*)
- Symptom: nervousness
- Signs:
  - diminished body weight
  - exophthalmos ("bulging eyes") due to periorbital connective deposition

cause ↑ T_4

wt loss

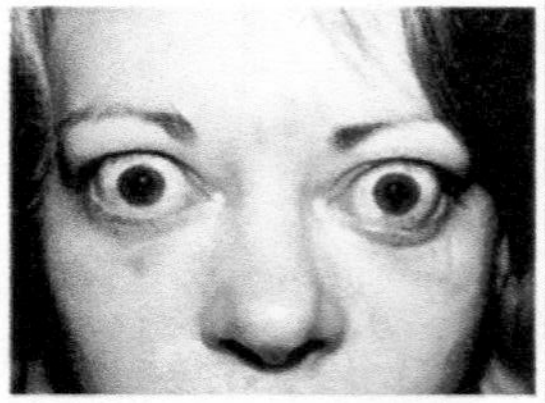

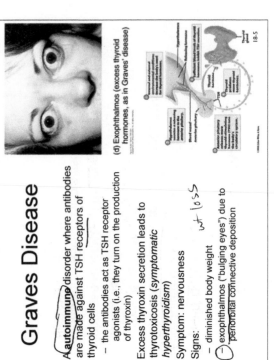

(d) Exophthalmos (excess thyroid hormones, as in Graves' disease)

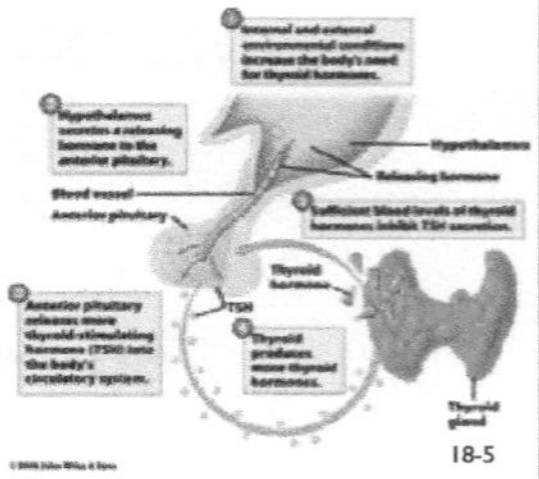

18-5

Thyrotoxic Crisis ("Thyroid Storm")

- A very dangerous worsening of the thyrotoxic state
  - Now rare, but still dangerous
- Manifests as hyperthermia, tachycardia, nausea and vomiting, diarrhea, high-output heart failure, agitation, delirium
  - If untreated, patient can die within 48 hours
- Treatment
  - Prevent the patient from becoming hyperthyroid in the first place by blocking hormone production or ablating the gland (surgery or radiation therapy).

- cut, amputate excise.

18-5

Hypothyroidism

- Low levels of circulating thyroid hormone is the most common abnormal thyroid finding - it can be a primary abnormality, or appear secondary to another disorder:
  - Primary causes include Hashimoto disease (an autoimmune destruction of the thyroid gland)
  - Secondary causes include Toxic Thyroiditis from a bacterial infection of the thyroid and hypothyroidism as a complication of thyroid surgery

18-6

Myxedema

- Myxedema is a rare but serious form of severe hypothyroidism that results from prolonged insufficient thyroxin during adulthood
  - The "myxedema" comes from deposition of connective tissue fibers separated by excessive protein and mucopolysaccharides (these bind water, causing boggy edema)
  - It results in dry brittle hair, dry skin due to decreased perspiration and sebaceous gland secretion, lethargy, low basal metabolic rate (low temp and heart rate); patients gain weight easily

18-6

Myxedema Coma

- A CNS-cardiovascular complication of the disease presenting as hypothermia (no shivering), hypoventilation, hypotension, hypoglycemia, lactic acidosis, and a deterioration of mental status
  - It is a medical emergency, and if not promptly treated will result in permanent brain damage or death

18-6

Congenital Hypothyroidism (Cretinism)

- Congenital hypothyroidism results from inadequate thyroid hormone during intrauterine growth
- Signs and symptoms include lethargy, hypothermia, and bradycardia
- Because thyroid hormones have a synergistic effect on HGH effects, patient also has stunted growth, abdominal protrusion and umbilical hernia

18-6

Parathyroid Glands

- Parathyroid hormone (PTH) is secreted by the parathyroids when the plasma [Ca^{++}] is low
  - PTH increases absorption of Ca^{++} from the GI tract, reabsorption from the kidneys **and** stimulates the release of Ca^{++} from bone (osteoclastic activity)
  - The osteoclastic activity of PTH is a negative feedback with the osteoblastic activity of calcitonin (from the thyroid) and does not involve the pituitary

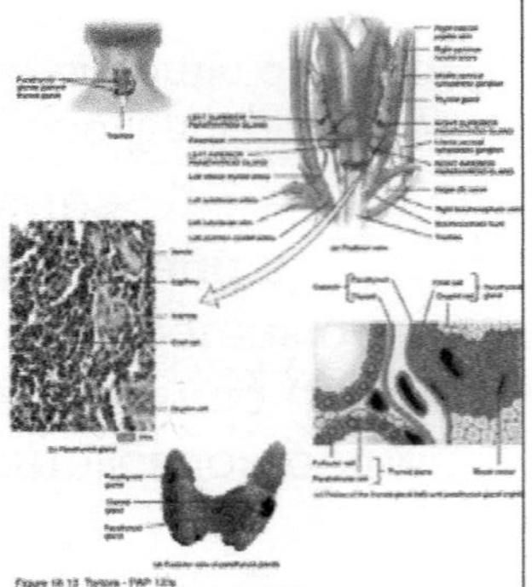

Figure 18.12 Tortora - PAP 12/e
Copyright © John Wiley and Sons, Inc. All rights reserved.

18-7

Hyperparathyroidism

- 80-85% of cases are caused by parathyroid adenomas, but it can also be caused by a compensatory response to hypocalcemia.
- Hyperparathyroidism causes:
  - Increase in demineralization of bone (osteoclastic activity)
  - Fragile bones with fractures and abnormal curvatures and bone pain
  - High plasma calcium levels can lead to a number of systemic problems.

18-7

Hypoparathyroidism

- Commonly caused by damage to the parathyroid glands during thyroid surgery
- Signs and symptoms include tetany (muscle spasms)
  - Due to low plasma [Ca^{++}] which lowers the threshold for nerve signals and muscle contraction
- Patients are treated with oral calcium and vitamin D
- Can cause hypoplastic dentin, bone deformation, and basal ganglia calcifications

18-7

Endocrine Pancreas

- Glucagon (alpha cells)
  - **Increases** blood glucose level
  - Acts on hepatocytes to convert glycogen to glucose
- Insulin (beta cells)
  - **Decreases** blood glucose levels
  - Speeds conversion of glucose to glycogen and accelerates facilitated diffusion of glucose into cells

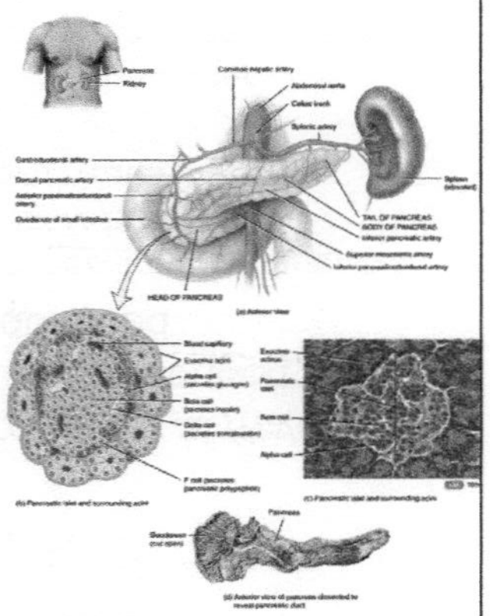

Figure 18.18 Tortora - PAP 12/e
Copyright © John Wiley and Sons, Inc. All rights reserved.

18-8

Diabetes Mellitus

- Type I: typically an immune disease of children, with destruction of the β-islets of the pancreas
- Type II: typically a complex multifactorial disease of adults
- Classical signs and symptoms include polydipsia, polyuria, and polyphagia
- Diagnosis is made by:
  - More than one fasting glucose level above 126 mg/dl
  - Two-hour glucose tolerance test ≥ 200 mg/dl
  - Random blood glucose > 200 mg/dl
  - Elevated levels of HbA_{1C}

18-8

Type I Diabetes Mellitus

- Genetic factor plus a “trigger” of some sort (virus, a food, chemical, drug). The exact mechanism is not known.
- As insulin producing β -cells are gradually destroyed by **islet cell antibodies, insulin levels fall and blood sugar levels rise.**
- Usually diagnosed under 30 years of age

18-8

Type II Diabetes Mellitus

- Of the nearly 16 million Americans with diabetes, 90-95% have type II. The genetic susceptibility is greater than type I but it is also triggered by environmental factors such as obesity.
- It usually develops after age 45
- The biggest problem in type II is insulin resistance at the cellular level
  - Body's cells do not respond to insulin made by the pancreas
  - Glucose accumulates in the blood but cannot be properly used by cells
- Almost all type II DM is associated with **metabolic syndrome**
  - hyperglycemia
  - hypertension
  - dyslipidemia
  - truncal (i.e. waist) obesity

18-8

Glycosylated Hemoglobin (HbA_{1c})

- Increased blood glucose plus insulin resistance, over a long period of time, leads to sugar being deposited on hemoglobin A molecules
- This is called HbA_{1c}
- Used to measure long term blood glucose control
- Should be around 5%

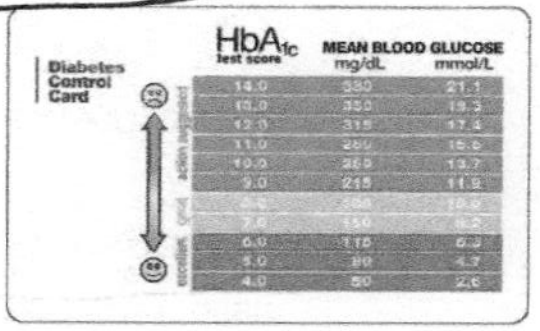
Diabetes Control Card
HbA1c test score
MEAN BLOOD GLUCOSE
mg/dL
mmol/L

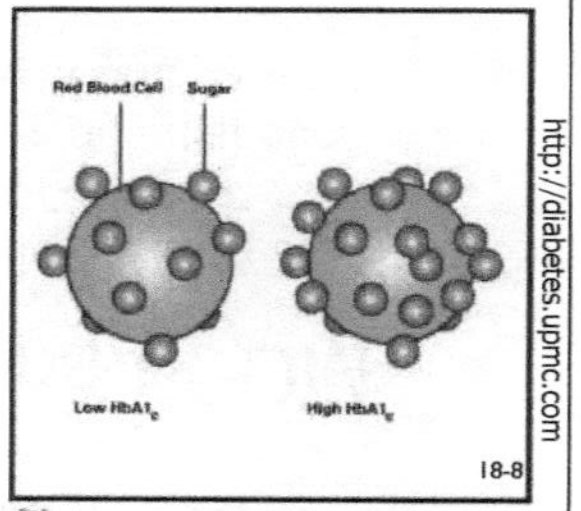
Red Blood Cell
Sugar
Low HbA1c
High HbA1c

http://diabetes.upmc.com

18-8

Blood Glucose < 60

Acute Complications of DM

- Hypoglycemia and insulin shock is a frequent occurrence in diabetics – especially those on insulin
  - Signs and symptoms of hypoglycemia is seen with levels < 60 mg/dL (infants < 30), and is related to activation of the sympathetic nervous system, cessation of glucose delivery to the brain, or both
  - It is usually rapid in onset. Patients are diaphoretic (sweaty) and appear weak, anxious, and confused
  - Treatment includes fast-acting carbohydrate solution (Coke, orange juice), intravenous infusions of dextrose containing fluids, or an injection of glucagon

18-9

Acute Complications of DM

- The other extreme is high blood sugar levels (often >300 mg/dl) which may precipitate a condition called **Diabetic ketoacidosis (DKA)**. DKA is due to a complete lack of insulin resulting in cells turning to fat for energy
  - Accumulation of keto acids (the by-products of fatty acid catabolism) leads to:
    - nausea, vomiting, irritability, and altered mental states (including coma)
    - the patient appears dehydrated with flushed, dry skin and mucous membranes
  - Treatment includes intravenous fluids, insulin, and K^+ replacement

18-9

B Glu > 300

Acute Complications of DM

- **Diabetic ketoacidosis (DKA)**
  - Due to a complete lack of insulin, type I diabetics catabolize fatty acids as a source of energy when glucose is unavailable
    - Keto acids are a by-product of fatty acid catabolism
  - Nausea, vomiting, comatose, irritable, general diabetic symptoms
  - Dry, hot, flushed skin and mucous membranes
  - Glucose level >300 mg/dl
  - Treatment: insulin, electrolyte and fluid replacement

18-9

B Glu > 700 w/o acidosis

Acute Complications of DM

- **Hyperosmolar hyperglycemic non-ketotic syndrome (HHNKS)** is a condition that manifests as extremely elevated blood glucose levels (>700 mg/dl), without acidosis.
  - **HHNKS** usually comes on slowly, most often in elderly patients with type II DM
  - It differs from DKA because of the presence of some small amount of insulin, so no ketosis develops
  - Blood sugars are > 700 mg/dl and dehydration can be severe

18-9

Chronic Complications of DM

- Microvascular Disease manifests as a thickening of the capillary basement membrane; leading to decreased perfusion of tissues
- Macrovascular Disease manifests as a 2-4 fold increase in heart disease
- Peripheral Neuropathy results from multiple metabolic, genetic, and environmental factors, with over 60-70% of patients showing some form of nerve damage
- Infections occur often in patients with diabetes
  - "Immunosuppressed"
  - Accounts for 60% of lower limb amputations
- Retinopathy: leading cause of new cases of blindness in adults 20-74
- Nephropathy: leading cause of death

18-10

Adrenal Glands

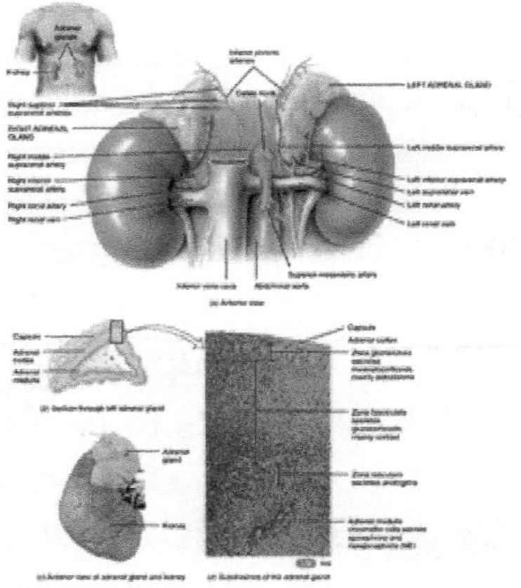

Figure 18.15 Tortora - PAP 12/e

18-11

Hormones of the Adrenal Cortex

- Glucocorticoids
  - **Cortisol** is the main player of the glucocorticoids
- Mineralocorticoids
  - **Aldosterone** is the main player of the mineralocorticoids
- A small amount of gonadocorticoids are made in the adrenal cortex (most are made in the gonads)

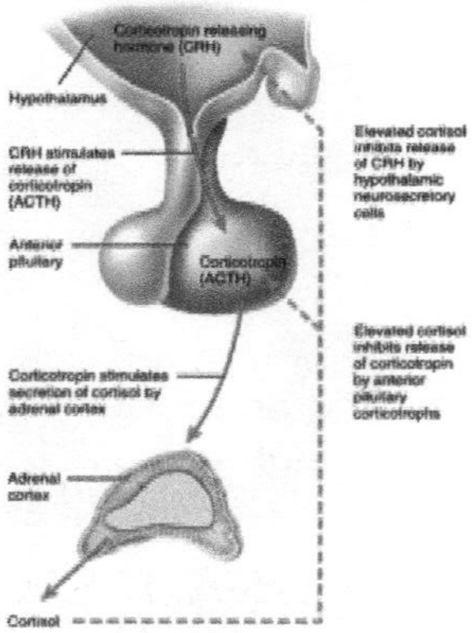
Corticotropin releasing hormone (CRH)
Hypothalamus
CRH stimulates release of corticotropin (ACTH)
Anterior pituitary
Corticotropin (ACTH)
Corticotropin stimulates secretion of cortisol by adrenal cortex
Adrenal cortex
Cortisol
Elevated cortisol inhibits release of CRH by hypothalamic neurosecretory cells
Elevated cortisol inhibits release of corticotropin by anterior pituitary corticotrophs

Figure 18.06 Tortora - PAP 12/e

18-11

Glucocorticoids

- The glucocorticoids **(cortisol) regulate metabolism** by promoting the breakdown of proteins and fats, and the formation of glucose (called gluconeogenesis, a catabolic activity)
- This raises blood glucose levels and helps the body **deal with stress**
- Glucocorticoids are powerful anti-inflammatory agents, and they also possess immune suppressive properties

18-11

Glucocorticoid Disorders

- **Cushing Disease/Syndrome**
  - **Excess cortisol** usually caused by a tumor of the adrenal gland or a tumor causing excess secretion of ACTH *cortisol?*
  - Cushing Syndrome develops from excess exogenous glucocorticoids *(fat? coming from outside the area?)*
  - Causes fat redistribution
    - Moon face, buffalo hump, and a hanging abdomen
  - Patients also exhibit slow wound healing, hyperglycemia, acne, osteoporosis, and susceptibility to infections

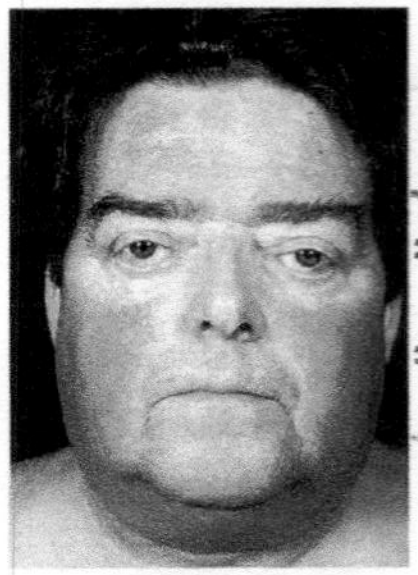

(e) Cushing's syndrome (excess glucocorticoids)

Figure 18.22e Tortora - PAP 12/e

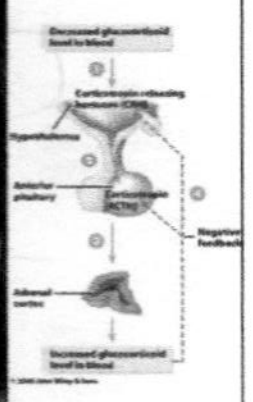

18-11

Mineralocorticoids

- Aldosterone is the body's main mineralcorticoid. It reegulates water and electrolytes (mainly Na^+ and K^+)
  - Aldosterone conserves Na^+ and H_2O but promotes the excretion of H^+ and K^+

keeps (Na^+ and H_2O) / *lose* (H^+ and K^+)

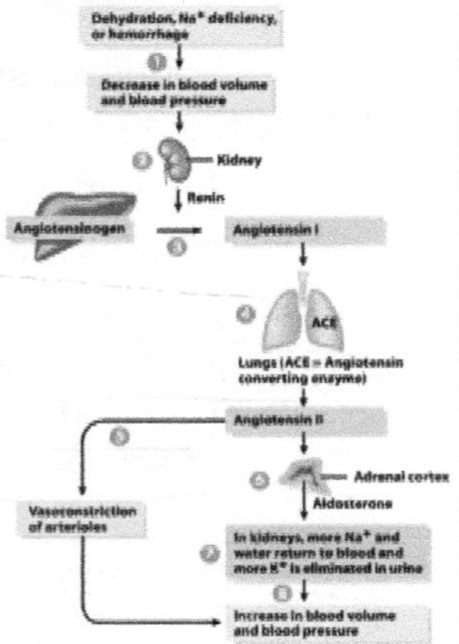

Dehydration, Na+ deficiency, or hemorrhage
Decrease in blood volume and blood pressure
Kidney
Renin
Angiotensinogen
Angiotensin I
ACE
Lungs (ACE = Angiotensin converting enzyme)
Angiotensin II
Adrenal cortex
Aldosterone
Vasoconstriction of arterioles
In kidneys, more Na+ and water return to blood and more K+ is eliminated in urine
Increase in blood volume and blood pressure

18-11

regulates urination with ADH

Mineralocorticoid Disorders

- **Conn disease (primary hyperaldosteronism)** results from excessive aldosterone secretion usually as the result of a tumor in the adrenal cortex.
  - The kidneys respond by conserving Na^+ and H_2O while wasting (excreting) K^+
  - Signs and symptoms include hypertension and hypokalemia from renal potassium wasting with its attendant neuromuscular irritability (twitching and cramps)

18-11

DeHydroEpiAndrosterone

Gonadocorticoid Disorders

Adrenal genital hormones

- **Adrenogenital Syndromes** are rare, congenital syndromes
  - Hypersecretion of weak androgens (DHEA)
    - In ♀: DHEA is masculinizing *androgenous*
      - deep voice & increased body hair
  - Hypersecretion of estrogens
    - In ♂: estrogens are feminizing *estrogenous?*
      - development of female secondary sex characteristics

18-11

Gonadocorticoid Disorders

- Adrenogenital Syndromes (more properly known as congenital adrenal hyperplasia), are a group of autosomal recessive conditions that lead to a deficiency of an enzyme needed to make cortisol
  - In an attempt to compensate, the pituitary produces high levels of ACTH which results in overproduction of certain intermediary androgens
    - these hormones have testosterone-like effects on the fetus and child leading to virilization

Th biological development of sex differences. secondarily.

18-11

Gonadocorticoid Disorders

- In ♀ virilization means that the clitoris is enlarged, and may resemble the male penis to the point that the sex of the child is questioned or mistaken
- ♂ may have enlarged penile size, but the problem may go undetected
  - During development the androgens may lead to early puberty, with a deep voice and increased body hair

18-11

Disorders of the Entire Adrenal Cortex

- **Addison Disease** results from the autoimmune destruction of the adrenal cortex
    - this leads to hyposecretion of **cortisol and aldosterone**
  - Signs and symptoms include weight loss, Na^+ loss and hyponatremia, K^+ retention and hyperkalemia, muscle weakness, dehydration, hypotension, and hypoglycemia

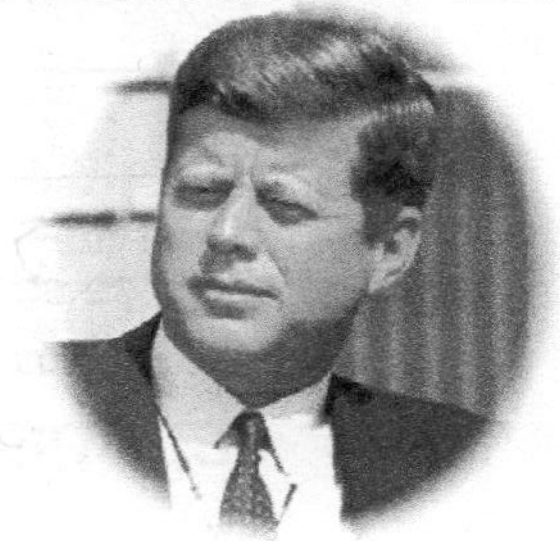

18-11

Adrenal Medulla

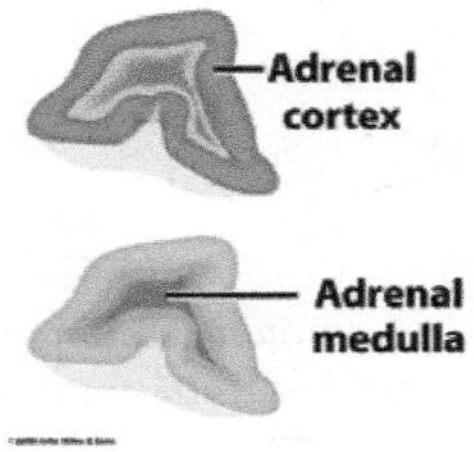
Adrenal cortex
Adrenal medulla

- The adrenal medullary secretions are part of the sympathetic nervous system
  - Secretes **epinephrine** and some **norepinephrine (catecholamines)**
  - Innervated by sympathetic preganglionics
  - Acts similar to a sympathetic postganglionic neuron
  - The secretions of the medulla duplicate and prolong the sympathetic response

18-12

Adrenal Medulla

- The adrenal medullary develops as a sympathetic "ganglia" – as such, its secretions are part of the sympathetic nervous system, epinephrine and some norepinephrine (catecholamines)
  - The secretions of the medulla duplicate and prolong the sympathetic "fight or flight" response (similar to a sympathetic postganglionic neuron)

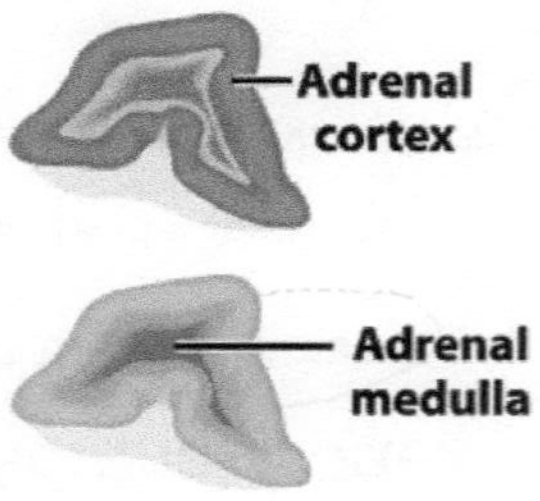
Adrenal cortex
Adrenal medulla

18-12

Adrenal Medulla Disorders

- **Pheochromocytoma** is a benign tumor of medullary cells, and is the only common disorder of this part of the gland.
  - Results in increased secretion of high levels of medullary catecholamines, producing an exaggerated (and often dangerous) sympathetic response.
  - Signs and symptoms include malignant hypertension, tachycardia, palpitations, and other dysrhythmias. Anxiety can sometimes be very severe and disconcerting

18-12

Unit 6
Chapter 10
Stress and Disease

Stress

- A person experiences stress when a demand exceeds a person's coping abilities.
- Stress begins with a stimulus that the brain perceives as stressful and in turn promotes adaptational and survival-related physiologic responses.
- These responses can become dysregulated and cause pathophysiology.

10-1

Stress

- Stressors
  - Physical or psychologic
  - Eustress vs. distress
- **Distress**: demand exceeds a person's coping abilities
- Stress in not an independent entity but a system of processes controlled by nature, intensity, and duration of the stressor

10-1

Stress

- Stress provoking factors include:
  - Environmental
    - Work, home, neighborhood
    - Major Life Events
    - Trauma, abuse
- Stress processes are an interaction between the brain and autonomic, immune, neural, and endocrine systems
- Designed for short term adaptation
- Chronic stress can lead to disorders compromising health

10-1

Physiologic and Behavioral Stress Responses

- Stress response is an interaction between:
  - Individual differences
    - Genes, development, experience
  - Behavioral responses
    - Fight or flight
    - Personal behavior: diet, smoking, drinking, exercise
  - Physiologic responses

10-1

The Stress Response
Adrenal Glands

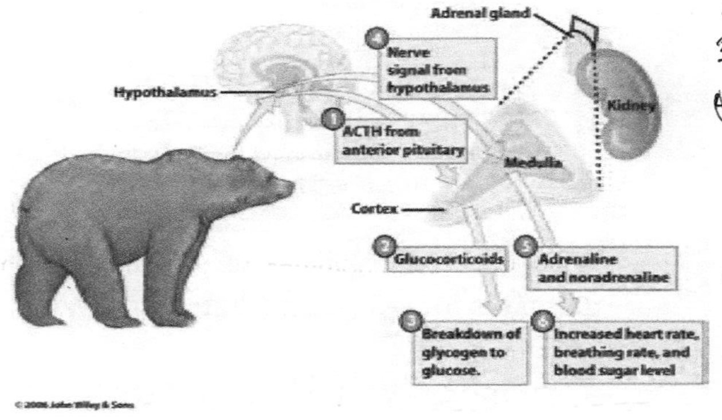

Adrenal gland
Hypothalamus
Nerve signal from hypothalamus
ACTH from anterior pituitary
Kidney
Medulla
Cortex
Glucocorticoids
Adrenaline and noradrenaline
Breakdown of glycogen to glucose.
Increased heart rate, breathing rate, and blood sugar level
© 2006 John Wiley & Sons

10-1

1. ACTH from ant pituitary
2. Glucocorticoids (adrenals
3. Glycogen → glucose
4. Nerve signal from hypothalmus
5 norepinephrine
6. ↑ rate resp + B Gluc

The Stress Response

- In the early 20th century, Hans Selye described general adaptation syndrome (GAS)
- General Adaptation Syndrome stages
  - **Alarm** stage
    - CNS and body defenses activated (epinephrine)
  - **Resistance** (adaptation) stage
  - **Exhaustion** stage
    - Continuous stress causes breakdown of compensatory mechanisms
    - Diseases result from continuous stress

10-2

The Alarm Stage

- Activation of the central nervous system
  - Sympathetic response
  - Norepinephrine
    - Increased cardiac output
    - Increase blood pressure
    - Promote hyperglycemia
    - Cause vasoconstriction of vessels in the skin, viscera, extremities, and kidneys
    - Cause vasodilation of vessels in the heart, skeletal muscles and the smooth muscle of the bronchi

10-2
10-3

The Resistance Stage

- Activation of the sympathetic nervous system causes the hypothalamus to stimulate the pituitary gland resulting in:
  - The adrenal cortex increases ACTH release
    - controls **aldosterone** and **cortisol**
  - The adrenal medulla secretes epinephrine and norepinephrine
  - The pituitary gland secretes **TSH**
  - Increased secretion of **HGH**
  - Increased release of **ADH** from the posterior pituitary

10-2
10-3

The Resistance Stage

- **Cortisol**
  - Increases protein catabolism, hyperglycemia, promotes gluconeogenesis in liver cells, and delays the healing process
  - Promotes lipolysis in adipose tissue (especially in the extremities), increases gastric secretion, anti-inflammatory effects
  - Although there is an increase in antibody formation, there is an **overall decrease in the immune response** (decline in lymphocytes)

10-2
10-3

The Resistance Stage

- **TSH**
  - Increased thyroxin (increased BMR)
- **Aldosterone**
  - Increases sodium and water retention
  - Increases blood volume and pressure
- **ADH**
  - Water retention
  - Increases blood volume and pressure

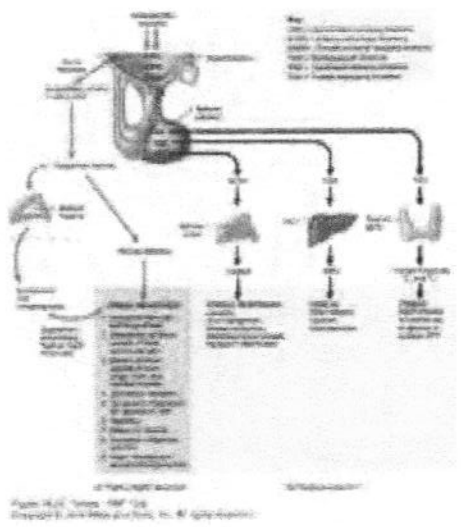

10-2
10-3

The Stress Response

Adrenal Glands
Liver
Thyroid

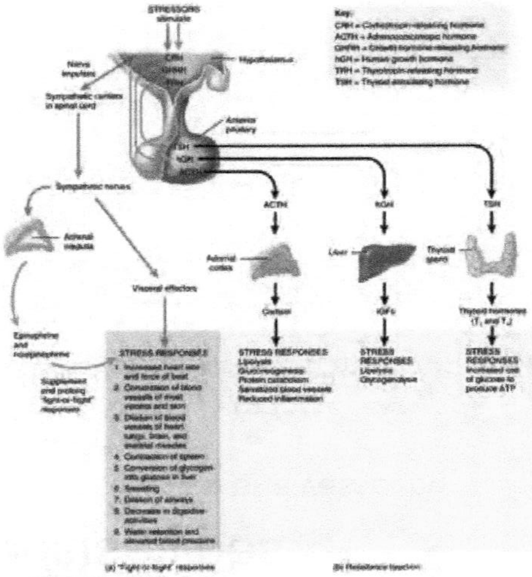

Figure 18.20 Tortora - PAP 12/e

10-2
10-3

Exhaustion Stage

- With continuous, **uncompensated** stress, **disease** can result
  - **Cardiovascular system**
    - coronary artery disease
    - hypertension
    - stroke
    - arrhythmias
  - **Muscular system**
    - tension headache
    - muscle contractions (spasms)
  - **Connective tissues**
    - rheumatoid arthritis
    - inflammatory diseases of connective tissues
      - e.g. myofascial pain syndrome

10-2
10-3

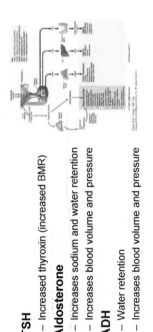

Unit 6
Chapter 23
Alterations of Cardiovascular Function

Vascular Disease

Thrombi, Emboli
Venous Disease
Arterial Disease

Thrombus

- A thrombus is a clot that forms in a blood vessel and remains attached
- Locations include veins, systemic and coronary arteries
- Cause: conditions encourage activation of the coagulation cascade
  - Roughing of vessel wall
  - Stasis or pooling of blood
  - Infectious agents

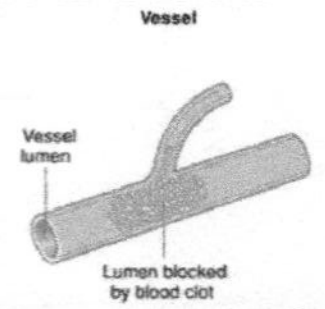

Vessel
Vessel lumen
Lumen blocked by blood clot

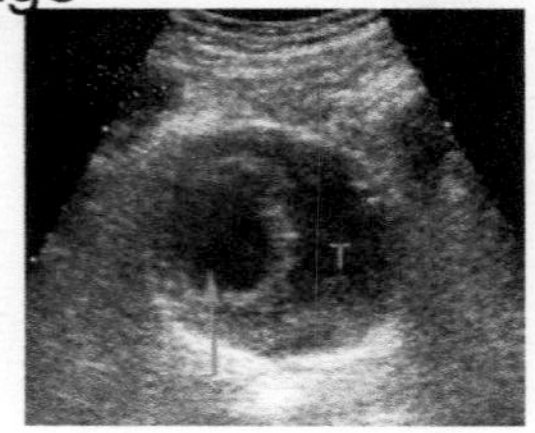

T

23-1

Thrombus

- Thrombophlebitis
  - thrombi form in veins (with associated inflammation)
- Thrombi of heart valves
  - due to endocardial inflammation or rheumatic fever
- Thrombi can occlude vessels and cause ischemia or infarction of organs

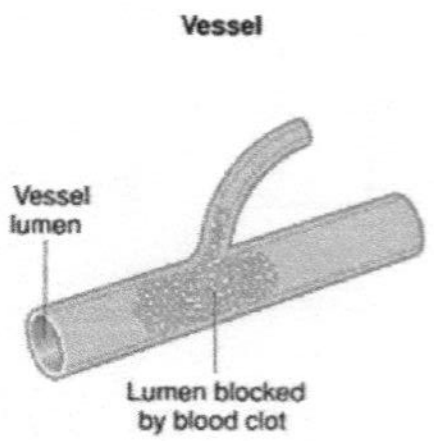

Vessel
Vessel lumen
Lumen blocked by blood clot

23-1

Embolus Types

- **Embolism (emboli)**: obstruction of a vessel by moving chunk of material
  - **Thromboemboli**
    - thrombi which break loose and travel to another site
  - **Air emboli**
    - air bubble from injection, punctured lung, or open vessel
  - **Fat emboli**
    - hip replacement surgery
    - broken bone
  - Plaque
    - atherosclerosis as described above

23-1

Embolus Sources

- **Pulmonary emboli**
  - usually arise from thrombophlebitis of veins in lower extremity
- **Systemic (arterial) emboli**
  - Originate in the left circulation
  - left heart
    - thrombi after myocardial infarction, endocarditis, or dysrhythmias
  - renal emboli
  - mesenteric emboli
  - coronary emboli
  - cerebral emboli

23-1

Thromboembolic Disease: Treatment

- Administration of anticoagulants to prevent clot formation
  - Aspirin
  - Heparin
  - Warfarin
- "Clot busters"
- Slow or stop thrombus growth
  - Aggressive reversal of risk factors

23-1

Diseases of the Veins

- **Varicose veins** are distended, tortuous, and palpable
- Varicose veins in the legs are caused by damage to one or more venous valves due to standing for extended periods of time and the contributing force of gravity
- A damaged valve permits back flow of blood **(venous incompetence)** and distended veins

23-2

Varicose Veins

- Because the vein becomes swollen and engorged, the surrounding tissues become edematous
- Varicose veins and valvular incompetence can progress to chronic venous insufficiency
  - Chronic pooling of blood leading to hypercoagulability, severe edema, cell death, and necrosis (**venous stasis ulcers**)

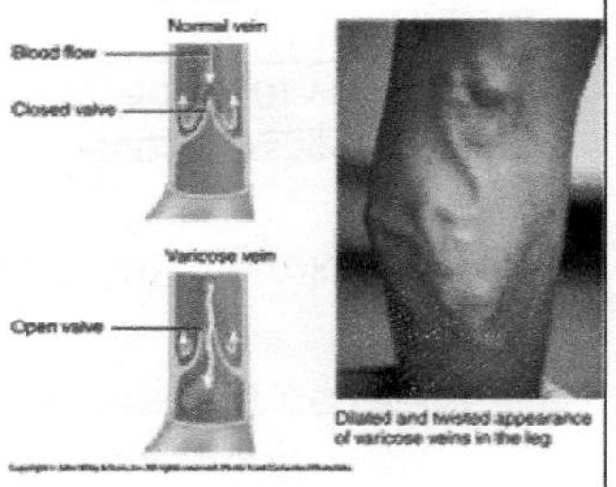
Normal vein
Blood flow
Closed valve
Varicose vein
Open valve
Dilated and twisted appearance of varicose veins in the leg

23-2

Venous Thrombi

- Why would venous thrombi be more common than arterial thrombi?
- With age, deep veins in the legs become very susceptible to thrombi
  - Deep vein thrombosis (DVT)
- DVT is very often asymptomatic, but can lead to pulmonary emboli
- Treatment
  - thrombolytics
  - anti-embolism stockings
  - avoid prolonged sitting / immobility

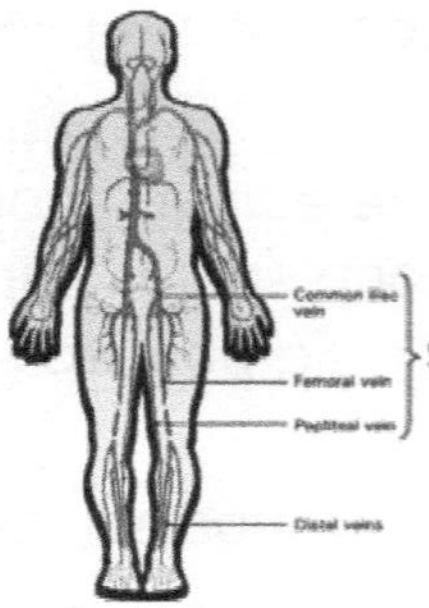
Common iliac vein
Femoral vein
Popliteal vein
Proximal veins
Distal veins

Wiley Handbook of Current and Emerging Drug Therapies

23-2

Arterial Disease

- **Hypertension** is caused by increased in cardiac output, total peripheral resistance or both:
  - Cardiac output: increase in heart rate or stroke volume
  - Peripheral resistance: increase in blood viscosity or reduction in vessel diameter, total length of vessels
- Types:
  - Primary, secondary, and complicated

23-3

Hypertension: Definition

Classification	Normal	Stage 1	Stage 2	Stage 3
Descriptive Category	Normal blood pressure (BP) (≤120 mmHg systolic and ≤80 mmHg diastolic) with rare elevations **and** no cardio-vascular disease (CVD) signs	Occasional or intermittent elevations of BP (140–160 mmHg systolic or 80–100 mmHg diastolic) **or** early CVD signs	Sustained BP elevations (140–160 mmHg systolic or 80–100 mmHg diastolic) **or** progressive CVD	Marked and sustained BP elevations (≥160 mmHg systolic or ≥100 mmHg diastolic) **or** advanced CVD
Cardiovascular risk factors (include age, sex, lipid levels, BMI, smoking, diabetes, and family history)	None or few	Several	Many	Many
Early disease markers (e.g., micro-albuminuria or exaggerated BP response to exercise/stress)	None	Usually present	Overtly present	Overtly present with progression
Target-organ disease (e.g., in the heart, arteries, kidneys, or eyes)	None	None	Early signs present	Overtly present with or without CVD events

Joint National Committee on Prevention, Detection, Evaluation, and Treatment of High Blood Pressure (JNC-7), 2003

23-3

Primary or "Essential" Hypertension

- In primary (also called essential or idiopathic) hypertension, the cause is unknown **(multifactorial).**
- 90-95% of hypertensive patients fall into this group
- Contributing factors:
  - Family history (polygenic), age, gender, race, diet, diabetes, obesity, cigarettes, heavy alcohol consumption

23-3

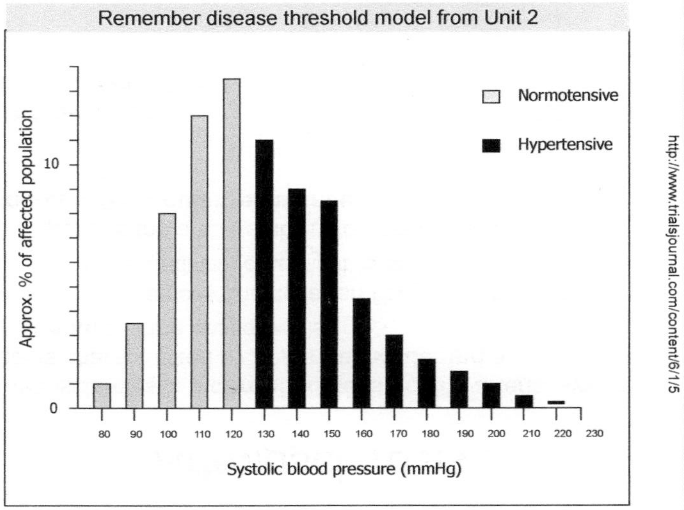

Remember disease threshold model from Unit 2
Approx. % of affected population
0
10
80
90
100
110
120
130
140
150
160
170
180
190
200
210
220
230
Systolic blood pressure (mmHg)
Normotensive
Hypertensive
http://www.trialsjournal.com/content/6/1/5

Secondary Hypertension

- Renal
  - Renal vascular stenosis, renin-producing tumors, renal failure, primary sodium retention
- Endocrine
  - Acromegaly, or thyroid or adrenal disorders
- Vascular
  - Arteriosclerosis, constriction of the aorta
- Pregnancy-induced hypertension (PIH)
  - Pre-eclampsia, eclampsia
- Stress
  - Epinephrine, norepinephrine, glucocorticoids (cortisol)

23-3

Complicated Hypertension

- Prolonged hypertension
  - Demonstrates pathologic effects *beyond* hemodynamic alterations
    - Vascular remodeling (smooth muscle hypertrophy)
    - Hypoperfusion: heart, kidneys, eyes and brain
  - Examples of problems: aneurysm rupture, arteriosclerosis, vessel occlusion, uremia, left ventricular enlargement

23-3

Treatments for Hypertension

- Non-pharmacologic c/o eliminating risk factors
- Pharmacologic:
  - Diuretics - decrease blood volume and cardiac output
  - Block the renin-angiotensin-aldosterone system
    - ACE inhibitors and angiotensin II rc blockers
  - Drugs which relax blood vessel smooth muscle
    - Ca^{++} channel blockers prevent calcium entry, which prevents smooth muscle contraction
    - β -blockers block catecholamines effects at β -adrenergic rcs

23-3

Orthostatic (Postural) Hypotension

- Decrease in systolic and diastolic arterial blood pressure upon standing from a reclining position
- The vasoconstrictive response to changing blood pressure and blood flow is inadequate, and dizziness results
- Causes: age, drugs (antihypertensive and antidepressant therapy), volume depletion, prolonged immobility (chronic illness), starvation, physical exhaustion

23-3

Aneurysms

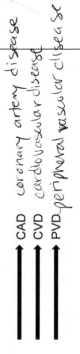

- An aneurysm is a dilation or pouching of a vessel wall or cardiac chamber.
- As tension increases, the wall becomes thinner.
- True aneurysms involve all three layers
  - Saccular or "berry" aneurysms
  - Fusiform aneurysms

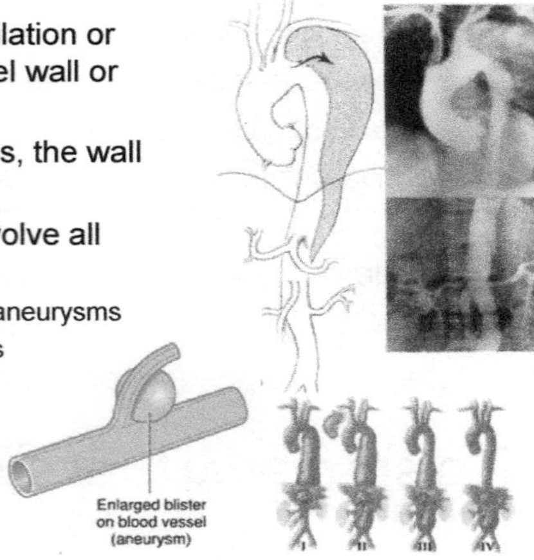
Enlarged blister on blood vessel (aneurysm)
I
II
III
IV

Haimovici's Vascular Surgery, 5e (Fifth Edition), (p 661-686)

23-4

Arteriosclerosis

- Arteriosclerosis is a **chronic disease** of the arterial system that is characterized by abnormal **hardening** and **thickening** of the vessel walls
- Smooth muscle cells and collagen fibers migrate into the tunica interna (intima), causing it to stiffen and thicken
- This restricts the artery's ability to change lumen size **(increased vascular resistance)**

- **Atherosclerosis** is a form of arteriosclerosis

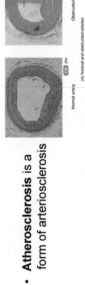

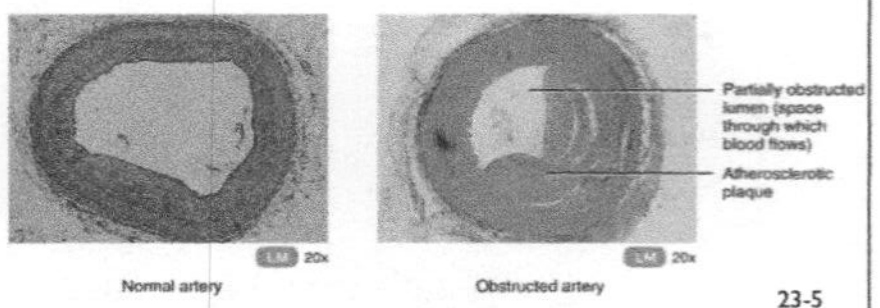
Partially obstructed lumen (space through which blood flows)
Atherosclerotic plaque
LM 20x
LM 20x
Normal artery
Obstructed artery

(A) Normal and obstructed arteries

23-5

Atherosclerosis

- **Atherosclerosis is a form of arteriosclerosis**
  - Thickening and hardening of the vessel walls are caused by deposits of intra-arterial fat (i.e. LDL cholesterol) and fibrin that harden over time
  - Atherosclerosis is not a single disease; it varies depending on location, age, and genetics

→ CAD coronary artery disease
→ CVD cardiovascular disease
→ PVD peripheral vascular disease.

23-5

Atherosclerosis

- Atherosclerosis is an **inflammatory** disease
- Stages:
  1. **Endothelial injury**
  2. **Fatty streak**
  3. **Fibrous plaque**
  4. **Complicated lesion**

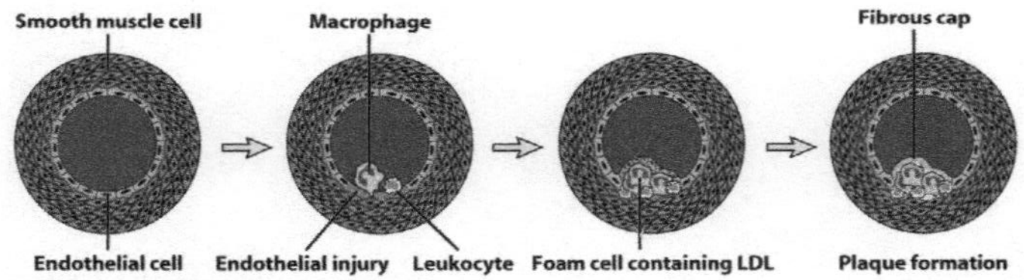

Smooth muscle cell
Macrophage
Fibrous cap
Endothelial cell
Endothelial injury
Leukocyte
Foam cell containing LDL
Plaque formation

Figure 8-44 Cell and Molecular Biology, 5/e (© 2008 John Wiley & Sons)

Karp G. *Cell & Molecular Biology*, 5e

23-5

Atherosclerosis
Step 1: Injury

- Chemical or mechanical injury begins the process
  - possible causes: smoking, high cholesterol, hypertension
- Endothelial cells
  - ↓ release of antithrombotic & vasodilating cytokines
  - ↑ release of inflammatory cytokines
    - TNF, interferon & interleukins
  - ↑ release of growth factors
    - smooth muscle proliferates

23-5

Progression of Atherosclerosis

- Macrophages adhere to the injured endothelium
  - release enzymes and toxic oxygen free radicals
  - free radicals oxidize low density lipoprotein (LDL)
  - this oxidized LDL is toxic to endothelial cells

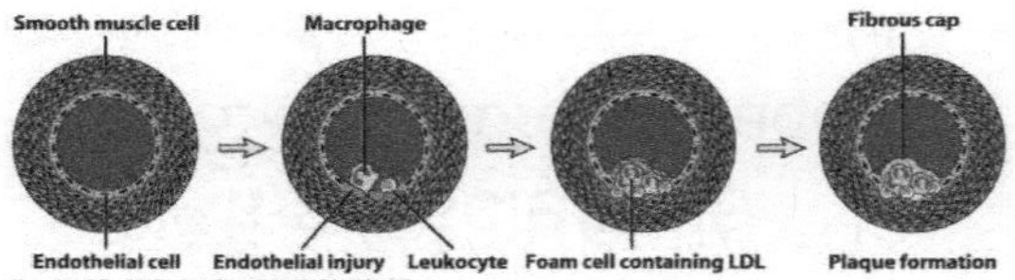

Smooth muscle cell
Macrophage
Fibrous cap
Endothelial cell
Endothelial injury
Leukocyte
Foam cell containing LDL
Plaque formation

Figure 8-44 Cell and Molecular Biology, 5/e (© 2008 John Wiley & Sons)

Karp G. *Cell & Molecular Biology*, 5e

23-5

Atherosclerosis
Step 2: Formation of the Fatty Streak

- Macrophages engulf oxidized LDL
- The macrophages filled with oxidized LDL are called **foam cells**
- **Fatty streak** is an accumulation of foam cells
  - these produce even more oxygen free radicals

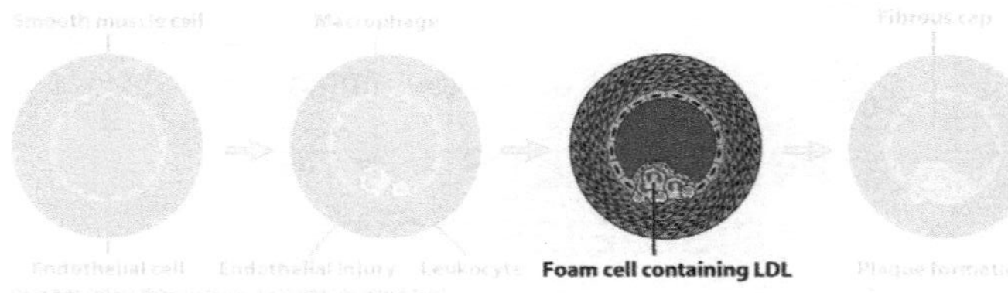

Foam cell containing LDL

Karp G. *Cell & Molecular Biology*, 5e

23-5

Atherosclerosis
Step 3: The Fibrous Plaque

- Under the influence of growth factors, smooth muscle cells proliferate
- Smooth muscle migrates over the fatty streak, forming a cap
- **Fibrous plaque** is formed

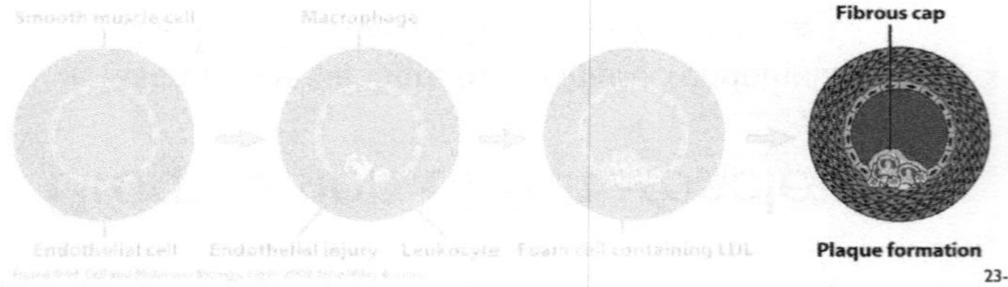

Fibrous cap
Plaque formation

Karp G. *Cell & Molecular Biology*, 5e

23-5

Atherosclerosis
Step 4: It's Complicated

- Fibrous plaques are not stable
  - ulcerations
  - calcifications
  - apoptosis causes rupture
- Platelets now have an adherence site and become activated
- This is called a **complicated lesion**

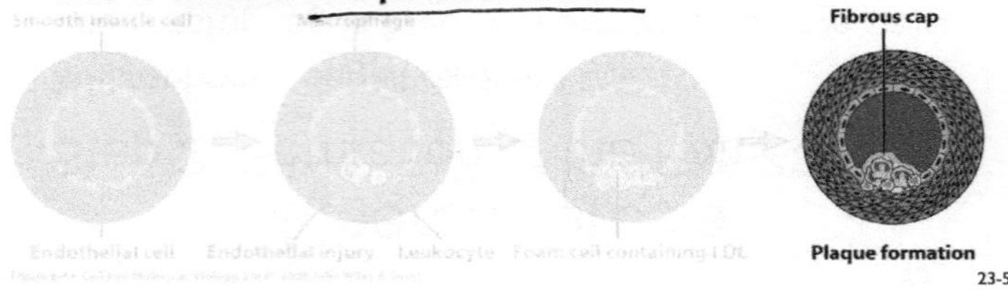

Fibrous cap
Plaque formation

Karp G. *Cell & Molecular Biology*, 5e

23-5

Peripheral Vascular Disease

Thromboangiitis Obliterans
(Buerger Disease)

- An inflammatory **autoimmune** disease of the peripheral arteries of the hands and feet resulting in the formation of **non-atherosclerotic lesions which obliterates the vessels**
- Causes pain and hair loss (not on their head) in **young men who smoke (tobacco) or even those who use smokeless tobacco**
- Progresses to ulcers & gangrenous lesions of fingers/toes

23-6

Raynaud Disease

- **Raynaud disease** is primary vasospastic disorder of unknown etiology causing episodic vasospasm in arteries of the fingers, and less commonly the toes (pallor/cyanosis)
- **Raynaud phenomenon** is the same thing, but it is secondary to other systemic diseases
  - Collagen vascular disease (scleroderma), smoking, pulmonary hypertension, and environmental factors (cold, prolonged exposure to vibrating machinery)

23-6

Raynaud Signs & Symptoms

- In Raynaud phenomenon/disease
  - Vasospasm causes **pallor**, **numbness**, and cold sensations in the digits
  - **Cyanosis** can also appear
  - There is a cycle of pallor, cyanosis (blue), then rubor (red) due to vasospasm, followed by relaxation pale?
  - The treatment is simply to remove the stimulus
    - e.g. **cold**, drugs, or treat the primary disease

23-6

Heart Disease

Heart Diseases

- Coronary artery disease (**CAD**)
  - Diminishes the myocardial blood supply
- Coronary artery disease can lead to:
  - Reversible myocardial ischemia **(angina)**
  - Irreversible myocardial infarction **(MI)** and death
  - **Both** inhibit the pumping ability of the heart (either temporarily or permanently) due to a lack of O_2 and nutrients

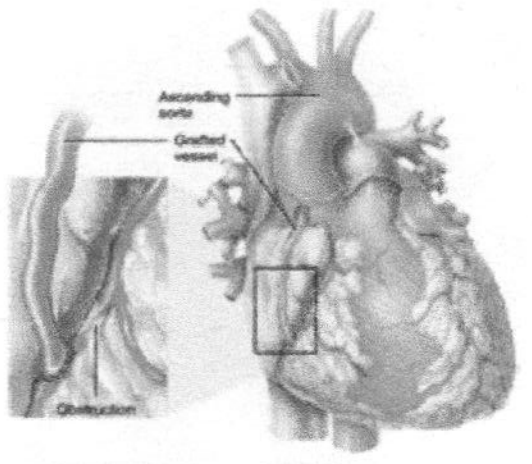

Ascending aorta
Grafted vessel
Obstruction

(B) Coronary artery bypass grafting (CABG)

23-7

Risk Factors for CAD

- Major:
  - Increased age
  - Family history
  - Male gender or female gender post menopause
- Modifiable:
  - Dyslipidemia
  - Hypertension
  - Cigarette smoking
  - Diabetes mellitus
  - Obesity/sedentary lifestyle
  - Atherogenic diet

23-7

Heart Diseases

- Myocardial ischemia
  - Most commonly caused by atherosclerosis
  - Mass of plaque, platelets, fibrin and debris eventually narrows the artery lumen
  - Vasoconstriction encourages symptoms
  - If the ischemia is **without** pain, it is referred to as **silent ischemia (especially in diabetics)**.

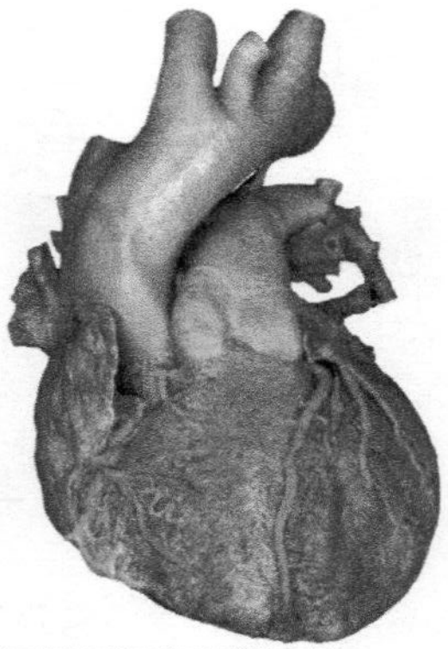

23-7

Myocardial Infarction

- Myocardial cells become ischemic within 10 seconds of a coronary blockage
  - cells remain viable for 20 minutes
- If the arteries cannot compensate for lack of oxygen, myocardial infarction is the result
- Myocardial infarction is death of heart muscle tissue

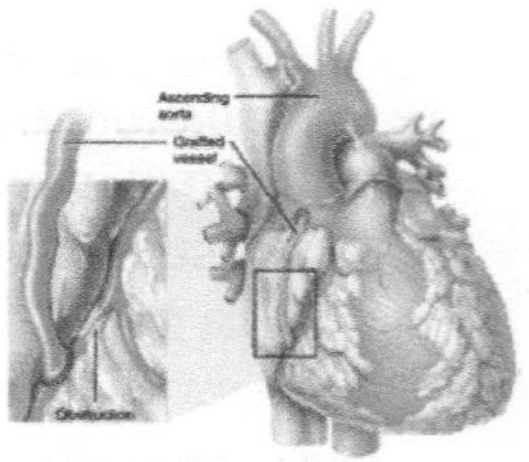
Ascending aorta
Grafted vessel
Obstruction

(B) Coronary artery bypass grafting (CABG)

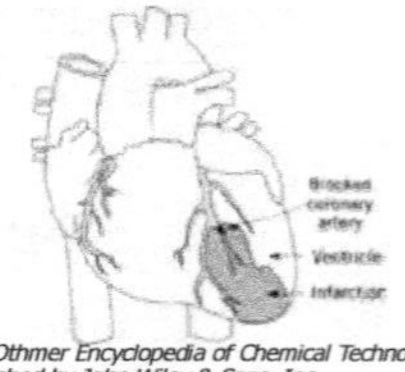
Blocked coronary artery
Ventricle
Infarction

Kirk-Othmer Encyclopedia of Chemical Technology
Published by John Wiley & Sons, Inc.

23-7

	Angina	MI
Cause	Temporary ischemia	Irreversible ischemia Necrosis
ECG	Normal, transient ST depression T wave inversion	Abnormal pronounced Q wave
Plasma Enzyme Levels	Normal	↑ creatine kinase-myocardial bound (CK-MB) ↑ lactate dehydrogenase (LDH) ↑ alanine transaminase (ALT) ↑ aspartate aminotransferase (AST) positive troponin I
Pain Relief and Treatment	Rest Nitroglycerin Beta-blockers Calcium antagonists	Narcotics Anticoagulant therapy ACE inhibitors Beta blockers Surgery

23-7

Complications of an MI

- The complications of an MI are variable and depend on the location and extent of necrosis
- Complications:
  - **Dysrhythmias**, pulmonary congestion, reduced myocardial contractility, inflammation of the pericardium, pain, fever, pleural effusion, pulmonary emboli, and strokes

23-7

Disorders of the Heart Wall

Pericardium
Myocardium
Endocardium

Pericardial Disease

- **Acute pericarditis** is when pericardial membranes become inflamed, and may produce an exudate
- It is usually a local manifestation of another disorder
- Signs and symptoms
  - "Pleuritic" chest pain
    - Chest pain which worsens with respiratory movements
    - Pericardial "friction rub" (sounds like scratchy sandpaper heard on auscultation of the lungs and heart)
  - Treatment is with analgesics and NSAIDs

The image cannot be displayed. Your computer may not have enough memory to open the image, or the image may have been corrupted. Restart your computer, and then open the file again. If the red x still appears, you may have to delete the image and then insert it again.

23-8

Pericardial Disease

- **Pericardial effusion**
  - An accumulation of fluid (transudate or exudate) in the pericardial cavity accompanying all types of pericarditis.
    - transudate: pressure filtration without capillary injury
    - exudate: inflammatory fluid
- Signs and symptoms depend on severity and range from mild, pleuritic chest pain to compression of the heart causing reduced cardiac output, hypotension, and even death

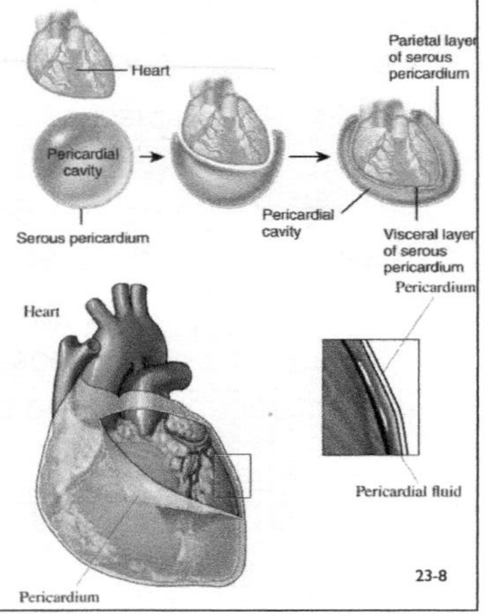

Heart
Pericardial cavity
Serous pericardium
Pericardial cavity
Parietal layer of serous pericardium
Visceral layer of serous pericardium
Pericardium
Heart
Pericardial fluid
Pericardium

23-8

Cardiac Tamponade

- In situations of severe trauma, like a steering wheel to the chest at high speeds (MVA), a large pericardial effusion of fluid or blood can lead to a serious compression of the heart called **cardiac tamponade**
  - Tamponade occurs whenever the pressure from the pericardial fluid equals the diastolic filling pressure
- **Which chamber(s) would be affected first?**
  - Increased venous pressure, edema, hepatomegaly, decreased stroke volume
- Treatment consists of an emergency **pericardiocentesis**
  - Aspiration of the excessive pericardial fluid
  - Fluid analysis can identify the cause of effusion

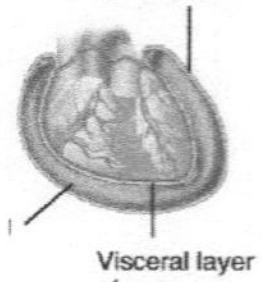
Parietal layer of serous pericardium
Visceral layer of serous pericardium

23-8

Constrictive Pericarditis

- Fibrous scarring with possible calcification of the pericardium causes the visceral and pericardial layers to adhere to one another
- Similar to tamponade, but demonstrates a slower "**insidious**" onset and progression
  - ½ idiopathic
  - TB, post-surgery, viral, acute pericarditis
- The heart becomes constricted and reduces the cardiac output
- Surgical removal of the pericardium may be required

23-8

Cardiomyopathies

- Diseases that affect the myocardium
- Often the results of infarction, longstanding hypertension, infections, toxins, connective tissue diseases, proliferative disorders or nutritional deficiencies
- Categories:
  - Ischemic
  - Hypertrophic
  - Restrictive
  - Dilated

23-9

Cardiomyopathies

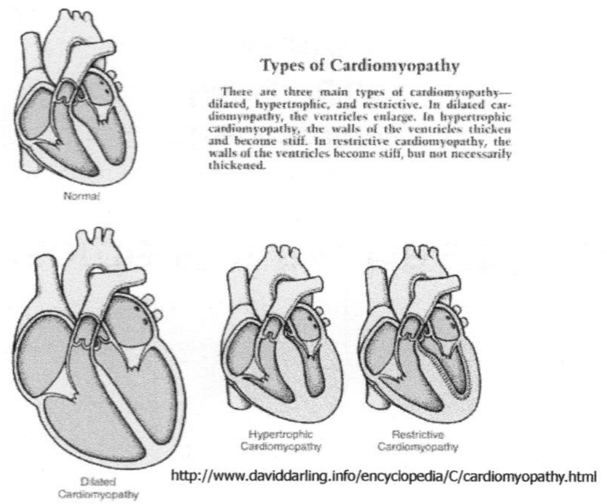
Types of Cardiomyopathy
There are three main types of cardiomyopathy—dilated, hypertrophic, and restrictive. In dilated cardiomyopathy, the ventricles enlarge. In hypertrophic cardiomyopathy, the walls of the ventricles thicken and become stiff. In restrictive cardiomyopathy, the walls of the ventricles become stiff, but not necessarily thickened.
Normal
Dilated Cardiomyopathy
Hypertrophic Cardiomyopathy
Restrictive Cardiomyopathy

http://www.daviddarling.info/encyclopedia/C/cardiomyopathy.html

23-9

Cardiomyopathies

- **Hypertrophic**
  - Thickening of the myocardium, often a result of hypertension and valve disease
- **Restrictive**
  - Due to infiltrative disease
  - The ventricular walls are excessively rigid and impede ventricular filling
  - No thickening of myocardium
  - Another common cause of heart failure in many under-developed countries
- **Dilated.** (Ischemic most common type)
  - Remodeling due to overfilling and weak myocardial contractions
  - Enlarging of heart without thickening of myocardium
  - Often the end result of the other cardiomyopathies mentioned above.

23-9

Endocardium Disorders

Valvular Stenosis

- When any valve orifice is **constricted** or narrowed
- The stenosis increases the workload of the chamber behind the valve and causes myocardial hypertrophy
- Caused by calcification or degeneration of a valve

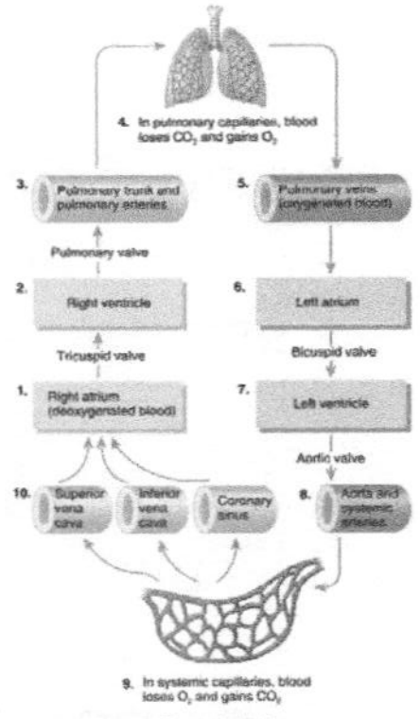

Pulmonary valve
Right ventricle
Tricuspid valve
Left atrium
Bicuspid valve
Left ventricle
Aortic valve
Coronary sinus

(b) Diagram of blood flow

23-10

Valvular Stenosis

- **Left-sided valvular disease most common**
  - **Aortic stenosis (AS)** presents with a low stroke volume, left ventricular hypertrophy, and a systolic murmur
  - **Mitral stenosis (MS)** presents with left atrial dilation and pulmonary hypertension
    - most commonly caused by acute rheumatic fever. 2-3X more common in women than men.
    - Diastolic murmur

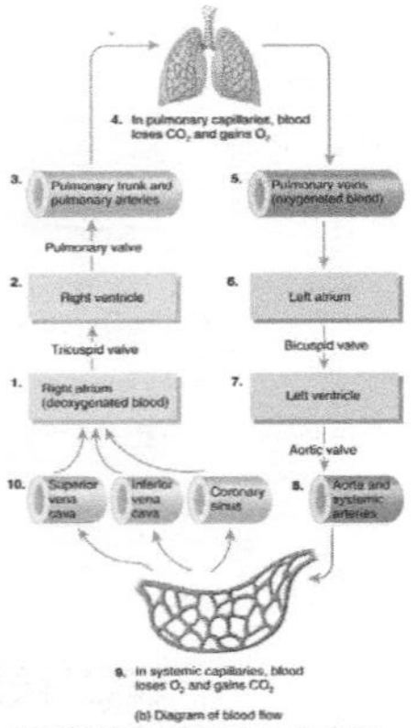

Pulmonary valve
Right ventricle
Tricuspid valve
Left atrium
Bicuspid valve
Left ventricle
Aortic valve
Coronary sinus

(b) Diagram of blood flow

23-10

Valvular Regurgitation

- Also called valvular insufficiency or incompetence
- When the cusps/leaflets of the valves fail to close, it permits backflow of blood during systole
  - The increased workload of pumping the blood "twice" causes myocardial hypertrophy
- All four valves can be affected, but the valves on the **left** are most common

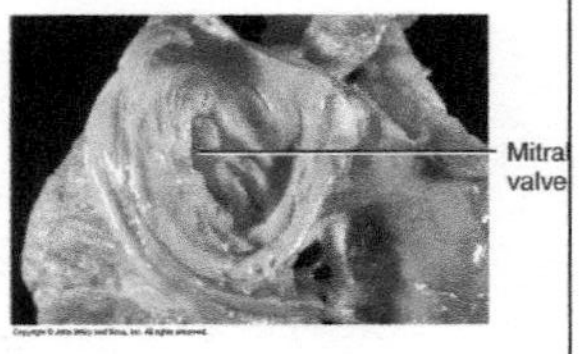

Mitral valve

23-10

Valvular Regurgitation

- **Aortic regurgitation (AR)** presents with a widened pulse pressure, dyspnea, throbbing peripheral pulse, & **diastolic** murmur (blood backflows during diastole). Dysrhythmias and endocarditis are common complications.
- **Mitral regurgitation (MR)** presents with pulmonary HTN, **systolic murmur** (blood backflows during systole), and left and right ventricle failure.
- **Tricuspid regurgitation (TR)** presents with right heart failure, edema, and a **systolic murmur** (blood backflows during systole).

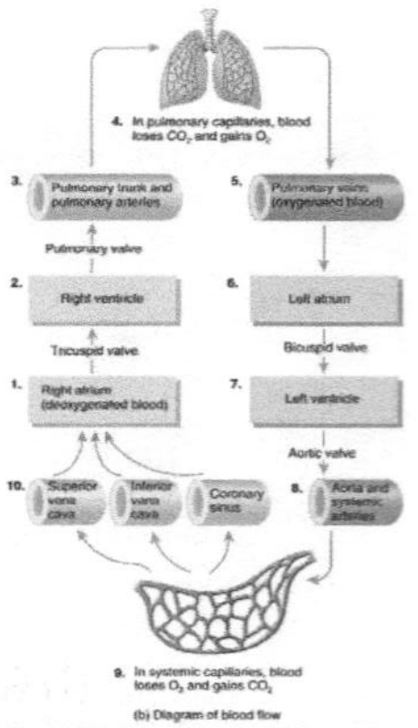

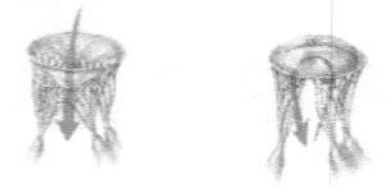

23-10

Mitral Valve Prolapse (MVP)

- **MVP** is an **autosomal dominant** disorder where the anterior and posterior mitral cusps prolapse into the left atrium during left ventricular systole.
- Usually asymptomatic
- It can cause endocarditis, chest pain, and dysrhythmias
- In severe cases, signs and symptoms are similar to those of mitral regurgitation.

23-10

Rheumatic Heart Disease (RHD)

- RHD is hypersensitivity reaction (type II) that occurs in about 1-3% of cases of untreated strep throat infections.
  - β-hemolytic group A streptococcal infection (*Streptococcus pyogenes*)
- It manifests as a systemic inflammatory attack on the heart and many other tissues in the body
  - CANCER: Carditis, Arthritis, Nodules, Chorea, Erythema Marginatum (characteristic rash)

23-11

Rheumatic Heart Disease

- Rheumatic heart disease is the heart component of rheumatic fever.
- Pathophysiology
  - Carditis of all three layers of the **heart wall**
  - Inflammation of the **endocardium**
  - Vegetative growths on **valves** and granulomas in the myocardium

23-11

Rheumatic Heart Disease

- The manifestations of RHD include
  - Fever
  - Lymphadenopathy
  - Chorea
  - Truncal rash (*erythema marginatum*)
  - High anti-streptolysin O titer, leukocytosis, elevated C-reactive protein, and ECG abnormalities
- Many of these are due to the prior history of strep infection or a general inflammatory response

23-11

Infective Endocarditis

- Is an inflammation of the endocardium
- Caused by Streptococci, Staphylococci, viruses, fungi, or Rickettsiae that enter the bloodstream
- Pathophysiological risk factors
  - Prior endothelial damage to valves, mitral valve, prolapse, prosthetic valves, septal defects, microbial colonization to damaged valve, adherence of microbes to form endocardial vegetations
  - **IV drug abuse by far the most common risk factor**

23-11

Infective Endocarditis

- Manifestations include fever, cardiac murmur, positive blood cultures, ECG abnormalities
- Treatment
  - Long-term anti-microbial therapy
  - Prophylactic antibiotics for procedures that increase risk bacteremia
    - For example, dental procedures place patients at risk

23-11

Dysrhythmias

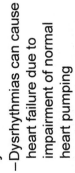

- Classified by abnormalities of rate or rhythm
  - Dysrhythmias can cause heart failure due to impairment of normal heart pumping
    - Hypotension, dizziness, chest pain, feeling of impending doom

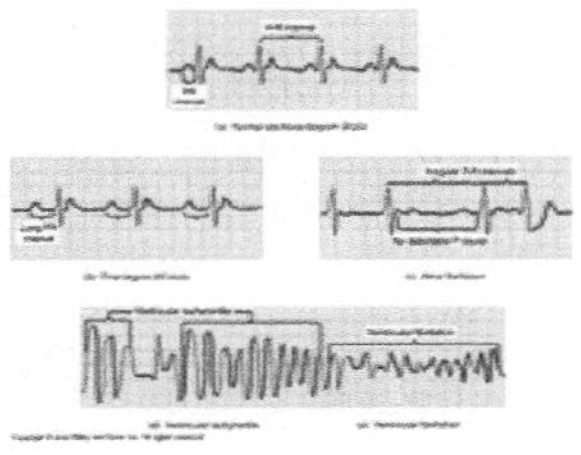

23-12

Dysrhythmias

- **Normal Sinus Rhythm (NSR)**
  - 1. SA node and atrial depolarization (P wave)
  - 2. Pause (PR interval)
  - 3. AV node then ventricular depolarization (QRS)
  - T wave
- **Tachycardia**
  - >100 bpm
- **Bradycardia**
  - <50 bpm

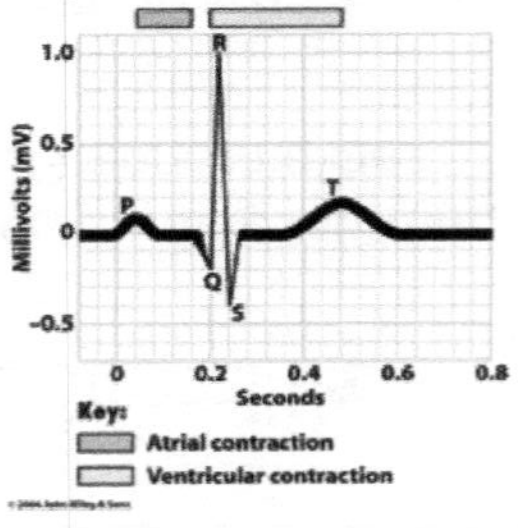

Millivolts (mV)
1.0
0.5
0
-0.5
P
R
Q
S
T
0
0.2
0.4
0.6
0.8
Seconds
Key:
Atrial contraction
Ventricular contraction

23-12

Dysrhythmias

- Atrial fibrillation / atrial flutter
  - Decreased ventricular filling leads to 20% drop in cardiac output
  - Blood clot embolisms are a risk
  - Treated by cardioversion or with "watchful waiting"

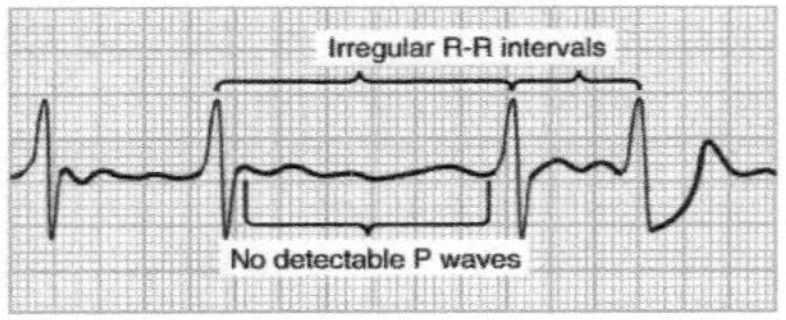

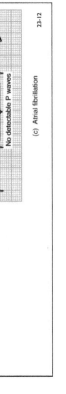

Irregular R-R intervals
No detectable P waves

(c) Atrial fibrillation

23-12

Dysrhythmias

- **Ventricular Tachycardia (VT)**
  - Refers to any rhythm faster than 100 b/m arising distal from the AV bundle
  - Usually hemodynamically unstable and required immediate treatment (usually cardioversion) – electrical pulse to restart ♡ to a normal rythm

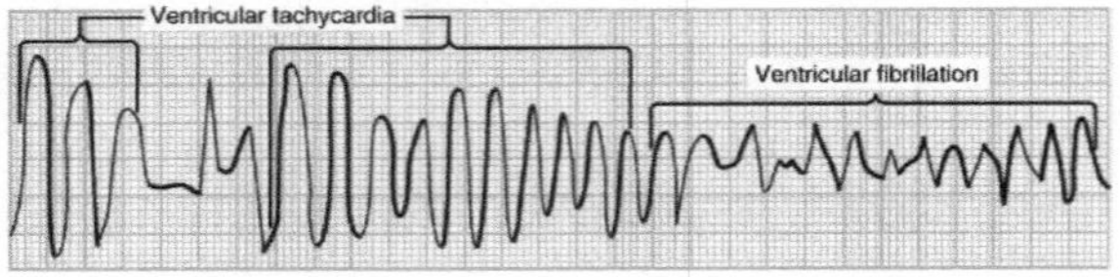

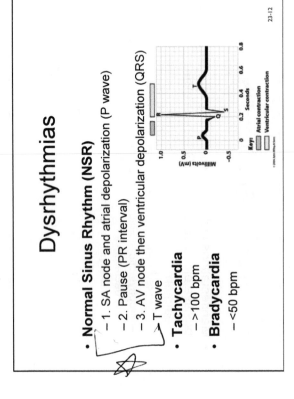

Ventricular tachycardia
Ventricular fibrillation

(d) Ventricular tachycardia (e) Ventricular fibrillation

23-12

Heart Failure

- A dysfunction of cardiac muscle contractility that results in inadequate cardiac output and hypoperfusion of tissues
- Failure of ventricle is failure of the pump
- Left sided (most common)
  - *congestive heart failure* (CHF)
- Right sided (less common)
  - *cor pulmonale*

23-13

Heart Failure

Congestive (Left-Sided) Heart Failure

- Failure of the left ventricle leads to disorders of the lungs and pulmonary vessels
- Fatigue
- Dyspnea
- Pulmonary edema, orthopnea, and a cough with frothy, blood-tinged discharge
- Cyanosis
- Rales (crackles)

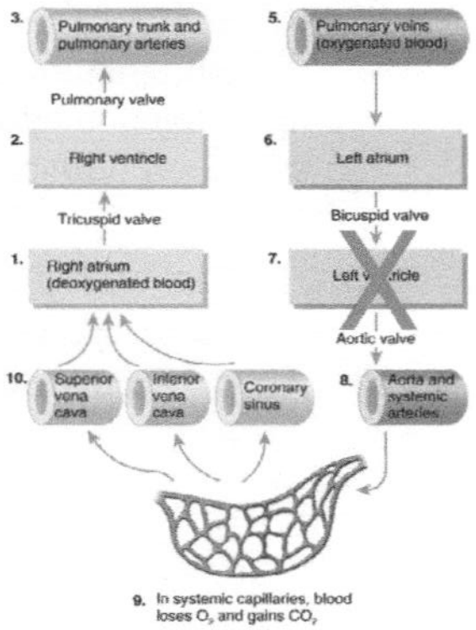
3. Pulmonary trunk and pulmonary arteries
Pulmonary valve
2. Right ventricle
Tricuspid valve
1. Right atrium (deoxygenated blood)
10. Superior vena cava
Inferior vena cava
Coronary sinus
5. Pulmonary veins (oxygenated blood)
6. Left atrium
Bicuspid valve
7. Left ventricle
Aortic valve
8. Aorta and systemic arteries
9. In systemic capillaries, blood loses O_2 and gains CO_2

(b) Diagram of blood flow

23-13

Heart Failure

Cor Pulmonale (Right-Sided Heart Failure)

- Cor pulmonale is often the result of pulmonary diseases causing pulmonary hypertension
- Blood likes to flow from higher pressure to low pressure, not the other way around

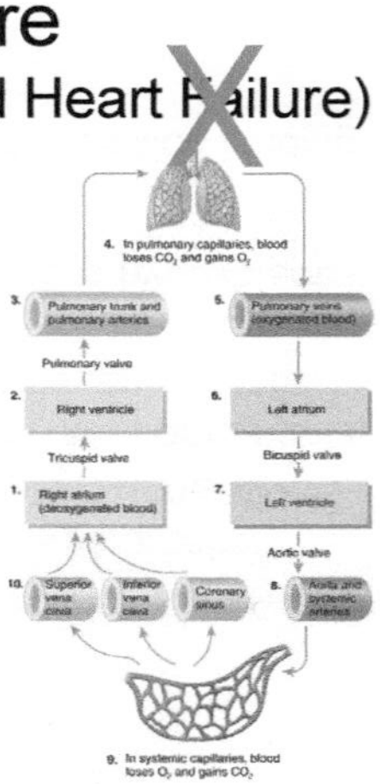

(b) Diagram of blood flow

23-13

Heart Failure

Cor Pulmonale (Right-Sided Heart Failure)

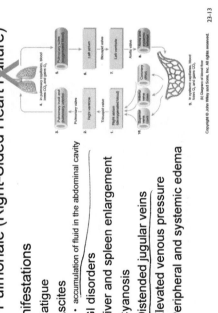

- Manifestations
  - Fatigue
  - Ascites
    - accumulation of fluid in the abdominal cavity
  - GI disorders
  - Liver and spleen enlargement
  - Cyanosis
  - Distended jugular veins
  - Elevated venous pressure
  - Peripheral and systemic edema

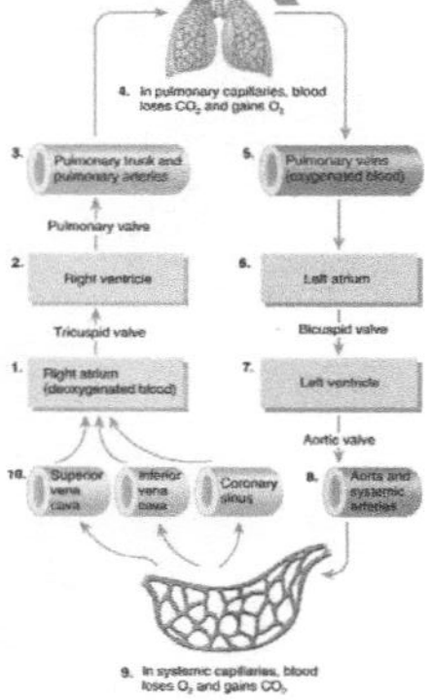

(b) Diagram of blood flow

23-13

Shock, Multiple Organ Dysfunction Syndrome (MODS)

hypovolemia - ↓ blood volume circulating the body.

Hypovolemic Shock
Normal Homeostatic Mechanisms

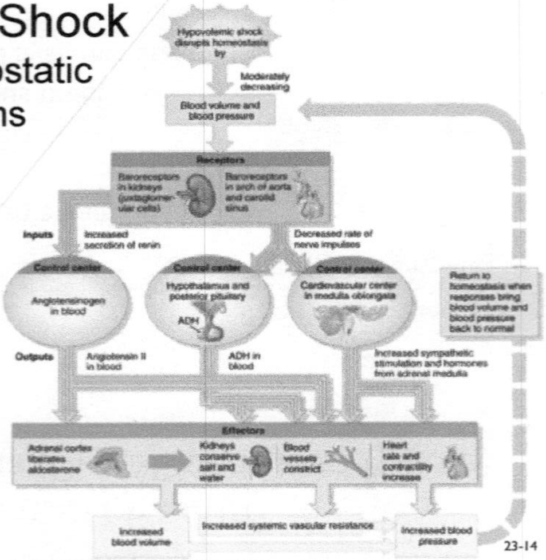

Hypovolemic shock disrupts homeostasis by
Moderately decreasing
Blood volume and blood pressure
Receptors
Baroreceptors in kidneys (juxtaglomerular cells)
Baroreceptors in arch of aorta and carotid sinus
Inputs
Increased secretion of renin
Decreased rate of nerve impulses
Control center
Angiotensinogen in blood
Control center
Hypothalamus and posterior pituitary
ADH
Control center
Cardiovascular center in medulla oblongata
Return to homeostasis when responses bring blood volume and blood pressure back to normal
Outputs
Angiotensin II in blood
ADH in blood
Increased sympathetic stimulation and hormones from adrenal medulla
Effectors
Adrenal cortex liberates aldosterone
Kidneys conserve salt and water
Blood vessels constrict
Heart rate and contractility increase
Increased blood volume
Increased systemic vascular resistance
Increased blood pressure

23-14

Shock

- Anything that causes hypoperfusion of the vital organs causes shock, and will **progress to death unless there is compensation** for the abnormalities.
- General symptoms: "feel sick", weak, cold, hot, nauseated, dizzy, confused, thirsty, and short of breath
- Clinical signs: decreased blood pressure, decreased cardiac output, and decreased urinary output

23-14

Types of Shock

- **Cardiogenic Shock**
  - Pure and simple, the heart isn't working
    - Ischemia, MI, myocardial or pericardial infections, dysrhythmias are all causes
- **Hypovolemic Shock**
  - Is insufficient intravascular fluid volume from loss of whole blood, blood plasma, interstitial fluid, or fluid sequestration outside the arterial vasculature

23-14

Types of Shock

- **Neurogenic (or Vasogenic) Shock** slack.
  - widespread vasodilation from parasympathetic overstimulation and sympathetic understimulation.
  - Causes include trauma to the spinal cord or medulla, depressive drugs, anesthetic agents, and severe emotional stress and pain.
  - Persistent vasodilation causing relative hypovolemia
- **Anaphylactic shock**
  - a widespread type I hypersensitivity reaction leading to vasodilation
    - Also causing relative hypovolemia

23-14

Types of Shock

- **Septic shock**
  - Bacteremia
  - **Endotoxins and exotoxins** cause the host to initiate a severe inflammatory process leading to widespread vasodilation and vascular collapse
    - Also causing relative hypovolemia

23-14

Multiple Organ Dysfunction Syndrome

- Inflammatory responses are triggered damaging the vascular endothelium
- Endothelium leaks fluid and protein into interstitial space resulting in hypotension and hypoperfusion
- Damaged endothelium activates platelets and tissue thromboplastin leading to systemic microvasculature coagulation that may lead to DIC
- Complement, coagulation, and kinin systems are activated leading to a hyperinflammatory and hypercoagulative state
  - Interstitial edema, cardiovascular instability, endothelial damage, and clotting abnormalities
- Decreased O_2 delivery to tissues
- Hypermetabolism starts as a compensatory mechanism but leads to consumption of needed O_2 to cells

Multiple Organ Dysfunction Syndrome

- Most common cause of mortality in intensive care units
- Progressive dysfunction of two or more organ systems resulting from an uncontrolled inflammatory response to a severe illness or injury.
- Most common cause is sepsis and septic shock
- Other triggers include severe trauma, burns, acute pancreatitis, obstetric complications, major surgery, circulatory shock, some drugs, and gangrenous or necrotic tissue

23-15

Multiple Organ Dysfunction

- Clinical Manifestations: Often a predictable clinical pattern
- Initial event
  - After inciting event, patient develops a low-grade fever, tachycardia, dyspnea, altered mental status, and hyperdynamic and hypermetabolic states.
  - Lung often first organ to fail resulting in tachypnea, pulmonary edema with crackles and hypoxemia
- 7-10 days
  - Beginning of liver and renal failure
    - Jaundice, abdominal distention, hepatic encephalopathy
    - Oliguria, uremia, and edema

23-15

Multiple Organ Dysfunction

- 14-24 days
  - Liver and renal failure progresses
  - GI system involvement with damage to the gut mucosa
    - Bacteria and toxins move into the portal and systemic systems
- Hematologic and myocardial failure follow
- Death may occur from 14 days to several weeks after inciting event
- **Mortality 30% to 100%**

23-15

Unit 6
Chapter 31
Alterations of Cardiac Function in Children

Fetal Circulation

- The developing fetus has special circulatory requirements because their lungs, kidneys and digestive tract are non-functional
- The fetus derives its oxygen and nutrients and eliminates wastes through the maternal blood supply by way of the placenta
- Normally, there is no maternal/fetal mixing
- The fetus is dependant on capillary exchange

24-1

Fetal Circulation

- Placenta
- Umbilical vein
- *Ductus venosus* between umbilical vein and inferior vena cava (bypasses the liver)
- Inferior vena cava to heart
  - *Foramen ovale* (bypasses the lungs)
  - *Ductus arteriosus* (bypasses the lungs)
- Aorta
- Umbilical arteries

24-1

Fetal Circulation

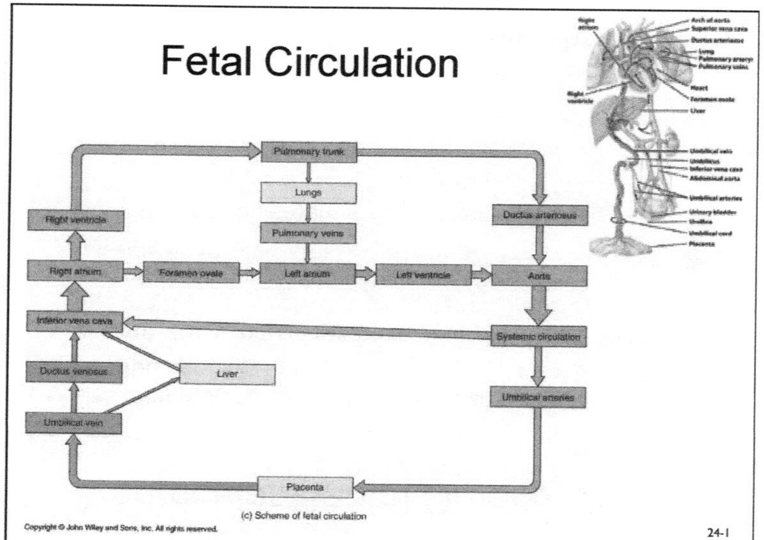

Pulmonary trunk
Lungs
Pulmonary veins
Right ventricle
Ductus arteriosus
Right atrium
Foramen ovale
Left atrium
Left ventricle
Aorta
Inferior vena cava
Systemic circulation
Ductus venosus
Liver
Umbilical arteries
Umbilical vein
Placenta

(c) Scheme of fetal circulation

24-1

Fetal vs Adult Circulation

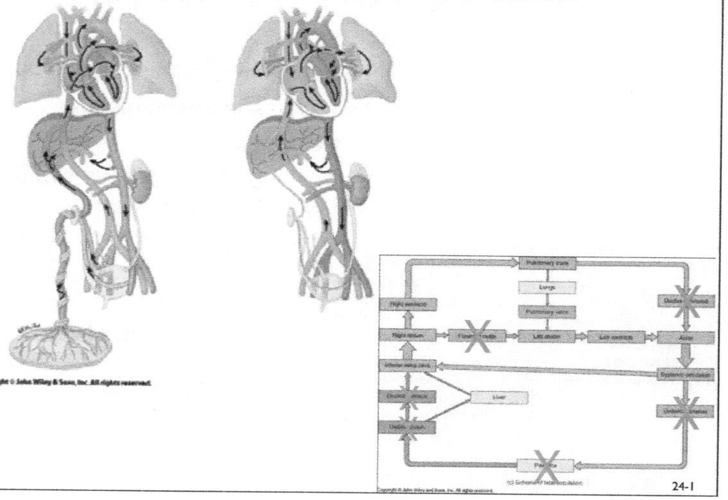

24-1

Congenital Heart Defects

- Numerous causes
- The most critical time is embryonic week 3 to week 8 (timed from conception)
- Right-to-left shunts result in hypoxia and cyanosis
- Left-to-right shunts result in overload of pulmonary hypertension and right heart failure

24-1

Patent Ductus Arteriosus

- Defined as failure of the ductus arteriosus to close within the first few weeks of life
- This increases the pressure in the pulmonary truck and overworks the ventricles
- Blood flows from the aorta (higher pressure) to lower pressure pulmonary artery ("left-to-right shunt")
- Patients present with a murmur and pulmonary vascular obstructive disease

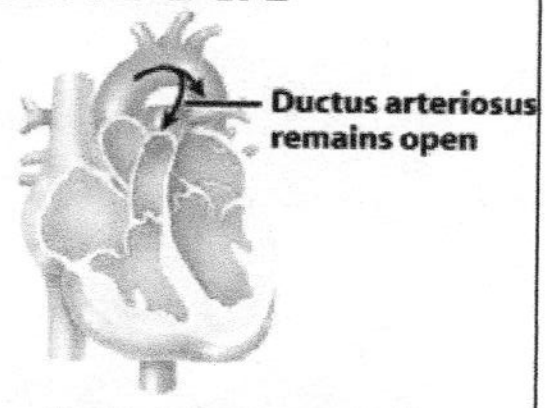

Ductus arteriosus remains open

Patent ductus arteriosus

R ♡ failure. + pulmoney hypertension.

24-1

Atrial Septal Defect (ASD)

- Failure of the interatrial septum to properly form
- Incidence 1/4000
- Left-to-right shunt
  - –Cardiomegaly and pulmonary vascular congestion will be a result

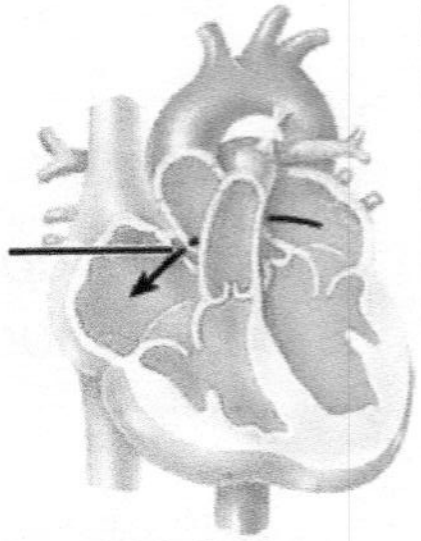

Atrial septal defect

24-1

Patent Foramen Ovale (PFO)

- In about 27% of people, the foramen ovale fails to close
- Not a congenital heart defect, because the foramen ovale is a normal structure
- Usually asymptomatic

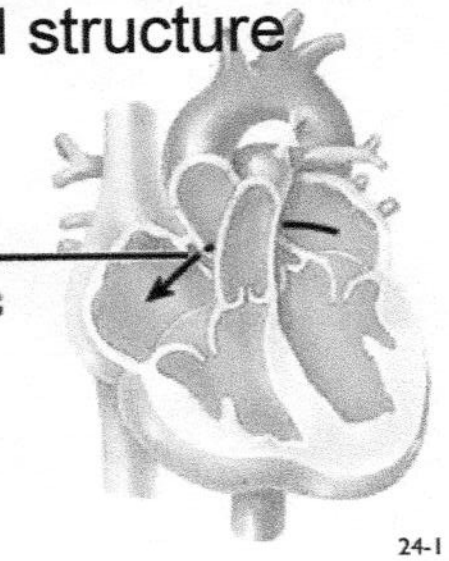
Foramen ovale fails to close

24-1

Ventricular Septal Defect (VSD)

- Defect in the intraventricular septum
- Most common type of congenital heart defect (3/1000 people)
- In large VSDs, pressures become equal, blood flows into the right ventricle due to systemic pressures, and large amounts of blood flow into the pulmonary vessels
- Contributes to enlargement of the left ventricle

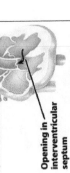

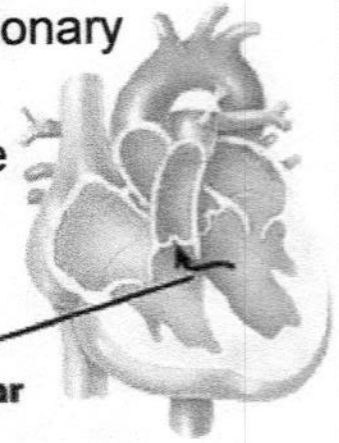
Opening in interventricular septum

Ventricular septal defect

24-1

Tetralogy of Fallot

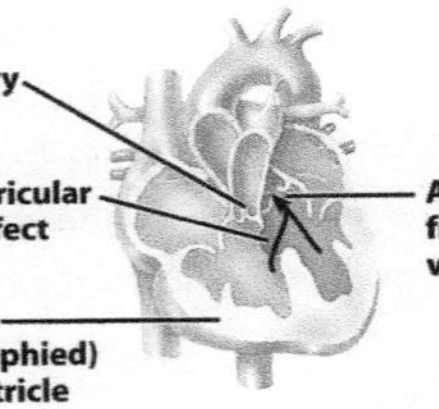
Stenosed pulmonary valve
Interventricular septal defect
Enlarged (hypertrophied) right ventricle
Aorta emerges from both ventricles

Tetralogy of Fallot

1. Pulmonary valve stenosis
   - blocks normal blood flow to lungs
2. Overriding aorta
   - emerges from both ventricles
3. Ventricular septal defect
4. Right ventricular hypertrophy

- The patient is often kept alive only because of mixing of blood in what turns out to be a common ventricle

24-2

Coarctation of the Aorta

- Congenital malformation causing narrowing of the aorta
- If the defect occurs near the ductus arteriosus, it will cause increased blood flow to the head and upper extremities and a decrease blood flow in the lower extremities
- Left heart failure is a potential result

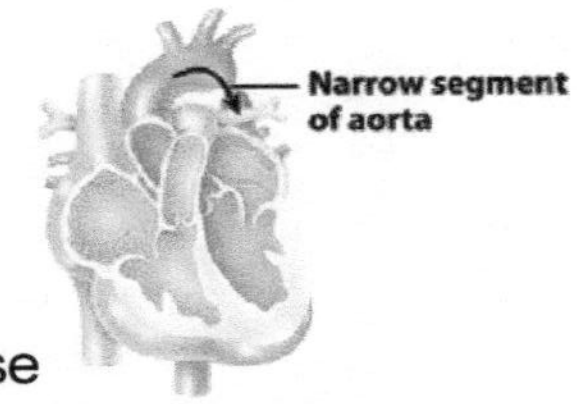
Narrow segment of aorta

Coarctation of the aorta

24-2

Transposition of the Great Vessels

- Transposition is a switch between the pulmonary and the systemic circulation
  - aorta emerges from the right ventricle
  - pulmonary artery emerges from the left ventricle
- Two completely separate pump systems where the blood never mixes
  - right side pumps blood from body back to body
  - left side pumps blood from lungs back to lungs
- Obviously, without septal defects to allow some mixing of blood, this would be incompatible with life

24-2

UNIT 7

Study Guide Objectives – Introductory Pathophysiology (HTHS 2230)

Unit 7

Chapter 26 – Alterations of Pulmonary Function

1. Explain the signs of pulmonary disease: dyspnea, cough, abnormal sputum, hemoptysis, abnormal breathing patterns, hypo/hyperventilation, cyanosis, clubbing and pain. (pp. 678-680)

2. Compare and contrast hypercapnia and hypoxemia. Define, and give examples of, ventilation/perfusion mismatch. (pp. 680-681)

3. Explain the pathophysiology of pneumothorax and atelectasis. (pp. 682-684, 685)

4. Give examples of the different forms of pleural effusion: transudative effusion, exudative effusion, empyema and hemothorax. (p. 684)

5. Classify diseases of the bronchial tree: bronchiectasis and bronchiolitis. (pp. 685-686)

6. List the causes of, and the steps that lead to, pulmonary edema. (pp. 686-687)

7. Explain the pathophysiology of acute respiratory distress syndrome. (pp. 687-689)

8. Discuss the pathophysiology of asthma. (pp. 689-691)

9. Give the key features and etiology of chronic obstructive pulmonary disease. (pp. 691-694)

10. Name the common respiratory tract infections and their signs, symptoms, and causes: pneumonia, tuberculosis, and bronchitis. (pp. 694-698)

11. Classify the pulmonary vascular diseases: pulmonary embolism, pulmonary artery hypertension, and cor pulmonale. (pp. 698-700)

Chapter 28 – Structure and Function of the Renal and Urologic Systems

1. State the principles of kidney function that underlie urinalysis. Explain how proteinuria, blood urea nitrogen, creatinine and glomerular filtration rate are used to diagnose kidney dysfunction. (pp. 736-737)

Chapter 29 – Alterations of Renal and Urinary Tract Function

1. Classify the urinary tract obstructions: upper and lower. Explain the pathophysiology of kidney stones. (pp. 741-747)
2. Compare and contrast clinical features of infections in the urinary system (cystitis and pyelonephritis). (pp. 747-750)
3. Classify and explain the pathophysiology of glomerulonephritis. (pp. 750-753)
4. Explain the pathophysiology of nephrotic syndrome. (pp. 753-754)
5. Explain the pathophysiology of acute renal failure to include causes, phases of urinary output, and diagnostic tests. (pp. 754-756)
6. Describe the pathophysiology and treatment of chronic kidney disease. (pp. 756-758; 760-761)
7. Name the ways in which kidney failure impacts other organ systems. (pp. 758-760)

Chapter 34 – Alterations of Digestive Function

1. Name the common signs and general causes of gastrointestinal dysfunction: anorexia, nausea, vomiting, retching, constipation, diarrhea, and gastrointestinal bleeding. Name the causes of the symptom of abdominal pain. (pp. 894-898)

2. Classify the disorders of gastrointestinal mobility: dysphagia, gastroesophageal reflux disease, hiatal hernia, pyloric obstruction, intestinal obstruction, and ileus. (pp. 898-903)

3. Explain the causes, signs and symptoms of gastritis. (p. 903)

4. Describe the pathophysiology of peptic ulcer disease. Classify peptic ulcer disease by location, causes, and treatments. (pp. 903-907)

5. Describe the causes and treatments for the common malabsorption syndromes resulting from pancreatic insufficiency, lactase deficiency and bile salt deficiency. (pp. 907-908)

6. Compare and contrast the inflammatory bowel diseases: ulcerative colitis and Crohn disease. (pp. 908-910)

7. State the pathophysiologic features of gluten-sensitive enteropathy (celiac disease). (Chapter 35, pp. 944-946)

8. Name the features of diverticular disease, and its treatments. (p. 910)

9. Explain the pathophysiology of appendicitis. (p. 910)

10. Compare and contrast the nutritional disorders: obesity, anorexia nervosa, bulimia nervosa, and starvation. (pp. 912-915)

11. State the clinical features and causes of liver disorders: portal hypertension, cirrhosis, hepatic encephalopathy, and jaundice. (pp. 915-916)

12. Discuss the causes of ascites. (pp. 916-917)

13. Compare and contrast the viral hepatides (A-C). (pp. 919-921)

14. Name common disorders of the gallbladder: cholelithiasis and cholecystitis. (pp. 923-924)

15. State the causes and signs of pancreatitis. (pp. 924-925)

Unit 7
Chapter 26
Alterations of Pulmonary Function

Pulmonary Disease: Signs and Symptoms

- **Dyspnea** Difficulty breathing
  - Also known as shortness of breath (SOB) ! not the expletive! :)
  - Breathlessness, air hunger, labored breathing
  - Caused by increased airway resistance
  - Symptom: breathing is uncomfortable
  - Signs: flared nostrils and use of accessory muscles

26-1

Pulmonary Disease: Signs and Symptoms

- **Coughing**
  - A protective reflex that cleans airways with an explosive expiration to remove foreign particles.
  - Should it be suppressed?

    only if it's nasty :(

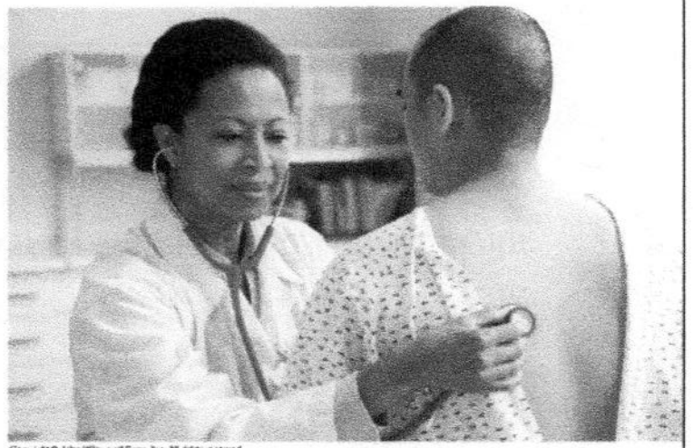
Copyright © John Wiley and Sons, Inc. All rights reserved.

26-1

Pulmonary Disease: Signs and Symptoms

- **Abnormal sputum**
  - Sputum is mucus mixed with substances in lower respiratory tract (the passengers on the **mucociliary escalator**)
  - Changes (color, consistency, odor, and amount) provide information about a disease and disease progression

26-1

Pulmonary Disease: Signs and Symptoms

- blood **Hemoptysis**
  - –Coughing up blood or bloody secretions
    - Usually bright red (mixing air and red blood cells keeps them oxygenated)
    - Localized infection or inflammation has damaged the bronchi or alveolar-capillary membrane

26-1

Brainstem Control of Respiration

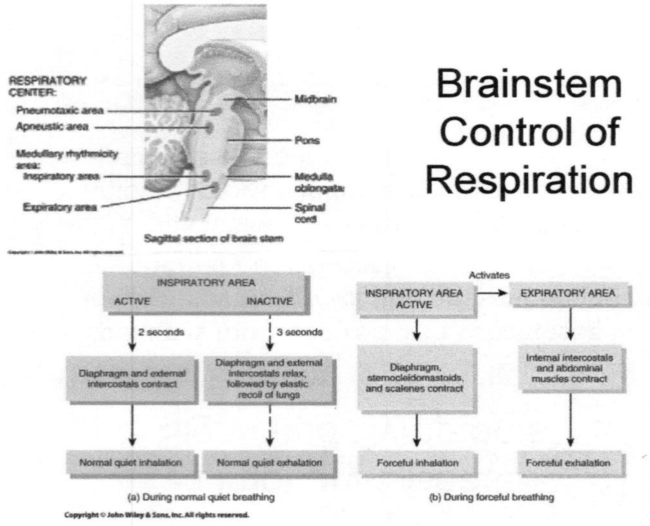

RESPIRATORY CENTER:
Pneumotaxic area
Apneustic area
Medullary rhythmicity area:
Inspiratory area
Expiratory area
Midbrain
Pons
Medulla oblongata
Spinal cord
Sagittal section of brain stem
INSPIRATORY AREA
ACTIVE
INACTIVE
2 seconds
3 seconds
Diaphragm and external intercostals contract
Diaphragm and external intercostals relax, followed by elastic recoil of lungs
Normal quiet inhalation
Normal quiet exhalation
(a) During normal quiet breathing
Activates
INSPIRATORY AREA ACTIVE
EXPIRATORY AREA
Diaphragm, sternocleidomastoids, and scalenes contract
Internal intercostals and abdominal muscles contract
Forceful inhalation
Forceful exhalation
(b) During forceful breathing
Copyright © John Wiley & Sons, Inc. All rights reserved.

26-1

Chemoreceptor Reflex

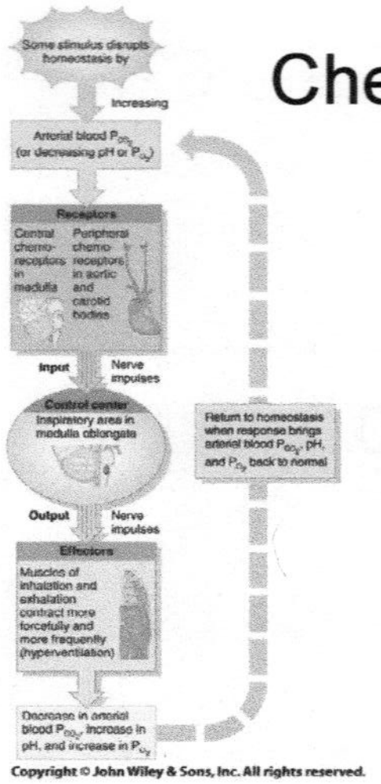

Some stimulus disrupts homeostasis by
Increasing
Arterial blood P_{CO_2} (or decreasing pH or P_{O_2})
Receptors
Central chemoreceptors in medulla
Peripheral chemoreceptors in aortic and carotid bodies
Input
Nerve impulses
Control center
Inspiratory area in medulla oblongata
Output
Nerve impulses
Effectors
Muscles of inhalation and exhalation contract more forcefully and more frequently (hyperventilation)
Decrease in arterial blood P_{CO_2}, increase in pH, and increase in P_{O_2}
Return to homeostasis when response brings arterial blood P_{CO_2}, pH, and P_{O_2} back to normal
Copyright © John Wiley & Sons, Inc. All rights reserved.

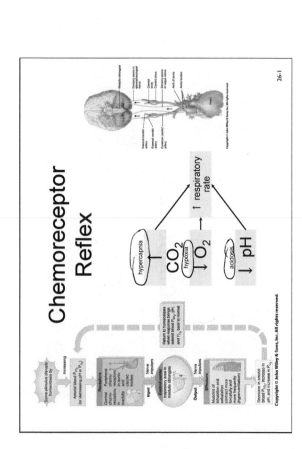

hypercapnia
↑ CO_2
hypoxia
↓ O_2 → ↑ respiratory rate
acidosis
↓ pH

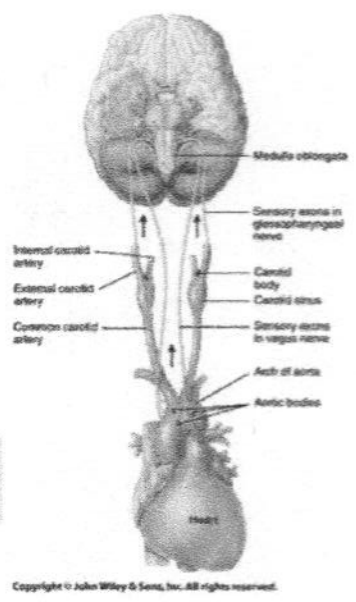

26-1

Kussmaul Respiration
(Hyperpnea) excess breathing

- Decrease in blood pH (increase in plasma ↑ $[H^+]$) causes hyperventilation
- Results in:
  - –increased respiratory rate
  - –large increase in tidal volume
  - –no expiratory pause

26-1

Cheyne-Stokes Respiration

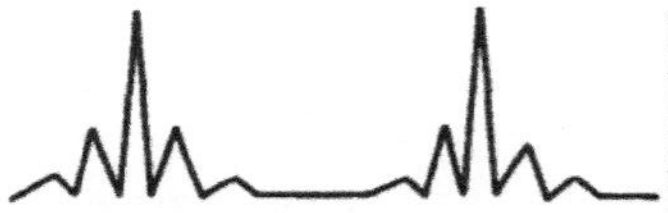

Cherniak NS & Longobardo GS. Abnormalities in respiratory rhythm. In: *Handbook of Physiology* 2011.

- Breathing fluctuates
  - periods of apnea or hypopnea alternating with periods of hyperpnea
- Occurs in about half of patients with congestive heart failure or neurological disease including stroke
- More common during sleep

26-I

Hypoventilation Hyperventilation

- **Hypoventilation**: alveolar gas exchange insufficient for metabolic demands
  - ↑ P_{CO2}
  - respiratory acidosis
- **Hyperventilation**: alveolar gas exchange greater than metabolic demands
  - ↓ P_{CO2} ↑ H^+ ions?
  - respiratory alkalosis
  - causes: anxiety, head injury, pain, ↓ P_{O2}

26-I

Pulmonary Disease: Signs and Symptoms

- **Cyanosis**
  - Bluish discoloration of mucous membranes and the skin caused by increased amounts of deoxygenated hemoglobin
    - O_2 saturation is a measure of how many oxygen binding sites on hemoglobin are occupied
    - normal:
      - O_2 saturation 97-99% in arterial blood
      - O_2 saturation 75% in venous blood
    - cyanosis
      - O_2 saturation < 85% in arterial blood

26-I

Pulmonary Disease: Signs and Symptoms Clubbing

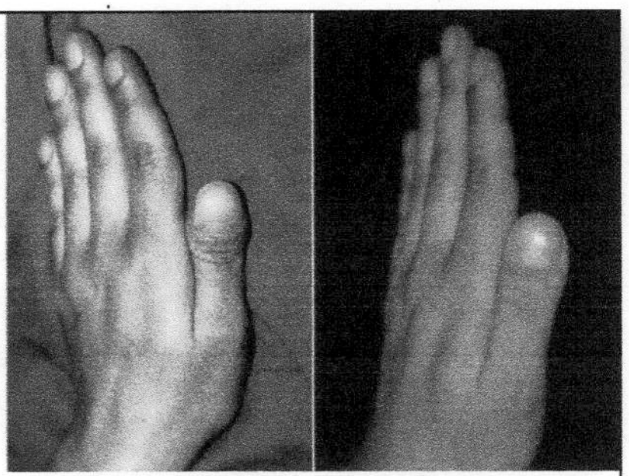

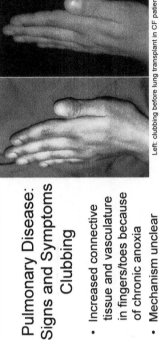

Left: clubbing before lung transplant in CF patient
Right: after transplant, clubbing gone
Augarten A *et al.*, *Pediatr Pulmonol* **34**:378, 2002.

- Increased connective tissue and vasculature in fingers/toes because of chronic anoxia
- Mechanism unclear
  - probably due to some sort of chemical signaling
  - prostaglandins, ferritin, bradykinin, estrogen, platelet-derived growth factor, hepatocyte growth factor and growth hormone have all been suggested

26-I

Pulmonary Disease: Signs and Symptoms

- **Pleuritic Pain**: Sharp, stabbing pain associated with breathing
  - From disorders affecting the pleurae, airways, and chest wall

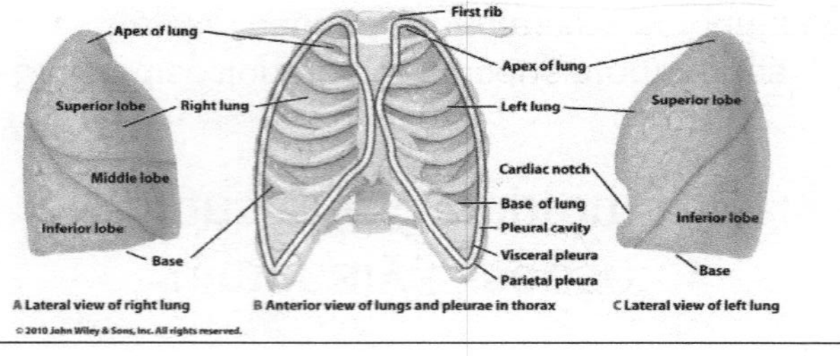

Apex of lung
Superior lobe
Right lung
Middle lobe
Inferior lobe
Base
First rib
Apex of lung
Left lung
Cardiac notch
Base of lung
Pleural cavity
Visceral pleura
Parietal pleura
Superior lobe
Inferior lobe
Base

A Lateral view of right lung B Anterior view of lungs and pleurae in thorax C Lateral view of left lung

26-1

Ventilation-Perfusion Coupling

- **Pulmonary ventilation** ($\dot{V}$): amount of air (in liters) entering lungs per minute
  - $\dot{V}_A$: amount of air (in liters) entering alveoli per minute
- **Perfusion** ($\dot{Q}$): amount of blood that flows through the lung capillaries each minute
- Ventilation-perfusion coupling: The matching of pulmonary blood flow to oxygen
  - under hypoxic conditions, pulmonary blood vessels constrict
  - forces or shunts blood to areas of higher oxygen

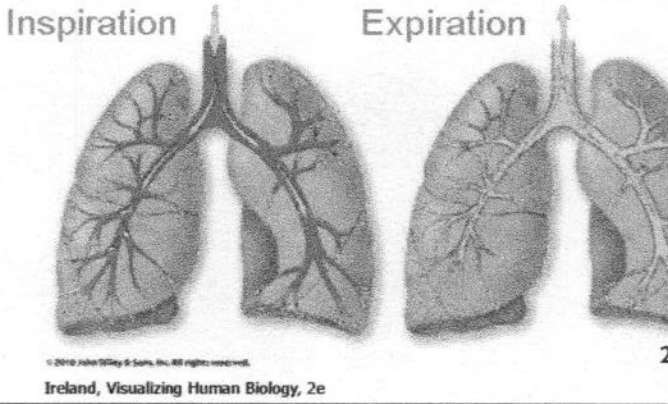

Inspiration
Expiration

Ireland, Visualizing Human Biology, 2e

26-2

Ventilation-Perfusion Coupling

- In healthy individuals:
  - $\dot{V}_A$ = 4.5 L/min
  - $\dot{Q}$ = 5.0 L/min
- Ideally, the ventilation/perfusion ratio ($\dot{V}_A/\dot{Q}$) is about 1
- If no air enters lungs, $\dot{V}_A/\dot{Q}$ = zero
  - blood flows but no gas exchange takes place
- If air enters lungs but blood does not flow, $\dot{V}_A/\dot{Q} = \infty$
  - for example, if blood clot lodges in lung (**pulmonary embolism**)
  - blood is not oxygenated and cannot release waste CO_2

26-2

Hypercapnia

Blood [CO_2] too high

- Depression of respiratory center by drugs
- Diseases of the medulla
  - respiratory centers of brainstem affected by infection or trauma
- Problem with phrenic nerve innervation
  - polio, amyotrophic lateral sclerosis, spinal cord injury
- Diseases of the neuromuscular junction
  - myasthenia gravis, muscular dystrophy
- Thoracic cage trauma or congenital deformity
- Large airway obstruction
  - tumors, apnea
- Physiologic dead space
  - emphysema

26-2

↓ O_2 in blood

Hypoxemia

Blood $[O_2]$ too low

- Problem with oxygen delivery to alveoli
  - reduced P_{O2}
  - reduced ventilation of alveoli ($\dot{V}_A$)
- Problem with oxygen moving across the alveolar-capillary membrane
  - $\dot{V}_A/\dot{Q}$ mismatch
  - blockage in alveolar-capillary (A-C) membrane
- Problem with blood arriving to be oxygenated

26-2

Hypoxemia

Pathophysiology which makes blood $[O_2]$ too low

- Problem with oxygen delivery to alveoli
  - reduced P_{O2}: high altitude, low O_2 content in air, suffocation (pollution)
  - reduced ventilation of alveoli ($\dot{V}_A$): brain damage, chest wall restriction, airway obstruction, chronic obstructive pulmonary disease (emphysema, chronic asthma)
- Problem with oxygen moving across the alveolar-capillary membrane
  - $\dot{V}_A/\dot{Q}$ mismatch: asthma, bronchitis, pneumonia, acute respiratory distress syndrome, atelectasis, pulmonary embolism
  - blockage in A-C membrane: edema, fibrosis, emphysema
- Problem with blood arriving to be oxygenated
  - cardiac defects, arteriovenous malformations in lung

26-2

lung collapse.

Pneumothorax

- If air can leak into the pleural cavity, then thoracic cavity cannot develop a pressure difference
- No pressure difference, and surface tension (even with surfactant) takes over and causes the delicate alveolar-capillary membrane to collapse in on itself
- When this happens all over the lung, the entire lung collapses and **pneumothorax** results
- This is a special case of the more general term **atelectasis**, any abnormal structure in the alveoli of the lung

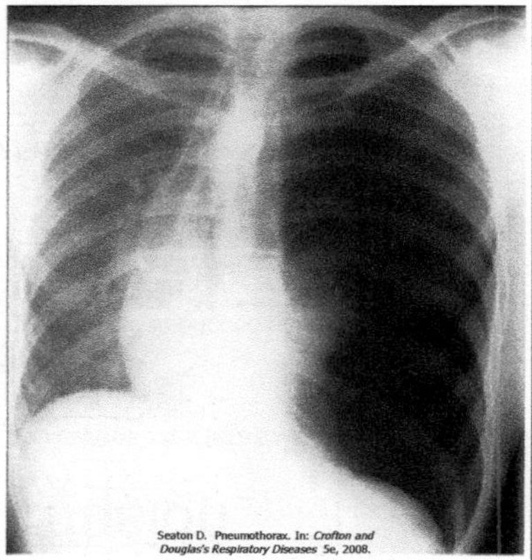

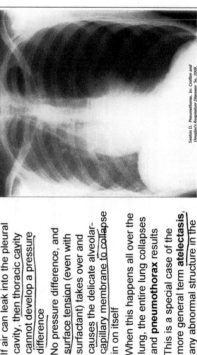

Seaton D. Pneumothorax. In: *Crofton and Douglas's Respiratory Diseases* 5e, 2008.

26-3

Atelectasis

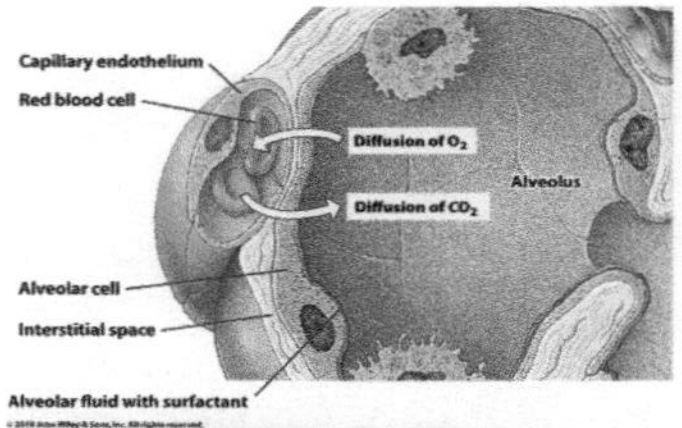

Capillary endothelium
Red blood cell
Diffusion of O_2
Diffusion of CO_2
Alveolus
Alveolar cell
Interstitial space
Alveolar fluid with surfactant

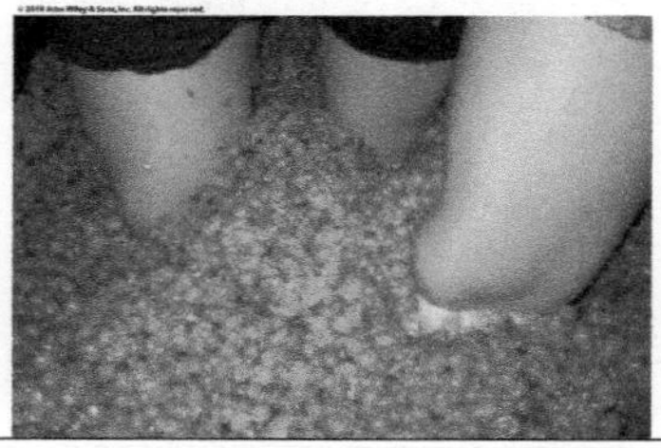

- **Atelectasis** is any abnormal structure in the alveoli
- If the alveoli resemble a bunch of grapes, then atelectasis is what happens when the grapes are smashed
- External respiration depends critically on the normal structure of alveoli
- Obviously, atelectasis interferes with gas exchange

26-3

Pleural Effusion

Swollen lung.

- Any abnormal or excess liquid in the alveoli interferes with external respiration → dyspnea
- **Transudative effusion**
  - increase in hydrostatic pressure or decrease in oncotic pressure in capillary (i.e. Starling forces that promote edema)
  - this is the mechanism of **pulmonary edema** in, for example, congestive heart failure
- **Exudative effusion**
  - increase in capillary permeability that allows blood cells and/or plasma proteins to leak into alveoli
  - **Empyema**
    - pus (i.e. neutrophils and dead invaders)
  - **Hemothorax**
    - blood
  - **Chylothorax**
    - chyle (lymph and fats)

26-4

Bronchiectasis

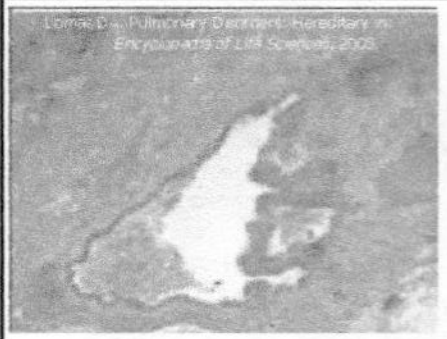

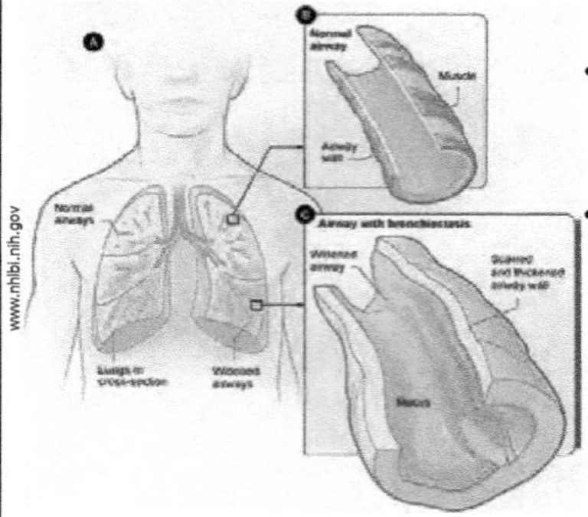
Normal airway
Muscle
Airway wall
Airway with bronchiectasis
Widened airway
Scarred and thickened airway wall
Mucus
Normal airways
Lungs in cross-section
Widened airways

www.nhlbi.nih.gov

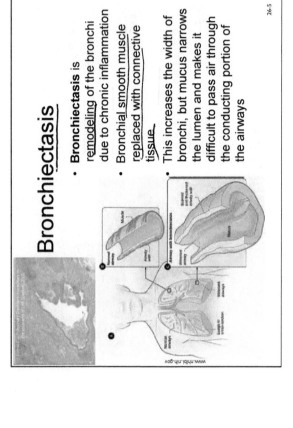

- **Bronchiectasis** is remodeling of the bronchi due to chronic inflammation
- Bronchial smooth muscle replaced with connective tissue
- This increases the width of bronchi, but mucus narrows the lumen and makes it difficult to pass air through the conducting portion of the airways

26-5

Bronchiectasis in Cystic Fibrosis

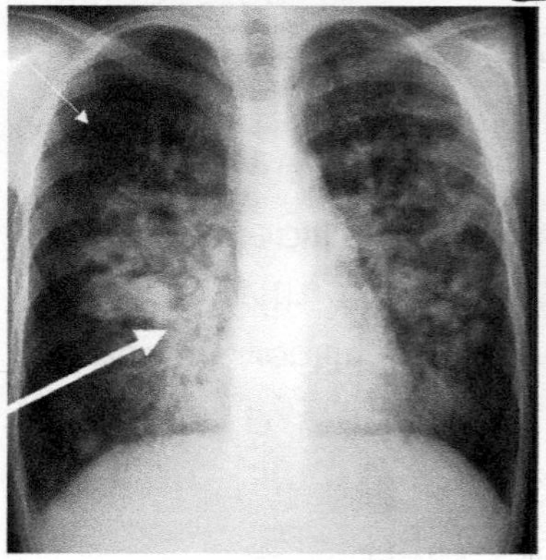

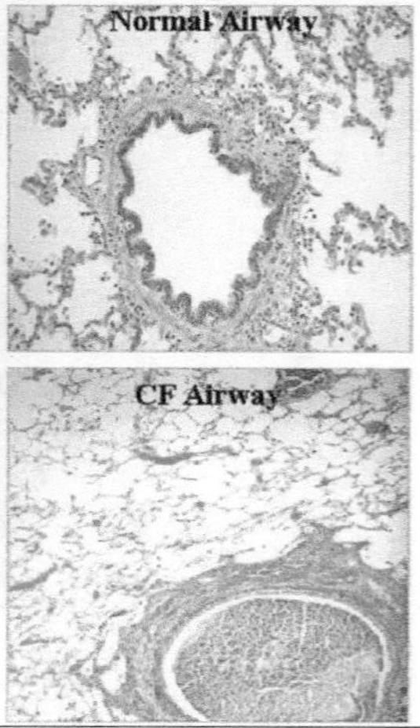
Normal Airway
CF Airway

Davies JC *et al.* Cystic Fibrosis in: *Encyclopedia of Life Sciences*, 2005.

26-5

Bronchiolitis

- Bronchiolitis is chronic inflammation of the bronchioles
- Like bronchiectasis, fibrous connective tissue replaces functional tissue (such as smooth muscle)
- Narrowing of bronchiole lumen

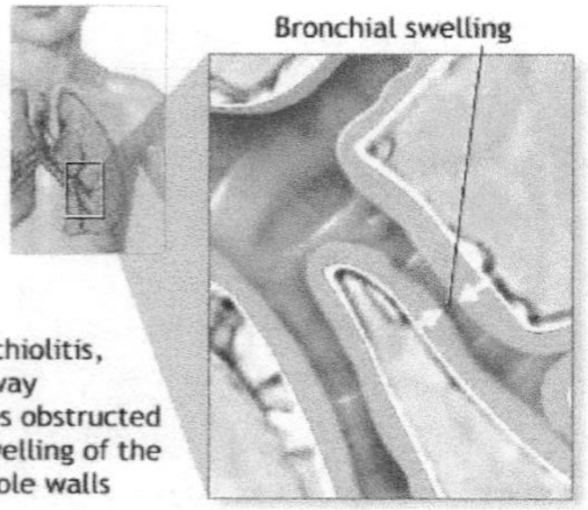
Bronchial swelling

In bronchiolitis, the airway becomes obstructed from swelling of the bronchiole walls

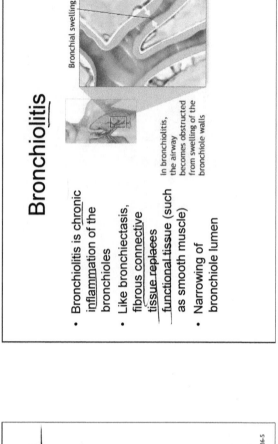

Medline Plus, www.nlmi.nih.gov

26-5

Pulmonary Edema

Heart disease
Valvular dysfunction
Coronary artery disease
Left ventricular dysfunction

↓

Increased pressure in left atrium

↓

Increased pulmonary capillary hydrostatic pressure

↓

Pulmonary edema

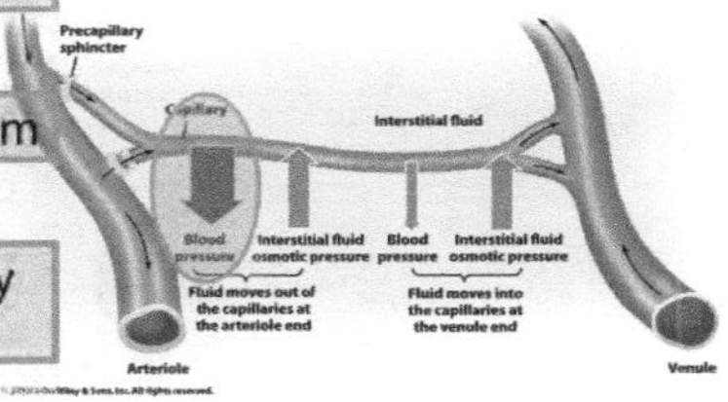

Precapillary sphincter
Capillary
Interstitial fluid
Blood pressure
Interstitial fluid osmotic pressure
Blood pressure
Interstitial fluid osmotic pressure
Fluid moves out of the capillaries at the arteriole end
Fluid moves into the capillaries at the venule end
Arteriole
Venule

26-6

Pulmonary Edema

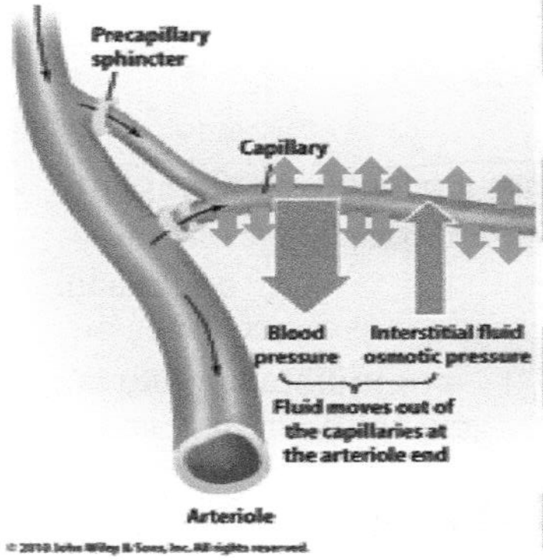

Precapillary sphincter
Capillary
Blood pressure
Interstitial fluid osmotic pressure
Fluid moves out of the capillaries at the arteriole end
Arteriole
© 2010 John Wiley & Sons, Inc. All rights reserved.

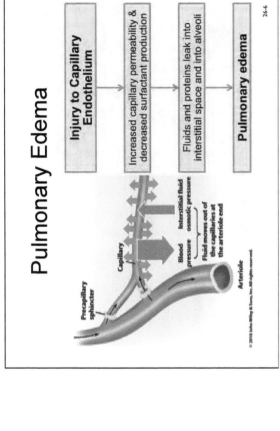

Injury to Capillary Endothelium

↓

Increased capillary permeability & decreased surfactant production

↓

Fluids and proteins leak into interstitial space and into alveoli

↓

Pulmonary edema

26-6

Pulmonary Edema

Blockage of lymphatic vessels

↓

Fluid not removed from interstitial space

↓

Fluid accumulates in interstitial space

↓

Pulmonary edema

26-6

Acute Respiratory Distress Syndrome (ARDS)

- ARDS is the most severe manifestation of acute lung injury in adults
  - also occurs in children
- All disorders that result in ARDS acutely injure the **alveolar-capillary (A-C) membrane**, causing severe pulmonary edema and markedly reduced compliance (elastic properties) of the lung

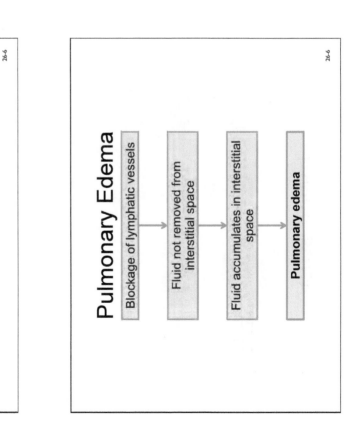

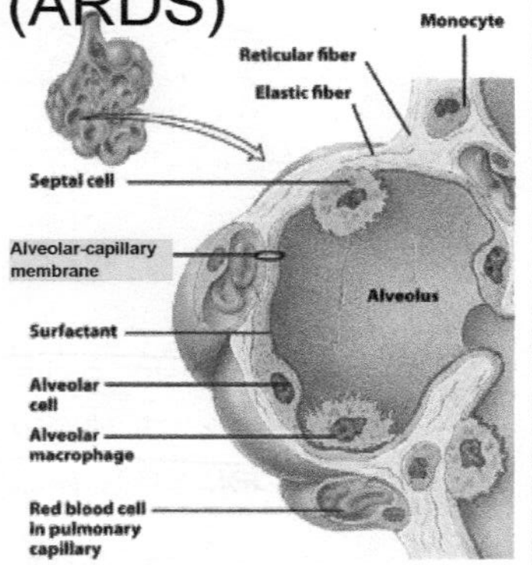

Monocyte
Reticular fiber
Elastic fiber
Septal cell
Alveolar-capillary membrane
Alveolus
Surfactant
Alveolar cell
Alveolar macrophage
Red blood cell in pulmonary capillary

Section through an alveolus showing its cellular components

26-7

ARDS: Step 1

- Neutrophils release a battery of inflammatory mediators
  - Proteolytic enzymes, O_2 free radicals, and proinflammatory cytokines
- This leads to pulmonary vasoconstriction, vascular occlusion, and pulmonary hypertension

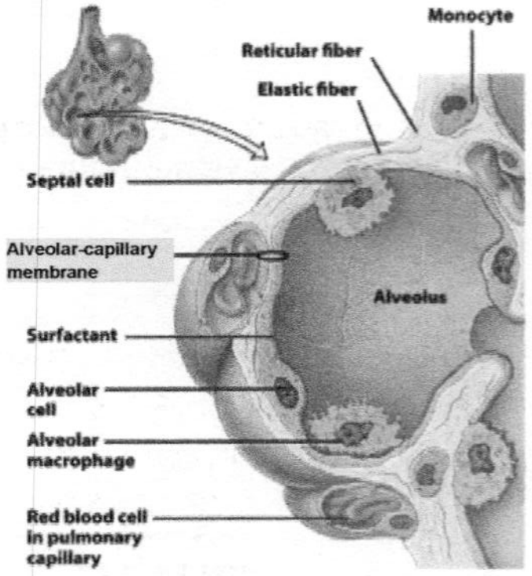

Monocyte
Reticular fiber
Elastic fiber
Septal cell
Alveolar-capillary membrane
Alveolus
Surfactant
Alveolar cell
Alveolar macrophage
Red blood cell in pulmonary capillary

Section through an alveolus showing its cellular components

26-7

ARDS: Step 2

- The damaged alveolar epithelial barrier breaks, allowing flooding of the alveolar space and making it difficult or impossible for oxygen to diffuse into the capillaries

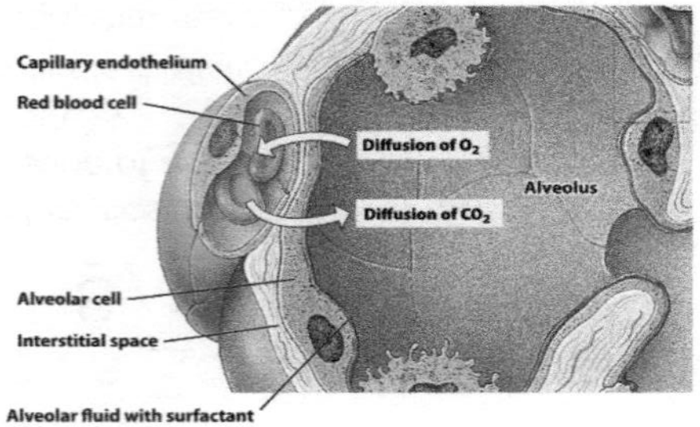

Capillary endothelium
Red blood cell
Diffusion of O_2
Diffusion of CO_2
Alveolus
Alveolar cell
Interstitial space
Alveolar fluid with surfactant

26-7

ARDS: Step 3

- Edema overwhelms type II alveolar cells (septal cells)
  - these cells make surfactant to reduce lung surface tension
  - now they cannot make enough surfactant to compensate for the huge amounts of liquid
  - surface tension of liquid causes the delicate alveoli to collapse

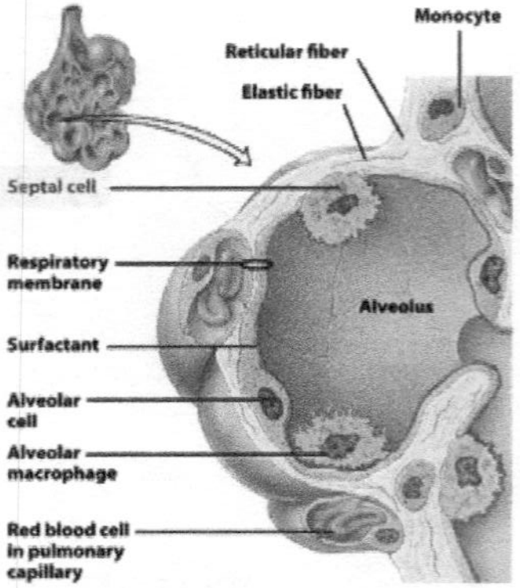

Monocyte
Reticular fiber
Elastic fiber
Septal cell
Respiratory membrane
Alveolus
Surfactant
Alveolar cell
Alveolar macrophage
Red blood cell in pulmonary capillary

Section through an alveolus showing its cellular components

26-7

ARDS: Step 4

- Protein and enzymes make a jelly-like substance called the **hyaline membrane**
- The figure below shows alveoli filled with hyaline membrane
  - not much gas exchange can take place
- ARDS requires treatment with mechanical ventilation

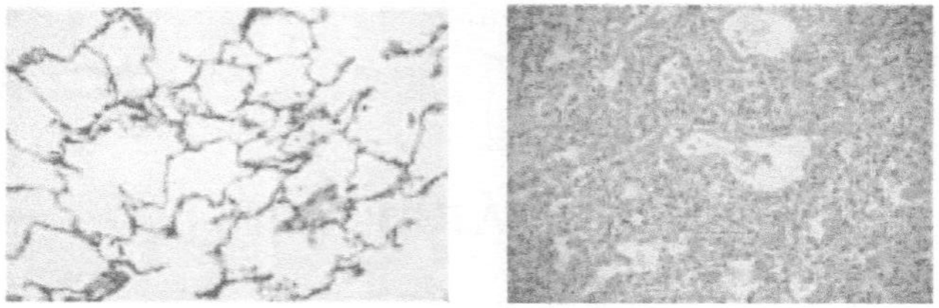

Lomas DA. Pulmonary Disorders: Hereditary in: *Encyclopedia of Life Sciences*, 2005.

26-7

Asthma

- More common in the young
- Manifestations
  - Dyspnea, prolonged expiration with expiratory wheezing, early nonproductive cough, tachycardia, tachypnea, and acidosis
- Treatment
  - Inhaled bronchodilators
    - decrease smooth muscle spasm
  - anti-inflammatory agents (glucocorticoids and leukotriene receptor blockers)
    - decrease production, release or binding of inflammatory mediators

26-8

Asthma

- More common in the young
- Manifestations
  - Dyspnea, prolonged expiration with expiratory wheezing, early nonproductive cough, tachycardia, tachypnea, and acidosis
- Treatment
  - Inhaled bronchodilators
    - decrease smooth muscle spasm
  - anti-inflammatory agents (glucocorticoids and leukotriene receptor blockers)
    - decrease production, release or binding of inflammatory mediators

26-8

Chronic Obstructive Pulmonary Disease (COPD)

- Signs/symptoms and treatments for chronic bronchitis and emphysema are very similar
- Therefore, both called COPD
- Signs/symptoms of COPD
  - exercise intolerance, dyspnea, wheezing, productive cough, hypoxemia causing polycythemia and cyanosis, pulmonary hypertension, and congestive heart failure

26-9

Emphysema

- Enlargement and destruction of alveoli (lung remodeling), loss of elasticity, and trapping of air
- Cigarette smoking always results in emphysema
  - chemicals in cigarette smoke inhibit a key lung enzyme called **α_1-antitrypsinase**
  - α_1-antitrypsinase blocks **neutrophil elastase** and prevents it from breaking down elastin
  - in the absence of α_1-antitrypsinase, elastase breaks down the elastic connective tissue of the alveolar wall, replacing it with non-elastic, fibrous connective tissue (**alveolar remodeling**)
  - patients with a mutation causing **α_1-antitrypsinase deficiency** (1/1500 persons of European descent) have syndrome where this occurs spontaneously, in absence of cigarette smoke

26-9

Emphysema

- Signs and symptoms
  - Dyspnea
  - Late developing cough
  - Tachypnea
  - Prolonged expiration
  - Pulmonary hypertension
  - Barrel chest
- Ironically, inspiration is intact, but ability to expire is reduced
  - Loss of elastin makes lungs less elastic
  - Lungs become over-inflated
  - Muscles in chest wall forced to work harder to expel air

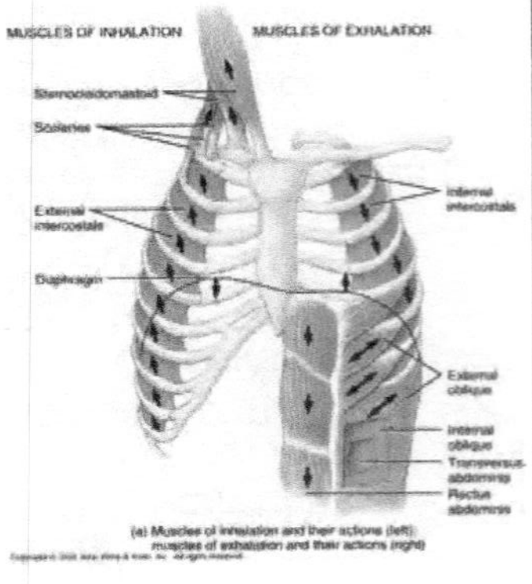

MUSCLES OF INHALATION
MUSCLES OF EXHALATION
Sternocleidomastoid
Scalenes
External intercostals
Diaphragm
Internal intercostals
External oblique
Internal oblique
Transversus abdominis
Rectus abdominis

26-9

Emphysema
Change in Expiratory Ability

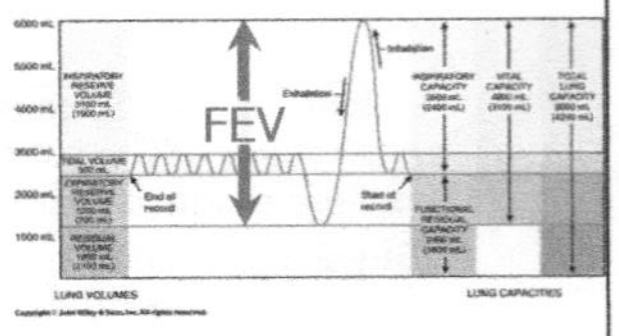

FEV

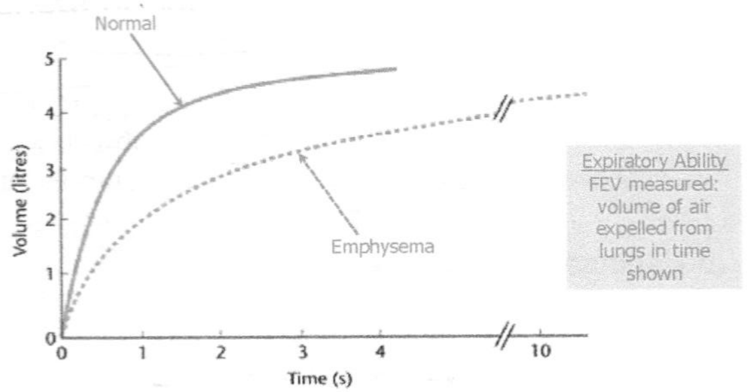

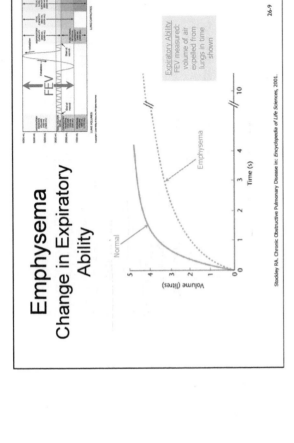

Normal
Emphysema
Volume (litres)
Time (s)
0
1
2
3
4
5
10
Expiratory Ability
FEV measured: volume of air expelled from lungs in time shown

Stockley RA. Chronic Obstructive Pulmonary Disease in: *Encyclopedia of Life Sciences*, 2001.

26-9

Chronic Obstructive Pulmonary Disease: CT

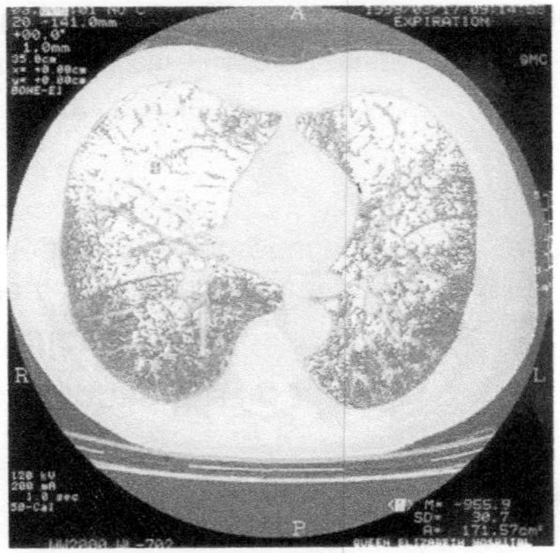

Stockley RA. Chronic Obstructive Pulmonary Disease in: *Encyclopedia of Life Sciences*, 2001.

26-9

Chronic Bronchitis

- In chronic bronchitis, the obstruction is caused by inflammation and thickening of the respiratory mucus membranes, ciliary impairment, accumulation of mucus and pus
- We don't see lung remodeling unless emphysema is also present   no remodeling
- Causes: cigarette smoking, air pollutants, infections

26-9

Treatment of COPD

- Treatment is virtually the same for emphysema and chronic bronchitis
  - Smoking cessation
  - Antibiotics:
    - given prophylactically because of patient's susceptibility to infection
  - Bronchodilators
  - Anti-inflammatory drugs: glucocorticoids
    - leukotriene inhibitors (e.g. Singulair™) less effective
  - O_2 administration

26-9

Pneumonia

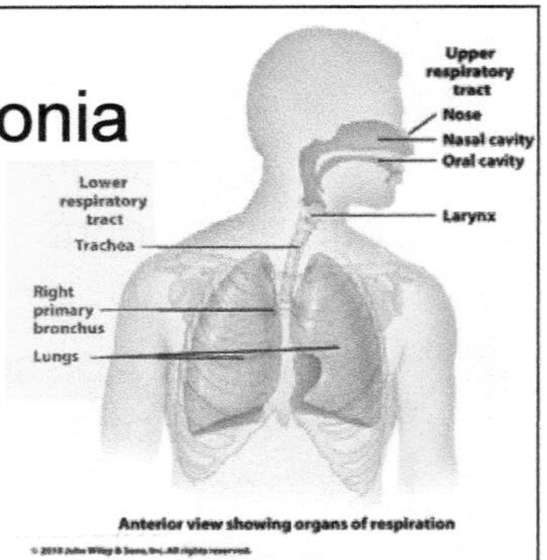
Upper respiratory tract
Nose
Nasal cavity
Oral cavity
Larynx
Lower respiratory tract
Trachea
Right primary bronchus
Lungs
Anterior view showing organs of respiration

- Acute infection of the **lower respiratory tract**
  - Caused by rickettsiae, mycoplasma, and other bacteria; fungi and viruses are also implicated
- **Community-acquired**
  - *Streptococcus pneumoniae*
  - *Mycoplasma pneumoniae* ("walking pneumonia")

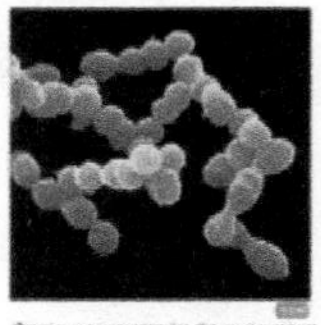

26-10

Pneumonia

- **Hospital-acquired** (nosocomial infection)
  - *Staphylococcus aureus* and *Klebsiella pneumoniae*
  - Occurs in patients with COPD or patients with a viral respiratory illness
- Pneumonia of immunocompromised individuals
  - Fungal pneumonia (*Pneumocystis jiroveci*) often seen in AIDS patients
    - Old name: *Pneumocystis carinii*
    - Often still called "PCP" (*P. carinii* pneumonia) for this reason

26-10

Pneumonia

- Organisms reach the lungs by:
  - inspiration or aspiration of oropharyngeal secretions
  - via the circulation (systemic infection, sepsis, or needle contamination)
- Normal lung defenses (cough reflex, mucociliary clearance and phagocytosis) become inadequate or compromised
  - e.g. cilia of the mucociliary escalator paralyzed by chemicals in cigarette smoke or preexisting COPD

26-10

Pneumonia

- In most individuals **susceptibility**, not **exposure**, is the overriding factor
  - The pathogen is not contained
  - Toxins are released that damage bronchial mucus membranes and alveolar-capillary membranes
  - Exudative edema and debris fill the bronchioles and ventilation/perfusion ($\dot{V}_A/\dot{Q}$) mismatch results in **shunting**

26-10

Pneumonia

- Signs and symptoms
  - Often a productive cough
  - Pleuritic chest pain, chills, malaise
  - Inspiratory crackles
  - Evidence of infiltrates on x-ray is the key diagnostic feature

26-10

Pneumonia

- Treatment depends on where the disease was acquired, the causative organism, and the severity of the disease
  - Antibiotics, supplemental oxygen, and in severe cases mechanical ventilation

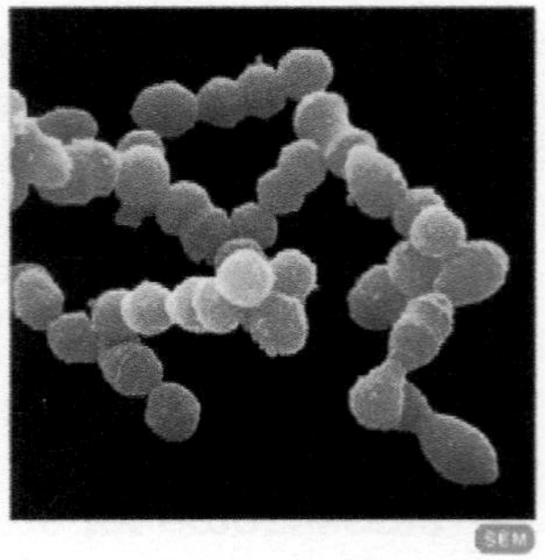
SEM

Streptococcus pneumoniae, the most common cause of pneumonia

26-10

Tuberculosis

- Infection caused by *Mycobacterium tuberculosis*, an acid-fast bacillus that affects the lungs
- Incidence is increasing due to drug-resistant strains and possibly related to HIV infections
- Emigration, crowded institutional settings, substance abuse and poor access to medical care also contribute

26-10

Tuberculosis

- Transmitted in airborne droplets
- Once in the lungs, the bacteria multiply and cause nonspecific lung inflammation
- The organism can also migrate to the lymphatics
- Neutrophils and macrophages wall off the colonies and form granulomas (**tubercles**)
- Cells within the tubercles die and form a cheese-like material (**caseous necrosis**)

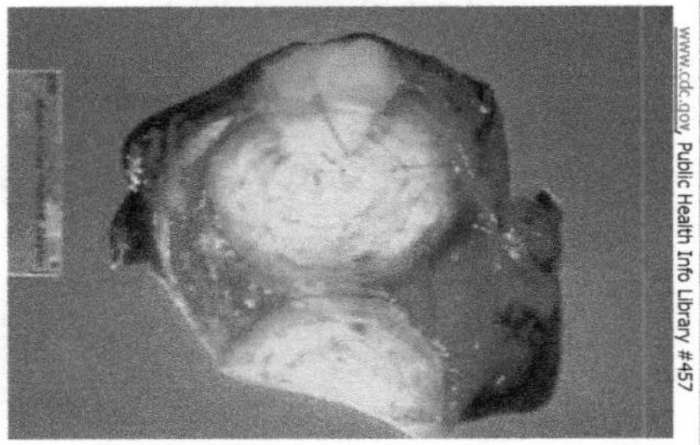

www.cdc.gov, Public Health Info Library #457

26-10

Tuberculosis

- The surviving bacteria become isolated by collagenous scar tissue
- This allows the bacteria to remain dormant
- Because TB is slow-growing, patients may be asymptomatic until the disease is well advanced
- Symptoms
  - fatigue, weight loss, lethargy, loss of appetite, fever, purulent sputum, and "night sweats"

26-10

Tuberculosis

- A positive tuberculin skin test (PPD) indicates exposure, not the presence or absence of active disease.
- Bacille Calmette-Guérin (BCG) "vaccination" interferes with interpretation of PPD
- Chest x-rays and sputum cultures contribute to the diagnosis and monitoring of the disease.
- Treatment is with antibiotics
  - A four-drug regimen is not uncommon
  - Lengthy course

26-10

Pulmonary Vascular Disorders

- Pulmonary Embolism (PE)
- Pulmonary Hypertension (HTN)
- Cor Pulmonale

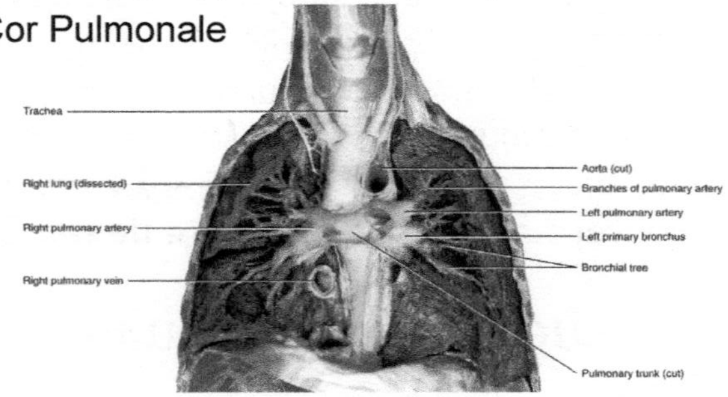

Trachea
Right lung (dissected)
Right pulmonary artery
Right pulmonary vein
Aorta (cut)
Branches of pulmonary artery
Left pulmonary artery
Left primary bronchus
Bronchial tree
Pulmonary trunk (cut)

(c) Pulmonary circulation into the lungs

26-11

Pulmonary Embolism

- Caused by an embolus obstructing the pulmonary artery
  - e.g. deep venous thrombosis, fatty embolus, air, microclots
- Signs and symptoms
  - tachypnea, dyspnea, pleuritic chest pain, systemic hypotension, and shock
- $\dot{V}_A/\dot{Q}$ mismatch results in **alveolar dead space**
  - $\dot{Q} \rightarrow$ zero so $\dot{V}_A/\dot{Q} \rightarrow \infty$
- Risk factors include those for a hypercoagulable state
  - Obesity, sedentary life style, birth control, smoking
- Treatment includes avoiding venous stasis and using anticoagulant and fibrinolytic agents

26-11

Pulmonary Hypertension

- Causes an elevated blood pressure in the pulmonary arteries
- Caused by: elevation of pulmonary arterial pressure due to increased left atrial pressure (as in congestive heart failure) or lung disease
- Manifested by: fatigue, chest pain, dyspnea with exercise, abnormal chest x-ray and abnormal electrocardiogram (showing ventricular hypertrophy)

26-11

Cor Pulmonale
(Pulmonary-Related Heart Disease)

- Right ventricular disease due to pulmonary hypertension
- Manifested by
  - chest pain
  - tricuspid murmur
  - pulmonary valve murmur

26-11

Unit 7
Chapter 28/29
Alterations of Renal and Urinary Tract Function

Glomerular Filtration & Urine Production

Net Filtration = $HP_{Blood} - OP_{Blood} - HP_{Capsular}$

Net Filtration = 55 – 30 – 15 = +10 mm Hg

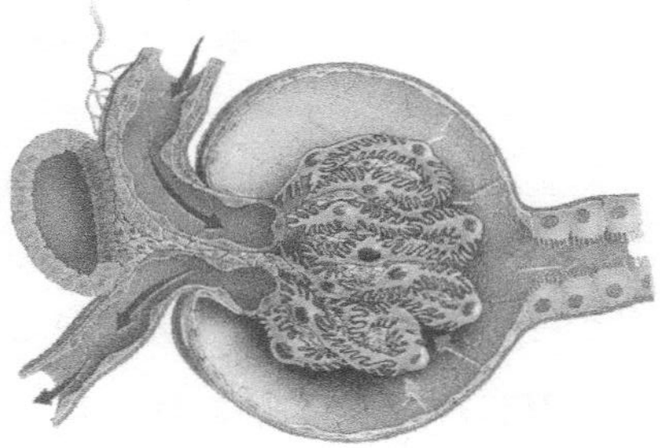

28-I

Net Filtration = $HP_{Blood} - OP_{Blood} - HP_{Capsular}$

Net Filtration = 55 – 30 – 15 = +10 mm Hg

	Total Amount in Plasma	Amount in 180 L of filtrate (/ day)	Amount in Urine (/day)
Water	3 L	180 L	1-2 L
Protein	200 g	10-20 g	0 g
Glucose	3 g	180 g	0 g
Urea	1 g	54 g	25 g
Creatinine	0.3 g	1.4 g	1.4 g

28-I

Net Filtration = $HP_{Blood} - OP_{Blood} - HP_{Capsular}$

Net Filtration = 55 – 30 – 15 = +10 mm Hg

Altering Urine Production

- Without compensation, how would someone's filtration rate change if they had high blood pressure?
- What about low blood pressure?
- Increased blood concentration (i.e. of Na^+)
  - Decreased urine production
- Increased ambient temperature
  - Decreased urine production
- Diuretics
  - Increased urine production

28-I

Renal Threshold

- If the filtrate concentration of a substance cannot be reabsorbed fast enough, then the renal threshold of that substance will be reached and the substance will spill into the urine.
- Example:
  - The renal threshold of glucose is 180-200 mg/dl. When this level is exceeded, the glucose will begin to show up in the urine.

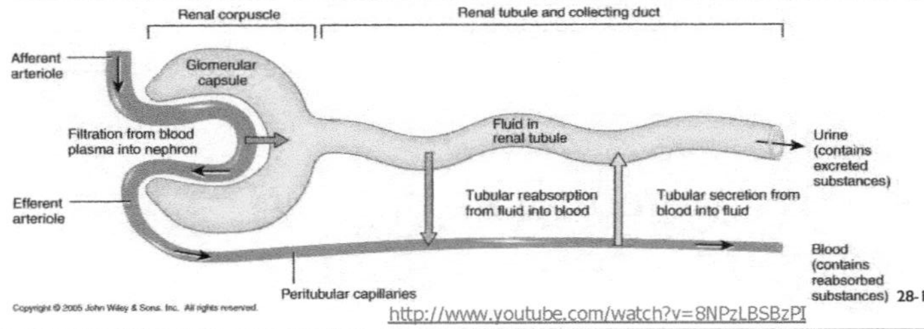
Renal corpuscle
Renal tubule and collecting duct
Afferent arteriole
Glomerular capsule
Filtration from blood plasma into nephron
Fluid in renal tubule
Urine (contains excreted substances)
Efferent arteriole
Tubular reabsorption from fluid into blood
Tubular secretion from blood into fluid
Blood (contains reabsorbed substances)
Peritubular capillaries

http://www.youtube.com/watch?v=8NPzLBSBzPI

28-I

Tests of Kidney Function

Proteinuria

- Remember that albumin (molecular weight 68 kDa) is the most abundant plasma protein
- The glomerular filter theoretically blocks passage of anything < 10 kDa
- In reality, some protein leaks through
- The tubular system has a limited capacity for protein reabsorption and is easily overwhelmed
- More protein leakage than can be reabsorption results in **proteinuria**
- This usually indicates microscopic damage to the glomeruli

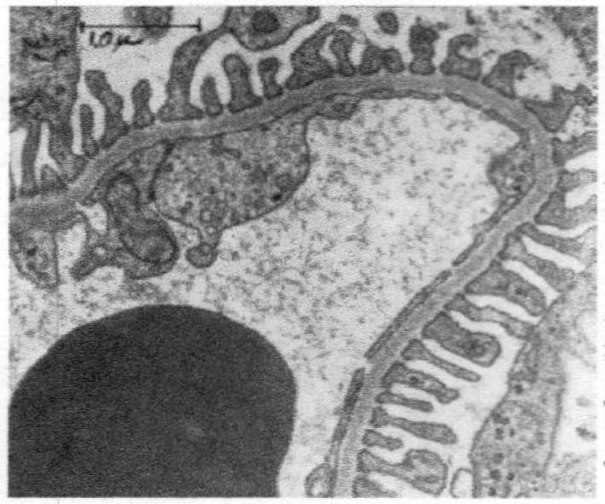

Farquhar MG. Glomerular capillary of normal rat kidney. http://cellimages.ascb.org

28-I

Tests of Kidney Function

Blood Urea Nitrogen (BUN)

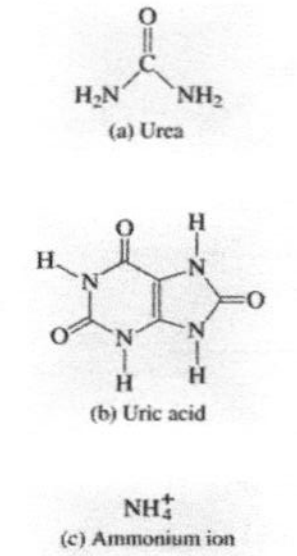
(a) Urea
(b) Uric acid
(c) Ammonium ion

Figure 19-16 Concepts in Biochemistry, 3/e © 2006 John Wiley & Sons

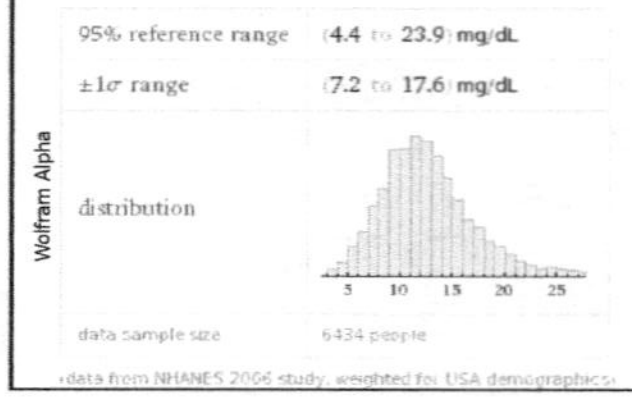
95% reference range (4.4 to 23.9) mg/dL
±1σ range (7.2 to 17.6) mg/dL
distribution
5 10 15 20 25
data sample size 6434 people
(data from NHANES 2006 study, weighted for USA demographics)

Wolfram Alpha

- Metabolism of the amino ($-NH_2$ or $-NH_3^+$) groups in proteins produces
  - urea ($H_2N-CO-NH_2$)
  - ammonia ($NH_3 + H_2O \rightarrow NH_4OH$)
  - related nitrogen-containing compounds
- These are collectively called **blood urea nitrogen**
- In kidney failure, these compounds are not cleared by the kidney (usually because of a decreased GFR) and build up in the blood

28-I

Tests of Kidney Function

Creatinine

- **Creatinine** is a waste product of muscle metabolism
- Creatinine levels are directly related to muscle mass
  - muscles use creatine phosphate as an energy source
  - creatinine is a by-product of this pathway
  - creatinine clearance rate can be measured
    - directly by taking blood and urine at intervals
    - approximately by measuring blood creatinine, then using an equation that gives an approximate value based on blood creatinine level, height, weight, and age
- Creatinine clearance rate normal values
  - men 97-137 mL/min
  - women 88-128 mL/min

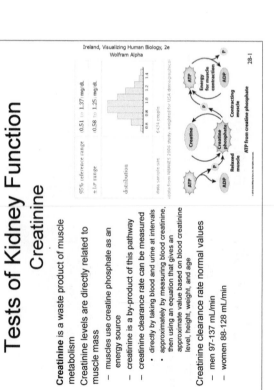

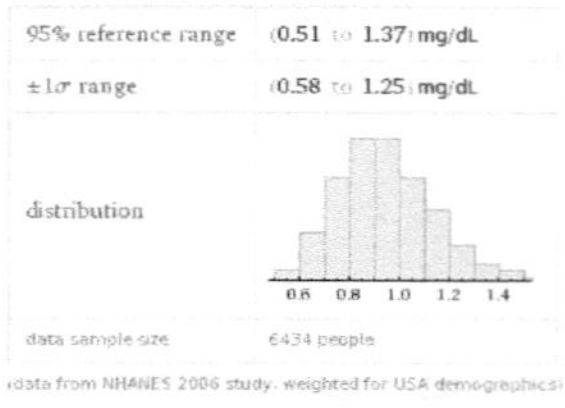
95% reference range (0.51 to 1.37) mg/dL
±1σ range (0.58 to 1.25) mg/dL
distribution
0.6 0.8 1.0 1.2 1.4
data sample size 6434 people
(data from NHANES 2006 study, weighted for USA demographics)

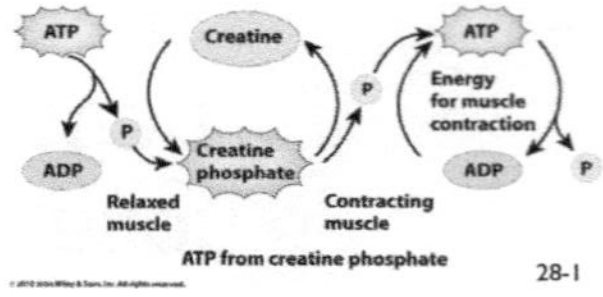
ATP
ADP
P
Creatine
Creatine phosphate
Relaxed muscle
Energy for muscle contraction
Contracting muscle
ATP from creatine phosphate

Ireland, Visualizing Human Biology, 2e
Wolfram Alpha

28-I

Tests of Kidney Function

Glomerular Filtration Rate

- This measures how much blood is filtered through the glomerulus and becomes filtrate (filtrate + tubular processing → urine)
- Normal > 90 mL / min
- Decreased in kidney disease
  - stage 1 (kidney damage with normal GFR): 90 mL / min
  - stage 2: 60-89 mL / min
  - stage 3: 30-59 mL / min
  - stage 4: 15-29 mL / min
  - stage 5 (kidney failure): < 15 mL / min

28-I

Urine

- Volume: 1-2 liters/day
- Color: variable shades of yellow
- Turbidity: clear
- Odor: variable
- pH: 5.0-6.5
  - varies widely due to diet & disease: can be 4.5-8.0
- Specific gravity: 1.005 -1.025
- Chemicals: water, urea, and small amounts of uric acid, creatinine, ketones, Na^+, K^+, bicarbonate

28-1

Urinalysis

- Complete urinalysis (U/A)
  - Biochemical ("Dipstick")
    - Absorbent pads specific to certain analytes
    - Detects possible presence of blood, bilirubin, glucose, albumin, bacteria, and white blood cells
  - Microscopic
    - Visualization of urinary sediment

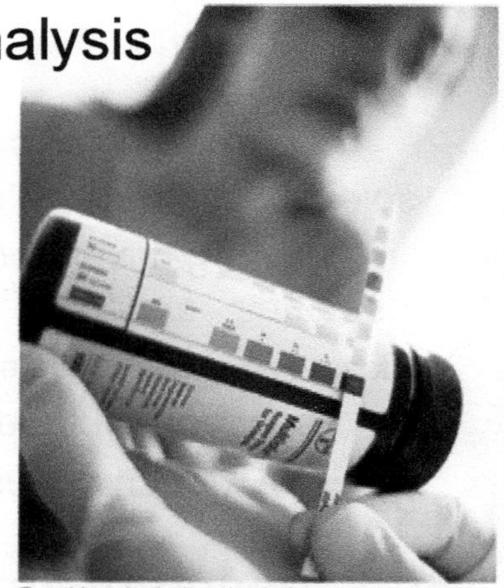
Test stick previously placed in urine is compared to a chart to detect abnormal constituents in urine

Ian Hooton/Photo Researchers, Inc.

28-1

Upper & Lower Urinary Tract Obstructions

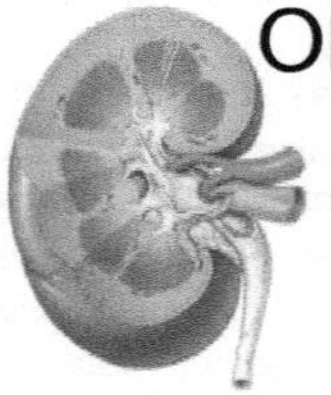

- Upper urinary tract obstruction
  - kidney
    - stones
    - blood vessel compression
    - tumor
    - scarring/fibrosis
  - ureter
    - stones
    - tumor
- Lower urinary tract obstruction
  - bladder
    - neurogenic bladder
  - urethra
    - urethral stricture
    - prostate enlargement (♂)
    - pelvic organ prolapse
    - obstruction of urethra

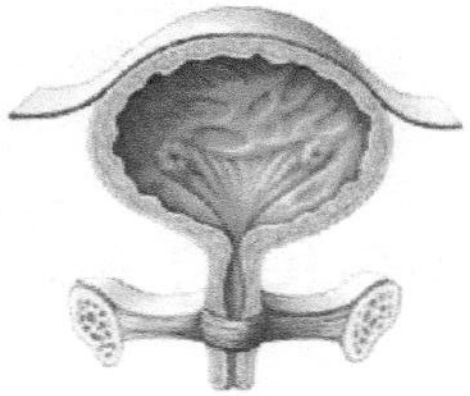

29-1

Renal Calculi (Kidney Stones)

- Caused by underlying disorders (infections, obstructions) increased dietary intake of specific chemicals (Ca^{++} and PO_4), high or low pH levels, and dehydration
  - Symptoms: **flank pain** radiating to the groin area, nausea, vomiting, and abdominal pain
  - Laboratory findings: high urine specific gravity, hematuria, possible crystals on microscopic exam
  - Diagnosed by performing an intravenous pyelogram (IVP)
  - Treatment: high fluid intake, stone extraction, stone fragmentation (laser or ultrasonic lithotripsy)
  - Can cause renal failure and predispose to infections

29-1

Renal Calculi (Kidney Stones)

- Caused by underlying disorders (infections, obstructions) increased dietary intake of specific chemicals (Ca^{++} and PO_4)) high or low pH levels, and dehydration
  - Symptoms: **flank pain** radiating to the groin area, nausea, vomiting, and abdominal pain
  - Laboratory findings: high urine specific gravity, hematuria, possible crystals on microscopic exam
  - Diagnosed by performing an intravenous pyelogram (IVP)
  - Treatment: high fluid intake, stone extraction, stone fragmentation (laser or ultrasonic lithotripsy)
  - Can cause renal failure and predispose to infections

29-1

Innervation of the Bladder

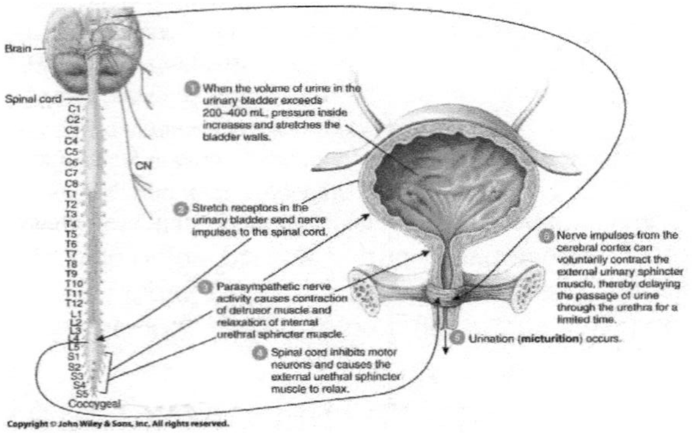

Brain
Spinal cord
C1
C2
C3
C4
C5
C6
C7
C8
T1
T2
T3
T4
T5
T6
T7
T8
T9
T10
T11
T12
L1
L2
L3
L4
L5
S1
S2
S3
S4
S5
Coccygeal
CN
1 When the volume of urine in the urinary bladder exceeds 200–400 mL, pressure inside increases and stretches the bladder walls.
2 Stretch receptors in the urinary bladder send nerve impulses to the spinal cord.
3 Parasympathetic nerve activity causes contraction of detrusor muscle and relaxation of internal urethral sphincter muscle.
4 Spinal cord inhibits motor neurons and causes the external urethral sphincter muscle to relax.
5 Urination (**micturition**) occurs.
6 Nerve impulses from the cerebral cortex can voluntarily contract the external urinary sphincter muscle, thereby delaying the passage of urine through the urethra for a limited time.

29-1

Neurogenic Bladder

- An **obstructive uropathy** caused by an interruption of the nerve supply to the bladder. Both CNS or spinal cord damage can be a cause.
  - Loss of upper motor neuron function in the primary neuron between the cortex and sacrum results in a patient's loss of **voluntary** voiding control
  - Loss of lower motor neurons in the peripheral nerves from the sacrum causes the patient to lose both **voluntary** and **involuntary** urination due to disruption of the sacral reflex.

29-1

Urinary Tract Infection

- Infection anywhere in the urinary tract
- *E. coli* is the main pathogen for UTIs
  - Other Gram-negative bacteria are also seen
- Caused by: surgery, catheters, diabetes, ptosis, prostatic hyperplasia, STDs
- Common in females, uncommon in males
  - Except for STDs which are equal in both sexes

29-2

Urinary Tract Infections (UTI)

- Symptoms:
  - Dysuria (burning urination, urgency and frequency)
  - Incontinence
  - Low back or flank pain

29-2

Cystitis

- May be an infectious or non-infectious inflammation
  - Obstruction, prostatitis, microorganisms
- Signs and symptoms
  - Painful, burning urination, frequency, urgency, hematuria (not always), and foul smelling and cloudy urine
- Laboratory findings
  - WBCs with/without bacteria

29-2

Pyelonephritis

- Again, infection is the usual etiology, but not always
  - Ascending microorganisms, urinary obstruction, condition that causes urinary reflux, or urine retention (organisms don't get flushed out)
- Signs and symptoms
  - Fever, chills, back pain, dysuria, frequency
- Laboratory findings
  - WBCs and WBC casts, with/without bacteriuria

29-2

Glomerulonephritis

- Group of diseases of the glomerulus that are caused by immune responses, toxins, vascular disorders and other systemic diseases.
- Hallmark of this disease is blood in the urine (**hematuria**)
- Damage occurs from the activation of the inflammatory process (complement, WBCs and fibrin)
- There can be antibodies to the glomerulus or antigen/antibody complexes that localize in the glomerular membrane wall.
- This inflammatory response changes the permeability of the glomerular membrane

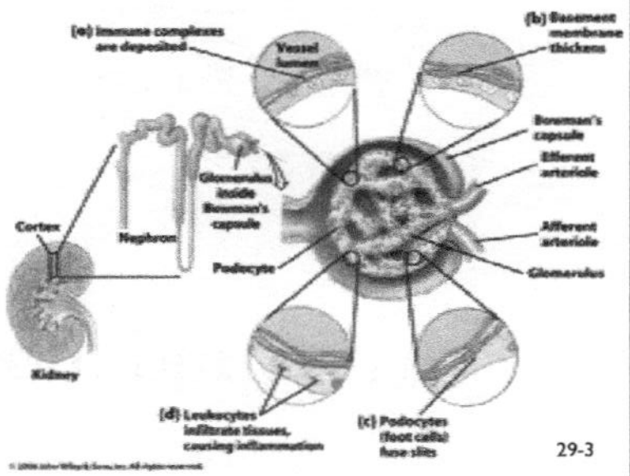

(a) Immune complexes are deposited
Vessel lumen
(b) Basement membrane thickens
Bowman's capsule
Efferent arteriole
Afferent arteriole
Glomerulus
Glomerulus inside Bowman's capsule
Nephron
Cortex
Kidney
Podocyte
(d) Leukocytes infiltrate tissues, causing inflammation
(c) Podocytes (foot cells) fuse slits

29-3

Glomerulonephritis

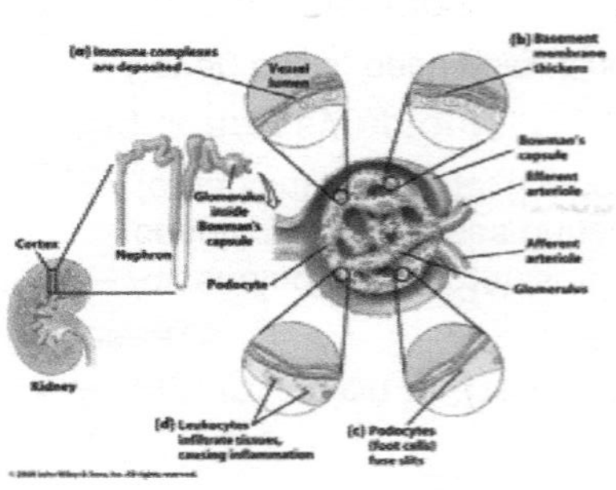
(a) Immune complexes are deposited
Vessel lumen
(b) Basement membrane thickens
Bowman's capsule
Efferent arteriole
Afferent arteriole
Glomerulus
Podocyte
Nephron
Cortex
Kidney
(d) Leukocytes infiltrate tissues, causing inflammation
(c) Podocytes (foot cells) fuse slits

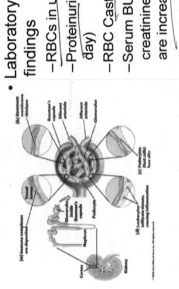

- Laboratory findings
  - RBCs in urine
  - Proteinuria (3-5 g/day)
  - RBC Casts
  - Serum BUN and creatinine levels are increased

29-3

Glomerulonephritis

- Common types
  - **Post-streptococcal (PSGN)**
  - Rapidly progressing (crescentic)
  - Membranoproliferative and minimal change disease (MCD)
  - IgA nephropathy (Berger's disease)

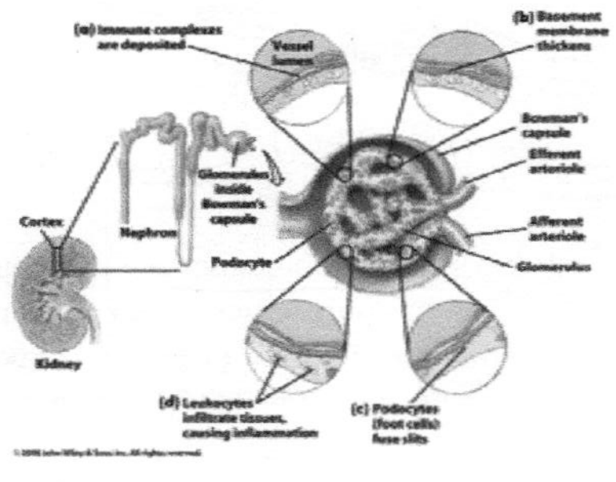
(a) Immune complexes are deposited
Vessel lumen
(b) Basement membrane thickens
Bowman's capsule
Efferent arteriole
Afferent arteriole
Glomerulus
Glomerulus inside Bowman's capsule
Podocyte
Nephron
Cortex
Kidney
(d) Leukocytes infiltrate tissues, causing inflammation
(c) Podocytes (foot cells) fuse slits

29-3

Nephrotic Syndrome

- Is a group of symptoms including protein in the urine (exceeding 3.5 gm/dL– from an increase in glomerular permeability), low blood protein levels, high cholesterol levels, and edema. The urine may also contain fat (lipiduria – visible under the microscope as fatty casts)
- Often the result of a different primary disease
  - Nephrotic syndrome secondary to toxemia of pregnancy, diabetes, systemic lupus erythromatosus (SLE), or glomerulonephritis

29-4

Nephrotic Syndrome

- Loss of the various blood products reduces the blood oncotic pressure, allows water to leave the capillaries, and encourages edema
  - remember from Unit 1 that low serum protein reduces the blood oncotic pressure and promotes edema
- Hyperlipidemia results from the liver's response to the hypoalbuminemia
- As the liver tries to restore the albumin level to normal, the liver also synthesizes lipoproteins

29-4

Acute Renal Failure

- **Pre-renal** (renal hypoperfusion)
  - Hypovolemia, shock, cardiac failure and hypotension
- **Intrarenal**
  - Renal ischemia, acute tubular necrosis, toxins, glomerulopathies, or malignancies
- **Post-renal** (urinary obstruction)
  - Tumors, stones, clots and outlet obstructions (benign prostatic hyperplasia or urethral structures)

Causes of Renal Failure →

(%)	White	Black	Asian
Diabetes	38	36	40
Glomerulonephritis	12	9	18
Pyelonephritis	6	3	4
Polycystic kidney disease	4	1	2
Hypertension	26	37	24
Renovascular disease	5	3	5
Cause unknown	5	3	5

Gokal R. Renal Failure. *Encyclopedia of Life Sciences*

29-5

Acute Renal Failure

- Renal failure is a rapid deterioration of renal function with an accompanying elevation of BUN and plasma creatinine
  - Uremia
- Phases:
  - Oliguria
    - begins ~1 day after hypotensive event and may last 1-3 weeks
  - Diuresis
  - recovery

29-5

Acute Tubular Necrosis (ATN)

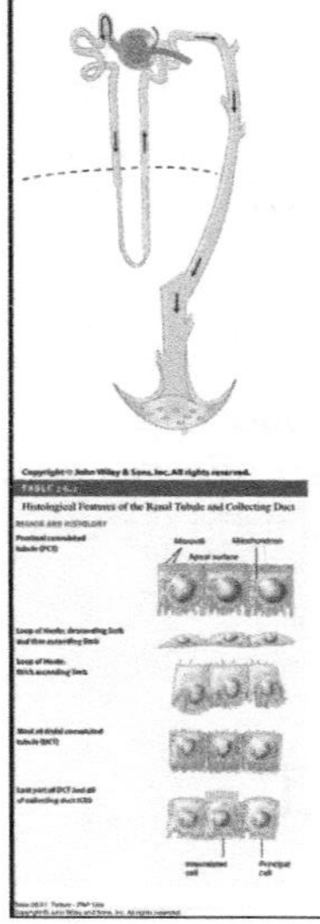

- Is the most common cause of acute renal failure
- Associated with sepsis, burns, trauma, or severe episode of hypotension (**acute decreases in renal perfusion**)
- Ischemia generates oxygen radicals and inflammatory mediators that cause swelling, injury, and necrosis of renal cells.
- One theory states that sloughed cells and cellular debris obstruct the tubules.

29-5

Chronic Renal Failure

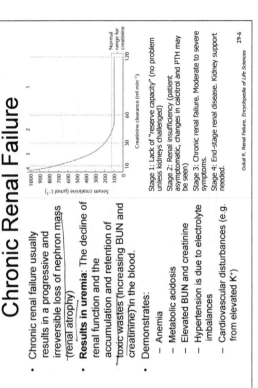

- Chronic renal failure usually results in a progressive and irreversible loss of nephron mass (renal atrophy)
- **Results in uremia**: The decline of renal function and the accumulation and retention of toxic wastes (increasing BUN and creatinine) in the blood.
- Demonstrates:
  - Anemia
  - Metabolic acidosis
  - Elevated BUN and creatinine
  - Hypertension is due to electrolyte imbalances
  - Cardiovascular disturbances (e.g. from elevated K^+)

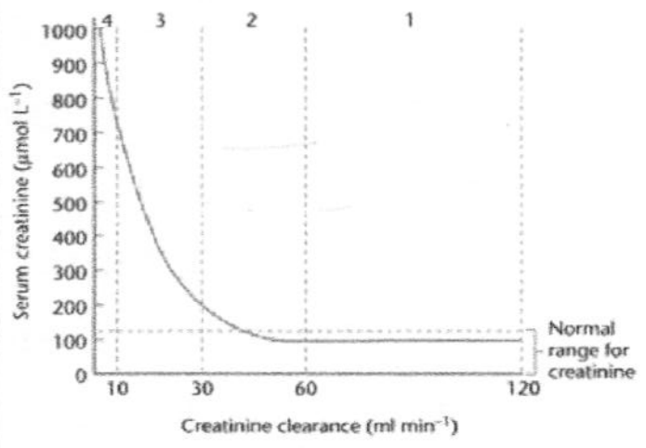

Serum creatinine (μmol L⁻¹)
Creatinine clearance (ml min⁻¹)
Normal range for creatinine
4
3
2
1

Stage 1: Lack of "reserve capacity" (no problem unless kidneys challenged)

Stage 2: Renal insufficiency (patient asymptomatic, changes in calcitrol and PTH may be seen)

Stage 3: Chronic renal failure. Moderate to severe symptoms.

Stage 4: End-stage renal disease. Kidney support needed.

Gokal R. Renal Failure. *Encyclopedia of Life Sciences*

29-6

Diabetic Nephropathy

- At right is a list of drugs used to treat diabetic nephropathy
- What do these drugs have in common?

they are all treating high osmotic pressure

ACE Inhibitors
Angiotensin II Receptor Antagonists
Diuretics
Calcium-channel blockers
Beta blockers
Alpha blockers

Source: "Diabetic Nephropathy", *Wiley Handbook of Current and Emerging Drug Therapies*

29-6

Systemic Effects of Uremia

- **Skeletal** – bone reabsorption
- **Cardiopulmonary** – hypertension
- **Neurologic** – encephalopathy (uremic toxins)
- **Endocrine** – decreased growth hormone
- **Hematologic** – reduced erythropoietin
- **GI** – retention of urochromes, urea, and acids
- **Immune** – cell-mediated immunity suppression
- **Reproduction** – sexual dysfunction, amenorrhea, infertility, decreased libido

29-7

Unit 7
Chapter 34
Alterations of Digestive Function

Gastrointestinal Signs and Symptoms
Anorexia

- *Orexis* (ο ρ ε ξ ι ς) is the Greek word for "yearning" or "desire"
- Therefore, **anorexia** is a lack of desire (in this case, desire to eat)
- This is a symptom, not to be confused with the disease **anorexia nervosa** (discussed later)
- Also see it in the names of hormones that stimulate eating (**orexins**) or inhibit eating (**anorexins**)

34-1

Gastrointestinal Signs and Symptoms Vomiting

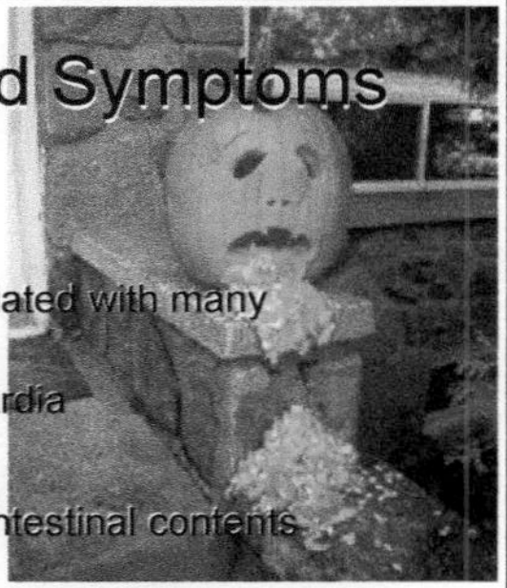

- **Nausea**
  - Symptom: subjective experience associated with many conditions
  - Signs: increased salivation and tachycardia
- **Vomiting**
  - Forceful emptying of the stomach and intestinal contents through the mouth
  - Stimuli initiate the vomiting reflex (in the **area postrema** of the medulla)
    - Area postrema (floor of 4th ventricle) has no blood-brain barrier: responds to chemicals, pain, GI distention
- **Retching**
  - Strong involuntary effort to vomit
  - Deep inspiration, abdominal muscles contract, upper esophageal sphincter remains closed

34-1

Gastrointestinal Signs and Symptoms Constipation

- Constipation is difficult or infrequent defecation
- Anything that reduces bowel motility can cause constipation
- Daily fecal output should average 150 mL / day
  - about 100 mL / day of water, rest solid material
- Less output than this is constipation, but daily output is highly variable
  - the normal ranges from 2 evacuations per day up to one per week (!)

Defined as two of the following that occur at least ¼ of the time for 12 weeks during the previous year:

1. straining
2. lumpy or hard stools
3. sensation of incomplete evacuation
4. manual maneuvers used to defecate
5. sensation of blockage/ obstruction
6. fewer than 3 bowel movements per week

34-1

Gastrointestinal Signs and Symptoms Diarrhea

- Increased frequency of defecation and an increase in the fluidity and volume of the feces
  - Osmotic
    - non-absorbable substance draws water into the lumen
    - the Joy of GoLytely™ and Fleet Phosphosoda™
  - Secretory
    - excess mucosal secretion due to bacterial toxins (*Cholera, Shigella*) or neoplasms
  - Motility
    - diarrhea due to surgical resection

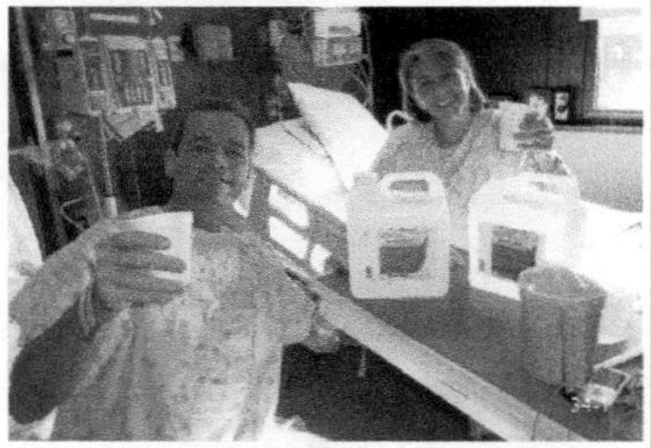

34-1

Gastrointestinal Signs and Symptoms Abdominal Pain

- Parietal pain
  - from parietal peritoneum
  - usually well-localized and sharp because these nerves travel with skin nerves from the same area
- Visceral pain
  - distension, inflammation, ischemia
  - poorly localized, dull pain
- Referred pain
  - e.g. gallbladder pain, if intense, is referred to the back, between scapulae

34-1

Gastrointestinal Signs and Symptoms Gastrointestinal Bleeding

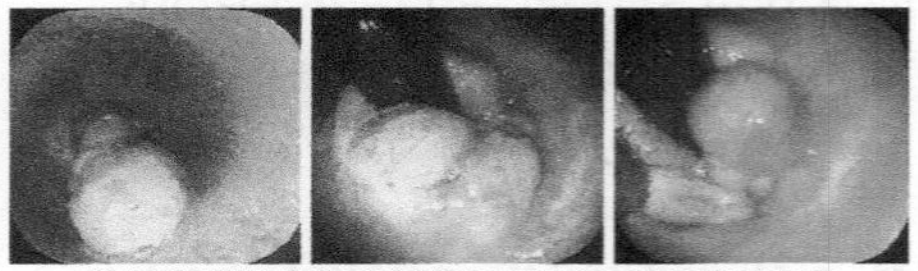

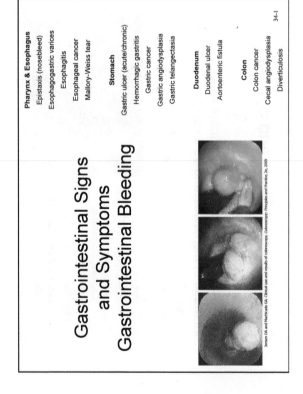

Jensen DA and Machicado GA. Clinical use and results of colonoscopy. *Colonoscopy: Principles and Practice*, 2e, 2009

Pharynx & Esophagus
Epistaxis (nosebleed)
Esophagogastric varices
Esophagitis
Esophageal cancer
Mallory-Weiss tear

Stomach
Gastric ulcer (acute/chronic)
Hemorrhagic gastritis
Gastric cancer
Gastric angiodysplasia
Gastric telangectasia

Duodenum
Duodenal ulcer
Aortoenteric fistula

Colon
Colon cancer
Cecal angiodysplasia
Diverticulosis

34-1

Gastrointestinal Motility
Dysphagia

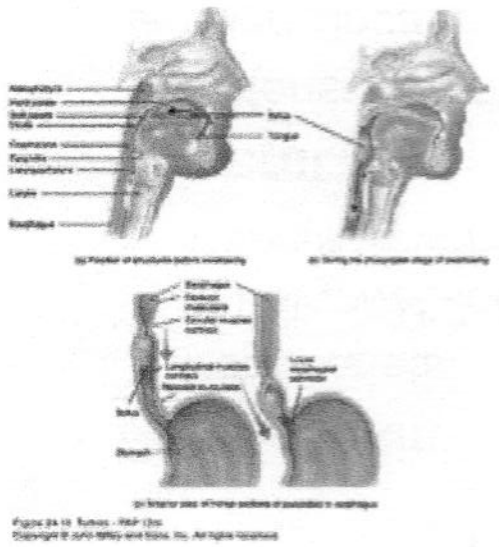

- Difficulty swallowing due to an obstruction or a disorder that affects esophageal motility
  - includes both voluntary and involuntary processes
- **Achalasia**
  - loss of cells in the autonomic ganglia in the wall of the esophagus
  - results in a dilated esophagus with absent peristalsis and a lower esophageal sphincter that doesn't open

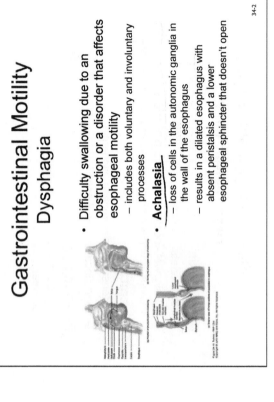

34-2

Gastrointestinal Motility
Dysphagia

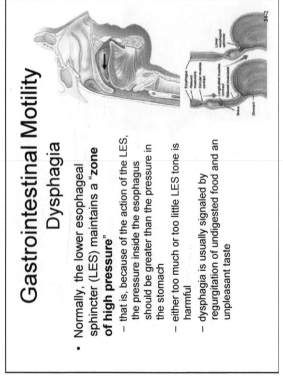

- Normally, the lower esophageal sphincter (LES) maintains a "**zone of high pressure**"
  - that is, because of the action of the LES, the pressure inside the esophagus should be greater than the pressure in the stomach
  - either too much or too little LES tone is harmful
  - dysphagia is usually signaled by regurgitation of undigested food and an unpleasant taste

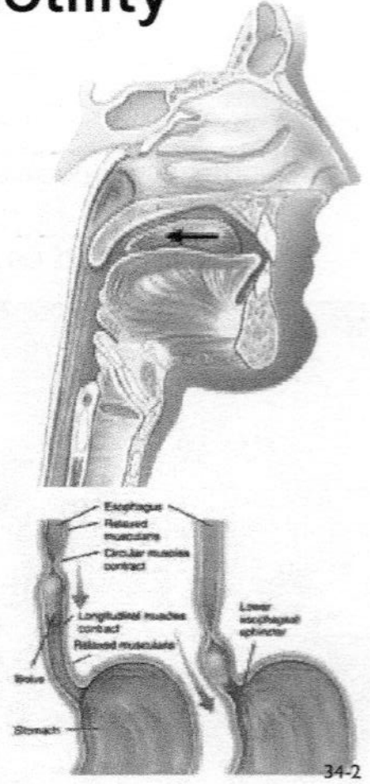

34-2

Peristalsis

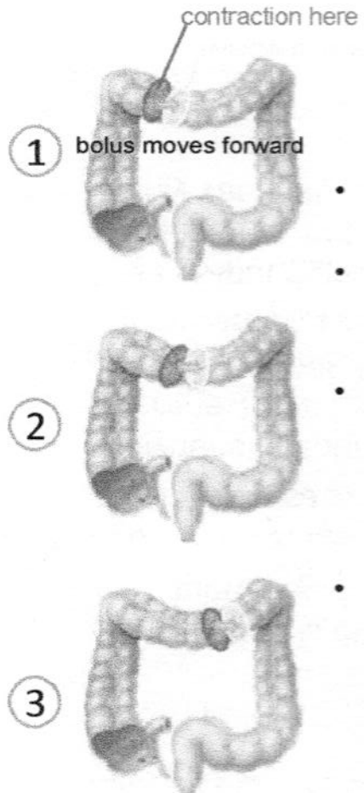

contraction here
1
bolus moves forward
2
3

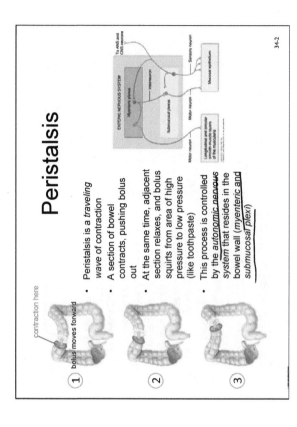

- Peristalsis is a *traveling wave* of contraction
- A section of bowel contracts, pushing bolus out
- At the same time, adjacent section relaxes, and bolus squirts from area of high pressure to low pressure (like toothpaste)
- This process is controlled by the *autonomic nervous system* that resides in the bowel wall (*myenteric and submucosal plexi*)

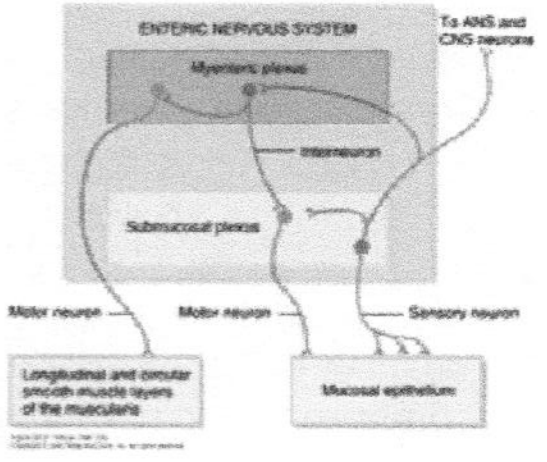

ENTERIC NERVOUS SYSTEM
To ANS and CNS neurons
Myenteric plexus
Interneuron
Submucosal plexus
Motor neuron
Motor neuron
Sensory neuron
Mucosal epithelium

34-2

GI Motility

- Laxatives act by increasing GI motility
- Increased motility means faster transit time from mouth to anus and therefore less absorption of water and nutrients
- Factors that increase bowel motility
  - chyme volume (↑ volume, ↑ motility)
  - chemical composition (chemicals that increase electrical or muscular activity ↑ motility)
  - osmolarity (substances such as sugar alcohols are not absorbed and "draw" water from bloodstream into intestinal lumen)

34-2

Motility Disorders
Gastroesophageal Reflux Disease (GERD)

- Two possible signs (either or both):
  1. Transient relaxations of the lower esophageal sphincter
     - Like "yawning" of the LES
  2. Decreased acid clearance from peristalsis failure
- Caused by:
  - High intraabdominal pressure – i.e. obesity
  - Sliding hiatal hernia acts as a fluid trap for acid
  - Ulcers (delay in gastric emptying)
  - Drugs

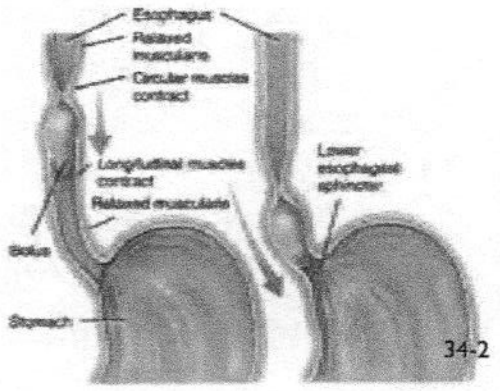

34-2

Motility Disorders
Hiatal Hernia

- A **hiatal hernia** is the protrusion of the upper stomach through the diaphragm into the thorax
  - Weak diaphragm muscles
  - Short esophagus
- Can lead to dysphagia, heartburn, reflux, and frequent epigastric pain
- Treatment
  - decrease meal size
  - remain upright after eating
  - **Nissen fundoplication**
    - making a muscular collar or ring from the stomach

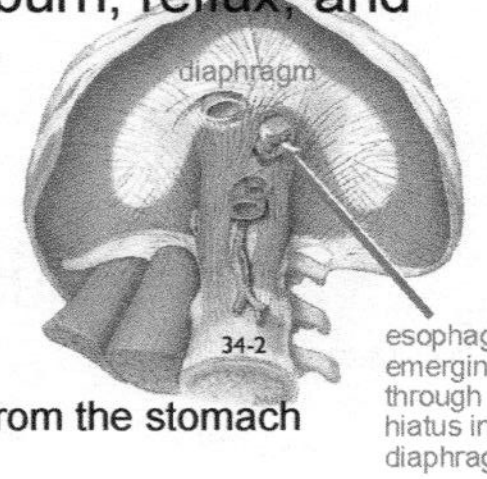
diaphragm
34-2
esophagus emerging through the hiatus in the diaphragm

Motility Disorders
Pyloric Obstruction

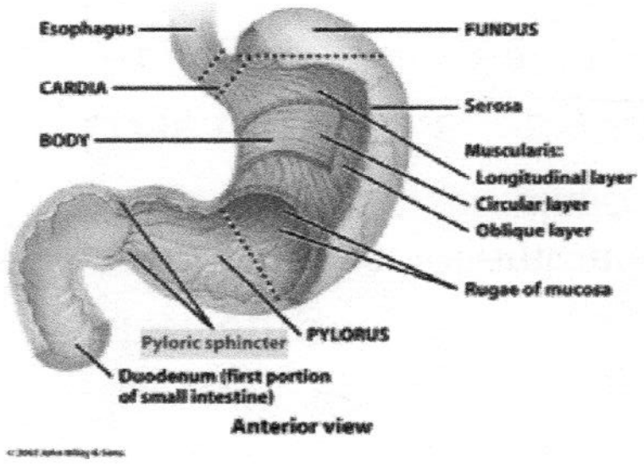
Esophagus
CARDIA
BODY
FUNDUS
Serosa
Muscularis:
Longitudinal layer
Circular layer
Oblique layer
Rugae of mucosa
Pyloric sphincter
PYLORUS
Duodenum (first portion of small intestine)
Anterior view

- Also called **gastric outlet obstruction**
- Obstruction in the pyloric region, between the body of the stomach and the duodenum
- Newborns:
  - smooth muscle hyperplasia (pyloric stenosis)
- Adults:
  - Ulcers or tumors

34-2

Motility Disorders
Intestinal Obstruction

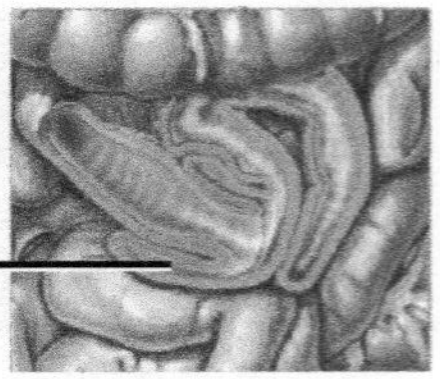

- **Volvulus** or torsion (twisting)
- **Intussusception** (telescoping)
- Foreign bodies
- **Herniation** (passing through a muscle layer when it isn't supposed to)
- Tumor growth
- Formation of strictures
- Physiological causes
  - electrolyte imbalances
  - drugs

34-2

Motility Disorders
Ileus

- Paralytic ileus is a failure of bowel motility after surgery
  - anesthetics, inflammation, opioids, and sympathetic stimulation contribute to ileus
- Loss of blood supply in a bowel segment
  - peristalsis stops at this point
- Loss of neurons in enteric ganglia
  - also stops peristalsis in a bowel segment

34-2

Gastritis vs. Peptic Ulcer Disease

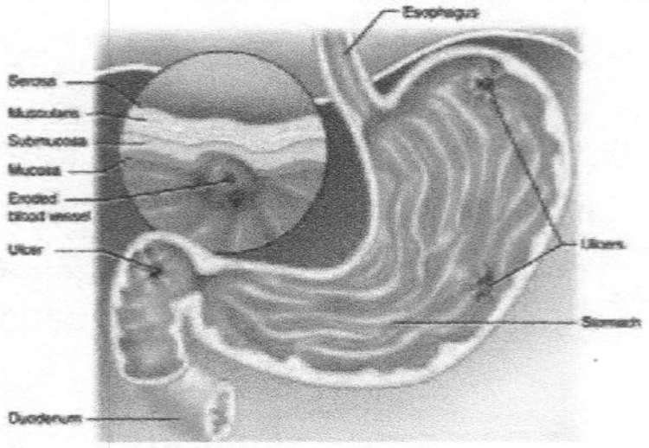
Esophagus
Serosa
Muscularis
Submucosa
Mucosa
Eroded blood vessel
Ulcer
Ulcers
Stomach
Duodenum

- **Gastritis** is an inflammatory disorder of the gastric mucosa and is usually superficial.
- **Peptic ulcer disease (PUD)** refers to an ulceration that exposes the submucosa to gastric secretions (acid and pepsin)
  - Acid and enzymes cannot distinguish between the meat you eat and the meat that is you, and **autodigestion** results

- Either disease results from an imbalance in:
  - Aggressive factors
    - acid production
    - pepsin production
    - histamine (inflammation)
  - Defensive factors
    - mucus
    - bicarbonate
    - blood flow

34-3
34-4

Acute Gastritis

- Inflammation of the gastric mucosa over a wide area
- Symptoms:
  - vague abdominal discomfort
  - epigastric tenderness

- Conditions which promote gastritis
  - uremia
  - trauma
  - stress

- Drugs which promote gastritis
  - non-steroidal anti-inflammatories (NSAIDs)
    - aspirin, acetaminophen, ibuprofen
    - inhibit prostaglandin synthesis
    - prostaglandins stimulate protective mucus
  - ethanol
  - histamine
  - digitalis

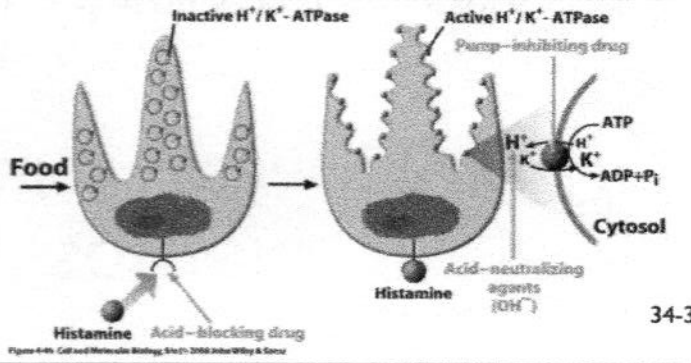
Inactive H+/K+-ATPase
Active H+/K+-ATPase
Pump-inhibiting drug
Food
ATP
ADP+Pi
Cytosol
Histamine
Acid-blocking drug
Acid-neutralizing agents (OH−)

34-3

Chronic Gastritis

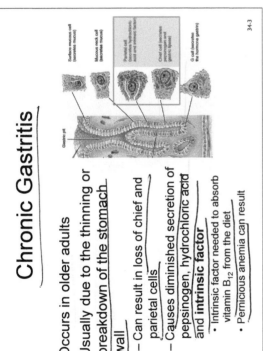

- Occurs in older adults
- Usually due to the thinning or breakdown of the stomach wall
  - Can result in loss of chief and parietal cells
  - Causes diminished secretion of pepsinogen, hydrochloric acid and **intrinsic factor**
    - Intrinsic factor needed to absorb vitamin B_{12} from the diet
    - Pernicious anemia can result

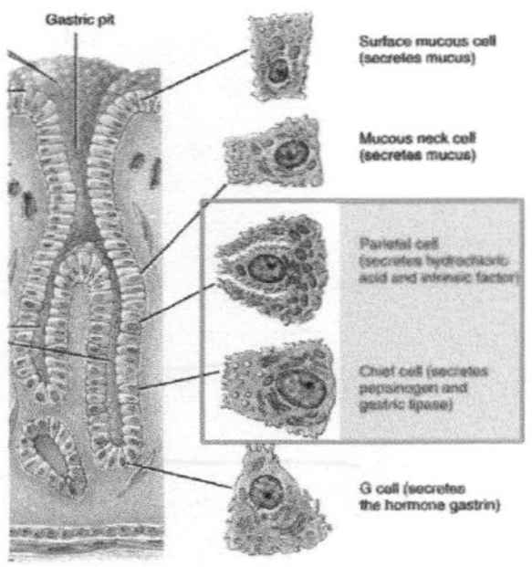

Gastric pit
Surface mucous cell (secretes mucus)
Mucous neck cell (secretes mucus)
G cell (secretes the hormone gastrin)

34-3

Peptic Ulcer Disease

- Peptic ulcer disease (PUD) refers to a discrete mucosal defect in the portions of the GI tract (gastric or duodenal) exposed to acid and pepsin secretion and leading to autodigestion
- Can be superficial or deep (hemorrhagic)
  - *H. pylori* bacteria cause more than 90% of duodenal ulcers and up to 80% of gastric ulcers
- Risks
  - smoking, persistent NSAID usage, stress or alcohol
- Prevalence percentage about matches age in years
  - i.e. about 20% at age 20, 30% at age 30, etc.

34-4

Peptic Ulcer Disease
Role of *Helicobacter pylori*

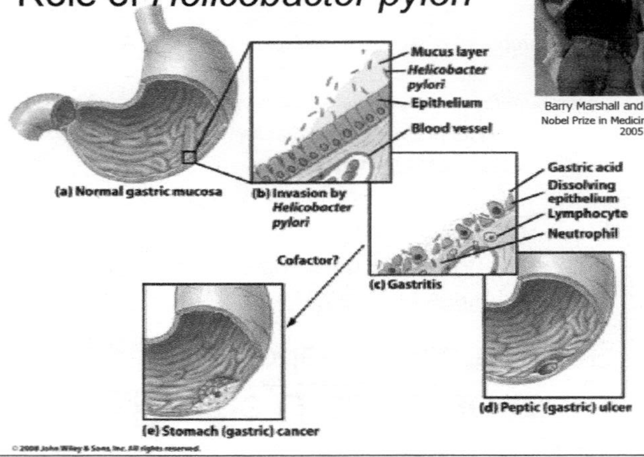

Mucus layer
Helicobacter pylori
Epithelium
Blood vessel
(a) Normal gastric mucosa
(b) Invasion by Helicobacter pylori
Cofactor?
(c) Gastritis
Gastric acid
Dissolving epithelium
Lymphocyte
Neutrophil
(d) Peptic (gastric) ulcer
(e) Stomach (gastric) cancer

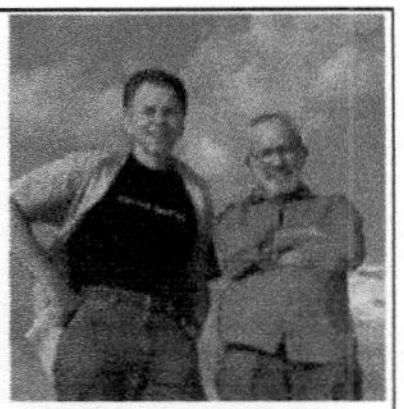

Barry Marshall and Robin Warren
Nobel Prize in Medicine or Physiology, 2005

34-4

Peptic Ulcer Disease
Gastric Ulcers

- Ulcers of the stomach
  - They usually occur in the **antral** region
  - The primary defect is an **increased permeability of the mucosa to H^+ ions** (*not* excess H^+ secretion)
  - Reflux of bile through a **defective pyloric sphincter** can also be a cause
  - Clinical presentation
    - pain-food-relief-pain
    - GI bleeding if not treated

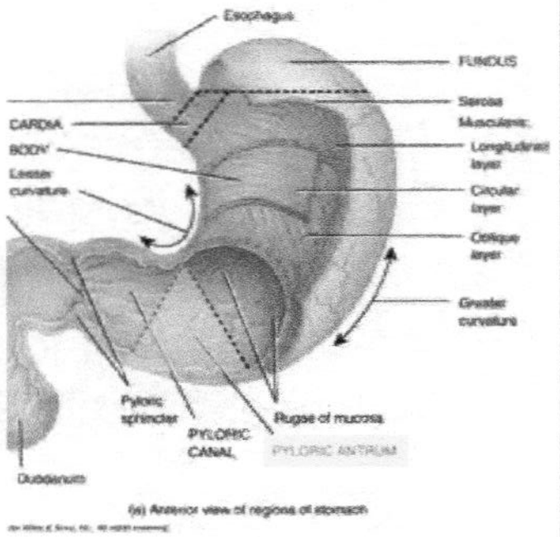

Esophagus
FUNDUS
CARDIA
BODY
Pyloric sphincter
PYLORIC CANAL
PYLORIC ANTRUM
Rugae of mucosa
Duodenum
(a) Anterior view of regions of stomach

34-4

Peptic Ulcer Disease
Duodenal Ulcers

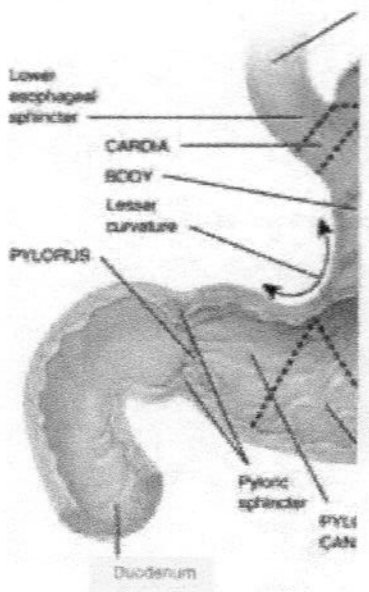

Lower esophageal sphincter
CARDIA
BODY
Lesser curvature
PYLORUS
Pyloric sphincter
Duodenum

- More common than gastric ulcers
- More common in men (2:1)
- More common at ages 25-50
- Contributing factors:
  - Increased acid
  - Decreased HCO_3^- and mucus
  - A larger number of acid-secreting cells
  - High gastrin levels
  - Rapid gastric emptying (abnormal acid-bicarbonate balance)
  - *H. pylori*, NSAIDs, toxins, and enzymes
- Treatment: relieve symptoms and find cause

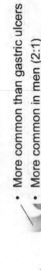

34-4

Malabsorption Syndromes

- Anything that interferes with digestion, absorption or transport of nutrients in the stomach or small intestines
- Can be caused by a variety of intestinal diseases (e.g. Crohn disease or parasitic infections), vascular problems, or resection of gastric or intestinal tissue
  - **Maldigestion → malabsorption**

34-5

Malabsorption Syndromes
Pancreatic Insufficiency

- Insufficient enzyme production by exocrine pancreas
  - Lipase, amylase, trypsin, or chymotrypsin
- Causes:
  - pancreatitis
  - pancreatic carcinoma
  - pancreatic resection
  - cystic fibrosis
- Fat maldigestion is the main problem
  - fatty stools and weight loss

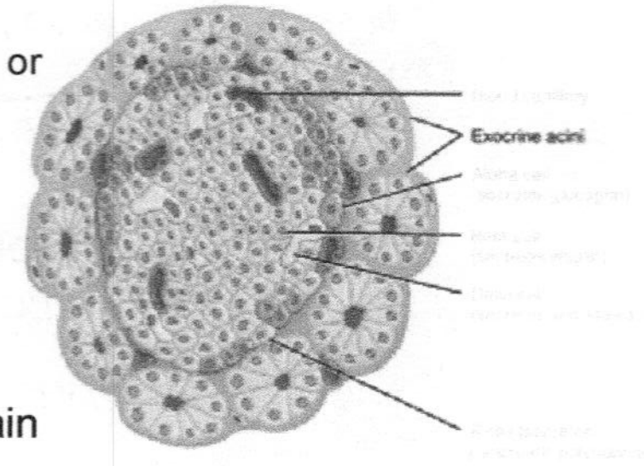

Exocrine acini

(b) Pancreatic islet and surrounding acini

34-5

Malabsorption Syndromes
Lactase Deficiency

- Lactase is the enzyme which breaks the milk sugar lactose into galactose and glucose
  - therefore, patients are **lactose intolerant**
- Bacteria are happy to take over the job of lactose fermentation
  - gas (cramping, pain, flatulence)
  - osmotic diarrhea

34-5

Malabsorption Syndromes
Bile Salt Deficiency

- Bile salts are needed to emulsify and absorb fats
- Caused by liver disease and bile obstruction
- Poor intestinal absorption causes
  - fatty stools
  - diarrhea
  - malabsorption of fat-soluble vitamins (A, D, K, E)
    - fat-soluble vitamins are much more susceptible to malabsorption than the water-soluble B and C vitamins
      - Vitamin A malabsorption → night blindness
      - Vitamin D malabsorption → decreased calcium absorption, bone pain, osteoporosis, fractures
      - Vitamin K malabsorption/non-production → deficiency in clotting factors II, VII, IX, and X → bleeding disorders, bruising
      - Vitamin E deficiency signs/symptoms not clear

34-5

Inflammatory Bowel Disease (IBD)
Ulcerative Colitis & Crohn Disease

- The signs and symptoms of ulcerative colitis and Crohn disease are very similar:
  - Abdominal pain
  - Bloody/mucus-filled diarrhea
- Patients demonstrate an increased risk of colon cancer
  - rule of thumb: anything that increases inflammation increases cancer risk

34-6

Inflammatory Bowel Disease (IBD)
Ulcerative Colitis

- Typically limited to the lower 1/3 of the colon
  - Sigmoid colon and rectum
- Ulcerations tend not to be as deep
  - Limited to the mucosa
- Treatment of ulcerative colitis is with broad-spectrum antibiotics, steroids, salicylates, immunosuppressants, and surgery

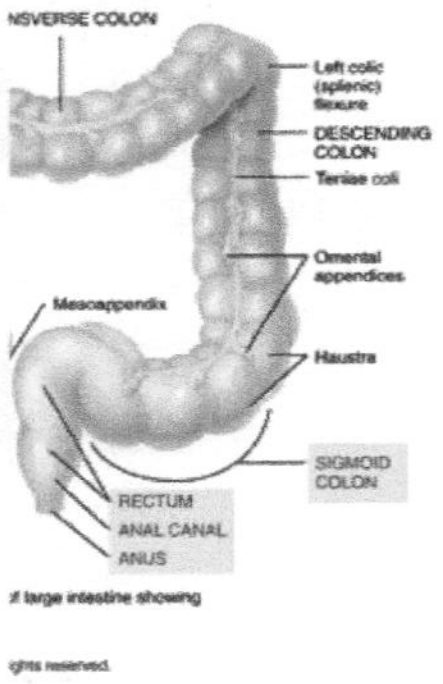
NSVERSE COLON
Left colic (splenic) flexure
DESCENDING COLON
Teniae coli
Omental appendices
Mesoappendix
Haustra
SIGMOID COLON
RECTUM
ANAL CANAL
ANUS
f large intestine showing
ghts reserved.

34-6

Inflammatory Bowel Disease (IBD)
Ulcerative Colitis

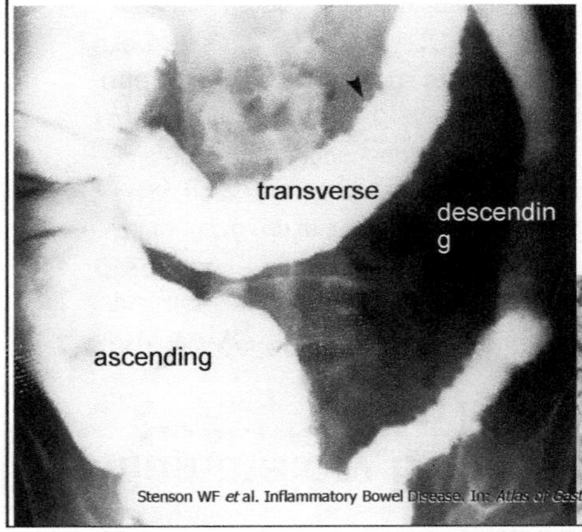
transverse
descendin
g
ascending

- In barium enema radiograph at left, note severe disease in descending colon and distal half of transverse colon
- polyps in ulcerative colitis can resemble precancerous polyps

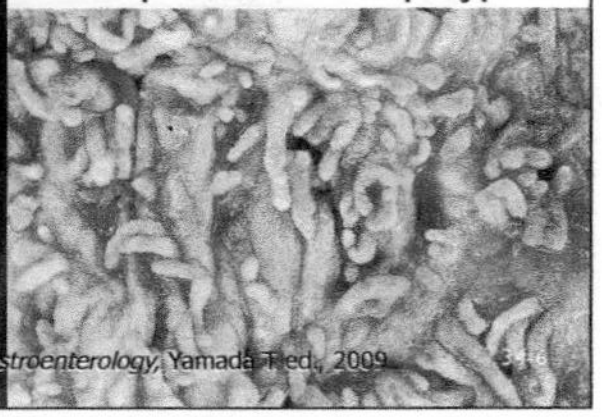

Stenson WF *et al.* Inflammatory Bowel Disease. In: *Atlas of Gastroenterology*, Yamada T ed., 2009

Inflammatory Bowel Disease (IBD)
Ulcerative Colitis

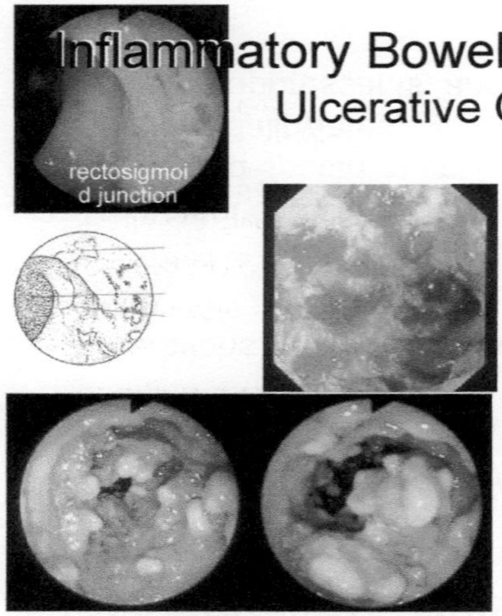
rectosigmoi
d junction

- Lesions can be erosions, or can be polyps
- Top left: rectum is inflamed (red areas) but sigmoid colon relatively healthy

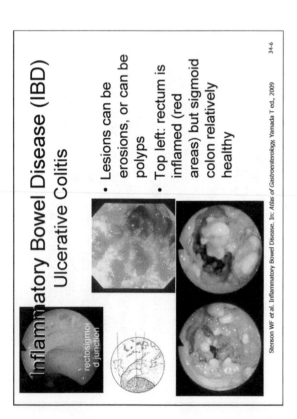

Stenson WF *et al.* Inflammatory Bowel Disease. In: *Atlas of Gastroenterology,* Yamada T ed., 2009

34-6

Inflammatory Bowel Disease (IBD)
Crohn Disease

- Formally called ileitis or granulomatous colitis
- Like ulcerative colitis, it is an **idiopathic inflammatory disorder** (unknown cause)
  - It tends to run in families (even more so than ulcerative colitis)
  - Age peak: 10–30 years
  - Gender distribution: equal
- Typically affects the distal ileum, but can cause inflammation anywhere in the GI tract from the mouth to the anus
  - "**Skip lesions**": inflammation of some areas but not others
  - Malabsorption of vitamin B_{12} and folic acid leads to anemia
  - Treatment is similar to ulcerative colitis

34-6

Inflammatory Bowel Disease (IBD)
Crohn Disease

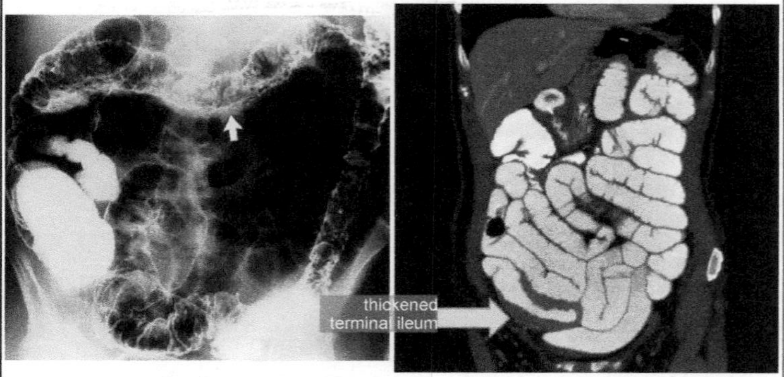
thickened
terminal ileum

Stenson WF *et al.* Inflammatory Bowel Disease. In: *Atlas of Gastroenterology,* Yamada T ed., 2009

34-6

Inflammatory Bowel Disease (IBD)
Crohn Disease

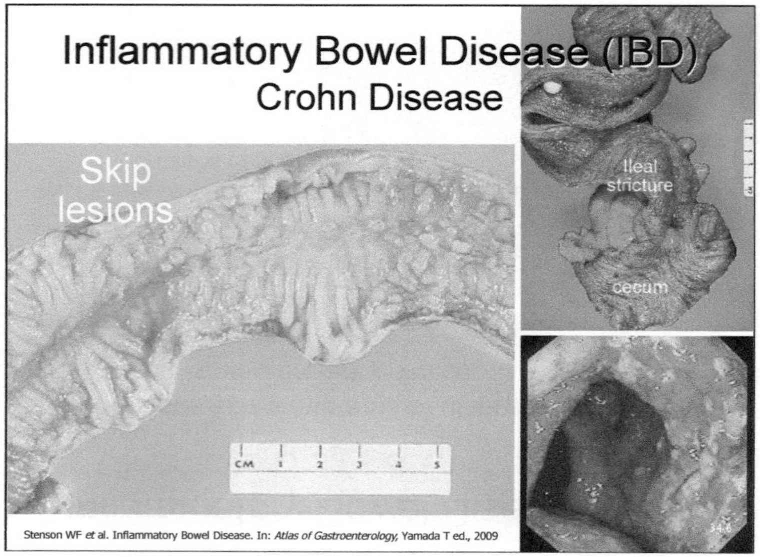
Skip
lesions
CM 1 2 3 4 5
Ileal
stricture
cecum

Stenson WF *et al.* Inflammatory Bowel Disease. In: *Atlas of Gastroenterology,* Yamada T ed., 2009

Gluten-Sensitive Enteropathy

- Also called **celiac disease**
- Gluten is the protein component in cereal grains (wheat, rye, barley, and malt)
- In these patients, gluten acts as a toxin causing loss of villous epithelium in the intestinal tract
- It occurs mainly in whites, and appears to be caused by a combination of dietary, genetic, and immunologic factors
- Children with this disease present with **failure to thrive**
- The patients will also exhibit malabsorption leading to rickets, bleeding, or anemia

34-7

Gluten-Sensitive Enteropathy

- The diagnosis is confirmed by performing a tissue biopsy
- The patient is put on a restrictive diet and given vitamin D, iron, and folic acid supplements
- Celiac crisis is severe malabsorption resulting in diarrhea, dehydration, and protein loss

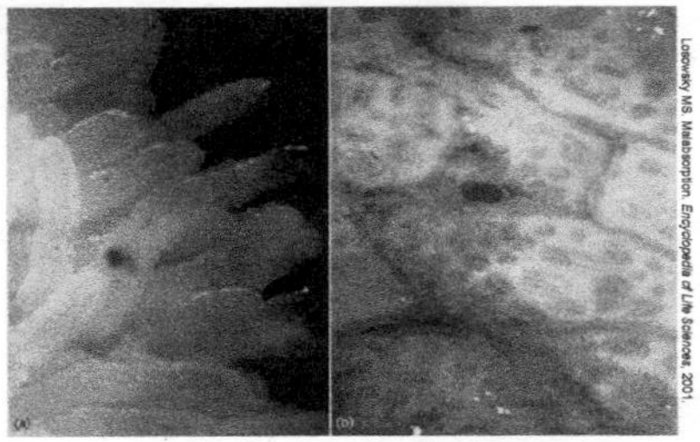

Normal villi Absent villi in Celiac Disease

Losowsky MS. Malabsorption. *Encyclopedia of Life Sciences*, 2001.

34-7

Diverticulitis

- Diverticula are herniations of mucosa through the muscle layers of the colon wall, especially the sigmoid colon
  - Having diverticula = **diverticulosis**
  - Inflamed diverticula = **diverticulitis**

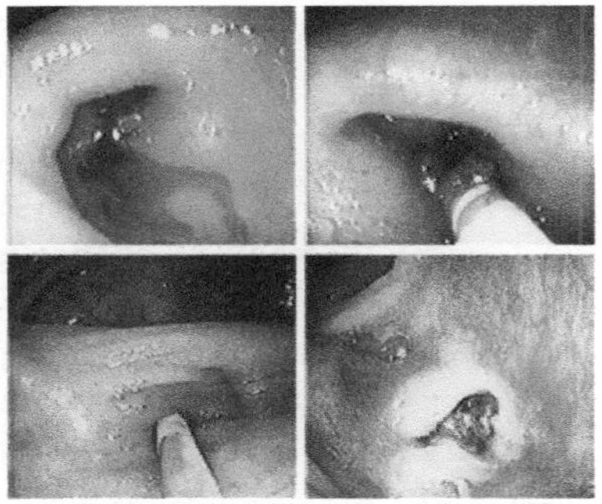

Jensen DA and Machicado GA. Clinical use and results of colonoscopy. Colonoscopy: Principles and Practice, 2e, 2009

34-8

Diverticulitis

- Occurs in the elderly who consume a diet lacking sufficient fiber and bulk, resulting in weakening of the colonic wall
- Signs and symptoms
  - constipation alternating with diarrhea
  - distention and flatulence
  - may progress to bowel obstruction and /or perforation
- Treatment
  - antibiotics
  - fiber
  - exercise

34-8

Appendicitis

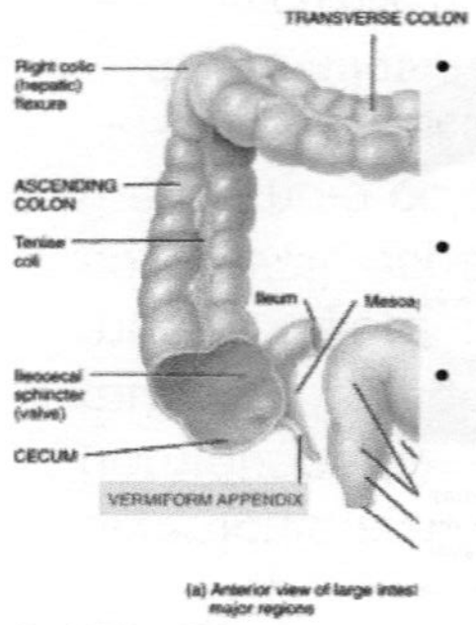
TRANSVERSE COLON
Right colic (hepatic) flexure
ASCENDING COLON
Teniae coli
Ileum
Ileocecal sphincter (valve)
CECUM
VERMIFORM APPENDIX

(a) Anterior view of large intestine showing major regions
Figure 24.22 Tortora - PAP 12/e

- Inflammation of the vermiform appendix (projection from the cecum)
- Possible causes include obstruction and infection
- Symptoms
  - diffuse epigastric pain
  - eventually becomes peri-umbilical
  - then localizes to the **RLQ: McBurney's point**
- Like diverticulitis, the most serious complication is peritonitis

34-9

Nutrition Disorders

- Obesity
  - Measured by **body mass index (BMI)**
    - $BMI = \frac{\text{weight in kg}}{(\text{height in m})^2}$
    - Most people don't know how to calculate this, so use a table or online calculator (http://www.nhlbisupport.com/bmi/)
    - Obesity defined as BMI > 120% of normal
  - Increased risk of cardiovascular disease, cancer, diabetes, breast, cervical, endometrial, prostatic, colon, rectal, and liver cancer
  - Causes: **excess caloric intake**, metabolic problems, number and size (adult onset) of adipose cells, genetics ("set-point"), diabetes, or psychological

34-10

Anorexia Nervosa

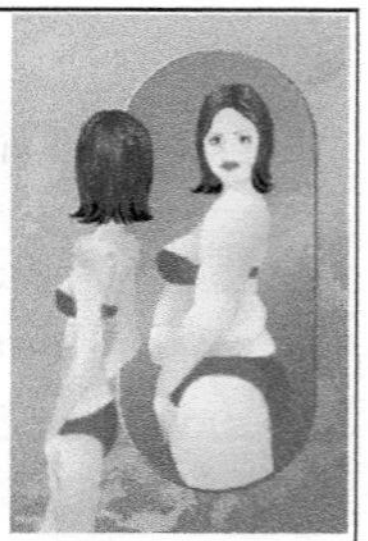

- A disorder of body image leads to starvation
- BMI less than 18
- Anorexic patients can lose 25-30% of their ideal body weight due to fat and muscle depletion
- Electrolyte imbalance may lead to cardiac failure
- The American Psychiatric Association's Diagnostic and Statistical Manual (DSM IV) Criteria for Anorexia are:
  - Refusal to maintain body weight – body weight less than 85% of that expected
  - Intense fear of gaining weight or becoming fat, even though underweight
  - Undue influence of body weight or shape on self-evaluation, or denial of the seriousness of the current low body weight
  - In post-menarchal females, the absence of at least three consecutive menstrual cycles

34-10

Bulimia Nervosa

- Can be a precursor to developing anorexia
- **Binge-purge-starve cycle**
  - **Binge eating**
  - **Purging** with vomiting, laxatives, diuretics or exercise
  - **Starvation**
- Continual vomiting of acidic chyme can cause pitted teeth, pharyngeal and esophageal inflammation, and tracheoesophageal fistulae
- DSM IV Criteria for Bulimia Nervosa
  - Eating, in a discrete period of time (e.g. within any 2 hour period), an amount of food that is definitely larger than most people would eat
  - A sense of lack of control over eating
  - Recurrent inappropriate compensatory behavior in order to prevent weight gain, such as self-induced vomiting; misuse of laxatives, diuretics, enemas, or other medications; fasting; or excessive exercise
  - Binging and inappropriate compensation occur, on average, at least twice a week for 3 months

34-10

Bulimia Nervosa

- DSM IV Criteria for Bulimia Nervosa
  - Eating, in a discrete period of time (e.g. within any 2 hour period), an amount of food that is definitely larger than most people would eat
  - A sense of lack of control over eating
  - Recurrent inappropriate compensatory behavior in order to prevent weight gain, such as self-induced vomiting; misuse of laxatives, diuretics, enemas, or other medications; fasting; or excessive exercise
  - Binging and inappropriate compensation occur, on average, at least twice a week for 3 months

Starvation

- 3-4 million people starve to death every year
  - Terri Schiavo lasted 13 days
  - Bobby Sands lasted 66 days in an Irish Prison in 1981
- Glycogen stores are depleted (glycogenolysis) and the body tries to produce glucose from non-carbohydrate molecules (gluconeogenesis)
- Once the body has used the glucose stores (long-term), it will use fat stores, and finally protein

Portal Hypertension

- **Hepatic portal vein** receives all nutrient-rich, oxygen-poor blood draining from GI tract
  - normal pressure 3 mmHg
  - in portal hypertension, pressure 10 mmHg
- Pathophysiology
  - **prehepatic**: clot, or narrowing of the portal vein
  - **intrahepatic**: liver disease interferes with blood flow
  - **posthepatic**: right heart failure

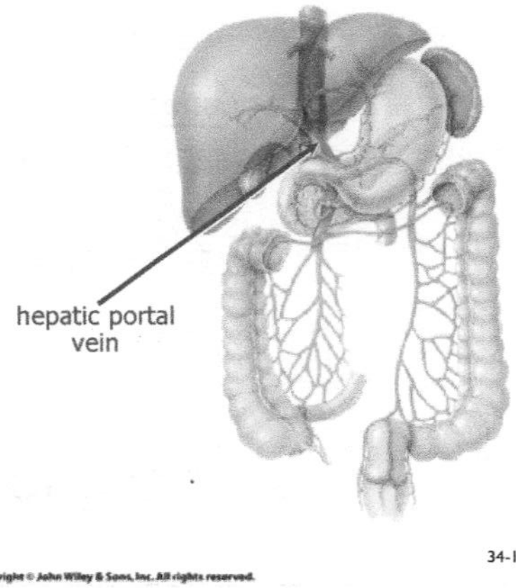
hepatic portal vein

Cirrhosis of the Liver

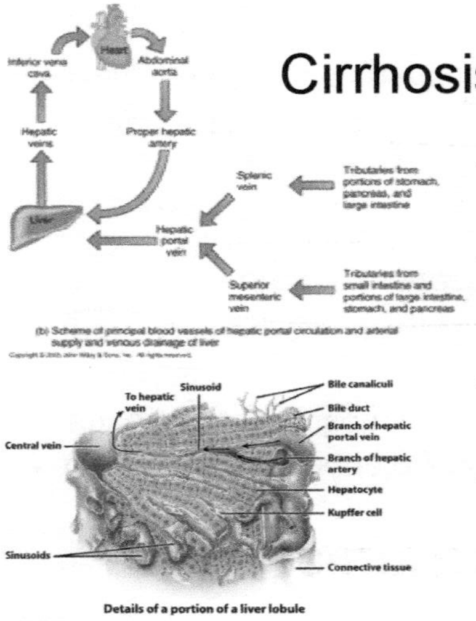
Inferior vena cava
Heart
Abdominal aorta
Hepatic veins
Proper hepatic artery
Liver
Hepatic portal vein
Splenic vein
Superior mesenteric vein
Sinusoid
To hepatic vein
Central vein
Sinusoids
Bile canaliculi
Bile duct
Branch of hepatic portal vein
Branch of hepatic artery
Hepatocyte
Kupffer cell
Connective tissue
Details of a portion of a liver lobule

- An irreversible inflammatory disease that disrupts liver structure
- There is decreased hepatic function due to nodular and fibrotic tissue synthesis (**hepatic fibrosis**)
- Biliary channels become obstructed and cause **portal hypertension**
- Due to hypertension, blood can be shunted away from the liver and hypoxic necrosis develops.

Cirrhosis of the Liver

- **Types**
  - **Alcoholic cirrhosis**
    - Oxidative damage to hepatocytes
  - **Biliary cirrhosis**
    - Primary biliary cirrhosis is an autoimmune disorder
    - Secondary biliary cirrhosis is caused by an obstruction
  - **Post-Necrotic**
    - It may follow viral hepatitis, dietary deficiencies, and a number of chronic diseases

34-11

Hepatic Encephalopathy

- Liver fails to adequately filter toxins, which then affect brain function
  - ammonia
- Increased permeability of the blood-brain barrier
- Astrocytes are most affected
  - these cells clean up the brain and die from ammonia toxicity
  - ammonia metabolized to glutamate, an excitatory transmitter which can lead to excitotoxicity
- Many other blood chemicals also involved

34-11

Hyperbilirubinemia

- **Heme to Bilirubin**
- **Three forms**
  - **Prehepatic**: before conjugation to become water soluble
    - Hemolytic jaundice (yellow pigmentation of the skin caused by hyperbilirubinemia)
  - **Hepatic**:
    - Hepatitis (viral or chemical)
    - Cirrhosis
  - **Post-hepatic** (after conjugation, it is now water-soluble)
    - Biliary obstruction

34-11

Circulation of Bile Salts

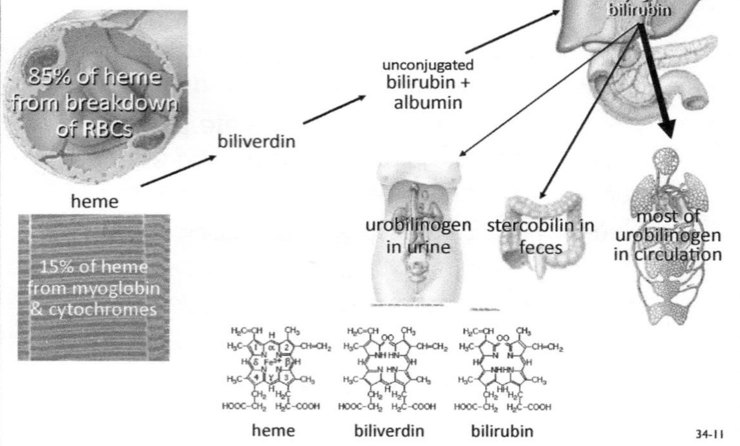

85% of heme from breakdown of RBCs
15% of heme from myoglobin & cytochromes
heme
biliverdin
unconjugated bilirubin + albumin
conjugated bilirubin
urobilinogen in urine
stercobilin in feces
most of urobilinogen in circulation
heme
biliverdin
bilirubin

34-11

Bile Obstruction

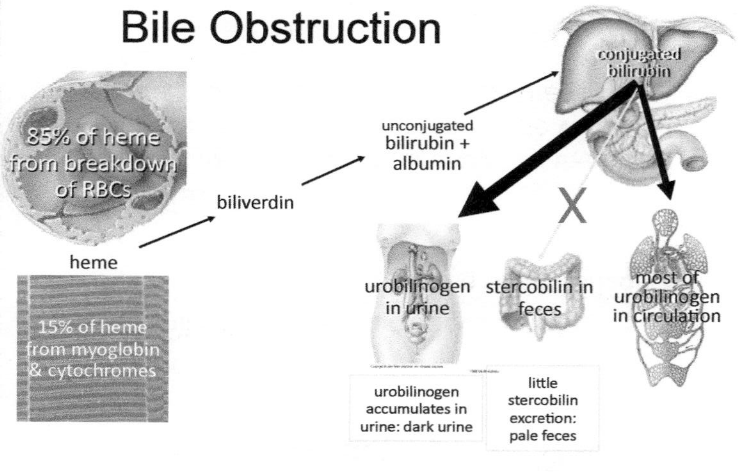
85% of heme from breakdown of RBCs
15% of heme from myoglobin & cytochromes
heme
biliverdin
unconjugated bilirubin + albumin
conjugated bilirubin
urobilinogen in urine
stercobilin in feces
X
most of urobilinogen in circulation
urobilinogen accumulates in urine: dark urine
little stercobilin excretion: pale feces

34-11

Jaundice

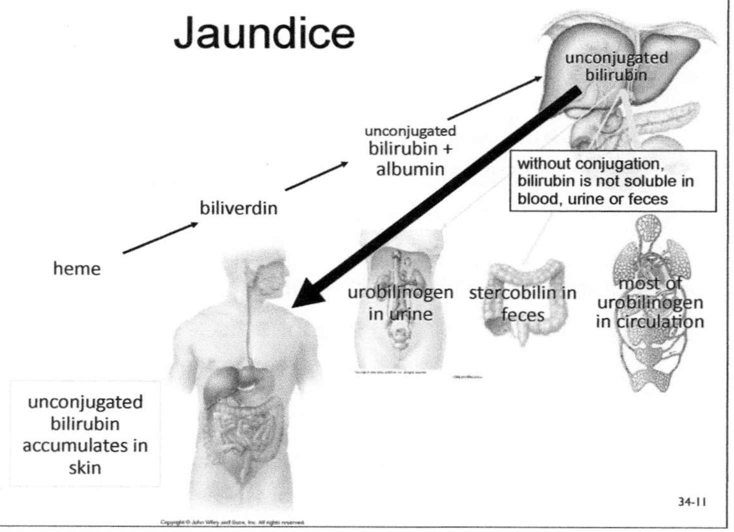
heme
biliverdin
unconjugated bilirubin + albumin
unconjugated bilirubin
without conjugation, bilirubin is not soluble in blood, urine or feces
urobilinogen in urine
stercobilin in feces
most of urobilinogen in circulation
unconjugated bilirubin accumulates in skin

34-11

Ascites

- Caused by
  - cirrhosis of the liver
  - heart failure
  - constrictive pericarditis
  - abdominal cancer
  - nephrotic syndrome
  - malnutrition (**kwashiorkor** or **marasmus**)
- Pathophysiology
  - portal hypertension
  - vasodilation
  - hepatocyte failure
  - sodium retention
- Fluid accumulates in peritoneal cavity

34-12

Viral Hepatitis

Infections caused by viruses that attack the liver

- Prodromal phase
  - From the time of exposure until jaundice appears
- Icteric phase
  - Yellow phase, painful swollen liver
- Recovery phase
  - Jaundice resolution (6-8 weeks)
- Patients with blood and body fluid associated hepatitis have a higher incidence of chronic hepatitis
- Laboratory tests:
  - Liver enzyme levels (ALT, AST)
  - Prolonged bleeding times and low serum albumin levels
- Immunology tests
  - Acute disease/recent infection-IgM
  - Exposure/immunity-IgG
  - Direct tests for the virus (HBV, HAV, HCV)

Alanine aminotransferase (ALT) and aspartate aminotransferase (AST) are enzymes located in liver cells that leak out into the general circulation when liver cells are injured.

34-13

Hepatitis Viruses

- Hepatitis A, B, C, D, E, F, G
- Hepatitis non A-E
  - Diagnosed through the exclusion of A-E
  - Wasn't it not too long ago that it was only non-A, non-B
- Other viruses can also cause hepatitis
  - **CMV & EBV**

34-13

Hepatitis A

- Pathology
  - Incubation period
    - Prodromal period is 14-45 days
  - Viral replication occurs in the liver
  - Virus is excreted through the biliary system into the feces
- Signs and symptoms
  - nausea and vomiting
  - loss of appetite
  - malaise
  - jaundice
  - diarrhea

34-13

Hepatitis B

- Incidence
  - 170 million people infected worldwide
  - At risk: homosexuals, IV drug users, prisoners, and health care workers
- Pathology
  - After initial inoculation (directly into the blood or through mucus membranes) the virus travels to the liver where it replicates in hepatocytes

34-13

Hepatitis B

- Prevention:
  - "universal precautions" for health care workers
  - Condoms, needle exchange, and methadone programs for IV drug users
  - HBV vaccine, three-dose series
  - Hepatitis B immunoglobulin (HBIG) or γ-globulin are hardly given anymore because of the success of the vaccine

34-13

Hepatitis C

- 300 million people affected worldwide
- Prior to testing many cases of transfusions and needle sticks resulted in Hepatitis C infection
  - Not sure about sexual transmission, though many prostitutes who are HBV^+ are also HCV^+
- The prevalence of the disease in IV drug abusers is 80-90% seropositivity

34-13

Gallbladder Disorders

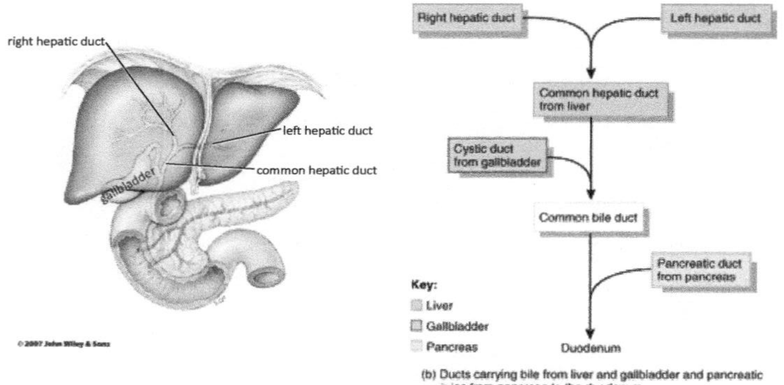

right hepatic duct
left hepatic duct
common hepatic duct
gallbladder
© 2007 John Wiley & Sons
Right hepatic duct
Left hepatic duct
Common hepatic duct from liver
Cystic duct from gallbladder
Common bile duct
Pancreatic duct from pancreas
Key:
Liver
Gallbladder
Pancreas
Duodenum

(b) Ducts carrying bile from liver and gallbladder and pancreatic juice from pancreas to the duodenum

34-14

Gallbladder Disorders

- Most gallbladder problems arise from one of two disorders:
  - **Cholecystitis**: Infection and inflammation of the common bile duct
  - **Cholelithiasis**: Obstruction of biliary drainage from gallstones
- **Cholelithiasis**: gallstone formation
  - There are two principal types of gallstones
    - Cholesterol stones
    - Pigmented stones (associated with cirrhosis)
  - Risks
    - Obesity, middle-age, female, and diseases of the gallbladder, pancreas, or ileum

34-14

Gallbladder Disorders

- Cholesterol stones form in bile that is saturated with cholesterol
- Theories include:
  - An enzyme defect in the formation of bile salts
  - Increased cholesterol synthesis
  - Decreased secretion of bile acids to emulsify fats
  - Combinations of all the above
- Signs and Symptoms
  - Heartburn/epigastric discomfort
  - RUQ abdominal pain (biliary colic)
  - Intolerance eating fatty food
  - Jaundice
  - Leukocytosis (especially if infection develops)
- Treatment
  - **Laparoscopic cholecystectomy**
  - Alternative: administration of stone-dissolving medicines

34-14

Pancreatitis

- Inflammation of the pancreas
- Caused by inflammation or injury to pancreatic ducts and cells causing a leakage of pancreatic enzymes
- Gallstones can cause obstruction of the pancreatic ducts which then damages pancreatic tissue
- Leaking enzymes cause autodigestion of the pancreas and surrounding tissues

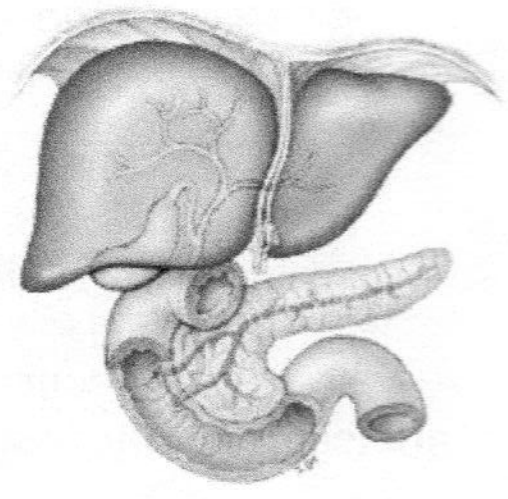

34-15

Pancreatitis

- Toxic enzymes can also be released into the bloodstream and injure other vital organs
- Signs and symptoms include:
  - Epigastric pain radiating to the back
  - Fever and leukocytosis
  - Hypotension and hypovolemia
    - Enzymes increase vascular permeability
  - Normally, there is little amylase in the serum (20-100 U/mL)
    - Pancreatitis causes leakage of digestive enzymes into the blood, and serum amylase level rises
    - Also increases serum lipase levels

34-15

UNIT 8

Study Guide Objectives – Introductory Pathophysiology (HTHS 2230)

Unit 8

Chapter 37 – Alterations of Musculoskeletal Function

1. Compare and contrast the different types of fractures: open, closed, comminuted, linear, oblique, spiral, impacted, transverse, greenstick, and transchondral. Relate the terms pathological and stress fracture. (pp. 978-979)
2. Describe the process of bone healing following a fracture. (p. 980)
3. Differentiate between subluxation, dislocation, and avulsion. (pp. 981-982)
4. Compare and contrast strains and sprains. (p. 982)
5. Characterize tendinopathy, epicondylopathy, and bursitis. (pp. 982-983)
6. Describe the pathophysiology of rhabdomyolysis, malignant hyperthermia, and compartment syndrome. Relate the development of myoglobinuria in the disorders rhabdomyolysis and malignant hyperthermia. (pp. 984-986)
7. Describe the pathophysiology of osteoporosis. (pp. 986-993)
8. Compare and contrast rickets and osteomalacia. (pp. 993-994)
9. Describe the pathophysiology and clinical features of Paget disease of the bone. (p. 994)
10. Characterize osteomyelitis. (p. 995)
11. Describe the pathophysiology and important features of osteoarthritis. (pp. 996-998)
12. State the pathophysiology and important features of rheumatoid arthritis. Compare and contrast rheumatoid arthritis and osteoarthritis. (pp. 999-1002)
13. State the pathophysiology and features of gout. (pp. 1005- 1007)
14. Compare the common types of secondary muscle dysfunction: contracture, stress-induced muscle tension, and disuse atrophy. (pp. 1007-1008)
15. Characterize fibromyalgia. (pp. 1008-1009)

Chapter 32 – Alterations of the Reproductive Systems

1. Review the factors which trigger puberty. (p. 776) Explain the signs and etiology of delayed and precocious puberty. (pp. 799-800)
2. Explain the pathophysiology of alterations in the female reproductive cycle: primary dysmenorrhea, primary amenorrhea, and secondary amenorrhea. (p. 801)
3. Characterize the possible reasons for dysfunctional uterine bleeding. (p. 802)
4. Describe the pathophysiology of polycystic ovarian syndrome. (pp. 803-804)
5. Name the signs and symptoms of premenstrual disorders (premenstrual syndrome and premenstrual dysphoric disorder). (pp. 804-805)
6. Discuss the various sites in which infection and inflammation can occur in the female reproductive system: pelvic inflammatory disease, vaginitis, cervicitis, and vulvovestibulitis. Describe manifestations of each. (pp. 805-808)
7. Compare and contrast the benign and proliferative conditions of the female reproductive tract: endometriosis, cervical cancer, and ovarian cancer. (pp. 812-816)
8. Characterize and compare benign and malignant changes in the breast. (pp. 839-855)
9. Classify the pathophysiology of disorders of the penis and urethra: urethritis, urethral stricture, phimosis and paraphimosis, Peyronie disease, and priapism. (pp. 819-821)
10. Describe the pathophysiologic features of disorders of the scrotum: varicocele, hydrocele, and spermatocele. (pp. 822-823)
11. Compare the disorders of the testes and epididymis: cryptorchidism, testicular torsion, orchitis, epididymitis, and testicular cancer. (pp. 823-826)
12. Compare and contrast benign prostatic hyperplasia, prostatitis, and prostate cancer. (pp. 826-836)
13. Discuss the pathophysiology of common bacterial infections of the reproductive tract: gonorrhea, chlamydia, syphilis, and bacterial vaginosis. (pp. 856-859)
14. Describe the clinical features and pathophysiology of viral infections of the reproductive tract: genital herpes and human papillomavirus (HPV). (pp. 856-859)
15. Characterize the parasitic infections of the reproductive tract: trichomoniasis, scabies, and pediculosis pubis. (pp. 856-859)

Unit 8
Chapter 37
Alterations of Musculoskeletal Function

Bone Fractures

- Pathological
  - Bone breaks because of an underlying disease that has weakened the bone
  - Cancer and osteoporosis are examples
- Stress
  - Bone placed under extreme or unusual forces
  - Motor vehicle accident, falls, sports injuries are examples

37-I

Bone Fracture Classification

- Open
  - Broken bone end protrudes through skin
- Closed
  - No penetration of skin
- Comminuted
  - Multiple bone fragments
- Linear
  - Along long axis of bone
- Oblique
  - At an angle to long axis of bone
- Impacted
  - Fragments pushed into each other

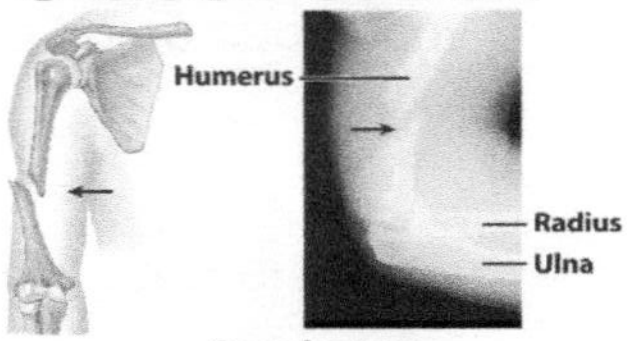
Humerus
Radius
Ulna
Open fracture

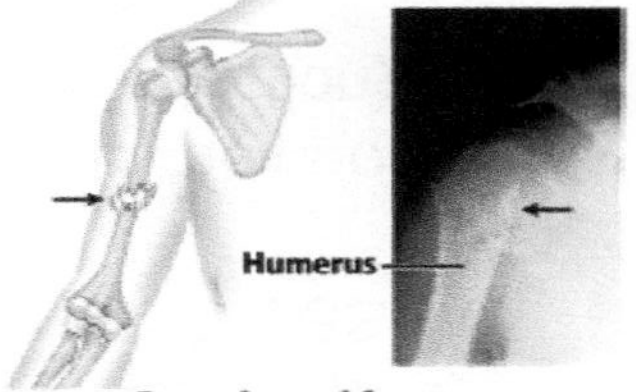
Humerus
Comminuted fracture

37-I

Bone Fracture Classification

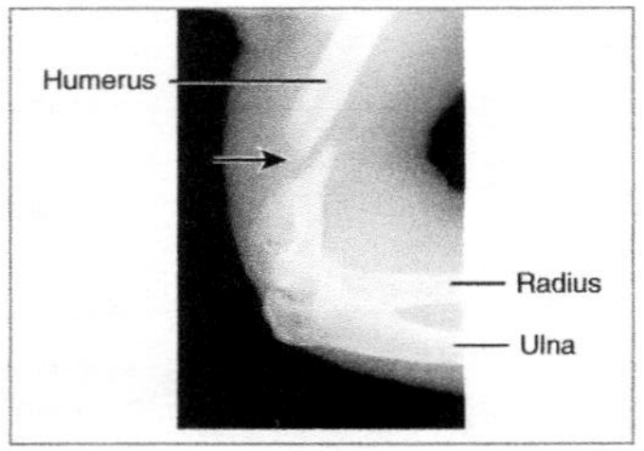
Humerus
Radius
Ulna

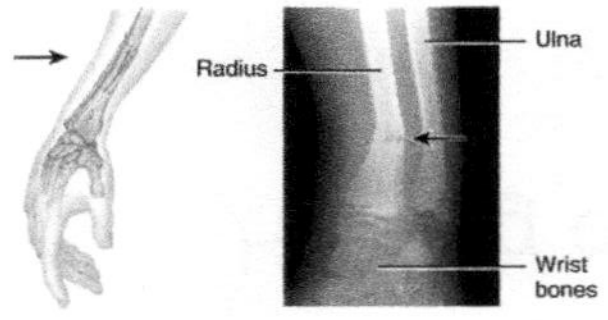
Radius
Ulna
Wrist bones
Greenstick fracture

- Spiral
  - Break forms twisted line
  - Torque on bone
  - Spiral fracture of tibia is a common ski injury
- Transverse
  - Across the long axis
- Greenstick
  - Partial break
- Transchondral
  - Through cartilage or growth plate

37-I

Healing of Fractures

- Realign bone fragments to their normal anatomic position (bone reduction)
  - –closed manipulation
  - –traction
  - –surgery: open reduction / internal fixation (ORIF)
- Splint or cast the fracture
  - –Hold it in place so bone union can occur
    - Plaster or fiberglass

37-2

Healing of Fractures

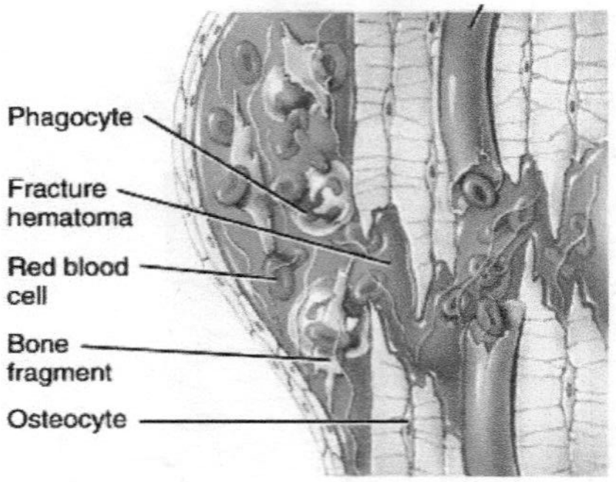

Phagocyte
Fracture hematoma
Red blood cell
Bone fragment
Osteocyte

1 Formation of fracture hematoma

- Fracture hematoma
  - –6-8 hours after injury
  - –Result of blood vessels breaking in the periosteum and the osteons

37-2

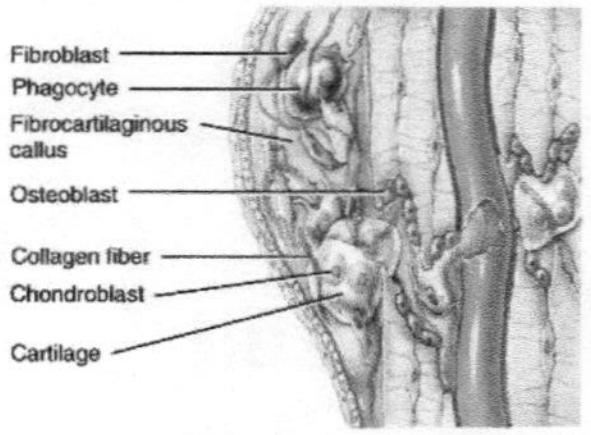

Fibroblast
Phagocyte
Fibrocartilaginous callus
Osteoblast
Collagen fiber
Chondroblast
Cartilage

2 Fibrocartilaginous callus fomation

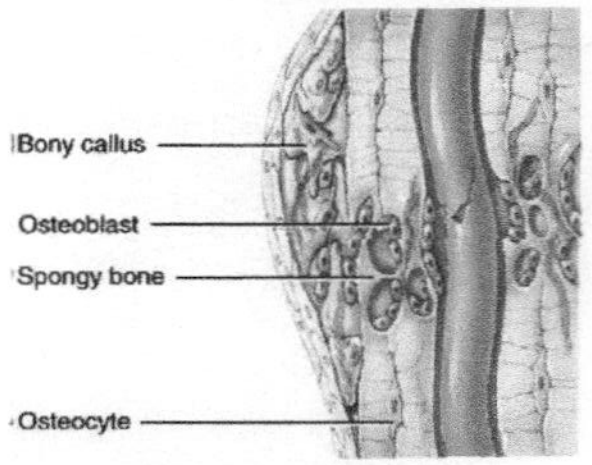

Bony callus
Osteoblast
Spongy bone
Osteocyte

3 Bony callus formation

Healing of Fractures

- **Callus** formation
  - –Takes from weeks up to 6 months
  - –Phagocytes remove cellular debris
  - –Osteoblasts synthesize collagen and matrix which mineralizes into a callus.

37-2

Healing of Fractures

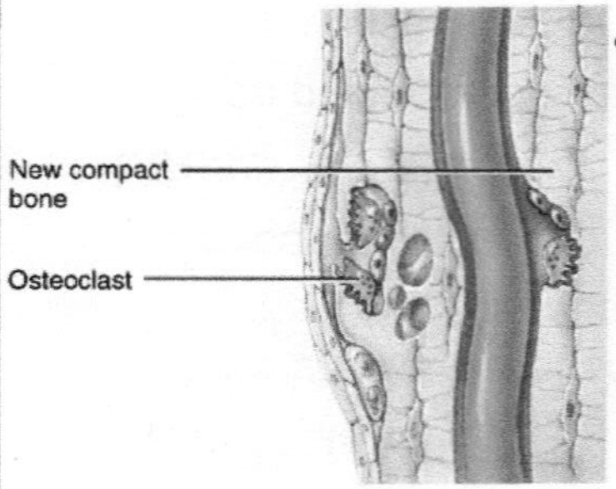

New compact bone
Osteoclast

4 Bone remodeling

- **Remodeling**
  - –Several months
  - –Callus is replaced with trabeculae (spongy bone)
  - –Spongy bone is replaced with compact bone

37-2

Skeletal System Stress

- Subluxation
  - Partial loss of contact between articular surfaces
- Dislocation
  - Complete loss of contact between articular surfaces

37-3

Skeletal System Stress

- **Sprain**
  - A partial tear of a **ligament** (at a joint)
  - Common in the wrist, elbow, ankle and knee
- **Strain**
  - A partial tear of a muscle or its tendon (which can also transverse a joint)
  - Sudden forced motion causing the muscle to become stretched beyond its normal capacity (local muscle damage)
- **Avulsion**
  - Separation of a tendon or ligament from its bony attachment

37-4

Skeletal System Stress

- **Tendinopathy** is any disease of a tendon
  - Slow to heal
  - Normal, organized collagen replaced with weaker, disorganized collagen
- **Epicondylopathy** is a type of tendinopathy, where it attaches to a bony epicondyle such as those on the humerus, radius, and ulna
  - Tennis elbow (lateral epicondylopathy)
  - Golfer's elbow (medial epicondylopathy)

37-5

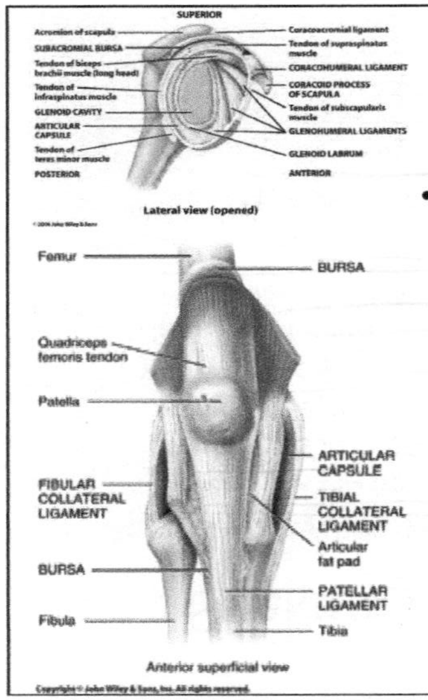
SUPERIOR
Lateral view (opened)
Femur
BURSA
Quadriceps femoris tendon
Patella
ARTICULAR CAPSULE
FIBULAR COLLATERAL LIGAMENT
TIBIAL COLLATERAL LIGAMENT
Articular fat pad
BURSA
PATELLAR LIGAMENT
Fibula
Tibia
Anterior superficial view

Skeletal System Stress

- **Bursitis**
  - Inflammation of the bursae
  - Usually caused by repeated trauma such as forceful rubbing of the bursa
  - Septic bursitis is caused by a wound infection
  - Shoulders, elbows, and knees are most common sites
    - Prepatellar, trochanteric, olecranon, subacromial

37-5

Skeletal System Stress

- **Rhabdomyolysis**
  - Rapid breakdown of muscle due to severe muscle damage
    - Muscle injury
    - Electric shock
    - Heat stroke
    - Drugs (especially statins, cholesterol-lowering drugs)
    - Malignant hyperthermia
  - Release of intracellular contents
    - Oxygen-carrying protein of muscle (myoglobin) found in urine (**myoglobinuria**)
    - Creatine kinase (CK)
    - Potassium

37-6

Skeletal System Stress

- **Malignant hyperthermia**
  - Genetic disease that causes a very rapid rise in body temperature in susceptible individuals exposed to certain anesthetics
  - The fever of malignant hypertension can itself be deadly, but if the patient survives, they may succumb to the overwhelming rhabdomyolysis
- **Myoglobinuria**
  - Dark urine (only 200 g of muscle damage required)
  - Causes acute renal failure due to precipitated myoglobin obstructing the renal tubules

37-6

Skeletal System Stress

- **Compartment syndrome**
  - Result of increased pressure with a muscle compartment
  - Fibrous, deep fascia surrounds muscle tissue and separates the muscles into compartments.
  - Increased pressure in a compartment results in diminished capillary blood flow, tissue hypoxia, and necrosis.

37-6

Osteoporosis

- A disease in which bone tissue is normally mineralized, but the density is decreased and the bone lacks structural integrity
- Bone densitometry used to measure

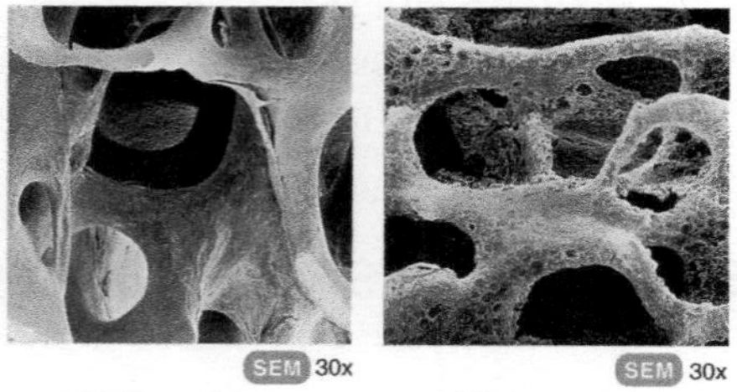
SEM 30x
SEM 30x
(a) Normal bone (b) Osteoporotic bone

37-7

Osteoporosis

- Potential causes include
  - Decreased levels of estrogen and testosterone
  - Decreased activity level
  - Inadequate levels of vitamin D, vitamin C, or Mg^{++}
- Usually asymptomatic until fractures occur

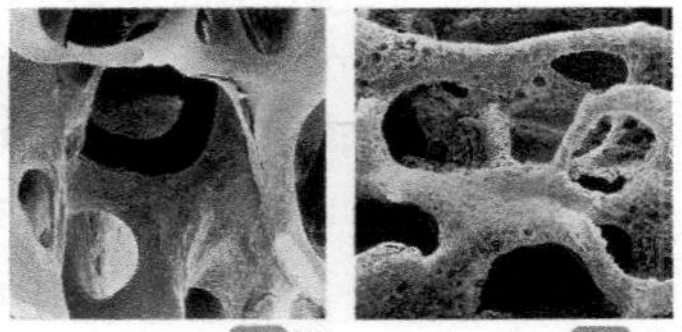
SEM 30x
SEM 30x
(a) Normal bone (b) Osteoporotic bone

37-7

Vitamin D Deficiency

- **Osteomalacia** (adulthood) and **rickets** (children) are diseases that result in inadequate or delayed mineralization of osteoid.
- Deficiency of vitamin D lowers absorption of calcium from the intestines
- Osteoid is laid down, but calcification does not occur (soft bones)
- Signs and symptoms include pain, bone fractures (e.g. hip fracture), vertebral collapse, and bony malformations

37-8

Paget Disease of Bone
(PDB, or Osteitis Deformans)

- The cause is unknown (Idiopathic) but it results in a state of increased metabolic activity (excessive bone remodeling)
- Manifested by disorganized, thickened but soft bones
- Most often affects the axial skeleton
  - Vertebrae, skull and pelvis
- Thickened bones can cause abnormal bone curvatures, brain and nerve compression, impaired motor function, and deafness

37-9

Osteomyelitis

- Bone infection; most often caused by a staphylococcal infection (*S. aureus*)
- An open wound is most common, but it can also be caused by a blood-borne infection
- Acute and chronic inflammation, fever, pain and necrotic bone
- Treatment: antibiotics, debridement, surgery, and hyperbaric oxygen therapy

37-10

The Arthropathies

- Represent a group of diseases which destroy the joints
- Differentiated by:
  - The presence or absence of synovial membrane inflammation
  - The presence or absence of systemic signs and symptoms
  - The findings from synovial fluid analysis

37-11

Osteoarthritis

- Degenerative joint disease
- Osteoarthritis is an atypical inflammatory process
- The primary defect is loss of articular cartilage, leaving underlying bone unprotected.
- This results in sclerosis of the underlying bone and formation of bone spurs (**osteophytes**)

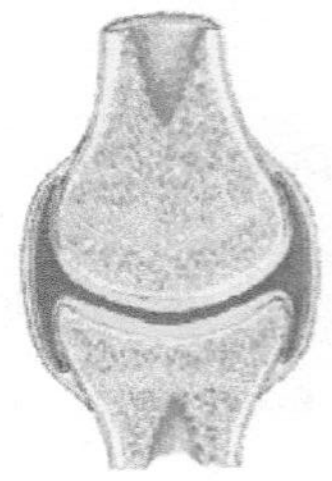

37-11

Osteoarthritis

- Signs and symptoms
  - Pain, stiffness, enlargement, tenderness, limited range of motion and deformity
- Joint fluid collected for analysis contains
  - Proteoglycan fragments from articular cartilage breakdown
- As the joint enlarges and is destabilized, subluxation can result

37-11

Rheumatoid Arthritis

- Chronic, systemic, inflammatory autoimmune disease
- The prototypical **inflammatory joint disease**
- Affects more women than men
- Signs and symptoms similar to osteoarthritis
  - Synovial fluid will be very different
- **Symmetric** arthritis
  - Morning joint stiffness lasting at least one hour
  - Swelling of soft tissue around 3 or more joints
  - Radiographic evidence of erosions in the joints of the hands

37-12

Rheumatoid Arthritis

- Presence of rheumatoid factors **(RF test)**
- Elevated **erythrocyte sedimentation rate (ESR)**
- Joint fluid presents with inflammatory exudate
- Nodules (necrotic areas) on the bones

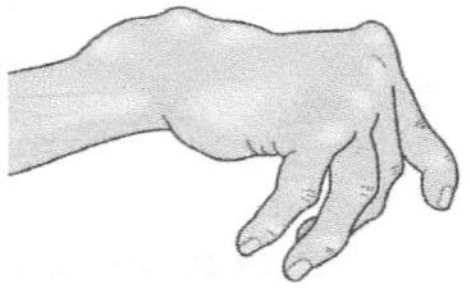

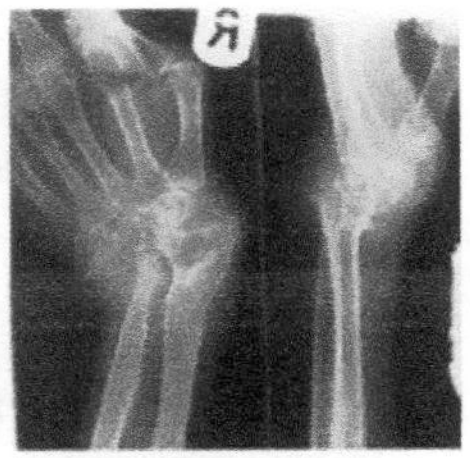

Figure 10.3 Rheumatoid arthritis affecting the wrist joint.
Lecture Notes Orthopaedics and Fractures, 4/e

37-12

Gout and Gouty Arthritis

- Abnormal metabolism of purine nucleotides (adenine, guanine) resulting in accumulation and elevation of uric acid in the blood (**hyperuricemia**) and body fluids
- High levels of uric acid eventually precipitate out of solution, forming crystal deposits
  - **gouty arthritis** in the joints
  - connective tissues throughout the body
- These uric acid crystals trigger the acute inflammatory response

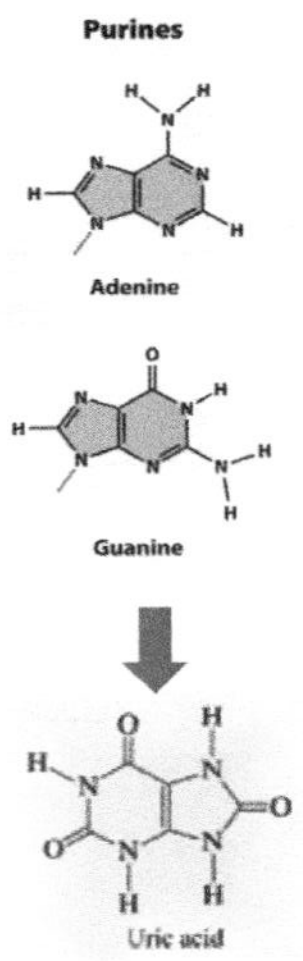
Purines
Adenine
Guanine
Uric acid

37-13

Gout and Gouty Arthritis

- Subcutaneous nodules that form from crystal deposition are called **tophi** (urate crystal granuloma)
- Uric acid stones often form in the kidney
- People with gout have 1000x greater risk of developing kidney stones

37-13

Secondary Muscle Dysfunction

- Muscular symptoms arising from a variety of causes, some unrelated to the muscle itself
- Examples include:
  - Contractures
  - Stress-induced muscle tension
  - Disuse atrophy

37-14

Contractures

- Physiologic Contractures
  - Muscle fiber shortening without an action potential
    - For example, malignant hyperthermia
  - Caused by failure of the calcium pump to replace calcium in the sarcoplasmic reticulum
  - Caused by heat, illness, or drugs
- Pathologic Contractures
  - Muscle fiber shortening caused by muscle spasm or weakness
  - For example, muscular dystrophy or spinal cord injury
  - Heel cord contractures after spinal injuries and muscular dystrophy are examples as well

37-14

Stress-Induced Muscle Tension

- Neck stiffness, back pain, clenching teeth, hand grip, and headache
- Caused by an increased activity of the reticular activating system (RAS); chronic anxiety

37-14

Secondary Muscle Dysfunction

- **Disuse atrophy**
  - Reduction in muscle the normal size of muscle cells due to **prolonged inactivity and muscular deconditioning**
    - Bed rest, trauma, casting, or nerve damage
  - Treatment:
    - Isometric movements and muscle-lengthening exercises

37-14

Fibromyalgia

- Chronic **non-inflammatory** musculoskeletal syndrome
- Diffuse, chronic pain
- Vague symptoms: increased sensitivity to touch, fatigue, and sleep disturbances. Often misdiagnosed as chronic fatigue syndrome.
- "**Tender points**" in are found in predictable patterns
- Etiology is unknown: suspects include viral illness, certain medications, physical or emotional trauma

37-15

Unit 8
Chapter 32
Alterations of the Reproductive Systems

Puberty Is Triggered by Complex Interactions

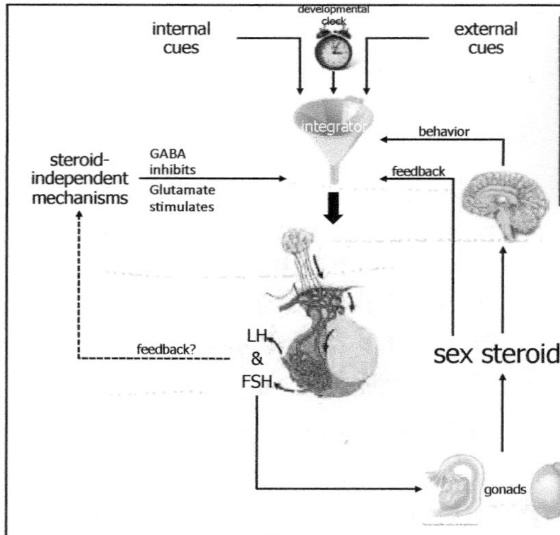
internal cues
developmental clock
external cues
integrator
behavior
feedback
steroid-independent mechanisms
GABA inhibits
Glutamate stimulates
feedback?
LH & FSH
sex steroids
secondary sex characteristics
gonads

Adapted from figure 1 of:
Sisk CL and Foster DL. *Nature Neuroscience* 7:1040, 2004

32-1

Delayed Puberty

- Diagnosed if no signs of secondary sexual characteristics at:
  - 13 in girls, 14 in boys
- 95% of cases are a physiologic "constitutional" delay
  - Hormone levels are normal
  - Hypothalamic – pituitary- gonadal pathway is intact
  - Tends to be familial and gender related; more common in boys
- The other 5% are caused by disruption of the hypothalamic – pituitary (FSH & LH) – gonadal pathway or a systemic disease

32-1

Early (Precocious) Puberty

- Onset of puberty before:
  - 6 in black girls, 7 in white girls, 9 in boys
  - More common in girls
  - Most cases are idiopathic
- Newer theories
  - Obesity-related
  - Better nutrition

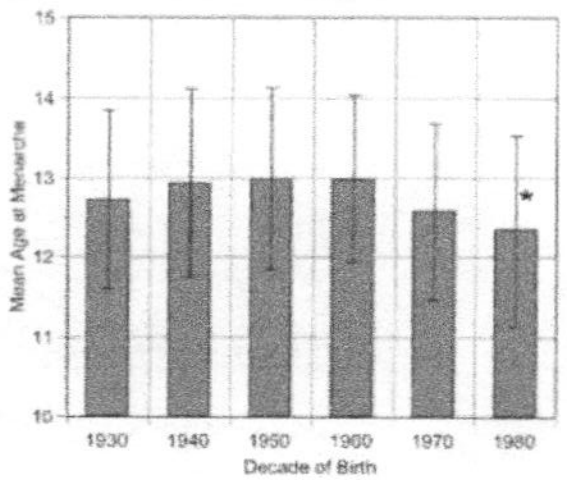
Mean Age at Menarche
15
14
13
12
11
10
1930
1940
1950
1960
1970
1980
Decade of Birth
*

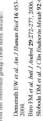

Fig. 1. Mean age at menarche (±SD) in 371 Fels Longitudinal Study girls, by decade of birth. An asterisk indicates mean age at menarche is significantly different from the reference group (1930 birth decade).

Demerath EW *et al. Am J Human Biol* 16:453-457, 2004.
Biro FM *et al. Intl J Androl* 29:272-277, 2006.
Sloboda DM *et al. J Clin Endocrin Metab* 92:46-50, 2007.

32-1

Female Reproductive Pathophysiology

The Female Reproductive Cycle

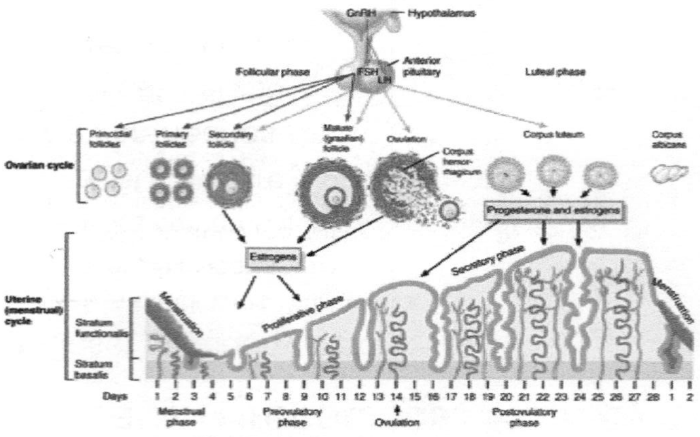
GnRH
Hypothalamus
Follicular phase
FSH
LH
Anterior pituitary
Luteal phase
Ovarian cycle
Primordial follicles
Primary follicles
Secondary follicle
Mature (graafian) follicle
Ovulation
Corpus hemorrhagicum
Corpus luteum
Corpus albicans
Estrogens
Progesterone and estrogens
Uterine (menstrual) cycle
Stratum functionalis
Stratum basalis
Menstruation
Proliferative phase
Secretory phase
Menstruation
Days
1 2 3 4 5 6 7 8 9 10 11 12 13 14 15 16 17 18 19 20 21 22 23 24 25 26 27 28 1 2
Menstrual phase
Preovulatory phase
Ovulation
Postovulatory phase

(a) Hormonal regulation of changes in the ovary and uterus

Figure 28.24a Tortora - PAP 12/e

32-2

Dysmenorrhea (Painful Menses)

- Primary dysmenorrhea
  - Not related to a pelvic disease
  - Excessive endometrial prostaglandin secretion during the uterine cycle
  - Decreases with age
  - Symptoms include backache, pelvic pain, vomiting, diarrhea, syncope, and headache (latter symptoms are due to prostaglandins acting systemically)
- Treatment: oral contraceptives and prostaglandin inhibitors

32-2

Dysmenorrhea (Painful Menses)

- Secondary dysmenorrhea
  - Is caused by an underlying pelvic disease
  - Pelvic inflammatory disease, endometriosis, and adhesions
  - May occur at any time in the menstrual cycle

32-2

Amenorrhea

- Primary amenorrhea
  - Lack of menarche and development of secondary sexual characteristics by age 14
  - Lack of menses even with sex characteristics by 16
- Secondary amenorrhea is the absence of menstruation for three or more cycles or six months in women who have previously menstruated
  - Pregnancy is the most common cause
  - Dramatic weight loss, excessive exercise, overproduction of prolactin

32-2

Dysfunctional Uterine Bleeding

- Is abnormal uterine bleeding from disturbances of the menstrual cycle – usually anovulation
- DUB is a diagnosis of exclusion
- Failure to ovulate due to age, stress, or endocrinopathy are the most common causes
- Common: someone in the symphony is out of tune: progesterone/estrogen imbalance leading to incomplete sloughing of endometrium
- Occurs mostly in adolescents and perimenopausal

32-3

Polycystic Ovarian Syndrome

- PCOS is the most common endocrine disturbance in the US (5-10%), usually affecting younger women
- It is familial, and is the leading cause of anovulation, and thus infertility

1. Hypertension
2. Dyslipidemias
3. Hyperinsulinemia
   - Leads to increased levels of androgens

- It manifests as polycystic ovaries, infertility, hirsuitism (abnormal hairiness), acne, thyroid disease, Cushing syndrome, and often progresses to diabetes mellitus

32-4

Premenstrual Syndrome

- Cyclic physical, psychologic, or behavioral changes that impair interpersonal relationships and/or activities
- Occurs in the luteal phase
- Results from abnormal tissue response to the normal fluctuations of the menstrual cycle (> 200 symptoms)
- Premenstrual dysphoric disorder (PMDD) is effectively treated by antidepressants (SSRIs)
  - *dysphoria* is the set of emotional disturbances in the disease
  - the effectiveness of SSRIs suggests a disorder of decreased synaptic levels of serotonin

32-5

Pelvic Inflammatory Disease

- PID is an acute, inflammation of the upper genital tract (uterus, uterine tubes, and/or ovaries)
- Often caused by sexually transmitted infections
  - Frequently initiated by gonorrhea and chlamydia
  - Considered a "polymicrobial" infection

32-6

Pelvic Inflammatory Disease

- Complications:
  - Tubonecrosis, pelvic adhesions, infertility, ectopic pregnancy, and chronic pelvic pain
- Signs and symptoms: purulent vaginal discharge and severe pelvic tenderness

32-6

Vaginal Infections

- Vaginitis is an infection/inflammation of the vagina commonly caused sexually transmitted pathogens, bacterial vaginosis, and *Candida albicans*
- Bacterial vaginosis (BV) is associated with an imbalance in the bacteria that are normally found in a women's vagina
  - BV is associated with bacterium of the *Gardnerella* species, and there is a characteristic "fishy smell"

32-6

Vaginal Infections

- Normally the acidic nature of the vagina provides some protection; maintained by cervical secretions and normal flora.
- Alteration of the vaginal pH may predispose a women to infection
  - Use of soaps, hygiene sprays, douching, deodorant pads or tampons

32-6

Vulvovestibulitis

- Also referred to as vulvitis or vestibulitis.
- Inflammation of the skin (dermatitis) of the vulva and often the perianal area
- It is commonly caused by contact with soaps, detergents, lotions, hygienic sprays, menstrual pads, perfumed toilet paper, or tight-fitting, nonabsorbent clothes
- It can also be caused by vaginal infections and STIs that spread to the labia

32-6

Cervicitis

- Is an inflammation of the cervix
- Mucopurulent cervicitis (MPC) usually caused by one or more STIs
  - Causes the cervix to become red and edematous
  - Mucopurulent exudate drains from the cervical opening
  - Signs and symptoms include pelvic pain, bleeding, and dysuria
  - Laboratory ID is followed by antibiotic therapy

32-6

Endometriosis

- Functioning endometrial tissue outside the uterus
- Associated with early menarche, infertility, frequent menstruations, pelvic pain, and nulliparity
- Theories
  - Depressed $T_{cytotoxic}$ cells tolerate ectopic tissue
  - Backflow of menstrual tissue (retrograde menstruation)
  - Spread of endometrial cells through the blood and lymphatics

32-7

Endometriosis

- Ectopic tissues respond to hormonal stimulation
- Bleeding causes pain and possibly pelvic adhesions
- Sites:
  - Ovaries, peritoneal surfaces, uterus, bladder, uterine tubes and uterine ligaments
- Is often clinically confused with early PID

32-7

Cervical Cancer

- Causes and risk factors
  - Human papilloma virus, other sexually transmitted diseases, early sexual activity, multiple sex partners, smoking, diet, and vitamin deficiencies
- Signs and symptoms
  - Pain and abdominal swelling, post-menopausal bleeding
- Testing
  - Pap smear and HPV testing

32-7

Ovarian Cancer

- Risk factors
  - not well understood
  - sibling with ovarian or breast cancer
  - nulliparity
- Mortality rates are still very high because of scarcity of early symptoms and the lack of a good screening test

32-7

Benign Breast Disease

- Manifested by palpable lumps in the breast that fluctuate with the menstrual cycle
- Types: cystic, fibrous, and epithelial proliferative
- Treatment: cyst drainage, surgical excision, and pain relief
- Although it doesn't increase cancer risk, it can make diagnosis more difficult

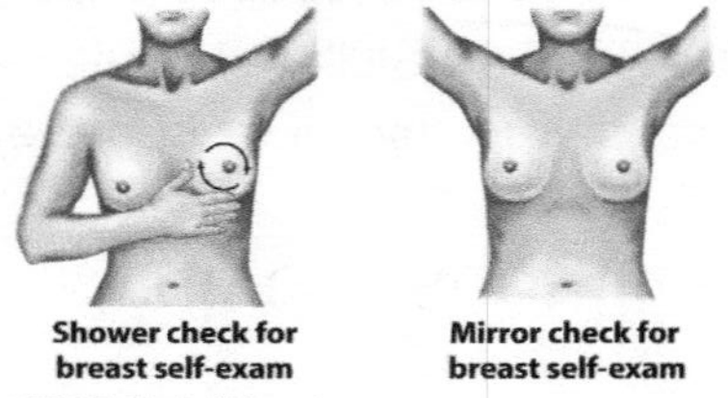
Shower check for breast self-exam
Mirror check for breast self-exam

Ireland, *Visualizing Human Biology*, 2e

32-8

Breast Cancer

- Lung and breast cancer are the 2 major cancers
- Lifetime risk is 1 in 8; rates have leveled off since 1987
- Multifactorial disease
  - Hormonal: long term estrogen exposure appears to increase risk (hormone replacement therapy, early menarche, nulliparity, late menopause, certain "high dose" oral contraceptives)
  - Familial: 2-3x higher risk if a primary relative
  - Environmental: Ionizing radiation, high fat diet
  - Reproductive: the protective effect of an early first full-term pregnancy

32-8

Male Reproductive Pathophysiology

Penile Disorders

- **Urethritis**
  - Inflammation of the urethra without bladder involvement
  - Usually caused by sexually transmitted infections
  - Nonsexual origins can be due to urologic procedures, insertion of foreign objects, anatomical abnormalities, or trauma
- **Urethral stricture**
  - Fibrotic narrowing of the urethra because of scarring
  - Trauma or untreated urethral infections

32-9

Penile Disorders

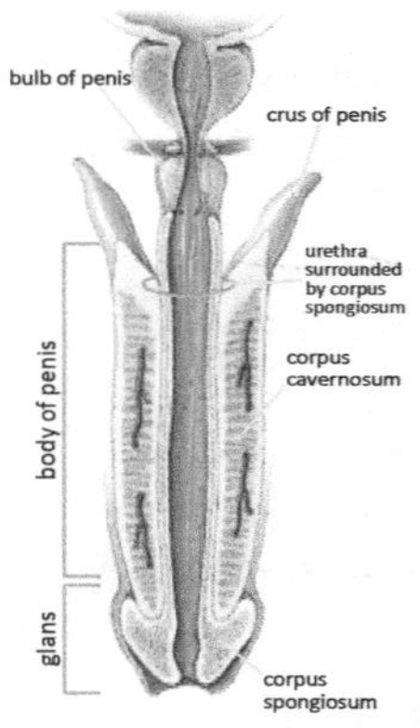

bulb of penis
crus of penis
urethra surrounded by corpus spongiosum
corpus cavernosum
body of penis
glans
corpus spongiosum

- **Phimosis**
  - Penile foreskin (prepuce) is "too tight"
  - Can't retract foreskin from the glans of the penis (distal to proximal)
- **Paraphimosis**
  - Foreskin is retracted and can't be reduced (proximal to distal) causing constriction around the penis
  - Most commonly caused by poor hygiene or chronic infections

32-9

Penile Disorders

- **Peyronie** (pā-rō-nē) **Disease**
  - "Bent-nail syndrome"
  - Slow development of fibrous plaques (thickening) in the erectile tissue of the corpus cavernosa causing a lateral curvature of the penis during erection
  - Occurs in middle-aged men and causes painful erections and intercourse
- **Priapism**
  - Prolonged penile erection, not associated with sexual arousal
  - Urologic emergency

32-9

Intrascrotal Disorders

- **Varicocele**
  - "Bag of worms"
  - Inflammation of the venous plexus in the spermatic cord
  - Caused by inadequate or absent valves in the spermatic veins
    - a "scrotal hemorrhoid"
  - Can interfere with spermatogenesis and cause infertility
  - 90% found on left side

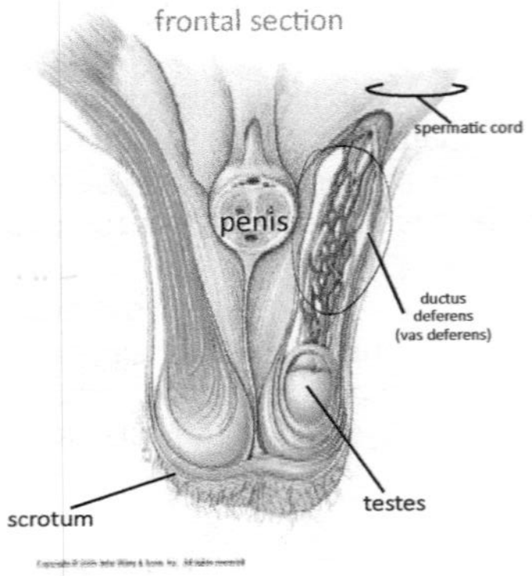
frontal section
spermatic cord
penis
ductus deferens (vas deferens)
scrotum
testes

32-10

Intrascrotal Disorders

- **Hydrocele**
  - Scrotal swelling due to collection of fluid within the tunica vaginalis
  - Imbalance between fluid secretion and reabsorption
  - Neonates: due to late closure of the tunica vaginalis (communicating hydrocele)
  - Use of transillumination for diagnosis

32-10

Intrascrotal Disorder

- **Spermatocele**
  - Cyst located between the head of the epididymis and the testis
  - Is usually asymptomatic or causes just mild discomfort
  - Milky fluid and does not cover the entire anterior scrotal surface

32-10

Intrascrotal Disorders

- **Cryptorchidism** (cryptorchism)
  - Failure of the testes to descend into the scrotum
  - Caused by a developmental delay, mechanical factor, or a deficiency in gonadotropin stimulation
  - Untreated cases can lead to **infertility** or **neoplastic** susceptibility (50 times greater)

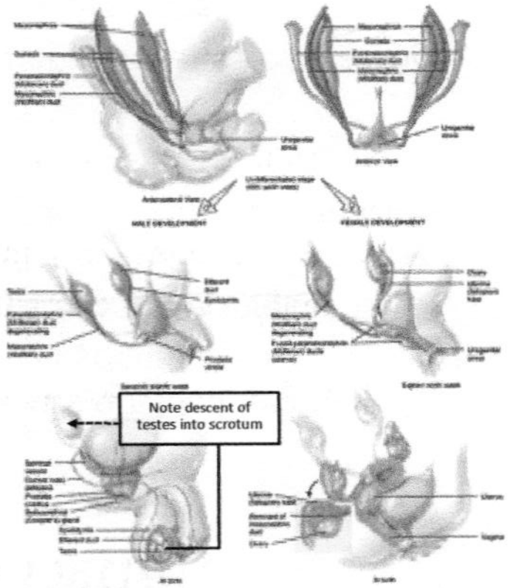
Note descent of testes into scrotum

Figure 28.27 Tortora - PAP 12/e

32-11

Intrascrotal Disorders

- **Testicular Torsion**
  - Rotation of spermatic cord
  - This interrupts blood supply by twisting the arteries and veins
  - Onset can be spontaneous (winter syndrome), or due to trauma or heavy physical exertion
  - Symptoms: tender, high-riding testis, thickened spermatic cord and absent cremasteric reflex
  - Must be surgically repaired within 6 hours

32-11

Intrascrotal Disorders

- **Epididymitis**
  - Inflammation of epididymis; usually due to a sexually transmitted microorganism in young males
  - Microorganisms ascend through vas deferens
  - Can cause abscess formation and scarring
  - Can be caused by chemical inflammation from the reflux of sterile urine into the ejaculatory duct.

32-11

Intrascrotal Disorders

- **Testicular Cancer**
  - Rare (1%), but most common tumors in young adult men; 95% cure rate
  - 90% are germ-cell tumors
  - Due to the population manifesting the disease, it is believed that high levels of androgens contribute to the carcinogenesis.
  - Dull gradual pain gives the patient a dull ache or a "testicular heaviness" sensation.

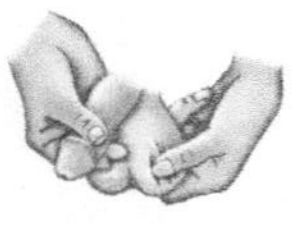

Shower check for testicular self-exam

Ireland, *Visualizing Human Biology*, 2e

32-11

Benign Prostatic Hyperplasia

- Enlarged prostate compresses the prostatic urethra and causes bladder outflow obstruction
- Symptoms: urge to urinate frequently, **delay starting urination**, and decreased force of the urinary system
- Treatment: removal of hyperplastic tissue, drugs to relax the smooth muscle, or drugs to interrupt prostate gland hormone secretions

32-12

Prostatitis

- Inflammation of the prostate
- Similar symptoms to BPH
- Caused by:
  - Ascending infection
  - Recurrent UTIs
- Can cause fibrosis of the prostate

32-12

Prostatic Cancer

- 29% of all cancer deaths in men
  - Rarely < 40 years-old
- Many men harbor undetected prostate cancer foci
  - 15-30% at age 50 and 80% at age 80
- 95% of prostate neoplasms are peripheral **adenocarcinomas**
- Prostatic cancer is asymptomatic until its advanced stages; symptoms are similar to BPH
- Test: ultrasound, digital exam, and PSA blood test

32-12

STIs (STDs)

- Caused by bacterial, viral, protozoan, parasitic, and fungal agents
- The increased rate of STIs is due to increased premarital sex, increased divorce rate, multiple sexual partners, and bisexuality (e.g. increased sexual partners and exposure)
- Generally, the viral STIs are considered incurable

32-13

Sexually transmitted diseases Table 18.2

Common name	Scientific name	Classification	Symptoms	Treatment
Chlamydia	*Chlamydia trachomatis*	Bacterial (can only reproduce inside body cells)	Usually asymptomatic, may cause urethritis in males; leads to pelvic inflammatory disease in females	Antibiotics
Gonorrhea or "the clap"	*Neisseria gonorrhoeae*	Bacterial	Urethritis with excess pus discharge; may be asymptomatic in females, leading to sterility	Antibiotics
Syphilis	*Treponema pallidum*	Bacterial (spiral bacterium)	Primary stage results in a painless open sore or chancre; secondary stage is a rash, fever, and joint pain; tertiary stage results when organs begin to degenerate	Antibiotics in primary or secondary stage
Genital herpes	Type II herpes simplex virus (HSV)	Virus	Painful blisters on the external genitals of males and females, with possible internal blistering in females	Incurable, but outbreaks can be controlled with anti-inflammatory drugs
Genital warts	Human papillomavirus (HPV)	Virus	Cauliflower growths on the external genital area and internal growths in females; can also appear on or around the anus	Incurable; warts can be removed cryogenically
Trichomoniasis	*Trichomonas vaginalis*	Protozoan	Foul-smelling discharge and itching in females	Prescription drug metronidazole

Ireland, *Visualizing Human Biology*, 2e

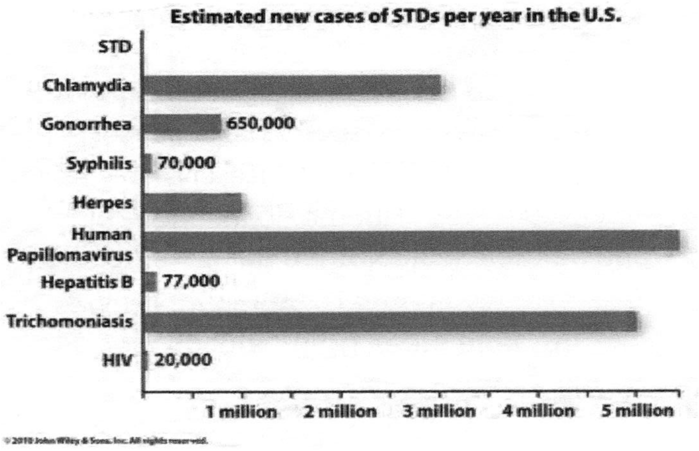
Estimated new cases of STDs per year in the U.S.
STD
Chlamydia
Gonorrhea
650,000
Syphilis
70,000
Herpes
Human Papillomavirus
Hepatitis B
77,000
Trichomoniasis
HIV
20,000
1 million
2 million
3 million
4 million
5 million

Ireland, *Visualizing Human Biology*, 2e

32-13

Gonorrhea

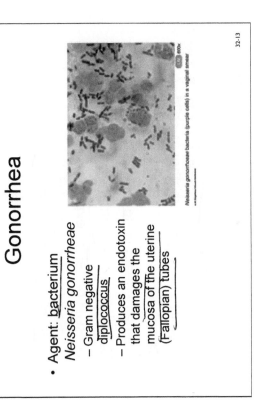

- Agent: bacterium *Neisseria gonorrheae*
  - Gram negative diplococcus
  - Produces an endotoxin that damages the mucosa of the uterine (Fallopian) tubes

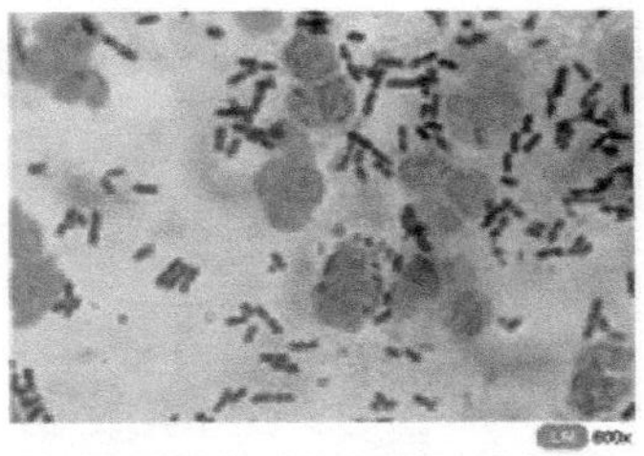

Neisseria gonorrhoeae bacteria (purple cells) in a vaginal smear

32-13

Gonorrhea

- Manifestations
  - urethritis/cervicitis (mucopurulent discharge)
  - anorectal infection
  - pharyngitis
  - conjunctivitis
  - may be asymptomatic
- Complications include
  - epididymitis, lymphangitis, salpingitis, infertility, disseminated blood infection, neonatal blindness
- Treatment is with antibiotics
  - antibiotic resistance is becoming more common

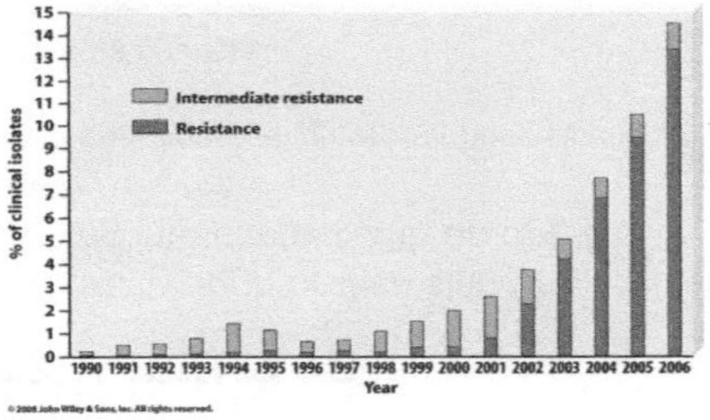
Intermediate resistance
Resistance
% of clinical isolates
Year
1990 1991 1992 1993 1994 1995 1996 1997 1998 1999 2000 2001 2002 2003 2004 2005 2006

Black, *Microbiology: Principles & Explorations*, 7e

32-13

Syphilis

- Agent: bacterium *Treponema pallidum*
  - Gram-negative helical bacterium (spirochete)
  - moves in corkscrew fashion
  - not found in environment
    - must multiply within a living host, difficult to culture and isolate in the laboratory
    - organism rapidly destroyed by heat, cold or drying

32-13

Syphilis
Primary Infection

- Sexual transmission occurs through broken skin or mucus membranes coming into contact with an open lesion
  - endothelial cell thickening from aggregation of lymphocytes and macrophages
  - this painless lesion is called a *chancre*
    - may occur internally and never be detected
    - develops 10-90 days after infection (average 21)
- 1/3 of individuals contacting active lesions will acquire the disease
- Other modes of transmission
  - Congenital
  - IV drug use (rare)

32-13

Syphilis
Secondary Stage

- If untreated, ¼ of cases will progress to the secondary stage
- The **secondary stage** is characterized by the systemic dissemination of the organism
  - Lymphadenopathy, malaise, fever, pharyngitis, skin rash
- Skin lesions will last up to 8 weeks, but relapses can occur up to 4 years

32-13

Syphilis
Tertiary Stage

- Usually occurs 10-30 years after the secondary stage
- Patients exhibit neurological, cardiac and cutaneous involvement
  - Large skin lesions (*gummas*)
  - Degeneration of spinal cord (*neurosyphilis*)
  - Mimics meningitis (thickening of the meninges)
  - Destruction of elastic tissue of the aorta

32-13

Syphilis
Congenital Infections

- Syphilis passes from mother to child
- Can occur staring at 18 weeks gestation
- Perinatal death in up to 40% of cases
- Bone, neural, and cutaneous abnormalities
- TORCH panel for expectant mothers
  - Toxoplasmosis, Other (HBV, syphilis), Rubella, Cytomegalovirus, Herpes simplex

32-13

Chlamydia

- Agent: *Chlamydia trachomatis*
  - obligate intracellular bacterium
  - Gram-negative coccus
- Exists as an extracellular elementary body
- Attaches to a receptor host cell and enters by endocytosis
- Once inside, it replicates and forms many elementary bodies

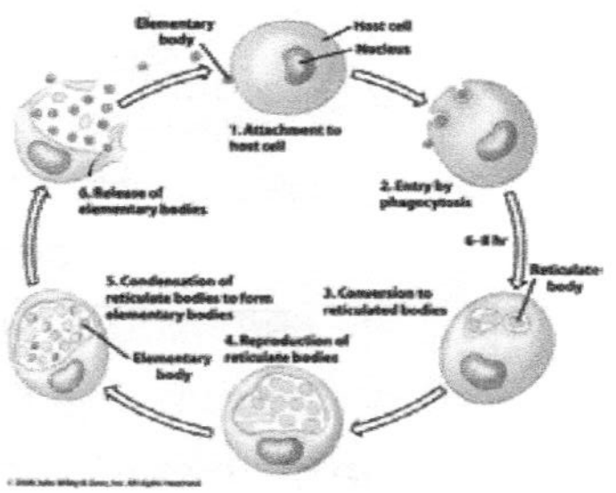

Black, *Microbiology: Principles & Explorations*, 7e

32-13

Chlamydia

- Most common bacterial STI
  - 3 million new cases per year in U.S.
- Manifests with purulent discharge, cervicitis, urethritis, prostatitis
  - In newborns, congenital infections cause conjunctivitis

32-13

Herpes Simplex I & II

- Agent: viruses *Herpes simplex type I* or *Herpes simplex type II*
  - Virus may remain dormant in posterior root ganglion or trigeminal ganglion for a lifetime
- 1 million new cases per year in U.S.
- Painful blister-like lesions on external genitalia and genital tract
- Treatment: Acyclovir (Zovirax or Valtrex)
- Complications
  - spontaneous abortions
  - neonatal morbidity and mortality from CNS infection

32-14

Condylomata Acuminata

- Genital warts
  - Caused by the human papilloma virus (HPV)
    - types HPV-6 and HPV-11
  - Appear several weeks to several months after contact
  - Soft, skin-colored single or clustered growths
  - Can cause cervical, anorectal, and penile cancers
  - High transmission rates

32-14

Association Between HPV and Cervical Cancer

- Agent: Human papilloma viruses
  - 150 related viruses
    - include those that cause warts on hands and feet
  - 40 types are STIs
    - some types cause genital warts
    - high-risk or oncogenic HPVs cause cancer
  - Persistent HPV infection causes essentially all cervical cancers
    - 12K diagnoses, 4K deaths per year in U.S.
    - 5% of all cancer worldwide
- Treatment: Gardisil or Cervarix
  - Gardisil vaccinates against
    - HPV-16 and -18 (cause 70% of cervical cancers)
    - HPV-6 and -11 (cause genital warts)
  - Cervarix also prevents persistent HPV-16 and -18 infections

32-14

Trichomoniasis

- *Trichomonas vaginalis*
- Sexually transmitted protozoan parasite
- Causes erythema of the vaginal wall, discharge (yellow-green), pruritis (itching), painful intercourse, and dysuria
- Diagnosed by performing a wet-prep of vaginal fluids

32-15

Scabies

- Agent: human itch mite *Sarcoptes scabiei*
- Burrows into upper layer of skin and lays eggs
- Causes intense itching and pimply rash
- Transmitted by direct contact
  - most scabies not caused by sexual contact
- Crusted scabies is a severe form that occurs in immunocompromised individuals
  - thick skin crusts contain mites and eggs
  - highly infectious and must be treated aggressively

32-15

Pediculosus Pubis

- Also called "crabs"
- *Phthirus pubis* (crab louse)
- Primarily transmitted sexually
  - Causes mild to severe pruritus
- Lice and nits are visible to the unaided eye

32-15